Laposata's
Laboratory Medicine

a LANGE medical book

Laposata's Laboratory Medicine

The Diagnosis of Disease in the Clinical Laboratory

Third Edition

Edited by

Michael Laposata, MD, PhD

Chairman
Department of Pathology
University of Texas Medical Branch
Galveston, Texas

New York   Chicago   San Francisco   Athens   Lisbon   Madrid
Mexico City   Milan   New Delhi   Singapore   Sydney   Toronto

Laposata's Laboratory Medicine: he Diagnosis of Disease in the Clinical Laboratory, hird Edition

1 2 3 4 5 6 7 8 9   DSS   23 22 21 20 19 18

ISBN 978-1-260-11679-3
MHID 1-260-11679-4

This book was set in Minion by MPS Limited.
The editors were Michael Weitz and Peter J. Boyle.
The production supervisor was Richard Ruzycka.
Project management was provided by Ruma Khurana, MPS Limited.
The cover designer was W2 Design.

Cataloging-in-publication data for this book is on file at the Library of Congress.

Library of Congress Cataloging-in-Publication Data
Names: Laposata, Michael, editor.
Title: Laposata's laboratory medicine : the diagnosis of disease in clinical
    laboratory / Michael Laposata, MD, PhD, Chairman, Department of Pathology,
    University of Texas Medical Branch, Galveston, Texas.
Other titles: Laboratory medicine (Laposata)
Description: Third edition. | New York : McGraw-Hill, 2018. | Includes
    bibliographical references and index.
Identifiers: LCCN 2018037655| ISBN 9781260116793 (paperback) | ISBN
    1260116794 (paperback)
Subjects: LCSH: Diagnosis, Laboratory. | BISAC: MEDICAL / Diagnosis.
Classification: LCC RB37 .L297 2018 | DDC 616.07/5—dc23

McGraw-Hill Education books are available at special quantity discounts to use as premiums and sales promotions or for use in corporate raining programs. To contact a representative, please visit the Contact Us pages at www.mhprofessional.com.

To Susan, with even more love than I had for you at the time of the previous edition

Contents

Authors

Yash P. Agrawal, MD, PhD
Chief of Chemistry, Toxicology, and Point of Care Testing, Rocky Mountain Regional Veterans Affairs Medical Center, University of Colorado School of Medicine, Denver, Colorado

David N. Alter, MD
Clinical/Chemical Pathologist, Spectrum Health/Michigan Pathology Specialists, Grand Rapids, Michigan

Fred S. Apple, PhD
Medical Director, Clinical Laboratories, Hennepin County Medical Center; Professor, Laboratory Medicine and Pathology, University of Minnesota School of Medicine, Minneapolis, Minnesota

Veerle Bossuyt, MD
Assistant Professor of Pathology, Yale School of Medicine, New Haven, Connecticut

Karin E. Finberg, MD, PhD
Assistant Professor of Pathology, Yale School of Medicine, New Haven, Connecticut

Ann M. Gronowski, PhD
Professor, Department of Pathology & Immunology and Obstetrics & Gynecology, Washington University School of Medicine, St. Louis, Missouri

Vipul Lakhani, MD
Assistant Professor of Medicine, Department of Medicine, Division of Endocrinology, Vanderbilt University Medical Center, Nashville, Tennessee

Michael Laposata, MD, PhD
Chairman, Department of Pathology, University of Texas Medical Branch, Galveston, Texas

Daniel D. Mais, MD
Clinical Pathology Associates, Department of Pathology, Baptist Health System, San Antonio, Texas

Stacy E.F. Melanson, MD, PhD
Assistant Professor of Pathology, Harvard Medical School; Associate Medical Director, Clinical Chemistry, Medical Director of Phlebotomy, Brigham and Women's Hospital, Boston, Massachusetts

Charles H. Muller, PhD, HCLD (AAB)
Director, Male Fertility Laboratory and Lecturer, Full-Time, Department of Urology and Biological Structure, University of Washington School of Medicine, Seattle, Washington

Mandakolathur R. Murali, MD
Director, Assistant Professor, Department of Clinical Immunology Laboratory, Massachusetts General Hospital, Harvard Medical School, Boston, Massachusetts

Robert D. Nerenz, PhD
Assistant Professor of Medicine, Pathology, and Laboratory Medicine, Geisel School of Medicine, Dartmouth University, Hanover, New Hampshire

James H. Nichols, PhD
Professor of Pathology, Microbiology and Immunology; Medical Director of Clinical Chemistry, Vanderbilt University School of Medicine, Nashville, Tennessee

Nicola J. Rutherford, PhD
Fellow in Clinical Chemisty, Department of Pathology, Microbiology, and Immunology, Vanderbilt University School of Medicine, Nashville, Tennessee

Daniel E. Sabath, MD, PhD
Associate Professor, Department of Laboratory Medicine; Adjunct Associate Professor, Department of Medicine (Medical Genetics); Head, Hematology Division, Department of Laboratory Medicine; Director of Hematology Laboratories, University of Washington Medical Center and Harborview Medical Center, Seattle, Washington

Susan L. Saidman, PhD
Associate Professor of Pathology, Harvard Medical School; Director, Histocompatibility Laboratory, Massachusetts General Hospital, Boston, Massachusetts

Mayukh K. Sarkar, PhD
Doctoral Clinical Laboratory Scientist, Department of Pathology, University of Texas Medical Branch, Galveston, Texas

Erin Schuler, PhD
Clinical Chemistry Fellow, Pathology and Laboratory Medicine, College of Medicine, University of Kentucky, Lexington, Kentucky

Eric D. Spitzer, MD, PhD
Associate Professor, Department of Pathology, Stony Brook University Medical Center, Stony Brook, New York

Paul Steele, MD
Medical Director, Clinical Associate Professor, Department of Pathology and Laboratory Medicine, Clinical Laboratories, Cincinnati Children's Hospital Medical Center, University of Cincinnati, Cincinnati, Ohio

Christopher P. Stowell, MD, PhD
Director, Blood Transfusion Service; Associate Professor of Pathology, Department of Pathology, Massachusetts General Hospital, Harvard Medical School, Boston, Massachusetts

Thomas P. Stricker, MD, PhD
Assistant Professor, Department of Pathology, Microbiology, and Immunology, Vanderbilt University School of Medicine, Nashville, Tennessee

Elizabeth M. Van Cott, MD
Director, Coagulation Laboratory; Medical Director, Core Laboratory, Massachusetts General Hospital; Associate Professor, Harvard Medical School, Boston, Massachusetts

Mark H. Wener, MD, ABIM, ABAI (CLI/DLI)
Professor, Departments of Laboratory Medicine & Medicine, University of Washington, Seattle, Washington

William E. Winter, MD
Professor, Department of Pathology, Immunology, and Laboratory Medicine, University of Florida College of Medicine, Gainesville, Florida

Alison Woodworth, PhD
Associate Professor, Pathology and Laboratory Medicine, College of Medicine, University of Kentucky, Lexington, Kentucky

Preface

In 2015, the National Academy of Medicine in the United States published a report on diagnostic error. The report from the committee, of which I was a member, concluded that virtually every adult American has been a victim of at least one diagnostic error, often with serious clinical consequences. Studies that followed the publication of the report estimated the number of deaths from diagnostic error in the United States to be on the order of 60,000 individuals per year.

The report investigated contributing factors to diagnostic error. One of the major difficulties identified was that the diagnostic specialty of laboratory medicine is too often left in the hands of the treating physician, without consistent or clinically valuable support from laboratory medicine specialists. This is unlike anatomic pathology and radiology, which provide diagnostic information to other specialties of medicine from individuals who have years of specialized training in their respective areas. The clinical laboratory test menu has become increasingly complex, expensive, and confusing to most physicians, especially with the introduction of much genetic information since the early 2000s. In most medical schools in the United States, and certainly in schools training nurses and other front-line health care providers, there is no course in laboratory medicine, and the laboratory medicine that is taught is usually not presented by experts who are knowledgeable about the operating parameters of clinical laboratory tests. The meanings of sensitivity, specificity, and predictive value of a positive or negative test are not part of the working knowledge of the treating physician. This is not the fault of these health care providers, but it does present a challenge to those creating curricula, about meeting current and future demands of health care practitioners. The diagnostic error committee noted that there is a substantial need for laboratory medicine education for all health care providers, beginning when they are students, as well as an increased number of specialists in laboratory medicine to help non-specialists in the selection of appropriate tests and in the interpretation of test results.

The National Academy of Medicine Committee also noted in their report that another major problem leading to diagnostic error is that treating doctors "do not know what they do not know." Too many physicians are confident in their knowledge about laboratory testing when, in fact, they should not be. The clinical significance of the result has become far more complex than most physicians understand because so much more is known about both diseases and the technical issues relevant to the tests. It is abundantly clear that most of the diagnostic errors made by treating physicians are initially unrecognized, and many are never recognized, by either the provider or the patient, and only brought to attention if an expert becomes involved in the case.

It is much easier, especially for a first-time learner, to have the most important material in a single field presented in one scholarly work. When I was a medical student, most comprehensive textbooks in laboratory medicine, many of which still exist, were written at a level for experts in the field. It was said frequently to me as a specialist in laboratory medicine, in the years prior to the publication of the first edition of this book, that the field of laboratory medicine was unlikely to become a part of general medical education unless there was a new textbook in the field that is comprehensive yet simple for medical students, clinical laboratory scientists, and health care professionals involved in patient care, including practicing physicians.

As this textbook enters its third edition, all of the chapters continue to improve in presentation of both the material and the content. The journey from the first edition of this book to this third edition has involved a quantum leap from each previous edition to the new one. As this textbook is translated into languages that allow it to serve the global community of laboratory medicine, it is my greatest hope to continue making each new edition far better than the last.

Michael Laposata
Galveston, Texas

Acknowledgments

I would first like to acknowledge all the expert chapter authors associated with this textbook. Many of them have been close professional friends for many years, and I am deeply honored to be a colleague of theirs. There are more than 300 years of collective experience in laboratory medicine among this highly distinguished group of authors. I extend my deepest thanks to those at McGraw-Hill who have been involved in the production of this book, now for three editions. I am delighted that this book has been included in the Lange series of medical books, which has such a proud tradition in medical education. It is especially exciting to watch the book grow into a global source of information in the field, with its translations into three languages from its original English version, with more to come. Thank you to all the translators and publishers outside the United States who have made this possible.

Clinical Laboratory Reference Values

The conventional units in this table are the ones most commonly used in the United States. Outside the United States, SI units are the predominant nomenclature for laboratory test results. The base units in the SI system related to laboratory testing that are found in this table include the mole (amount of substance), meter (length), kilogram (mass), second (time), and Celsius (temperature).

Reference ranges vary depending on the instrument and the reagents used to perform the test. Therefore, the reference ranges shown in this table are only close approximations to the adult reference ranges found in an individual clinical laboratory. For example, coagulation tests measured in seconds until a clot forms in the tube, such as the PT and the PTT, have reference ranges that are affected by both the instrument and the reagents used to perform the test. There are more than 100 possible combinations of coagulation instruments and reagents, and, therefore, there are at least 100 different reference ranges, which are mostly similar but not identical. The cutoff value for troponin for acute myocardial infarction is at the 99th percentile of a reference range which is also instrument and reagent dependent. In addition, it is important to understand that reference ranges can be significantly affected by age and sex.

The table contains information about selected drugs for which there is no reference range because they are not present in the circulation of those not taking the drug. However, drugs which are monitored have therapeutic levels, and some of these are included in the list of reference ranges. The therapeutic range for a drug is most often established by the concentration of the drug just prior to administration of the next dose. This is called the trough level. For other drugs, the therapeutic range refers to its range at peak concentration. This varies from drug to drug and is dependent upon many factors, such as absorption, distribution within the body, and metabolism of the drug. The table does not indicate whether the therapeutic level is a peak or a trough level.

Also listed in the table are selected compounds which are neither drugs nor laboratory tests, but are compounds which can be measured in the blood and, at some concentration, become toxic. For these listings, the compound is named and the word (toxic) is listed on the same line.

Conversion factors are provided in the table to allow the reader to convert conventional units to SI units and vice versa. The conversion of the conventional unit to SI unit requires a multiplication with the conversion factor, and conversion of the SI unit to the conventional unit requires division by the conversion factor.

The sample fluid is sometimes highly restrictive. For example, coagulation tests must be performed using plasma samples and serum samples are unacceptable. For other compounds, both plasma samples and serum samples may be acceptable. However, there may be differences, often minor, in the results obtained using plasma versus serum. Potassium is one such compound in which reference ranges may be different for plasma and serum. There is a significant movement away from the use of serum in favor of plasma. The principal reason for this is that extra time is required for samples to clot so that serum may be generated. A sample collected into a tube with an anticoagulant results in the generation of plasma rather than serum after the tube is centrifuged. The clotting step is omitted when plasma samples are prepared, and, therefore, the turnaround time for the performance of the test is shortened. In some circumstances, whole blood is used for analysis, but the number of tests performed using whole blood is very limited. Urine and other body fluids, such as pleural fluid and cerebrospinal fluid, are also used for testing. Some of the entries in the table are associated with a fluid other than plasma, serum, or whole blood.

	Specimen	Traditional Reference Interval	Traditional Units	Conversion Factor, Multiply →, ← Divide	SI Reference Interval	SI Units
Acetaminophen (therapeutic)	Serum, plasma	10–30	μg/mL	6.62	70–200	μmol/L
Acetoacetic acid	Serum, plasma	<1	mg/dL	0.098	<0.1	mmol/L
Acetone	Serum, plasma	<2.0	mg/dL	0.172	<0.34	mmol/L
Acetylcholinesterase	Red blood cells	5–10	U/mL	1	5–10	U/L
Activated partial thromboplastin time (APTT)	Whole blood	25–40	seconds	1	25–40	seconds
Adenosine deaminase[a]	Serum	11.5–25.0	U/L	0.017	0.20–0.43	μKat/L
Adrenocorticotropic hormone (ACTH) (see corticotropin)						
Alanine[b] (adult)	Plasma	1.87–5.88	mg/dL	112.2	210–661	μmol/day
Alanine aminotransferase (ALT, SGPT)[b]	Serum	10–40	U/L	1	10–40	U/L
Albumin[b]	Serum	3.5–5.0	g/dL	10	35–50	g/L
Alcohol (see ethanol, isopropanol, methanol)						
Alcohol dehydrogenase[a]	Serum	<2.8	U/L	0.017	<0.05	μKat/L
Aldolase[a,b]	Serum	1.0–7.5	U/L	0.017	0.02–0.13	μKat/L
Aldosterone[b] (upright)	Plasma	7–30	ng/dL	0.0277	0.19–0.83	nmol/L
Aldosterone	Urine, 24 h	3–20	μg/24 h	2.77	8–55	nmol/day
Alkaline phosphatase[b]	Serum	50–120	U/L	1	50–120	U/L
α_1-Acid glycoprotein	Serum	50–120	mg/dL	0.01	0.5–1.2	g/L
α_2-Macroglobulin	Serum	130–300	mg/dL	0.01	1.3–3.0	g/L
Alprazolam (therapeutic)	Serum, plasma	10–50	ng/mL	3.24	32–162	nmol/L
Aluminum	Serum, plasma	<6	ng/mL	37.06	0.0–222.4	nmol/L
Amikacin (therapeutic)	Serum, plasma	20–30	μg/mL	1.71	34–52	μmol/L
Amino acid fractionation:						
Alanine[b]	Plasma	1.87–5.89	mg/dL	112.2	210–661	μmol/L
α-Aminobutyric acid[b]	Plasma	0.08–0.36	mg/dL	97	8–35	μmol/L
Arginine[b]	Plasma	0.37–2.40	mg/dL	57.4	21–138	μmol/L
Asparagine[b]	Plasma	0.40–0.91	mg/dL	75.7	30–69	μmol/L
Aspartic acid[b]	Plasma	<0.3	mg/dL	75.1	<25	μmol/L
Citrulline[b]	Plasma	0.2–1.0	mg/dL	57.1	12–55	μmol/L
Cystine[b]	Plasma	0.40–1.40	mg/dL	83.3	33–117	μmol/L
Glutamic acid[b]	Plasma	0.2–2.8	mg/dL	67.97	15–190	μmol/L
Glutamine[b]	Plasma	6.1–10.2	mg/dL	68.42	420–700	μmol/L
Glycine[b]	Plasma	0.9–4.2	mg/dL	133.3	120–560	μmol/L
Histidine[b]	Plasma	0.5–1.7	mg/dL	64.5	32–110	μmol/L
Hydroxyproline[b]	Plasma	<0.55	mg/dL	76.3	<42	μmol/L
Isoleucine[b]	Plasma	0.5–1.3	mg/dL	76.24	40–100	μmol/L
Leucine[b]	Plasma	1.0–2.3	mg/dL	76.3	75–175	μmol/L
Lysine[b]	Plasma	1.2–3.5	mg/dL	68.5	80–240	μmol/L
Methionine[b]	Plasma	0.1–0.6	mg/dL	67.1	6–40	μmol/L

	Specimen	Traditional Reference Interval	Traditional Units	Conversion Factor, Multiply →, ← Divide	SI Reference Interval	SI Units
Ornithine[b]	Plasma	0.4–1.4	mg/dL	75.8	30–106	µmol/L
Phenylalanine[b]	Plasma	0.6–1.5	mg/dL	60.5	35–90	µmol/L
Proline[b]	Plasma	1.2–3.9	mg/dL	86.9	104–340	µmol/L
Serine[b]	Plasma	0.7–2.0	mg/dL	95.2	65–193	µmol/L
Taurine[b]	Plasma	0.3–2.1	mg/dL	80	24–168	µmol/L
Threonine[b]	Plasma	0.9–2.5	mg/dL	84	75–210	µmol/L
Tryptophan[b]	Plasma	0.5–1.5	mg/dL	48.97	25–73	µmol/L
Tyrosine[b]	Plasma	0.4–1.6	mg/dL	55.19	20–90	µmol/L
Valine[b]	Plasma	1.7–3.7	mg/dL	85.5	145–315	µmol/L
α-Aminobutyric acid[b]	Plasma	0.08–0.36	mg/dL	97	8–35	µmol/L
Amiodarone (therapeutic)	Serum, plasma	0.5–2.5	µg/mL	1.55	0.8–3.9	µmol/L
δ-Aminolevulinic acid	Urine	1.0–7.0	mg/24 h	7.626	8–53	µmol/day
Amitriptyline (therapeutic)	Serum, plasma	80–250	ng/mL	3.61	289–903	nmol/L
Ammonia (as NH_3)[b]	Plasma	15–50	µg/dL	0.714	11–35	µmol/L
Amobarbital (therapeutic)	Serum	1–5	µg/mL	4.42	4–22	µmol/L
Amoxapine (therapeutic)	Plasma	200–600	ng/mL	1	200–600	µg/L
Amylase[a,b]	Serum	27–130	U/L	0.017	0.46–2.21	µKat/L
Androstenedione,[b] male	Serum	75–205	ng/dL	0.0349	2.6–7.2	nmol/L
Androstenedione,[b] female	Serum	85–275	ng/dL	0.0349	3.0–9.6	nmol/L
Angiotensin I	Plasma	<25	pg/mL	1	<25	ng/L
Angiotensin II	Plasma	10–60	pg/mL	1	10–60	ng/L
Angiotensin-converting enzyme (ACE)[a,b]	Serum	8–52	U/L	0.017	0.14–0.88	µKat/L
Anion gap (Na^+)−(Cl^- + HCO_3^-)	Serum, plasma	8–16	mEq/L	1	8–16	nmol/L
Antidiuretic hormone (ADH, vasopressin) (varies with osmolality)	Plasma	1–5	pg/mL	0.926	0.9–4.6	pmol/L
Antiplasmin	Plasma	80–130	%	0.01	0.8–1.3	Fraction of 1.0
Antithrombin activity	Plasma	80–130	%	0.01	0.8–1.3	Fraction of 1.0
α_1-Antitrypsin	Serum	80–200	mg/dL	0.01	0.8–2.0	g/L
Apolipoprotein A[b]:						
Male	Serum	80–151	mg/dL	0.01	0.8–1.5	g/L
Female	Serum	80–170	mg/dL	0.01	0.8–1.7	g/L
Apolipoprotein B[b]:						
Male	Serum, plasma	50–123	mg/dL	0.01	0.5–1.2	g/L
Female	Serum, plasma	25–120	mg/dL	0.01	0.25–1.20	g/L
Arginine[b]	Plasma	0.37–2.40	mg/dL	57.4	21–138	µmol/L
Arsenic (As)	Whole blood	<23	µg/L	0.0133	<0.31	µmol/L
Arsenic (As) (chronic poisoning)	Whole blood	100–500	µg/L	0.0133	1.33–6.65	µmol/L
Arsenic (As) (acute poisoning)	Whole blood	600–9300	µg/L	0.0133	7.9–123.7	µmol/L

Continued next page—

	Specimen	Traditional Reference Interval	Traditional Units	Conversion Factor, Multiply →, ← Divide	SI Reference Interval	SI Units
Ascorbate, ascorbic acid (see vitamin C)						
Asparagine[b]	Plasma	0.40–0.91	mg/dL	75.7	30–69	μmol/L
Aspartate aminotransferase (AST, SGOT)[a,b]	Serum	20–48	U/L	0.017	0.34–0.82	μKat/L
Aspartic acid[b]	Plasma	<0.3	mg/dL	75.1	<25	μmol/L
Atrial natriuretic hormone	Plasma	20–77	pg/mL	1	20–77	ng/L
Barbiturates (see individual drugs; pentobarbital, phenobarbital, thiopental)						
Basophils (see complete blood count, white blood cell count)						
Benzodiazepines (see individual drugs; alprazolam, chlordiazepoxide, diazepam, lorazepam)						
Beryllium (toxic)	Urine	>20	μg/L	0.111	>2.22	μmol/L
Bicarbonate	Plasma	21–28	mEq/L	1	21–28	mmol/L
Bile acids (total)	Serum	0.3–2.3	μg/mL	2.448	0.73–5.63	μmol/L
Bilirubin:						
Total[b]	Serum	0.3–1.2	mg/dL	17.1	2–18	μmol/L
Direct (conjugated)	Serum	<0.2	mg/dL	17.1	<3.4	μmol/L
Biotin	Whole blood, serum	200–500	pg/mL	0.0041	0.82–2.05	nmol/L
Bismuth (therapeutic)	Whole blood	1–12	μg/L	4.785	4.8–57.4	nmol/L
Blood gases:						
Pco$_2$	Arterial blood	35–45	mm Hg	1	35–45	mm Hg
pH	Arterial blood	7.35–7.45	—	1	7.35–7.45	—
Po$_2$	Arterial blood	80–100	mm Hg	1	80–100	mm Hg
Blood urea nitrogen (BUN, see urea nitrogen)						
Brain natriuretic peptide (BNP)	Plasma	<100	pg/mL	1	<100	pg/mL
Bupropion (therapeutic)	Serum, plasma	25–100	ng/mL	3.62	91–362	nmol/L
C1 esterase inhibitor	Serum	12–30	mg/dL	0.01	0.12–0.30	g/L
C3 complement[b]	Serum	1200–1500	μg/mL	0.001	1.2–1.5	g/L
C4 complement[b]	Serum	350–600	μg/mL	0.001	0.35–0.60	g/L
CA125	Serum	<35	U/mL	1	<35	kU/L
CA19-9	Serum	<37	U/mL	1	<37	kU/L
CA15-3	Serum	<30	U/mL	1	<30	kU/L
CA27.29	Serum	<37.7	U/mL	1	<37.7	kU/L
Cadmium (nonsmoker)	Whole blood	0.3–1.2	μg/L	8.897	2.7–10.7	nmol/L
Caffeine (therapeutic, infants)	Serum, plasma	8–20	μg/mL	5.15	41–103	μmol/L
Calciferol (see vitamin D)						
Calcitonin	Serum, plasma	<19	pg/mL	1	<19	ng/L
Calcium, ionized	Serum	4.60–5.08	mg/dL	0.25	1.15–1.27	mmol/L
Calcium, total	Serum	8.2–10.2	mg/dL	0.25	2.05–2.55	mmol/L
Calcium, normal diet	Urine	<250	mg/24 h	0.025	<6.2	mmol/day
Carbamazepine (therapeutic)	Serum, plasma	8–12	μg/mL	4.23	34–51	μmol/L
Carbon dioxide	Serum, plasma, venous blood	22–28	mEq/L	1	22–28	mmol/L

	Specimen	Traditional Reference Interval	Traditional Units	Conversion Factor, Multiply →, ← Divide	SI Reference Interval	SI Units
Carboxyhemoglobin (carbon monoxide), as fraction of hemoglobin saturation:						
Nonsmoker	Whole blood	<2.0	%	0.01	<0.02	Fraction of 1.0
Toxic	Whole blood	>20	%	0.01	>0.2	Fraction of 1.0
β-Carotene	Serum	10–85	μg/dL	0.0186	0.2–1.6	μmol/L
Catecholamines, total (see norepinephrine)						
CEA, nonsmoker	Serum	<3	ng/mL	1	<3	μg/L
CEA, smoker	Serum	<5	ng/mL	1	<5	μg/L
Ceruloplasmin[b]	Serum	20–40	mg/dL	10	200–400	mg/L
Chloramphenicol (therapeutic)	Serum	10–25	μg/mL	3.1	31–77	μmol/L
Chlordiazepoxide (therapeutic)	Serum, plasma	0.7–1.0	μg/mL	3.34	2.3–3.3	μmol/L
Chloride	Serum, plasma	96–106	mEq/L	1	96–106	mmol/L
Chloride	CSF	118–132	mEq/L	1	118–132	mmol/L
Chlorpromazine (therapeutic, adult)	Plasma	50–300	ng/mL	3.14	157–942	nmol/L
Chlorpromazine (therapeutic, child)	Plasma	40–80	ng/mL	3.14	126–251	nmol/L
Chlorpropamide (therapeutic)	Plasma	75–250	mg/L	3.61	270–900	μmol/L
Cholesterol, high-density lipoproteins (HDL):						
Optimal	Plasma	>60	mg/dL	0.02586	>1.55	
Adequate	Plasma	40–60	mg/dL	0.02586	1.03–1.55	mmol/L
High risk for heart disease	Plasma	<40	mg/dL	0.02586	<1.03	mmol/L
Cholesterol, low-density lipoproteins (LDL)[b]:						
Optimal	Plasma	<100	mg/dL	0.02586	<2.59	mmol/L
Near optimal	Plasma	100–129	mg/dL	0.02586	2.59–3.34	mmol/L
Borderline high	Plasma	130–159	mg/dL	0.02586	3.37–4.12	mmol/L
High	Plasma	160–189	mg/dL	0.02586	4.15–4.90	mmol/L
Very high	Plasma	>190	mg/dL	0.02586	>4.90	mmol/L
Cholesterol total, adult:						
Desirable	Serum	<200	mg/dL	0.02586	<5.17	mmol/L
Borderline high	Serum	200–239	mg/dL	0.02586	5.17–6.18	mmol/L
High	Serum	>240	mg/dL	0.02586	>6.21	mmol/L
Cholesterol total, children:						
Desirable	Serum	<170	mg/dL	0.02586	4.4	mmol/L
Borderline high	Serum	170–199	mg/dL	0.02586	4.40–5.15	mmol/L
High	Serum	>200	mg/dL	0.02586	>5.18	mmol/L
Chromium	Whole blood	0.7–28.0	μg/L	19.2	13.4–538.6	nmol/L
Citrate	Serum	1.2–3.0	mg/dL	52.05	60–160	μmol/L
Citrulline[b]	Plasma	0.4–2.4	mg/dL	57.1	20–135	μmol/L
Clonazepam (therapeutic)	Serum	15–60	ng/mL	3.17	48–190	nmol/L

Continued next page—

	Specimen	Traditional Reference Interval	Traditional Units	Conversion Factor, Multiply →, ← Divide	SI Reference Interval	SI Units
Coagulation factor I (fibrinogen)	Plasma	150–400	mg/dL	0.01	1.5–4.0	g/L
Coagulation factor II (prothrombin)	Plasma	60–140	%	0.01	0.60–1.40	Fraction of 1.0
Coagulation factor V	Plasma	60–140	%	0.01	0.60–1.40	Fraction of 1.0
Coagulation factor VII	Plasma	60–140	%	0.01	0.60–1.40	Fraction of 1.0
Coagulation factor VIII	Plasma	50–200	%	0.01	0.50–2.00	Fraction of 1.0
Coagulation factor IX	Plasma	60–140	%	0.01	0.60–1.40	Fraction of 1.0
Coagulation factor X	Plasma	60–140	%	0.01	0.60–1.40	Fraction of 1.0
Coagulation factor XI	Plasma	60–140	%	0.01	0.60–1.40	Fraction of 1.0
Coagulation factor XII	Plasma	60–140	%	0.01	0.60–1.40	Fraction of 1.0
Cobalt	Serum	<1.0	µg/L	16.97	<17	nmol/L
Codeine (therapeutic)	Serum	10–100	ng/mL	3.34	33–334	nmol/L
Complete blood count (CBC):						
Hematocrit[b]:						
Male	Whole blood	41–50	%	0.01	0.41–0.50	Fraction of 1.0
Female	Whole blood	35–45	%	0.01	0.35–0.45	Fraction of 1.0
Hemoglobin (mass concentration)[b]:						
Male	Whole blood	13.5–17.5	g/dL	10	135–175	g/L
Female	Whole blood	12.0–15.5	g/dL	10	120–155	g/L
Hemoglobin (substance concentration, Hb [Fe]):						
Male	Whole blood	13.6–17.2	g/dL	0.6206	8.44–10.65	mmol/L
Female	Whole blood	12.0–15.0	g/dL	0.6206	7.45–9.30	mmol/L
Mean corpuscular hemoglobin (MCH), mass concentration[b]	Whole blood	27–33	pg/cell	1	27–33	pg/cell
MCH, substance concentration, Hb [Fe]	Whole blood	27–33	pg/cell	0.06206	1.70–2.05	fmol
Mean corpuscular hemoglobin concentration (MCHC), mass concentration	Whole blood	33–37	g Hb/dL	10	330–370	g Hb/L
MCHC, substance concentration, Hb [Fe]	Whole blood	33–37	g Hb/dL	0.6206	20–23	mmol/L
Mean cell volume (MCV)[b]	Whole blood	80–100	µm^3	1	80–100	fL
Platelet count	Whole blood	150–450	10^3 µL^{-1}	1	150–450	10^9 L^{-1}
Red blood cell count:						
Female	Whole blood	3.9–5.5	10^6 µL^{-1}	1	3.9–5.5	10^{12} L^{-1}
Male	Whole blood	4.6–6.0	10^6 µL^{-1}	1	4.6–6.0	10^{12} L^{-1}
Reticulocyte count[b]	Whole blood	25–75	10^3 µL^{-1}	1	25–75	10^9 L^{-1}
Reticulocyte count[b] (fraction)	Whole blood	0.5–1.5	% of RBCs	0.01	0.005–0.015	Fraction of RBCs
White blood cell count[b]	Whole blood	4.5–11.0	10^3 µL^{-1}	1	4.5–11.0	10^9 L^{-1}

	Specimen	Traditional Reference Interval	Traditional Units	Conversion Factor, Multiply →, ← Divide	SI Reference Interval	SI Units
Differential count[b] (absolute):						
Neutrophils	Whole blood	1800–7800	μL^{-1}	1	1.8–7.8	$10^9\,L^{-1}$
Bands	Whole blood	0–700	μL^{-1}	1	0.00–0.70	$10^9\,L^{-1}$
Lymphocytes	Whole blood	1000–4800	μL^{-1}	1	1.0–4.8	$10^9\,L^{-1}$
Monocytes	Whole blood	0–800	μL^{-1}	1	0.00–0.80	$10^9\,L^{-1}$
Eosinophils	Whole blood	0–450	μL^{-1}	1	0.00–0.45	$10^9\,L^{-1}$
Basophils	Whole blood	0–200	μL^{-1}	1	0.00–0.20	$10^9\,L^{-1}$
Differential count[b] (number fraction):						
Neutrophils	Whole blood	56	%	0.01	0.56	Fraction of 1.0
Bands	Whole blood	3	%	0.01	0.03	Fraction of 1.0
Lymphocytes	Whole blood	34	%	0.01	0.34	Fraction of 1.0
Monocytes	Whole blood	4	%	0.01	0.04	Fraction of 1.0
Eosinophils	Whole blood	2.7	%	0.01	0.027	Fraction of 1.0
Basophils	Whole blood	0.3	%	0.01	0.003	Fraction of 1.0
Copper[b]	Serum	70–140	µg/dL	0.1574	11.0–22.0	µmol/L
Coproporphyrin	Urine	<200	µg/24 h	1.527	<300	nmol/day
Corticotropin[b] (08:00)	Plasma	<120	pg/mL	0.22	<26	pmol/L
Cortisol, total[b]:						
Time of day:						
8:00	Plasma	5–25	µg/dL	27.6	138–690	nmol/L
16:00	Plasma	3–16	µg/dL	27.6	83–442	nmol/L
20:00	Plasma	<50% of 08:00	µg/dL	1	<50% of 08:00	nmol/L
Cortisol, free[b]	Urine	30–100	µg/24 h	2.76	80–280	nmol/day
Cotinine (smoker)	Plasma	16–145	ng/mL	5.68	91–823	nmol/L
C-peptide	Serum	0.5–3.5	ng/mL	0.333	0.17–1.17	nmol/L
Creatine, male	Serum	0.2–0.7	mg/dL	76.3	15.3–53.3	µmol/L
Creatine, female	Serum	0.3–0.9	mg/dL	76.3	22.9–68.6	µmol/L
Creatine kinase (CK)[a]	Serum	50–200	U/L	0.017	0.85–3.40	µKat/L
CK-MB fraction	Serum	<6	%	0.01	<0.06	Fraction of 1.0
Creatinine[b]	Serum, plasma	0.6–1.2	mg/dL	88.4	53–106	µmol/L
Creatinine	Urine	1–2	g/24 h	8.84	8.8–17.7	mmol/day
Creatinine clearance, glomerular filtration rate	Serum, urine	75–125	mL/min/1.73 m²	0.00963	0.72–1.2	mL/s/m²
C-telopeptide:						
Men	Serum, plasma	60–700	pg/mL	1	60–700	pg/mL
Premenopausal women	Serum, plasma	40–465	pg/mL	1	40–465	pg/mL
Cyanide (toxic)	Whole blood	>1.0	µg/mL	38.4	>38.4	µmol/L

Continued next page—

	Specimen	Traditional Reference Interval	Traditional Units	Conversion Factor, Multiply →, ← Divide	SI Reference Interval	SI Units
Cyanocobalamin (see vitamin B_{12})						
Cyclic adenosine monophosphate (cAMP)	Plasma	4.6–8.6	ng/mL	3.04	14–26	nmol/L
Cyclosporine (toxic)	Whole blood	>400	ng/mL	0.832	>333	nmol/L
Cystine[b]	Plasma	0.40–1.40	mg/dL	83.3	33–117	μmol/L
D-dimer[b]	Plasma	Negative (<500)	ng/mL	1	Negative (<500)	ng/mL
Dehydroepiandrosterone (DHEA) (unconjugated, male)[b]	Plasma, serum	180–1250	ng/dL	0.0347	6.2–43.3	nmol/L
Dehydroepiandrosterone sulfate (DHEA-S) (male)[b]	Plasma, serum	10–619	μg/dL	0.027	0.3–16.7	μmol/L
Desipramine (therapeutic)	Plasma, serum	50–200	ng/mL	3.75	170–700	nmol/L
Diazepam (therapeutic)	Plasma, serum	100–1000	ng/mL	0.00351	0.35–3.51	μmol/L
Digoxin (therapeutic)	Plasma	0.5–2.0	ng/mL	1.281	0.6–2.6	nmol/L
Disopyramide (therapeutic)	Plasma, serum	2.8–7.0	mg/L	2.95	8–21	μmol/L
Doxepin (therapeutic)	Plasma, serum	150–250	ng/mL	3.58	540–890	nmol/L
Electrolytes:						
Chloride	Serum, plasma	96–106	mEq/L	1	96–106	mmol/L
Carbon dioxide (CO_2)	Serum, plasma, venous blood	22–28	mEq/L	1	22–28	mmol/L
Potassium	Plasma	3.5–5.0	mEq/L	1	3.5–5.0	mmol/L
Sodium[b]	Plasma	136–142	mEq/L	1	136–142	mmol/L
Eosinophils (see complete blood count, white blood cell count)						
Epinephrine (supine)	Plasma	<50	pg/mL	5.46	<273	pmol/L
Epinephrine[b]	Urine	<20	μg/24 h	5.46	<109	nmol/day
Erythrocyte count (see complete blood count, red blood cell count)						
Erythrocyte sedimentation rate (ESR)[b]	Whole blood	0–20	mm/h	1	0–20	mm/h
Erythropoietin	Serum	5–36	mU/mL	1	5–36	IU/L
Estradiol (E2, unconjugated),[b] female:						
Follicular phase	Serum	20–350	pg/mL	3.69	73–1285	pmol/L
Midcycle peak	Serum	150–750	pg/mL	3.69	551–2753	pmol/L
Luteal phase	Serum	30–450	pg/mL	3.69	110–1652	pmol/L
Postmenopausal	Serum	<59	pg/mL	3.69	<218	pmol/L
Estradiol (unconjugated),[b] male	Serum	<20	pg/mL	3.67	<184	pmol/L
Estriol (E3, unconjugated), males and nonpregnant females, varies with length of gestation	Serum	<2	ng/mL	3.47	<6.9	nmol/L
Estrogens (total),[b] female:						
Follicular phase	Serum	60–200	pg/mL	1	60–200	ng/L
Luteal phase	Serum	160–400	pg/mL	1	160–400	ng/L

	Specimen	Traditional Reference Interval	Traditional Units	Conversion Factor, Multiply →, ← Divide	SI Reference Interval	SI Units
Postmenopausal	Serum	<130	pg/mL	1	<130	ng/L
Estrogens (total),[b] male	Serum	20–80	pg/mL	1	20–80	ng/L
Estrone (E1),[b] female:						
Follicular phase	Plasma, serum	100–250	pg/mL	3.69	370–925	pmol/L
Luteal phase	Plasma, serum	15–200	pg/mL	3.69	55–740	pmol/L
Postmenopausal	Plasma, serum	15–55	pg/mL	3.69	55–204	pmol/L
Estrone (E1),[b] male	Plasma, serum	15–65	pg/mL	3.69	55–240	pmol/L
Ethanol (ethyl alcohol) (legal intoxication—2 levels listed)	Serum, whole blood	>80 / >100	mg/dL	0.2171	>17.4 / 21.7	mmol/L
Ethosuximide (therapeutic)	Plasma, serum	40–100	µg/mL	7.08	283–708	µmol/L
Ethylene glycol (toxic)	Plasma, serum	>30	mg/dL	0.1611	>5	mmol/L
Everolimus (therapeutic)	Whole blood	3–15	ng/mL	1.04	5–16	nmol/L
Fatty acids (nonesterified)	Plasma	8–25	mg/dL	0.0354	0.28–0.89	mmol/L
Fecal fat (as stearic acid)	Stool	2.0–6.0	g/day	1	2–6	g/day
Felbamate (therapeutic)	Serum, plasma	30–60	µg/mL	4.2	126–252	µmol/L
Ferritin[b]	Plasma	15–200	ng/mL	1	15–200	µg/L
α-Fetoprotein[b]	Serum	<10	ng/mL	1	<10	µg/L
Fibrinogen	Plasma	150–400	mg/dL	0.01	1.5–4.0	g/L
Fibrin breakdown products (fibrin split products)	Serum	<10	µg/mL	1	<10	mg/L
Folate (folic acid)	Red blood cells	166–640	ng/mL	2.266	376–1450	nmol/L
Folate (folic acid)	Serum	5–25	ng/mL	2.266	11–57	nmol/L
Follicle-stimulating hormone (FSH),[b] female:						
Follicular phase	Serum	1.37–9.9	mIU/mL	1	1.3–9.9	IU/L
Ovulatory phase	Serum	6.17–17.2	mIU/mL	1	6.1–17.2	IU/L
Luteal phase	Serum	1.09–9.2	mIU/mL	1	1.0–9.2	IU/L
Postmenopausal	Serum	19.3–100.6	mIU/mL	1	19.3–100.6	IU/L
FSH[b] male	Serum	1.42–15.4	mIU/mL	1	1.4–15.4	IU/L
FSH[b] female	Urine	2–15	IU/24 h	1	2–15	IU/day
FSH[b] male	Urine	3–12	IU/24 h	1	3–11	IU/day
Fructosamine[b]	Serum	1.5–2.7	mmol/L	1	1.5–2.7	mmol/L
Gabapentin (therapeutic)	Serum, plasma	2–20	µg/mL	5.84	12–117	µmol/L
Gastrin (fasting)	Serum	<100	pg/mL	1	<100	ng/L
Gentamicin (therapeutic)	Serum	6–10	µg/mL	2.1	12–21	µmol/L
Glucagon[b]	Plasma	20–100	pg/mL	1	20–100	ng/L
Glucose[b]	Serum, plasma	70–110	mg/dL	0.05551	3.9–6.1	mmol/L
Glucose	CSF	50–80	mg/dL	0.05551	2.8–4.4	mmol/L
Glucose-6-phosphate dehydrogenase	Red blood cells	10–14	U/g of Hb	0.0645	0.65–0.90	U/mol of Hb

Continued next page—

	Specimen	Traditional Reference Interval	Traditional Units	Conversion Factor, Multiply →, ← Divide	SI Reference Interval	SI Units
Glutamic acid[b]	Plasma	0.2–2.8	mg/dL	67.97	15–190	µmol/L
Glutamine	Plasma	6.1–10.2	mg/dL	68.42	420–700	µmol/L
γ-Glutamyltransferase (GGT; γ-glutamyl transpeptidase)[b]:						
Female	Serum	<30	U/L	0.017	0.51	µKat/L
Male	Serum	<50	U/L	0.017	<0.85	µKat/L
Glycerol (free)[b]	Serum	<1.5	mg/dL	0.1086	<0.16	mmol/L
Glycine[b]	Plasma	0.9–4.2	mg/dL	133.3	120–560	µmol/L
Glycated hemoglobin (hemoglobin A1, A1c):						
Whole blood	Whole blood	4–5.6	% of total Hb	1	4–5.6	Fraction of total Hb
Gold (therapeutic)	Serum	100–200	µg/dL	0.05077	5.1–10.2	µmol/L
Growth hormone, adult (GH, somatotropin)[b]	Plasma, serum	<10	ng/mL	1	<10	µg/L
Haloperidol (therapeutic)	Serum, plasma	5–20	ng/mL	2.6	13–52	nmol/L
Haptoglobin[b]	Serum	40–180	mg/dL	0.01	0.4–1.8	g/L
Hematocrit (see complete blood count)						
Hemoglobin (see complete blood count)						
Hemoglobin A1c (see glycated hemoglobin)						
Hemoglobin A2[b]	Whole blood	2.0–3.5	% total Hb		2.0–3.5	Fraction of 1.0
Hemoglobin F[b] (fetal hemoglobin in adult)	Whole blood	<2	%	0.01	<2	Fraction of 1.0
Histidine[b]	Plasma	0.5–1.7	mg/dL	64.5	32–110	µmol/L
Homocysteine (total)	Plasma, serum	4–12	µmol/L	1	4–12	µmol/L
Homovanillic acid[b]	Urine	<8	mg/24 h	5.489	<45	µmol/day
Human chorionic gonadotropin (hCG) (nonpregnant adult female)	Serum	<3	mIU/mL	1	<3	IU/L
β-Hydroxybutyric acid	Serum	0.21–2.81	mg/dL	96.05	20–270	µmol/L
5-Hydroxyindoleacetic acid (5-HIAA)	Urine	<25	mg/24 h	5.23	<131	µmol/day
17α-Hydroxyprogesterone,[b] female:						
Follicular phase	Serum	15–70	ng/dL	0.03	0.4–2.1	nmol/L
Luteal phase	Serum	35–290	ng/dL	0.03	1.0–8.7	nmol/L
Postmenopausal	Serum	<70	ng/dL	0.03	<2.1	nmol/L
17α-Hydroxyprogesterone,[b] male	Serum	27–199	ng/dL	0.03	0.8–6.0	nmol/L
Hydroxyproline	Plasma	<0.55	mg/dL	76.3	<42	µmol/L
5-Hydroxytryptamine (see serotonin)						
Ibuprofen (therapeutic)	Serum, plasma	10–50	µg/mL	4.85	49–243	µmol/L
Imipramine (therapeutic)	Serum, plasma	150–250	ng/mL	3.57	536–893	nmol/L
Immunoglobulin A (IgA)[b]	Serum	50–350	mg/dL	0.01	0.5–3.5	g/L
Immunoglobulin D (IgD)	Serum	0.5–3.0	mg/dL	10	5–30	mg/L

	Specimen	Traditional Reference Interval	Traditional Units	Conversion Factor, Multiply →, ← Divide	SI Reference Interval	SI Units
Immunoglobulin E (IgE)	Serum	10–179	IU/mL	2.4	24–430	µg/L
Immunoglobulin G (IgG)[b]	Serum	600–1560	mg/dL	0.01	6.0–15.6	g/L
Immunoglobulin M (IgM)[b]	Serum	54–222	mg/dL	0.01	0.5–2.2	g/L
Insulin	Plasma	5–20	µU/mL	6.945	34.7–138.9	pmol/L
Inhibin A:						
Males	Serum	1.0–3.6	pg/mL	1	1.0–3.6	ng/L
Female, early follicular	Serum	5.5–28.2	pg/mL	1	5.5–28.2	ng/L
Female, late follicular	Serum	19.5–102.3	pg/mL	1	19.5–102.3	ng/L
Female, midcycle	Serum	49.9–155.5	pg/mL	1	49.9–155.5	ng/L
Female, midluteal	Serum	13.2–159.6	pg/mL	1	13.2–159.6	ng/L
Female, postmenopausal	Serum	1.0–3.9	pg/mL	1	1.0–3.9	ng/L
Insulin C-peptide (see C-peptide)						
Insulin-like growth factor[b]	Serum	130–450	ng/mL	1	130–450	µg/L
Ionized calcium (see calcium)						
Iron (total)[b]	Serum	60–150	µg/dL	0.179	10.7–26.9	µmol/L
Iron-binding capacity	Serum	250–400	µg/dL	0.179	44.8–71.6	µmol/L
Isoleucine[b]	Plasma	0.5–1.3	mg/dL	76.24	40–100	µmol/L
Isoniazid (therapeutic)	Plasma or serum	1–7	µg/mL	7.29	7–51	µmol/L
Isopropanol (toxic)	Plasma, serum	>400	mg/L	0.0166	>6.64	mmol/L
Lactate (lactic acid)	Arterial blood	3–11.3	mg/dL	0.111	0.3–1.3	mmol/L
Lactate (lactic acid)	Venous blood	4.5–19.8	mg/dL	0.111	0.5–2.2	mmol/L
Lactate dehydrogenase (LDH, LD)	Serum	50–200	U/L	1	50–200	U/L
Lamotrigine (therapeutic)	Serum, plasma	2.5–15	µg/dL	3.91	10–59	µmol/L
Lead (toxic)	Whole blood	>5	µg/dL	0.0483	>0.24	µmol/L
Leucine[b]	Plasma	1.0–2.3	mg/dL	76.3	75–175	µmol/L
Leukocyte count (see complete blood count, white blood cell count)						
Levetiracetam (therapeutic)	Serum, plasma	12–46	µg/mL	5.88	71–270	µmol/L
Lidocaine (therapeutic)	Serum, plasma	1.5–6.0	µmL g/mL	4.27	6.4–25.6	µmol/L
Lipase[a]	Serum	0–160	U/L	0.017	0–2.72	µKat/L
Lipoprotein(a) (Lp(a))	Serum, plasma	10–30	mg/dL	0.01	0.1–0.3	g/L
Lithium (therapeutic)	Serum, plasma	0.6–1.2	mEq/L	1	0.6–1.2	mmol/L
Lorazepam (therapeutic)	Serum, plasma	50–240	ng/mL	3.11	156–746	nmol/L
Luteinizing hormone (LH),[b] female:						
Follicular phase	Serum	2.0–15.0	mIU/L	1	2.0–15.0	IU/L
Ovulatory peak	Serum	22.0–105.0	mIU/L	1	22.0–105.0	IU/L
Luteal phase	Serum	0.6–19.0	mIU/L	1	0.6–19.0	IU/L
Postmenopausal	Serum	16.0–64.0	mIU/L	1	16.0–64.0	IU/L
Luteinizing hormone (LH),[b] male	Serum	2.0–12.0	mIU/L	1	2.0–12.0	IU/L

Continued next page—

	Specimen	Traditional Reference Interval	Traditional Units	Conversion Factor, Multiply →, ← Divide	SI Reference Interval	SI Units
Lymphocytes (see complete blood count, white blood cell count)						
Lysine[b]	Plasma	1.2–3.5	mg/dL	68.5	80–240	µmol/L
Lysozyme (muramidase)	Serum	4–13	mg/L	1	4–13	mg/L
Magnesium[b]	Serum	1.5–2.5	mg/dL	0.4114	0.62–1.03	mmol/L
Manganese	Whole blood	10–12	µg/L	18.2	182–218	nmol/L
Maprotiline (therapeutic)	Plasma, serum	200–600	ng/mL	1	200–600	µg/L
MCH (see complete blood count)						
MCHC (see complete blood count)						
Meperidine (therapeutic)	Serum, plasma	0.4–0.7	µg/mL	4.04	1.6–2.8	µmol/L
Mercury	Whole blood	0.6–59.0	µg/L	4.99	3.0–294.4	nmol/L
Metanephrines (total)[b]	Urine	<1.0	mg/24 h	5.07	<5	µmol/day
Methadone (therapeutic)	Serum, plasma	100–400	ng/mL	0.00323	0.32–1.29	µmol/L
Methanol (toxic)	Whole blood, serum	>1.5	mg/L	0.0312	>0.05	mmol/L
Methemoglobin	Whole blood	<0.24	g/dL	155	<37.2	µmol/L
Methemoglobin	Whole blood	<1.0	% of total Hb	0.01	<0.01	Fraction of total Hb
Methionine[b]	Plasma	0.1–0.6	mg/dL	67.1	6–40	µmol/L
Methsuximide (therapeutic)	Serum, plasma	10–40	µg/mL	5.29	53–212	µmol/L
Methyldopa (therapeutic)	Serum, plasma	1–5	µg/mL	4.73	5–24	µmol/L
Metoprolol (therapeutic)	Serum, plasma	75–200	ng/mL	3.74	281–748	nmol/L
Mexthotrexate:						
Toxic 24 h after dose	Serum, plasma	≥10	µmol/L	1	≥10	µmol/L
Toxic 48 h after dose	Serum, plasma	≥1	µmol/L	1	≥1	µmol/L
Toxic 72 h after dose	Serum, plasma	≥0.1	µmol/L	1	≥0.1	µmol/L
β_2-Microglobulin	Serum	<2	µg/mL	85	<170	nmol/L
Monocytes (see complete blood count, white blood cell count)						
Morphine (therapeutic)	Serum, plasma	10–80	ng/mL	3.5	35–280	nmol/L
Muramidase (see lysozyme)						
Mycophenolic acid (therapeutic)	Serum, plasma	1.3–3.5	µg/mL	3.12	4–11	µmol/L
Naproxen (therapeutic)	Plasma, serum	>50	µg/mL	4.34	>217	µmol/L
Neutrophils (see complete blood count, white blood cell count)						
Niacin (Vitamin B$_3$, nicotinic acid)	Plasma, serum	0.50–8.45	ug/mL	7.3	3.65–61.69	µmol/day
Nickel	Whole blood	1.0–28.0	µg/L	17	17–476	nmol/L
Nicotine (smoker)	Plasma	0.01–0.05	mg/L	6.16	0.062–0.308	µmol/L
Norepinephrine[b]	Plasma	110–410	pg/mL	5.91	650–2423	nmol/L
Norepinephrine[b]	Urine	15–80	µg/24 h	5.91	89–473	nmol/day
Nortriptyline (therapeutic)	Serum, plasma	50–150	ng/mL	3.8	190–570	nmol/L

	Specimen	Traditional Reference Interval	Traditional Units	Conversion Factor, Multiply →, ← Divide	SI Reference Interval	SI Units
N-telopeptide (BCE, bone collagen equivalents):						
Men	Serum	5.4–24.2	nmol BCE/L	1	5.4–24.2	nmol BCE/L
Premenopausal women	Serum	6.2–19.0	nmol BCE/L	1	6.2–19.0	nmol BCE/L
Ornithine[b]	Plasma	0.4–1.4	mg/dL	75.8	30–106	µmol/L
Osmolality[b]	Serum	275–295	mOsm/kg H_2O	1	275–295	mmol/kg H_2O
Osmolality	Urine	250–900	mOsm/kg H_2O	1	250–900	mmol/kg H_2O
Osteocalcin[b]	Serum	3.0–13.0	ng/mL	1	3.0–13.0	µg/L
Oxalate	Serum	1.0–2.4	mg/L	11.4	11–27	µmol/L
Oxazepam (therapeutic)	Serum, plasma	0.2–1.4	µg/mL	3.49	0.7–54.9	µmol/L
Oxycodone (therapeutic)	Plasma, serum	10–100	ng/mL	3.17	32–317	nmol/L
Oxygen, partial pressure (Po_2)	Arterial blood	80–100	mm Hg	1	80–100	mm Hg
Pantothenic acid (see vitamin B_5)						
Parathyroid hormone:						
Intact[b]	Serum	10–50	pg/mL	1	10–50	ng/L
N-terminal specific[b]	Serum	8–24	pg/mL	1	8–24	ng/L
C-terminal (mid-molecule)	Serum	0–340	pg/mL	1	0–340	ng/L
Pentobarbital (therapeutic)	Serum, plasma	1–5	µg/mL	4.42	4.0–22	µmol/L
Pepsinogen I[h]	Serum	28–100	ng/mL	1	28–100	µg/L
pH (see blood gases)						
Phenobarbital (therapeutic)	Serum, plasma	15–40	µg/mL	4.31	65–172	µmol/L
Phenylalanine[b]	Plasma	0.6–1.5	mg/dL	60.5	35–90	µmol/L
Phenytoin (therapeutic)	Serum, plasma	10–20	µg/mL	3.96	40–79	µmol/L
Phosphatase, tartrate-resistant acid	Serum	1.5–4.5	U/L	0.017	0.03–0.08	µkat/L
Phosphorus (inorganic)[b]	Serum	2.3–4.7	mg/dL	0.3229	0.74–1.52	mmol/L
Phosphorus (inorganic)[b]	Urine	0.4–1.3	g/24 h	32.29	12.9–42.0	mmol/day
Plasminogen	Plasma	80–120	%	0.01	0.80–1.20	Fraction of 1.0
Plasminogen activator inhibitor activity	Plasma	3–56	mIU/mL	1	3–56	IU/L
Platelet count (see complete blood count, platelet count)						
Porphobilinogen deaminase	Red blood cells	>7.0	nmol/s/L	1	>7.0	nmol/(s L)
Potassium	Plasma	3.5–5.0	mEq/L	1	3.5–5.0	mmol/L
Prealbumin—transthyretin	Serum, plasma	18–45	mg/dL	0.01	0.18–0.45	g/L
Pregnanediol,[b] female:						
Follicular phase	Urine	<2.6	mg/24 h	3.12	<8	µmol/day
Luteal phase	Urine	2.3–10.6	mg/24 h	3.12	8–33	µmol/day
Pregnanediol,[b] male	Urine	0–1.9	mg/24 h	3.12	0–5.9	µmol/day
Pregnanetriol[b]	Urine	<2.5	mg/24 h	2.97	<7.5	µmol/day

Continued next page—

	Specimen	Traditional Reference Interval	Traditional Units	Conversion Factor, Multiply →, ← Divide	SI Reference Interval	SI Units
Primidone (therapeutic)	Serum, plasma	12 May	µg/mL	4.58	23–55	µmol/L
Procainamide (therapeutic)	Serum, plasma	10 Apr	µg/mL	4.23	17–42	µmol/L
Progesterone,[b] female:						
Follicular phase	Serum	0.1–0.7	ng/mL	3.18	0.5–2.2	nmol/L
Luteal phase	Serum	2.0–25.0	ng/mL	3.18	6.4–79.5	nmol/L
Progesterone,[b] male	Serum	0.13–0.97	ng/mL	3.18	0.4–3.1	nmol/L
Prolactin (nonlactating subject)	Serum	1–25	ng/mL	1	1–25	µg/L
Proline[b]	Plasma	1.2–3.9	mg/dL	86.9	104–340	µmol/L
Propoxyphene (therapeutic)	Serum	0.1–0.4	µg/mL	2.946	0.3–1.2	µmol/L
Propanolol (therapeutic)	Serum, plasma	50–100	ng/mL	3.86	190–386	nmol/L
Protein (total)[b]	Serum	6.0–8.0	g/dL	10	60–80	g/L
Protein C activity	Plasma	70–140	%	0.01	0.70–1.40	Fraction of 1.0
Protein electrophoresis (serum protein electrophoresis [SPEP]), fraction of total protein:						
Albumin	Serum	52–65	%	0.01	0.52–0.65	Fraction of 1.0
α_1-Globulin	Serum	2.5–5.0	%	0.01	0.025–0.05	Fraction of 1.0
α_2-Globulin	Serum	7.0–13.0	%	0.01	0.07–0.13	Fraction of 1.0
β-Globulin	Serum	8.0–14.0	%	0.01	0.08–0.14	Fraction of 1.0
γ-Globulin	Serum	12.0–22.0	%	0.01	0.12–0.22	Fraction of 1.0
Protein electrophoresis (SPEP), concentration:						
Albumin	Serum	3.2–5.6	g/dL	10	32–56	g/L
α_1-Globulin	Serum	0.1–0.4	g/dL	10	1–10	g/L
α_2-Globulin	Serum	0.4–1.2	g/dL	10	4–12	g/L
β-Globulin	Serum	0.5–1.1	g/dL	10	5–11	g/L
γ-Globulin	Serum	0.5–1.6	g/dL	10	5–16	g/L
Protein S activity	Plasma	70–140	%	0.01	0.70–1.40	Fraction of 1.0
Protein S free antigen	Plasma	80–160	%	0.01	0.80–1.60	Fraction of 1.0
Prothrombin time (PT)	Plasma	10–13	seconds	1	10–13	seconds
Protoporphyrin	Red blood cells	15–50	µg/dL	0.0177	0.27–0.89	µmol/L
Prostate-specific antigen (PSA)	Serum	0–4.0	ng/mL	1	0–4.0	µg/L
Pyridinium cross-links (deoxypyridinoline):						
Male	Urine	10.3–20	nmol/mmol creatinine	1	10.3–20	nmol/mmol creatinine
Premenopausal female	Urine	15.3–33.6	nmol/mmol creatinine	1	15.3–33.6	nmol/mmol creatinine
Pyridoxine (see vitamin B₆)						
Pyruvate (as pyruvic acid)	Whole blood	0.3–0.9	mg/dL	113.6	34–102	µmol/L
Quinidine (therapeutic)	Serum, plasma	2.0–5.0	µg/mL	3.08	6.2–15.4	µmol/L

	Specimen	Traditional Reference Interval	Traditional Units	Conversion Factor, Multiply →, ← Divide	SI Reference Interval	SI Units
Red blood cell count (see complete blood count)						
Red cell folate (see folate)						
Renin (normal-sodium diet)[b]	Plasma	1.1–4.1	ng/mL/h	1	1.1–4.1	ng/(mL h)
Reticulocyte count[b]	Whole blood	25–75	$10^3\ \mu L^{-1}$	1	25–75	$10^9\ L^{-1}$
Reticulocyte count[b] (fraction)	Whole blood	0.5–1.5	% of RBCs	0.01	0.005–0.015	Fraction of RBCs
Retinol (see vitamin A)						
Rheumatoid factor	Serum	<30	IU/mL	1	<30	kIU/L
Riboflavin (see vitamin B_2)						
Salicylates (therapeutic)	Serum, plasma	15–30	mg/dL	0.0724	1.08–2.17	mmol/L
Sedimentation rate (see erythrocyte sedimentation rate)						
Selenium	Whole blood	58–234	µg/L	0.0127	0.74–2.97	µmol/L
Serine[b]	Plasma	0.7–2.0	mg/dL	95.2	65–193	µmol/L
Serotonin (5-hydroxytryptamine)	Whole blood	50–200	ng/mL	0.00568	0.28–1.14	µmol/L
Sertraline (therapeutic)	Serum or plasma	10–50	ng/mL	3.27	33–164	nmol/L
SPEP (see protein electrophoresis)						
Sex hormone-binding globulin[b]	Serum	0.5–1.5	µg/dL	34.7	17.4–52.1	nmol/L
Sirolimus (therapeutic)	Whole blood	4–20	ng/mL	1.1	4–22	nmol/L
Sodium[b]	Plasma	136–142	mEq/L	1	136–142	mmol/L
Somatostatin	Plasma	<25	pg/mL	1	<25	ng/L
Somatomedin C (see insulin-like growth factor)						
Strychnine (toxic)	Whole blood	>0.5	mg/L	2.99	>1.5	µmol/L
Substance P	Plasma	<240	pg/mL	1	<240	ng/L
Sulfhemoglobin	Whole blood	<1.0	% of total Hb	0.01	<0.010	Fraction of total Hb
Tacrolimus (therapeutic)	Whole blood	3–20	ng/mL	1.24	4–25	nmol/L
Taurine[b]	Plasma	0.3–2.1	mg/dL	80	24–168	µmol/L
Testosterone,[b] male	Plasma, serum	300–1200	ng/dL	0.0347	10.4–41.6	nmol/L
Testosterone,[b] female	Plasma, serum	<85	ng/dL	0.0347	2.95	nmol/L
Theophylline (therapeutic)	Plasma, serum	10–20	µg/mL	5.55	56–111	µmol/L
Thiamine (see vitamin B_1)						
Thiocyanate (nonsmoker)	Plasma, serum	1–4	mg/L	17.2	17–69	µmol/L
Thiopental (therapeutic)	Plasma, serum	1–5	µg/mL	4.13	4–21	µmol/L
Thioridazine (therapeutic)	Plasma, serum	1.0–1.5	µg/mL	2.7	2.7–4.1	µmol/L
Thrombin time	Plasma	16–24	seconds	1	16–24	seconds
Threonine[b]	Plasma	0.9–2.5	mg/dL	84	75–210	µmol/L

Continued next page—

	Specimen	Traditional Reference Interval	Traditional Units	Conversion Factor, Multiply →, ← Divide	SI Reference Interval	SI Units
Thyroglobulin[b]	Serum	3–42	ng/mL	1	3–42	µg/L
Thyrotropin (thyroid-stimulating hormone, TSH)[b]	Serum	0.5–5.0	µIU/mL	1	0.5–5.0	mU/L
Thyroxine, free (FT$_4$)[b]	Serum	0.9–2.3	ng/dL	12.87	12–30	pmol/L
Thyroxine, total (T$_4$)[b]	Serum	5.5–12.5	µg/dL	12.87	71–160	nmol/L
Thyroxine-binding globulin (TBG),[b] as T$_4$ binding capacity	Serum	10–26	µg/dL	12.9	129–335	nmol/L
Tissue plasminogen activator	Plasma	<0.04	IU/mL	1000	<40	IU/L
Tobramycin (therapeutic)	Plasma, serum	5–10	µg/mL	2.14	10–21	µmol/L
Tocainide (therapeutic)	Plasma, serum	4–10	µg/mL	5.2	21–52	µmol/L
α-Tocopherol (see vitamin E)						
Topiramate (therapeutic)	Serum, plasma	5–20	µg/mL	2.95	15–59	µmol/L
Transferrin (siderophilin)[b]	Serum	200–380	mg/dL	0.01	2.0–3.8	g/L
Triglycerides[b]	Plasma, serum	10–190	mg/dL	0.01129	0.11–2.15	mmol/L
Triiodothyronine, free (FT$_3$)[b]	Serum	260–480	pg/dL	0.0154	4.0–7.4	pmol/L
Triiodothyronine, resin uptake[b]	Serum	25–35	%	0.01	0.25–0.35	Fraction of 1.0
Triiodothyronine, total (T$_3$)[b]	Serum	70–200	ng/dL	0.0154	1.08–3.14	nmol/L
Troponin I (cardiac)	Serum	0–0.4	ng/mL	1	0–0.4	µg/L
Troponin T (cardiac)	Serum	0–0.1	ng/mL	1	0–0.1	µg/L
Tryptophan[b]	Plasma	0.5–1.5	mg/dL	48.97	25–73	µmol/L
Tyrosine[b]	Plasma	0.4–1.6	mg/dL	55.19	20–90	µmol/L
Urea nitrogen (BUN)[b]	Serum	8–23	mg/dL	0.0357	2.9–8.2	mmol/L
Uric acid[b]	Serum	4.0–8.5	mg/dL	0.0595	0.24–0.51	mmol/L
Urobilinogen[b]	Urine	0.05–2.5	mg/24 h	1.693	0.1–4.2	µmol/day
Valine[b]	Plasma	1.7–3.7	mg/dL	85.5	145–315	µmol/L
Valproic acid (therapeutic)	Plasma, serum	50–150	µg/mL	6.93	346–1040	µmol/L
Vancomycin (therapeutic)	Plasma, serum	10–20	µg/mL	0.69	6.9–13.8	µmol/L
Vanillylmandelic acid (VMA)[b]	Urine	2.1–7.6	mg/24 h	5.046	11–38	µmol/day
Vasoactive intestinal polypeptide	Plasma	<50	pg/mL	1	<50	ng/L
Verapamil (therapeutic)	Plasma, serum	100–500	ng/mL	2.2	220–1100	nmol/L
Vitamin A (retinol)[b]	Serum	30–80	µg/dL	0.0349	1.05–2.80	µmol/L
Vitamin B$_1$ (thiamine)	Whole blood	2.5–7.5	µg/dL	29.6	74–222	nmol/L
Vitamin B$_2$ (riboflavin)	Plasma, serum	4–24	µg/dL	26.6	106–638	nmol/L
Vitamin B$_5$ (pantothenic acid)	Whole blood	0.2–1.8	µg/mL	4.56	0.9–8.2	µmol/L
Vitamin B$_6$ (pyridoxine)	Plasma	5–30	ng/mL	4.046	20–121	nmol/L
Vitamin B$_{12}$ (cyanocobalamin)[b]	Serum	160–950	pg/mL	0.7378	118–701	pmol/L
Vitamin C (ascorbic acid)	Plasma, serum	0.4–1.5	mg/dL	56.78	23–85	µmol/L
Vitamin D, 1,25-dihydroxyvitamin D	Plasma, serum	16–65	pg/mL	2.6	42–169	pmol/L

	Specimen	Traditional Reference Interval	Traditional Units	Conversion Factor, Multiply →, ← Divide	SI Reference Interval	SI Units
Vitamin D, 25-hydroxyvitamin D	Plasma, serum	14–60	ng/mL	2.496	35–150	nmol/L
Vitamin E (α-tocopherol)[b]	Plasma, serum	0.5–1.8	mg/dL	23.22	12–42	μmol/L
Vitamin K	Plasma, serum	0.13–1.19	ng/mL	2.22	0.29–2.64	nmol/L
von Willebrand factor (ranges vary according to blood type)	Plasma	70–140	%	0.01	0.70–1.40	Fraction of 1.0
Warfarin (therapeutic)	Plasma, serum	1.0–10	μg/mL	3.24	3.2–32.4	μmol/L
White blood cell count[b]	Whole blood	4.5–11.0	$10^3\ \mu L^{-1}$	1	4.5–11.0	$10^9\ L^{-1}$
White blood cell, differential count (see complete blood count)						
Xylose absorption test (25-g dose)[b]	Whole blood	>25 mg/dL	mg/dL	0.06661	>1.7	mmol/L
Zidovudine (therapeutic)	Plasma, serum	0.15–0.27	μg/mL	3.74	0.56–1.01	μmol/L
Zinc	Serum	50–150	μg/dL	0.153	7.7–23.0	μmol/L

The sample type listed under Specimen in this table shows the reference interval for that specimen type. Thus, if the specimen for a test is listed as serum, the reference interval shown is for serum specimens. For many tests listed with serum as the specimen type, plasma is also acceptable, often with a similar reference interval.

The normal ranges listed here are included as a helpful guide and are by no means comprehensive. The listed reference, unless noted, pertains to adults. Laboratory results are method dependent and can have intralaboratory variation. Conversion factors are not affected by age-related differences. This table is compiled from data in the following sources: (1) Tietz NW, ed. *Clinical Guide to Laboratory Tests*. 3rd ed. Philadelphia, PA: WB Saunders Co; 1995; (2) Laposata M. *SI Unit Conversion Guide*. Boston, MA: NEJM Books; 1992; (3) *American Medical Association Manual of Style: A Guide for Authors and Editors*. 9th ed. Chicago, IL: AMA; 1998:486–503. Copyright 1998, American Medical Association; (4) Jacobs DS, DeMott WR, Oxley DK, eds. *Jacobs & DeMott Laboratory Test Handbook with Key Word Index*. 5th ed. Hudson, OH: Lexi-Comp Inc; 2001; (5) Henry JB, ed. *Clinical Diagnosis and Management by Laboratory Methods*. 20th ed. Philadelphia, PA: WB Saunders Co; 2001; (6) Kratz A, et al. Laboratory reference values. *N Engl J Med*. 2006;351:1548–1563; (7) Burtis CA, ed. *Tietz Textbook of Clinical Chemistry and Molecular Diagnostics*. 5th ed. St. Louis, MO: Elsevier; 2012. This version of the table of reference ranges was reviewed and updated by Jessica Franco-Colon, PhD, and Kay Brooks.

[a]The SI unit katal is the amount of enzyme generating 1 mol of product per second. Although provisionally recommended as the SI unit for enzymatic activity, it has not been universally accepted. It is suitable to maintain use of U/L in these circumstances (conversion factor 1.0).

[b]For this analyte, there is sex or age dependence for the reference range. There may be several different normal ranges for different pediatric age groups. Consult your clinical laboratory for the local institution age-specific reference range. Pediatric reference values may also be found in Soldin SJ, Brugnara C, Wong EC, eds.; Hicks JM, editor emeritus. *Pediatric References Intervals*. 5th ed. (formerly *Pediatric Reference Ranges*). Washington, DC: AACC Press; 2005.

Amino Acid	3-Letter Code	1-Letter Code
Alanine	Ala	A
Cysteine	Cys	C
Aspartic acid or aspartate	Asp	D
Glutamic acid or glutamate	Glu	E
Phenylalanine	Phe	F
Glycine	Gly	G
Histidine	His	H
Isoleucine	Ile	I
Lysine	Lys	K
Leucine	Leu	L
Methionine	Met	M
Asparagine	Asn	N
Proline	Pro	P
Glutamine	Gln	Q
Arginine	Arg	R
Serine	Ser	S
Threonine	Thr	T
Valine	Val	V
Tryptophan	Trp	W
Tyrosine	Tyr	Y

Concepts in Laboratory Medicine

Michael Laposata

LEARNING OBJECTIVES

1. To understand the concepts of sensitivity, specificity, predictive value, prevalence, and incidence.
2. To learn the frequently encountered preanalytical variables that influence laboratory test results.
3. To identify the well-known interferences in many of the laboratory tests.
4. To understand the individual steps in specimen processing and handling.
5. To understand the guidelines for appropriate selection of laboratory tests.
6. To understand how cell injury and inflammation result in the generation of plasma markers of these processes.

CHAPTER OUTLINE

An understanding of the principles set forth in this chapter is essential for the appropriate selection of laboratory tests and the accurate interpretation of the test results.

ANALYTICAL AND STATISTICAL CONCEPTS IN DATA ANALYSIS

Ranges Used in the Interpretation of Test Results

In clinical practice, the laboratory test result is typically placed alongside a range of values for that test. In most cases, this is the reference range, which is often considered to be the normal range. It is important to understand that individuals with values inside the reference range may have subclinical disease, despite the presence of an apparently normal value. The reference range is dependent on the instrument and reagent used to perform the test. The reference ranges are ideally established inside the laboratory where the test is being performed. Reference ranges supplied by instrument and reagent manufacturers are not likely to correspond perfectly to ranges generated within an individual laboratory. This is because the population used to establish the range by the manufacturer and/or the instruments and reagents used by the manufacturer are likely to be different from those in an individual clinical laboratory.

The Reference Range

To obtain a reference range, individuals without disease and on no medications donate samples for testing. A distribution of these values, which should be numerous enough to be statistically reliable, is plotted. The data are not always distributed in a Gaussian pattern. Therefore, statistical methods that are nonparametric are used to identify the central 95% of values. This range, representing the middle 95% of results, is the reference range. As an indication that being outside the reference range does not always reflect the disease, 5% of normal healthy, nonmedicated individuals who donated samples for the reference range determination now fall outside of what has become the reference range for the test.

> To obtain a reference range, individuals without disease and on no medications donate samples for testing. The middle 95% of results is the reference range.

The Desirable Range

Several decades ago, the results for cholesterol testing demonstrated that individuals eating a high-fat diet showed high cholesterol levels that were associated with atherosclerotic vascular disease. When these apparently healthy, nonmedicated individuals provided samples for reference range determinations, the central 95% of values from this population provided an inappropriately high reference range. Therefore, the use of the classical reference range for selected laboratory tests in certain populations was not recommended. For that reason, desirable or prognosis-related ranges were developed. These are commonly established by groups of experts associating laboratory test results with clinical outcome.

Therapeutic Range

For certain medications, a therapeutic window exists to provide a target for a blood, plasma, or serum level for the medication. Values below the therapeutic range typically reflect an inadequate amount of medication, and values above the therapeutic range may be associated with a particular toxic effect. In some cases, the therapeutic range does not reflect the amount of medication in the blood, but instead reflects a therapeutic effect produced by the drug. For example, patients taking the drug warfarin are not monitored with warfarin levels in the blood. Instead, the warfarin decreases the level of coagulation factors, which results in a prolonged prothrombin time (PT), and a calculated value known as the international normalized ratio (INR). The therapeutic range of warfarin, therefore, is determined by its effect rather than its concentration in the blood.

Interpretations of Clinical Laboratory Test Results that Do Not Involve the Use of a Range

For certain laboratory tests, the presence of disease is associated with a value that is above a threshold. The use of troponin as a marker for myocardial infarction involves a threshold value, such that a level above the threshold is consistent with cardiac ischemia. Another prominent example is related to the detection of drugs of abuse. Any level above zero, as a threshold value, provides evidence for the ingestion of an illicit drug.

> For certain laboratory tests, the presence of disease is associated with a value that is above a threshold.

For laboratory tests that show too much variability to permit the use of a range or a threshold, an individual laboratory result for a specific patient can be compared with a result for that same patient that was generated previously. The longitudinal analysis of results over time can indicate the progression or regression of the disease.

The Need for a Diagnostic Cutoff

Figure 1–1 shows two populations of individuals and their results for a particular test. All of the individuals who do not have disease have a low value for the test, and all of the individuals with disease have a high value for the test. There is no overlap between groups in **Figure 1–1**. In **Figure 1–2**, a more commonly encountered situation is shown. There is overlap in laboratory values between individuals with disease and those without disease. This means that the diagnostic threshold will necessarily misclassify some patients to create false-positives, false-negatives, or both.

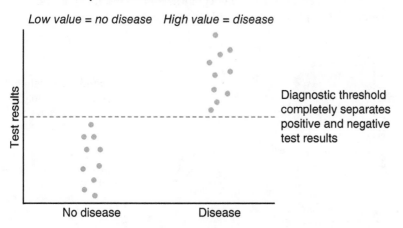

FIGURE 1–1   **A clinical situation in which the diagnostic threshold completely separates those with disease from those without disease.**

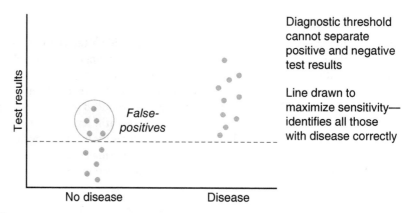

FIGURE 1–2   **A clinical situation in which a diagnostic threshold is selected to maximize sensitivity.**

The Definition of Sensitivity of a Laboratory Test

The population of individuals who have disease is the focus of sensitivity. The sensitivity of a laboratory test is its capacity to identify all individuals with disease. The threshold used in **Figure 1–2** maximizes sensitivity by placing all those with disease above the line. This placement of the diagnostic threshold would decrease the number of false-negatives (those with disease who fall below the line), because everybody with the disease would have a positive test result. However, there is a significant misclassification of individuals without disease. As the diagnostic threshold is lowered, an increasing number of patients without disease would be told they have a positive test result, and by implication, the disease in question. The formula for sensitivity is:

$$\frac{\text{true-positives}}{\text{true-positives} + \text{false-negatives}} \times 100$$

True-positives and false-negatives are groups with disease; as noted above, sensitivity focuses on those with disease.

The Definition of Specificity of a Laboratory Test

The population of individuals without disease is the focus of specificity. Specificity is a statistical term that indicates the effectiveness of a test to correctly identify those without disease. When used to describe a laboratory test, it does not refer to its ability to diagnose a "specific" disease among a group of related disorders. One could maximize specificity by raising the threshold shown in **Figure 1–3** to place all those without disease below the line. This would decrease the

> The sensitivity of a laboratory test is its capacity to identify all individuals with disease. Specificity is a statistical term that indicates the effectiveness of a test to correctly identify those without disease.

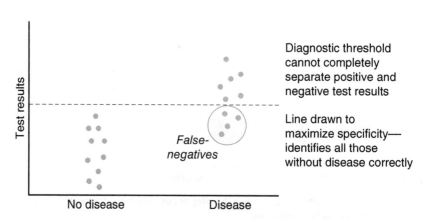

FIGURE 1–3   **A clinical situation in which a diagnostic threshold is selected to maximize specificity.**

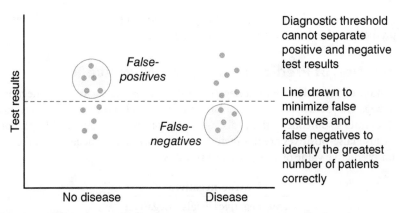

FIGURE 1–4 **A clinical situation in which a diagnostic threshold is selected to minimize the number of false-positives and false-negatives.**

number of false-positives because everyone without disease would have a negative test result. However, there would be a significant misclassification of the individuals with disease. As the diagnostic threshold is raised, an increasing number of patients with disease would be told they have a negative test result and, by implication, no disease. The formula for specificity is:

$$\frac{\text{true-negatives}}{\text{true-negatives} + \text{false-positives}} \times 100$$

True-negatives and false-positives are the groups without disease; as noted above, specificity focuses on those without disease.

The Identification of the Appropriate Value for the Diagnostic Threshold

For diseases that are serious and treatable, and for which a second confirmatory laboratory test exists, it is important to maximize sensitivity as in **Figure 1–2**. For example, for diagnosis of AIDS, it is better to have a few false-positives that can be subsequently correctly identified with a confirmatory test than to fail to identify individuals with HIV infection who might unknowingly infect others. However, for diseases that are serious and not curable, a false-positive result is catastrophic for the patient. For such diseases, such as pancreatic cancer, it is better to use the threshold shown in **Figure 1–3** for diagnosis because if individuals with disease are missed, it will have no effect on the treatment or outcome. When there are no compelling reasons to maximize either sensitivity or specificity, the threshold value should be established to minimize the total number of false-positives and false-negatives, as shown in **Figure 1–4**.

The Definition of Predictive Value of a Positive Test

The population of individuals with a positive test result is the focus of positive predictive value. The positive predictive value for a laboratory test indicates the likelihood that a positive test result identifies someone with disease. It should be noted that the predictive value of a positive test is greatly influenced by the prevalence of the disease in the area where testing is performed. As an example, a screening test for HIV infection is more likely to be confirmed as positive in an area where many individuals are infected with HIV, as opposed to a location where there is only a rare case of HIV infection. In the latter situation, most of the positive HIV tests in the initial evaluation of a patient are found to be false-positives by confirmatory tests. A high percentage of false-positives from a low prevalence disease, as shown in the following formula, decreases the predictive value of the positive test:

$$\frac{\text{true-positives}}{\text{true-positives} + \text{false-positives}} \times 100$$

The positive predictive value for a laboratory test indicates the likelihood that a positive test result identifies someone with disease. The negative predictive value for a laboratory test indicates the likelihood that a negative test result identifies someone without disease.

True-positives and false-positives are the groups with a positive test result; as noted above, positive predictive value focuses on those with a positive test.

The Definition of Predictive Value of a Negative Test

The population of individuals with a negative test result is the focus of the negative predictive value. The negative predictive value for a laboratory test indicates the likelihood that a negative test result identifies someone without disease. It is not greatly influenced by the prevalence of disease because false-positives are not included in the formula for negative predictive value. The formula for predictive value of a negative test result is:

$$\frac{\text{true-negatives}}{\text{true-negatives} + \text{false-negatives}} \times 100$$

True-negatives and false-negatives are the groups with a negative test result; as noted above, negative predictive value focuses on those with a negative test result.

The Difference Between Prevalence and Incidence

The prevalence of a disease reflects the number of existing cases in a population. It is usually expressed as a percentage of a certain population. Incidence refers to the number of new cases occurring within a period of time, usually 1 year. For example, in the United States, sore throat has a low prevalence because considering the size of the population there is a low percentage of individuals at a given time afflicted with sore throat. However, it has a high incidence because many new cases of sore throat appear each year.

Precision versus Accuracy

Precision refers to the ability to test one sample and repeatedly obtain results that are close to each other. This does not infer that the mean of these very similar numbers is the correct number (see **Figure 1–5**). Some analyses, which have great precision, are very inaccurate. The accuracy reflects the relationship between the number obtained and the true result. Thus, a sample could have high accuracy but low precision if it provides the correct answer but has substantial variability as the sample is repeatedly tested.

> Precision refers to the ability to test one sample and repeatedly obtain results that are close to each other. This does not infer that the mean of these very similar numbers is the correct number.

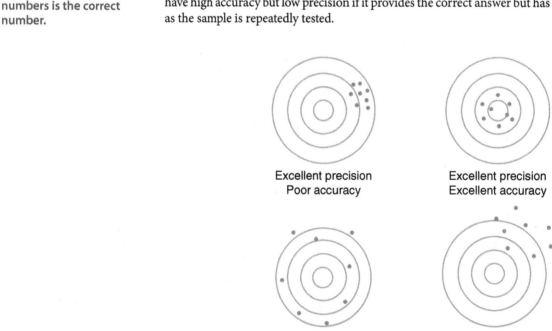

Excellent precision
Poor accuracy

Excellent precision
Excellent accuracy

Poor precision
Excellent accuracy

Poor precision
Poor accuracy

FIGURE 1–5 A series of "bulls-eye" illustrations that display excellent or poor precision and accuracy.

Analyzing Errors in Laboratory Performance

There are three phases of laboratory analysis. The first of these is the preanalytical phase. This time frame is from patient preparation for the laboratory test, through the time of sample collection, until the sample arrives in the laboratory. Most of the errors in laboratory test performance occur in this phase. Examples of preanalytical errors are inappropriate preparation of the patient, such as not fasting for a particular test in which fasting is required; ingesting drugs that will interfere with the laboratory tests; collection of the specimen in the wrong tube; delayed transport of the specimen to the laboratory; storage of the sample at an incorrect temperature; and collection of an inadequate amount of blood in vacuum tubes containing a fixed amount of anticoagulants. All these errors occur before the sample arrives for analysis and make it impossible, no matter how great the analytical precision within the laboratory, to provide a test result that truly reflects the patient's condition. The second phase is the analytical phase, which is the time that the sample is being analyzed in the laboratory. Errors can occur during this process, but they are much less common now because of the high level of automation of many laboratory instruments. Examples of analytical errors are incorrect use of the instrumentation and the use of expired reagents. The third phase of laboratory test performance is the postanalytical phase, which begins when the result is generated and ends when the result is reported to the physician. Examples of errors in this phase, which are more common than analytical errors but less common than preanalytical errors, are delay in time to enter a completed result into the laboratory information system and reporting results for the wrong patient.

Minimizing Errors in the Selection of Laboratory Tests

As the number of laboratory tests has increased in size, complexity, and cost, health care providers are highly challenged to select the correct tests, and only the correct tests, in pursuit of a diagnosis. One approach commonly implemented to assist physicians in correct test selection is the use of a reflex test algorithm. Tests are ordered by algorithm selection, such as selection of an algorithm to determine the cause of a prolonged PTT result. Using the algorithm, the clinical laboratory notes the results of the first test in the algorithm, and that result determines which test is performed next. For example, if the prolonged PTT is further evaluated with a PTT mixing study, a normal result would direct testing toward assays for factors VIII, IX, XI, and XII. An elevated result in the PTT mixing study, on the other hand, would direct testing toward an inhibitor in the PTT reaction, such as a lupus anticoagulant. Testing is continued within the algorithm until a diagnosis, which explains the prolonged PTT in this case, is identified.

Laboratory test selection is also made more difficult because many laboratory tests have synonyms, and many compounds have related forms. For example, the test most commonly known as the lupus anticoagulant is also called the lupus inhibitor, and the general term that includes the lupus anticoagulant and related entities is antiphospholipid antibody. Vitamin D has several isoforms that include 25-hydroxyvitamin D and 1,25-dihydroxyvitamin D. Incorrect laboratory test selection is a major source of medical error.

Minimizing Errors in the Interpretation of Laboratory Test Results

With thousands of tests on the clinical laboratory test menu, it is impossible for a health care provider to understand the clinical significance of an abnormality for each test. This has become particularly noteworthy with the introduction of tests for genetic alterations, because there are so many and the clinical significance of the alterations may not yet be well established. In some institutions, narrative interpretations of complex clinical laboratory evaluations are prepared by experts in the field. In most institutions, such narratives require a special request for completion, but an emerging concept is to provide narrative interpretations for all complex clinical laboratory evaluations automatically, as they are provided in radiology and in anatomic pathology. Misinterpretation of laboratory test results has been increasingly noted as a source of poor patient outcome.

PREANALYTICAL VARIABLES THAT AFFECT LABORATORY TEST RESULTS

The Effect of Age on Laboratory Tests

There are a number of laboratory tests that have different normal ranges for patients of different ages. This is particularly important in pediatrics. Newborns especially have many different normal ranges than adults or older children for substances in blood and other bodily fluids. For example, several of the coagulation factors do not reach adult levels for many months after birth. As a second well-known example, the cholesterol level rises with age.

The Effect of Gender on Laboratory Tests

Gender has a significant bearing on many laboratory tests. Testosterone and estradiol are obvious examples. In addition, among women there are variations in the serum concentration of various hormones throughout the menstrual cycle.

The Effect of Body Mass on Laboratory Tests

Muscle mass can affect the level of certain compounds, such as creatine kinase, in the blood. It is also known that there is an increase in the serum cholesterol level with obesity, because the cholesterol level is related to the amount of body fat.

Preparation of the Patient for Laboratory Testing

One of the most commonly encountered patient preparations is fasting, usually for 8 to 12 hours, depending on the test. The serum triglyceride level can be significantly affected by eating, and fasting is absolutely required. Another test for which fasting is required is the fasting blood glucose.

For certain laboratory tests, there are a number of special preparations of the patient that are necessary to provide the most clinically useful, accurate, and precise result. One of the most commonly encountered patient preparations is fasting, usually for 8 to 12 hours, depending on the test. The serum triglyceride level can be significantly affected by eating, and fasting is absolutely required. Another test for which fasting is required is the fasting blood glucose used in the evaluation of a patient for diabetes.

Patient Posture for Blood Collection

Patient posture may affect the result for certain tests. There is a lower plasma volume when the patient is upright because there is pooling of fluid in the dependent parts of the body when standing. When the patient is supine, there is a movement of fluid back into the circulation from the tissues. The extra volume in the circulation can dilute certain compounds in the blood. It is best to monitor the patient in the same postural position if the test result is affected by posture and if the values need to be compared with one another over time.

Differences in Test Results Between Samples of Venous, Arterial, and Capillary Blood

Venous blood may have a different concentration of a compound than arterial blood. The best examples are the blood gases that show marked differences between arterial and venous blood because of the exchange of gases in the lungs. There may also be a difference between capillary blood and arterial and venous blood. Blood glucose values may differ significantly in capillary (finger-stick) samples from venous or arterial blood.

INTERFERENCES IN LABORATORY TESTS

Analytical Interferences in Laboratory Testing

Interferences may result in falsely high or falsely low values, depending on the interfering substance and the particular test. Although there are many compounds that can interfere with the accurate and precise quantitation of a compound, there are three major interferences that must be considered when selecting and interpreting results of laboratory tests. These are hemolysis that makes plasma and serum red; elevated bilirubin that makes plasma and serum shades of orange, green, or brown; and lipemia that makes plasma and serum milky white. There are many drugs, particularly those that color the plasma and serum, that can produce significant analytical interference. Many automated laboratory tests are spectrophotometric, and therefore depend on measurable changes in the color of plasma or serum after a chemical reaction. This is why alterations in the color of the serum or plasma often interfere with laboratory test performance.

Impact of Drugs on Laboratory Test Results

Drugs can affect laboratory tests in two ways—as an interfering substance in the laboratory test only and by producing an effect in the body that alters a laboratory test result. For example, there are many drugs that will increase the PT in patients receiving warfarin (coumadin) by an in vivo potentiation or diminution of warfarin-induced anticoagulation. There are a number of drug effects, however, that alter the result of a particular test strictly in vitro, and do not change anything in vivo.

TEST SELECTION GUIDELINES

The Use of Screening Tests Before Esoteric Tests

Screening laboratory tests are typically inexpensive, easy-to-perform assays that indicate whether additional tests need to be performed to reach a diagnosis. Whenever possible, if a screening test is available, it should be used before the more expensive or time-consuming tests are performed. An example of the use of a screening test is the partial thromboplastin time (result within minutes/hours and at low cost) to assess a major portion of the coagulation cascade. Only if this value is elevated should tests be performed for PTT-related coagulation factor deficiencies (results within several hours and at high cost).

The Danger of Ordering Too Many Laboratory Tests

As noted in the discussion of the normal range, 5% of individuals who have no disease can fall outside of the reference range established by the central 95% of healthy individuals. Thus, if an individual without disease has 20 different tests, it is likely on a statistical basis that he/she will have 1 abnormal value (5% = 1 of 20). In medical practice, the abnormal test result for the normal patient often leads to further evaluation and raises suspicion for a disease that does not exist. Thus, by limiting the number of tests ordered for a patient to those relevant to the clinical presentation of the patient, one is less likely to encounter false-positive or false-negative results.

SPECIMEN PROCESSING AND HANDLING

The Importance of Turnaround Time

An accurate and precise laboratory test result provided after a decision has been made regarding patient management is of no value. Since results for all laboratory tests cannot be provided immediately, the physicians and laboratory personnel must decide on clinically relevant turnaround times for each laboratory test. In addition, if a patient is not discharged from the hospital because of a delay in laboratory testing, this may have a significant financial impact from unnecessary length of stay. All steps related to turnaround time, from ordering of the test to the reporting of the result, must be carefully analyzed and shortened as much as possible.

Tubes for Blood Collection

There are a number of different tubes into which blood may be collected. The tubes used for the vast majority of collections contain a vacuum to help draw the blood into the tube. The tops of the tubes have a different color depending on the contents of the tube prior to blood collection (**Table 1–1**). Several of the tubes contain anticoagulants to prevent the clotting of the blood in the tube.

There are three major interferences that must be considered when selecting and interpreting results of laboratory tests. These are hemolysis that makes plasma and serum red; elevated bilirubin that makes plasma and serum shades of orange, green, or brown; and lipemia that makes plasma and serum milky white.

TABLE 1-1   Cap Color and Contents of Tubes for Blood Collection

Cap Color	Contents
Red	Nothing—the sample clots and the product is serum
Light blue	Citrate anticoagulant
Purple (lavender)	EDTA anticoagulant
Green	Heparin anticoagulant
Red/Green with gel	No anticoagulant, but a gel is present that separates the serum or plasma and the cells after centrifugation
Gray	Fluoride (glycolysis inhibitor for optimum glucose measurements) with oxalate anticoagulant
Yellow	Acid-citrate-dextrose solution (ACD) that anticoagulates the blood and helps preserve the blood cells during processing
Dark blue	Nothing—but the tube is specially treated to permit accurate measurement of trace heavy materials

Clotted blood that is centrifuged to remove the clot and any cells is known as serum. Blood that has not been clotted and is then centrifuged to remove any cells is known as plasma.

Clotted blood that is centrifuged to remove the clot and any cells is known as serum. Blood that has not been clotted and is then centrifuged to remove any cells is known as plasma. For many laboratory tests, the same result is obtained in an assay if serum or plasma is used. However, this is often not the case. The clotting of the blood, for example, makes blood cell counts and coagulation tests impossible because the clotting factors are consumed in the clot and the blood cells become trapped in it. If the clotting of the blood to form serum is not absolutely necessary, tests can be performed with a shorter turnaround time using plasma because there is no requisite time to wait for the blood clot to form. The amount of anticoagulant in the light blue-top tube must be in a specific proportion to the blood volume in the tube, usually 9 parts blood to 1 part citrate solution. When an inadequate amount of blood is collected into a blue-top tube, the ratio of blood to anticoagulant is less than 9:1. This can result in spuriously high values for the PT and PTT tests. Thus, light blue-top tubes must be filled appropriately to obtain accurate results for clotting tests.

Timing of Blood Collection

Patients may have a need to present for phlebotomy at a certain time of the day if the parameter being measured has a diurnal variation in its concentration.

Dynamic tests involve the measurement of a patient response to a treatment or stimulus, and timing of collection is important in these studies. The oral glucose tolerance test, in which plasma glucose levels are measured after the oral ingestion of a glucose solution, is an example of such a test.

A third situation in which timing of sample collection is important is in therapeutic drug monitoring. The serum level of certain drugs is measured to determine if the concentration is within the therapeutic window. The serum level of a drug varies greatly as the drug is absorbed, distributed, and metabolized, so the timing of collection must be consistent. For the monitoring of many drugs, a "trough" level is obtained just before the next dose of the drug is administered.

EFFECTS OF CELL INJURY AND INFLAMMATION ON SELECTED LABORATORY TESTS

The Release of Plasma Markers of Organ Damage from Injured Cells

When cells are injured, components of the cells can leak out of the damaged or dead cells and make their way into the systemic circulation. This permits the measurement of these "marker" compounds in the serum or plasma as a test for injury to the organ. The most important features of plasma markers of cell injury are that (1) they are not rapidly removed from the circulation;

(2) they are relatively organ specific so that the damaged organ is identified; and (3) the compound is precisely and accurately measured in the clinical laboratory. A well-known example includes the release of the creatine kinase-MB fraction and troponin from myocardial cells injured by ischemia in myocardial infarction.

Markers of Inflammation and the Acute-Phase Response

The concentration of many plasma proteins changes significantly in patients with inflammation. Infections (even minor viral illnesses), autoimmune disorders, and many other conditions result in an increased concentration of proteins known as acute-phase reactants. Commonly used tests to assess the severity of inflammation, from whatever cause, are the erythrocyte sedimentation rate (ESR) and C-reactive protein (CRP). Examples of acute-phase reactant proteins include fibrinogen, which can rise as much as 10-fold over baseline, and von Willebrand factor, which can rise 2- to 3-fold over baseline. The rise in von Willebrand factor with inflammation can mask a deficiency of von Willebrand factor in patients with von Willebrand disease, and this highlights the need to obtain baseline values after an acute-phase response subsides for accurate diagnosis.

When cells are injured, components of the cells can leak out of the damaged or dead cells and make their way into the systemic circulation. This permits the measurement of these "marker" compounds in the serum or plasma as a test for injury to the organ.

The Serologic Diagnosis of Infectious Disease

It is not uncommon to suffer an infection with an organism that is not identifiable by Gram staining or other microscopic analysis and is not readily cultured. For these infections, the diagnosis is often made by identifying and measuring the amount of antibody produced in response to an antigen derived from the infectious agent. The antibody response typically takes several days to a week or two (dependent on past exposure) to emerge, and the appearance of IgM antibody before IgG occurs in most infections. This is why the presence of IgM antibody in a serologic test is likely to reflect an acute infection rather than past exposure. Serologic tests may also be designed to detect and measure an antigen associated with the infectious agent. This obviates the inherent delay in diagnosis of the infection of up to approximately 2 weeks while waiting for the antibody response to occur.

MOLECULAR TESTING

Overview

There is an increasing amount of genetic information used to establish a diagnosis, and there is limited understanding by the majority of practitioners about the genetic terminology which appears in the patient record. This section will attempt to clarify the terminology associated with the identification of genetic variations in tumors and in non-tumor tissue at both the gene level and at the level of the protein. This section will also present information about the genetic variations associated with poor responses to therapeutic drugs, also called pharmacogenomics. Finally, there will be a section to describe the molecular results from tests used to identify infectious organisms.

Genetic Structure and Function

Humans have more than 20,000 genes, and each human has many alterations when compared to a sequence established as normal. There are multiple reference sequences in use. The most frequently used reference is a "coding DNA reference sequence," and that is the reason why the changes at the DNA level are sometimes described starting with "c." The genetic sequence building blocks are four nucleotides—adenine (A), guanine (G), cytosine (C), and thymine (T). Individual genes contain segments called exons which code for a protein. The segments between the exons, which do not code for a protein, are called introns.

Genetic variations can result in the exchange of one nucleotide for another, the deletion of one or more nucleotides, the insertion of one or more nucleotides, or other complex changes. Most changes in an exon of a gene will result in a change in the amino acid sequence of the protein associated with that gene. Therefore, changes in the gene can result in the exchange of one amino acid for another, the deletion of one or more amino acids, the insertion of one or more amino acids, or if the change in the genetic code introduces a stop codon, protein synthesis will be truncated before synthesis is complete.

The commonly used term "mutation" is synonymous with "genetic variation" which is being increasingly used because patients are concerned about being designated as a "mutant." There is also confusion about the difference between mutation and polymorphism. A mutation is associated with disease, and is present in less than 1% of individuals. A polymorphism represents a genetic variation because it is different from the "normal" comparator genetic code, but it is not associated with a disease. A polymorphism is found in more than 1% of individuals. Mutations can arise spontaneously in any cell. When they appear in cells other than germ cells (eggs and sperm), they are called somatic mutations. For example, many mutations in tumors are somatic mutations because they are not present at birth. The opposite term is a germline mutation. As noted by the name, these mutations are in the patient's germ cells, and these mutations can be inherited. Importantly, even though mutations can be associated with disease, the effect of a mutation may remain silent or contribute to the development of active disease.

Genetic Variations/Mutations

When patients do not have a mutation for which they have been tested, the results in a patient report read "no mutation detected," "wild type," or "normal." The following example provides a description of an alteration in which there has been a substitution of one nucleotide for another. This results in a change of one amino acid. In this example, the colloquial name of the mutation is the factor V Leiden mutation, and there are numerous colloquial synonyms. One synonym is "activated protein C resistance mutation, Leiden type." The genetic variation that produces this mutation is a replacement of a guanine for an adenine at position 1691 within the gene. It is written as 1691G>A, and represents a single nucleotide variant (SNV), a term which is preferred over single nucleotide polymorphism (SNP). It is also written as c.1691G>A because the use of the "c" indicates that the change is at the DNA level. The change at this position in the gene results in a change in the amino acid at position 506 for the factor V protein. An arginine residue is substituted for by a glutamine residue. This is written as Arg506Gln using the three-letter code for an amino acid, or as R506Q using the one-letter code for an amino acid. Use of the three-letter code for an amino acid makes it much easier to identify the amino acid. For example, there are multiple amino acids which start with the letter A, and therefore these amino acids must have different single letter codes for identification. It is not clear, for example, why aspartic acid has a single letter amino acid code of D. Its three-letter code of Asp makes its identification much more obvious. A protein variation is also written as p.R506Q, to indicate that the change is at the level of the amino acid sequence of the protein.

The next example describes a genetic variation in which a single nucleotide has been deleted from the gene for the cystic fibrosis transmembrane regulator (CFTR). The colloquial name for this mutation is the Delta F508 mutation. At the genetic level, it is written as 1521_1523 del. This indicates that the nucleotides from position 1521 up to 1523 are deleted. The nucleotides which are deleted may be mentioned, and in this case, the genetic variation may be written as 1521_1523delCTT. The deletion of the nucleotide in the gene results in the deletion of the amino acid phenylalanine in the protein. Therefore, the protein designation using the three-letter amino acid code is Phe508del.

There are many other variants that can be present in the genome. A duplication occurs when one or more nucleotides are duplicated. When the nucleotides from position c.4375 to c.4385 are duplicated, the genetic variation is reported as c.4375_4385dup. When one or more nucleotides are inserted into a gene, the sequence of three nucleotides in the gene is altered. As an example, c.4375_4376insACCT indicates that four nucleotides were inserted between positions 4375 and 4376 in the gene. A number of more complex genetic variations are known to exist.

Clinical Studies—Tumor Genetics

When the DNA is extracted from non-tumor tissue of a patient, the genetic alterations described represent those found in the patient. However, DNA can be also be extracted from samples of carefully collected tumor tissue, and the genetic alterations described in those evaluations most often represent those found in the tumor tissue.

What follows is an example of a genetic variation found in many cancers in the BRAF gene. The BRAF-coded protein is part of a signaling pathway in cells that controls a number of important cell functions. Somatic mutations (i.e., not present in the germ cells) in the BRAF gene are common in several types of cancers including melanoma, and cancers of the colon and rectum, ovary, and thyroid gland. The results of these mutations produce a change in the signaling pathway in cells that leads to their uncontrolled growth. The mutation most commonly found in these cancers is one which replaces the amino acid valine with the amino acid glutamic acid at position 600. This is written as Val600Glu or V600E. Laboratory reports will typically state the presence or the absence of the BRAF mutation without description of the changes at the DNA or the protein level. Genetic information from tumors can lead to important information about choice of chemotherapeutic agents and patient prognosis. It is now common to assess mutations in dozens of different genes for a specific type of cancer. For example, a sample of breast cancer tissue can be analyzed to determine if there are genetic variations in six genes, including the genes for hereditary breast cancer known as BRCA1/2. Another available combination includes 17 genes to be evaluated in the assessment of treatment and prognosis for breast cancer patient. The analyses of these genes can involve targeted analysis for the presence of specific genetic alterations or the sequencing of small or large segments within the gene.

Mutations in the BRAF gene, also known as the BRAF proto-oncogene, can also appear in a variety of nonmalignant conditions. For example, at least two mutations in the BRAF gene have been found to cause Noonan syndrome. One change in the gene to produce Noonan syndrome results in replacement of the amino acid threonine with the amino acid proline at position 241. This is written as Thr241Pro. There is another mutation in the same gene which can also produce Noonan syndrome, and this variation is a replacement of the amino acid leucine with the amino acid phenylalanine at position 245 written as Leu245Phe.

A liquid biopsy is an assessment using a blood sample for circulating tumor cells or segments of DNA from tumor cells. It can be used to detect cancer early in the disease or to determine if a malignancy has recurred. Use of the blood samples rather than biopsies allows for more frequent evaluation of the patient and the detection of new molecular changes that occur with progression of the disease.

Clinical Studies—Whole Exome Sequencing (WES) and Whole Genome Sequencing (WGS)

When a patient evaluation does not lead to a diagnosis but does suggest an underlying genetic cause, it is possible to sequence the whole exome or the whole genome. This evaluation of the protein coding section of DNA sequences, that is WES, assesses only about 2 % of the DNA in human chromosomes, but this analysis identifies many mutations associated with disease. A whole exome sequence provides data on thousands of genes. WES can be performed on both tumor and non-tumor samples. The laboratory report from an exome analysis typically provides information on the number of genetic alterations found. One section names the specific deleterious mutations in disease genes related to the clinical phenotype which is submitted along with the sample. This genetic analysis would consider, for example, the presence of genetic variations associated with bleeding syndromes in a patient with a bleeding disorder. Another section lists variations within disease-related genes which have unknown clinical significance because it is not clear if the specific genetic variations are related to the clinical phenotype. Another section of the report lists mutations which are medically actionable but unrelated to clinical phenotype, which is bleeding in this example. New associations between mutations and specific diseases are appearing in the medical literature at a rapid rate. This has prompted the recommendation for whole exome and WGS (see below) that states "perform it once, but analyze it frequently."

The sequencing of both introns and exons, that is the whole genome, can also be performed. This analysis generates much more sequencing information because it covers 95% to 98% of the entire genome, and can, therefore, identify mutations outside of exons. WGS is an option, as is exome sequencing, when a diagnosis is elusive and it appears to have a genetic basis.

Currently, there is a debate over the benefits of WGS versus WES. The advantages of WES are largely less money and quicker turnaround time. WES reads only approximately 2% of the genome so the cost of performing the test is less. There is also less required data storage, and faster and less expensive data analyses. However, in WES, there are regions of the exome which are not sequenced, leading to missed identification of variants. The use of WGS allows for better identification of a number of complex genetic alterations, such as copy number variations and rearrangements, which are especially important in genetic analyses of tumors.

Clinical Studies—Pharmacogenomics

The terms pharmacogenomics and pharmacogenetics are often used interchangeably. Pharmacogenetics describes how a single gene variation influences the response to a single drug. Pharmacogenomics is a broader term. In this description, the two terms will be used interchangeably.

It has long been known that some individuals do not respond as expected to certain medications. For many of these individuals, the explanation is that a gene product associated with the metabolism of the drug causes the drug to be ineffective. In some cases, the gene codes for protein which metabolizes a drug into an active form. An example of this situation is the gene CYP2C19 which codes for a protein that is an enzyme which metabolizes the drug clopidogrel into its active form. The clopidogrel metabolite inhibits platelets at the ADP receptor. When the normal form of the gene is absent, it is known as a loss of function mutation because of the absence of the protein results in the patient being unable to generate the metabolite that is the active drug. Different mutations in the CYP2C19 gene can produce a gain of function. In patients with these mutations, clopidogrel is transformed more actively into its functional metabolite. In pharmacogenomics, the results are often but not always presented in the laboratory report as the allele, that is, the form of the gene which is present. It is uncommon in pharmacogenomics to present the molecular alteration associated with an individual allele. For example, a CYP2C19 allele known as *5 is associated with the replacement of a cytosine with a thymine at nucleotide position 1297 in the CYP2C19 gene (1297C>T). This results in CYP2C19 protein in which amino acid 433 has a tryptophan in place of an arginine (Arg433Trp). Despite knowledge of the change at the DNA level and at the protein level, the genetic description for this alteration is *X where the * indicates the allele which is present. For the drug–gene interaction between clopidogrel and CYP2C19, there are multiple loss of function alleles and one well-recognized gain of function allele. The normal allele, also called the wild–type allele for the CYP2C19 gene, is *1. All of the other alleles represent genetic variations leading to loss of function or gain of function. Importantly, clopidogrel can be replaced by two other drugs which inhibit platelets at the ADP receptor. Therefore, if a patient has a pharmacogenomic result that indicates an abnormal response to clopidogrel, the patient can receive a drug which is equally effective, though more expensive, to produce the desired clinical effect.

Clinical Studies—Molecular Testing for Infectious Disease

Identification of infectious agents can be completed within hours using molecular testing. The evaluation does not require isolation of the agent and growing it in culture, or testing it for a cytopathic effect, which can take days to weeks. Molecular-based techniques to determine if an infectious agent is present often able to assess for multiple infectious agents in one assay. Such testing ultimately assesses the resemblance of the DNA segments within the sample to known DNA sequences in microorganisms. The laboratory report indicates whether an agent of interest is detected or not. As an example where a single agent is targeted, a test can indicate if Zika virus DNA is detected. For a gastrointestinal virus panel performed to identify any of multiple agents causative for gastrointestinal illness, the laboratory report lists the agents which are detected.

CYTOGENETIC TESTING

Overview and Terminology

A karyotype allows for detection of gross alterations in chromosome size and in chromosome number. For example, cytogenetics allows for detection of chromosome breakage and transfer when two chromosomes break and the fragments rejoin with different chromosomes. In a cytogenetics report, the location of a gene on a chromosome is presented by first listing the number of the chromosome on which it is located, or the letter if it is on the X or Y chromosome.

Further localization is provided by the letter "p," which indicates the shorter arm of the chromosome, or by the letter "q" which indicates the longer arm of the chromosome. Further localization of a gene is provided by numbers that indicate first a region on the chromosome and then the band stained in the cytogenetic preparation which is closest to the gene of interest. For example, "7q31" indicates that the gene of interest is located on chromosome 7, on the long arm of the chromosome, within region 3, in band 1. Further information is provided by the terminology 7q31.1, which indicates that the gene is in sub-band 1 within band 1. (See Chapter 2 for the methodology used in the karyotype analysis.)

Genetic Variations Identified by Cytogenetics

When genetic variations are a result of the movement of large segments of a chromosome, the changes may be observed by reviewing the appearance of chromosomes in a karyotype analysis (see Chapter 2). A common variation visible by cytogenetics is a translocation. Translocations occur between non-homologous chromosomes. These are chromosomes that contain different genes. Homologous chromosomes, by comparison, are the pair of chromosomes, both of which have the same chromosome number, which are inherited as one from the mother and one from the father. Homologous chromosomes have the same genes, though the alleles for the genes may be different. When a piece of DNA moves from chromosome A to chromosome B, with no DNA from chromosome B transferring back to chromosome A, it is called a simple translocation. Alternatively, if a piece from chromosome B transfers to chromosome A, it is called a reciprocal translocation. If the amount switched between two chromosomes is the same, the translocation is balanced; and if the amount moving from one chromosome to another is larger than what is translocated back, the translocation is unbalanced.

As an example, a piece of chromosome 8 breaks off and translocates to chromosome 14. In this example, the location on chromosome 8 where the break occurred, is 8q24, and the location to which the piece is attached on chromosome 14 is 14q32. This translocation is reported as t(8;14)(q24;q32). Many such translocations are described in Chapter 13 involving hematologic malignancies. Several types of cancer are caused by acquired translocations. The "Philadelphia chromosome" found in chronic myelocytic leukemia is t(9;22)(q34;q11).

A translocation is only one of several cytogenetic changes. For example, pieces of chromosomes can be deleted. Deletion of a part of chromosome 5 which leads to cri-du-chat syndrome is reported as del(5). Extra chromosomes can arise. When a third chromosome of any type appears in a cell, the condition is known as trisomy. Transposition is an event in which a piece of a single chromosome breaks off and reattaches to the same chromosome in a different location. Crossing over occurs when genetic material is exchanged between homologous chromosomes during meiosis to produce recombinant chromosomes. Inversion is an event in which a piece of a chromosome breaks off, turns upside down, and reinserts itself in the same location. Duplication occurs when a piece of a chromosome is duplicated and remains present in the chromosome. There are other more complex cytogenetic changes that are known to occur.

Clinical Studies—Fluorescence In Situ Hybridization (FISH)

FISH involves the use of fluorescent probes to detect and localize specific DNA sequences on the chromosomes. For example, FISH analysis can be used to determine, using a probe for a gene on chromosome 21, the number of copies of chromosome number 21 which are present. Such an analysis is informative in an evaluation for Down syndrome. Using probes for two separate genes, FISH analysis can be used to determine if the two genes of interest are separated by a translocation or brought together by a translocation. FISH can also determine if a single gene has been disrupted by a translocation. (See Chapter 2 for the methodology used in FISH analysis.)

Clinical Studies—Comparative Genomic Hybridization (CGH) and Array CGH

A laboratory evaluation related to FISH is CGH, and the newer array CGH is more sensitive and specific than conventional CGH. This analysis determines whether there are gains or losses of either whole chromosomes or portions of a chromosome, and provides information on gene copy number variation. The most frequently identified candidates for CGH testing are patients with cancer, patients who have mental retardation of unknown etiology, and patients with congenital anomalies or dysmorphic features. (See Chapter 2 for the methodology used in CGH.)

SELF-ASSESSMENT QUESTIONS

1. Which of the following compounds is described in SI units?
   A. 4.3 g/dL albumin
   B. 0.6 mg/dL bilirubin
   C. 1.2 ng/mL digoxin
   D. 80 μmol/L creatinine

2. Which of the following blood collection vacuum tubes does not contain an anticoagulant?
   A. Blue top tube
   B. Purple top tube
   C. Red top tube
   D. Green top tube

3. Which of the following fluids is tested in the laboratory after producing a clot in the sample and removing the clot?
   A. Serum
   B. Cerebrospinal fluid
   C. Plasma
   D. Pleural fluid

4. Which of the following compounds is represented by desirable, borderline, and high ranges rather than a traditional reference range based on a Gaussian distribution of values?
   A. Sodium
   B. Hemoglobin
   C. Total cholesterol
   D. Thyroid-stimulating hormone

5. Which one of the following compounds has different ranges depending on the time of day because of diurnal variation?
   A. Total cortisol
   B. Total estrogens
   C. Prothrombin time
   D. Vitamin D

6. The range for the international normalized ratio (INR) is a
   A. Desirable range
   B. Reference range
   C. Therapeutic range
   D. Gender-specific range

7. When the diagnostic cutoff for a test is set to 100% sensitivity and there is overlap between the test results for those with and without disease, which of the following is true?
   A. There are no false-positives.
   B. False-positives are present.
   C. False-negatives are present.
   D. The percentage of true-positives is 100%.

8. Which of the following represents the correct definition for the predictive value of a negative test?
   A. (True-negatives/(true-negatives + false-positives)) × 100
   B. (True-positives/(true-positives + false-positives)) × 100
   C. (True-negatives/(true-negatives + false-negatives)) × 100
   D. (True-positives/(true-positives + false-negatives)) × 100

9. The result for a laboratory test repeated with the same sample of blood 10 times and an expected true value of 100 mg/dL shows a tight cluster of values between 300 and 305 mg/dL. Which of the following is true?
   A. The accuracy is excellent and the precision is poor.
   B. The precision is excellent and the accuracy is poor.
   C. Both the precision and the accuracy are excellent.
   D. Both the precision and the accuracy are poor.

10. Which one of the following hormones is least likely to be affected by gender?

    A. Testosterone
    B. Luteinizing hormone
    C. Estradiol
    D. Thyroid-stimulating hormone

11. Which is most likely to be elevated above its true baseline value if the patient does not fast for an appropriate period of time prior to sample collection?

    A. Glucose
    B. Creatinine
    C. Hemoglobin
    D. Prothrombin time

12. Which of the following is most likely to be used as a screening test that is often performed to determine the need for additional tests?

    A. Partial thromboplastin time (PTT)
    B. Factor VIII
    C. von Willebrand factor activity
    D. Genetic test for factor V Leiden

13. Which of the following compounds is released from injured cells, as opposed to being synthesized in normal-functioning organs?

    A. Albumin
    B. Immunoglobulin G (IgG)
    C. Troponin I
    D. Fibrinogen

14. The term Arg506Gln indicates which of the following?

    A. Glutamine is replaced by arginine at amino acid position 506 in the protein.
    B. Arginine and glutamine are deleted from the protein before and after amino acid number 506.
    C. Arginine is replaced by glutamine at amino acid position 506 in the protein.
    D. The genetic variation is the insertion of both arginine and glutamine at amino acid position 506 in the protein.

15. Pharmacogenomic testing for clopidogrel identifies on the laboratory report which of the following?

    A. DNA-associated nucleotide variations
    B. Allele variations
    C. Protein variations
    D. RNA associated nucleotide changes

FURTHER READING

den Dunnen JT, et al. HGVS recommendations for the description of sequence variants—2016 update. *Hum Mutat*. 2016;37:564–569.

Committee on Diagnostic Error in Health Care. In: Balogh EP, Miller BT, Ball JR, eds. *Improving Diagnosis in Health Care*. Washington, DC: National Academies Press; 2015:chap. 4.

Gornall AG. Basic concepts in laboratory investigation. In: Gornall AG, ed. *Applied Biochemistry of Clinical Disorders*. Philadelphia, PA: Harper and Row; 1980:chap 1.

Laposata M, Dighe AS. "Pre-pre" and "post-post" analytical error: high incidence patient safety hazards involving the clinical laboratory. *Clin Chem Lab Med*. 2007;45:712–719.

Laposata ME, Laposata M, Van Cott EM, Buchner DS, Kashalo MS, Dighe AS. Physician survey of a laboratory medicine interpretative service and evaluation of the influence of interpretations on laboratory test ordering. *Arch Pathol Lab Med*. 2004;128:1424–1427.

McPherson RA. Laboratory statistics. In: McPherson RA, Pincus MR, eds. *Henry's Clinical Diagnosis and Management by Laboratory Methods*. 21st ed. Philadelphia, PA: WB Saunders; 2006 [chapter 9].

Passiment E, Meisel JL, Fontanesi J, Fritsma G, Aleryani S, Marques M. Decoding laboratory test names: a major challenge to appropriate patient care. *J Gen Intern Med*. 2013;28:453–458.

Methods

Michael Laposata, James H. Nichols, Paul Steele,
Thomas P. Stricker, and Mayukh K. Sarkar

CHAPTER OUTLINE

No textbook in laboratory medicine would be complete without a description of methods used in the clinical laboratory. The methods described in this chapter are predominantly the common ones found in clinical laboratories. Each method description provides an overview of the basic concept of the assay, minimizing the details, while including clinically important information and a comment on the expense of the test and the complexity of the assay in the laboratory.

Some methods describe specific assays used almost exclusively in the clinical laboratory. For example, the PT and PTT are tests used for clinical assessment, with the goal to identify factor deficiencies in the coagulation cascade. Other methods are standard techniques used inside and outside the clinical laboratory. As an example, flow cytometry is a standard technique used in a variety of settings, and in this chapter it is shown how it is used in clinical laboratory testing.

Some tests are performed outside the laboratory in the vicinity of the patient. These tests are called "point-of-care tests," commonly abbreviated as POCT. This section contains illustrations for point-of-care testing for glucose and for point-of-care testing for a variety of compounds that can be detected by immunological methods (immunoassays).

There is rapid growth of testing in the clinical laboratory for genetic alterations. These laboratory studies are often highly complex and very expensive, and it is difficult for most clinical laboratories to perform them for these reasons. In addition, the clinical impact of many genetic alterations remains unknown. Therefore, it is not uncommon for a genetic test, especially an assay involving gene sequencing, to produce results that have no known clinical significance. Selected genetic methods for detection of mutations and for gene sequencing are illustrated in this chapter.

The expense assessment attached to each assay described in this chapter is an approximation, listed as low, moderate, or high. It should be understood that the charge for the test set by the institution operating the laboratory is usually proportional to the expense of the reagents, supplies, and labor required to perform the test. On occasion, however, there is a great disparity between the actual expense to perform the test and the amount charged by the institution for the assay. With this in mind, the expense estimation provided for each method in this chapter is more closely related to the actual cost of reagents, supplies, and labor in the laboratory, with the understanding that the amount charged for the test should be in the same range of low, moderate, or high—but it is not always the case.

Each method also has a descriptor to reflect whether it is manual, semiautomated, or highly automated. A comment has been added if microscopy is involved, as this makes any technique highly manual. It should be noted that for some methods, there is an option for manual performance or for using some level of automation. Manual methods are often less expensive. There is usually greater automation in the larger clinical laboratories because larger laboratories are more likely to have the test volume and the financial resources to justify the automated option. The term "semiautomated" indicates that there is a manual component associated with the use of an instrument that performs some steps of the analysis.

The turnaround time for an assay is not provided because it is impossible to know all of the elements associated with the turnaround time for a test within an individual institution. Broadly speaking, turnaround time is shorter for assays that are highly automated and less expensive, and longer for assays that are manual and highly expensive. It is important to understand that the turnaround time for an assay can be calculated using different starting points. For example, one starting point is the time a sample is collected. Another starting point is the time that a sample enters the laboratory. However, the most relevant starting time clinically, which predates the previous two starting times, is the time at which the physician orders the test. Similarly, there are different end points in the assessment of turnaround time. Most commonly, the end point is the time at which the result is reported by the laboratory into the laboratory information system. However, it is most important to know when the physician becomes aware of the result. This end point is extremely difficult to ascertain, and, therefore, virtually always the end point is considered to be the time at which the result is reported by the laboratory.

Finally, it should be noted what methods are not presented in this chapter. There are a number of methods that have been used progressively less over time, and in many institutions these assays are no longer performed at all in the clinical laboratory. These are numerous and include the radioimmunoassay (RIA), immunoelectrophoresis, lipoprotein electrophoresis, and the bleeding time. Also less frequently performed assays are not described in this chapter. Though this number of the infrequently used methods may be large, the number of tests performed using these methods account for a small percentage of the total tests performed in a typical hospital clinical laboratory.

Broadly speaking, the turnaround time is shorter for assays that are highly automated and less expensive, and longer for assays that are manual and highly expensive.

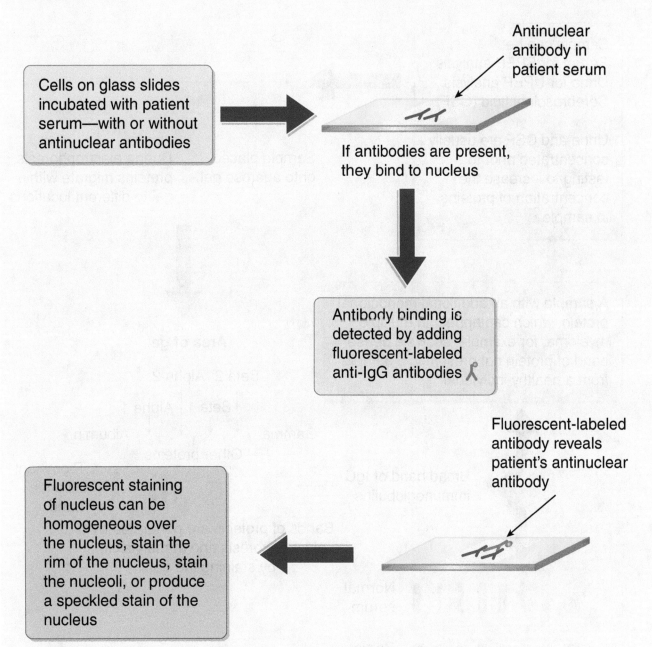

Antinuclear antibody (ANA) testing

To screen for autoimmune disorders by identifying antibodies which bind to the nucleus within cells in a specific pattern

Expense: Low   **Manual with microscopic evaluation**

Cells on glass slides incubated with patient serum—with or without antinuclear antibodies

Antinuclear antibody in patient serum

If antibodies are present, they bind to nucleus

Antibody binding is detected by adding fluorescent-labeled anti-IgG antibodies

Fluorescent-labeled antibody reveals patient's antinuclear antibody

Fluorescent staining of nucleus can be homogeneous over the nucleus, stain the rim of the nucleus, stain the nucleoli, or produce a speckled stain of the nucleus

If an antibody is detected, the patient's serum is progressively diluted until the staining is no longer detected. The final result includes the highest serum dilution producing a detectable response and the pattern of nuclear staining.

FIGURE 2–1

Protein electrophoresis (PEP)

To identify a monoclonal protein in blood, urine, or cerebrospinal fluid by separating it from normal proteins by electrophoresis

Expense: Moderate

Semiautomated

Sample can be:
Serum for SPEP analysis
Urine for UPEP analysis
Cerebrospinal fluid (CSF)

Urine and CSF are usually concentrated prior to testing to increase the concentration of proteins in sample

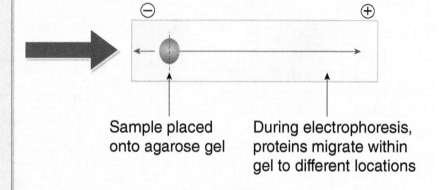

Sample placed onto agarose gel

During electrophoresis, proteins migrate within gel to different locations

A sample with an additional monoclonal protein, which can appear in multiple myeloma, for example, shows a dense band of protein not present in a sample from a healthy individual

Area of gel:

Beta 2   Alpha 2
Beta 1 | Alpha 1
Gamma   Albumin
Other proteins
Prominent albumin band

Broad band of IgG immunoglobulins

Bands of proteins are generated by electrophoresis and made visible by staining the gel

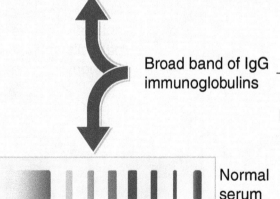

Normal serum

Serum from patient

Monoclonal protein

FIGURE 2–2

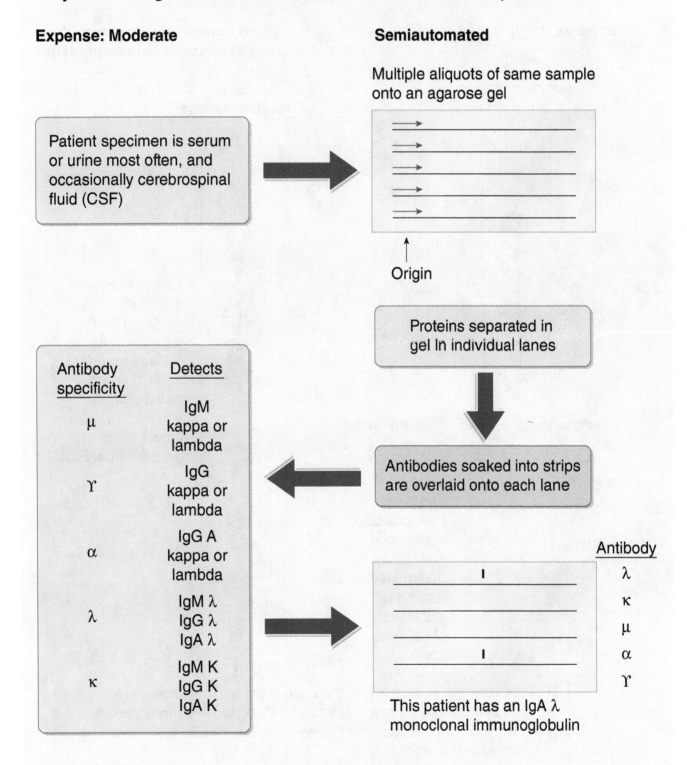

Immunofixation to identify monoclonal immunoglobulins

To identify the heavy chain and the light chain in a monoclonal immunoglobulin by determining the antibodies which bind to the monoclonal protein

Expense: Moderate

Semiautomated

Multiple aliquots of same sample onto an agarose gel

Origin

Patient specimen is serum or urine most often, and occasionally cerebrospinal fluid (CSF)

Proteins separated in gel In individual lanes

Antibodies soaked into strips are overlaid onto each lane

Antibody specificity	Detects
μ	IgM kappa or lambda
ϒ	IgG kappa or lambda
α	IgG A kappa or lambda
λ	IgM λ IgG λ IgA λ
κ	IgM K IgG K IgA K

Antibody

λ
κ
μ
α
ϒ

This patient has an IgA λ monoclonal immunoglobulin

FIGURE 2–3

Flow cytometry

To identify cell type and assess cell surface markers through the use of antigen-specific fluorescent antibodies

Expense: High

Much manual processing with moderately complex instrumentation

For identification of cell type

For assessment of cell surface markers

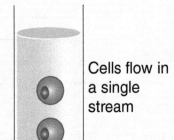

Cells flow in a single stream

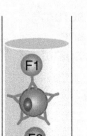

Laser beam of light onto cell → From amount of light scattered forward and to the side, cell size, shape, and granularity determined — leading to identification of cell type

Cell suspension mixed with antibodies to different cell surface markers — each of which has a unique fluorescent label (F1 is different from F2)

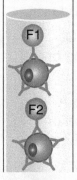

As cells flow in a stream within the instrument and are exposed to laser light, each fluorescent compound can be identified—fluorescent cells are positive for the cell surface marker with the specific fluorescent antibody to that surface marker

FIGURE 2–4

Nephelometry

To quantitate selected proteins and other compounds by measuring light scattering caused by antigen–antibody complexes

Expense: Moderate   **Semiautomated**

Sample of any body fluid is incubated with an antibody to the compound being measured

When the compound is present, antigen–antibody complexes form

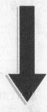

Antibody to the compound is the reagent added to the sample

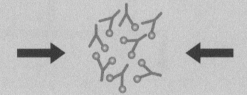

Antigen is compound being measured

The amount of scattered light is proportional to the amount of compound being measured

Antigen–antibody complexes scatter light from a beam of light shown through the sample

FIGURE 2–5

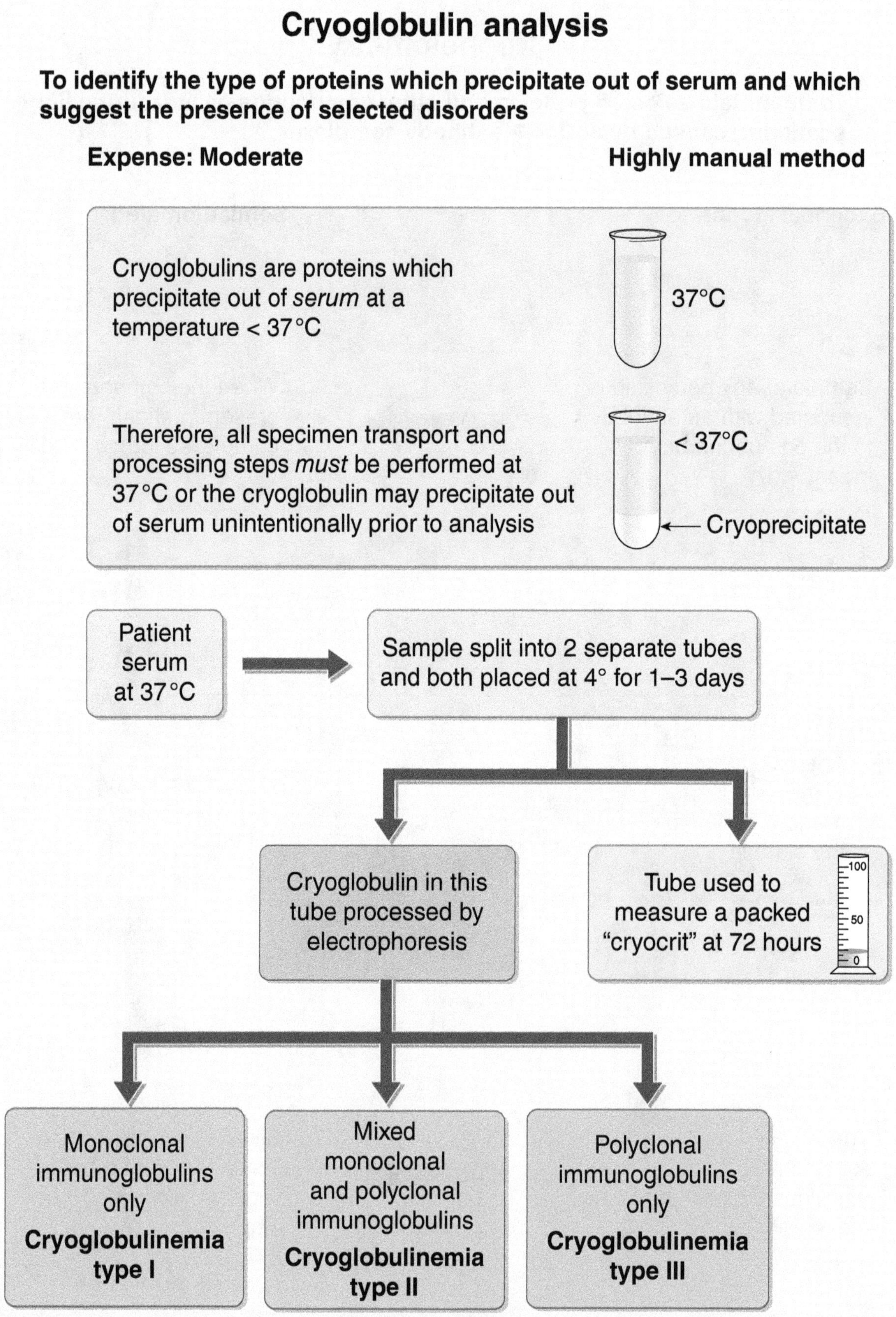

Cryoglobulin analysis

To identify the type of proteins which precipitate out of serum and which suggest the presence of selected disorders

Expense: Moderate　　　　　　　　　　　**Highly manual method**

Cryoglobulins are proteins which precipitate out of *serum* at a temperature < 37°C

37°C

Therefore, all specimen transport and processing steps *must* be performed at 37°C or the cryoglobulin may precipitate out of serum unintentionally prior to analysis

< 37°C

← Cryoprecipitate

Patient serum at 37°C

Sample split into 2 separate tubes and both placed at 4° for 1–3 days

Cryoglobulin in this tube processed by electrophoresis

Tube used to measure a packed "cryocrit" at 72 hours

Monoclonal immunoglobulins only
Cryoglobulinemia type I

Mixed monoclonal and polyclonal immunoglobulins
Cryoglobulinemia type II

Polyclonal immunoglobulins only
Cryoglobulinemia type III

FIGURE 2–6

Gram stain

To identify infectious organisms in many different sample types by fixing and staining the organisms and examining the material on a glass side microscopically

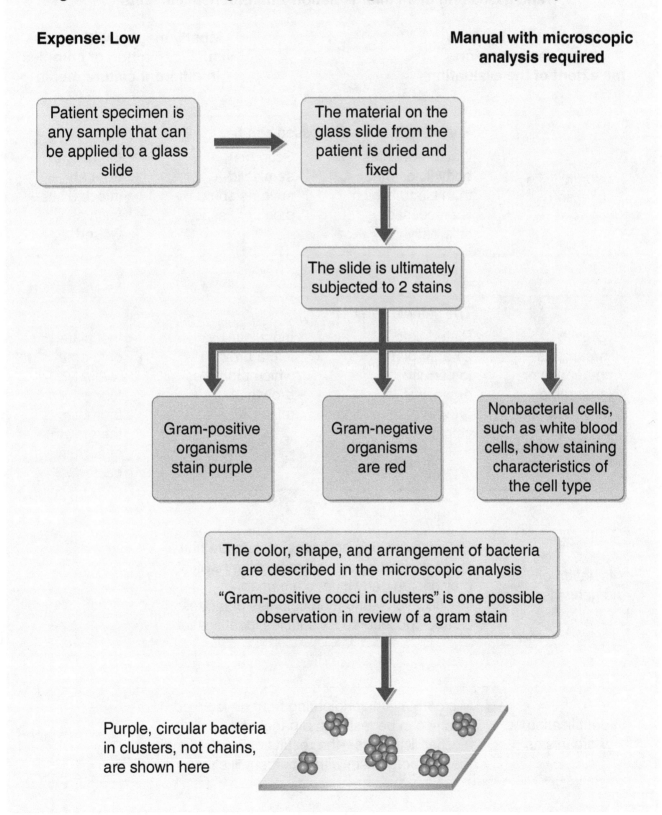

Expense: Low

Manual with microscopic analysis required

Patient specimen is any sample that can be applied to a glass slide

The material on the glass slide from the patient is dried and fixed

The slide is ultimately subjected to 2 stains

Gram-positive organisms stain purple

Gram-negative organisms are red

Nonbacterial cells, such as white blood cells, show staining characteristics of the cell type

The color, shape, and arrangement of bacteria are described in the microscopic analysis

"Gram-positive cocci in clusters" is one possible observation in review of a gram stain

Purple, circular bacteria in clusters, not chains, are shown here

FIGURE 2–7

Microbiologic culture and organism identification

To identify pathogenic organisms by growing them in culture and assessing them after isolation with biochemical tests

Expense: Moderate to high, depending on the extent of the evaluation

Mostly manual with much visual inspection of colonies in different culture media

Sample collection	The sample to be processed can be:		
	Liquid—such as body fluids other than blood, which is processed differently	Solid or semisolid—such as sputum, stool, or tissue	On a swab from an infected site—such as a wound

Growth of organisms—in aerobic or anaerobic environments	The sample can be:		
	Plated onto ≥1 agar plate to permit organisms to grow into colonies	Inoculated into a broth which promotes growth of microorganisms	Inoculated onto agar within a tube which promotes the growth of certain bacteria

Isolation of organisms	Colonies growing on agar surfaces are first characterized by colony morphology which provides an early clue to organism identification—and then colonies of interest can be subcultured for species identification

Identification of organisms	Microorganisms originating from an isolated colony can be tested in a panel of biochemical tests—the results of which identify the microorganism with a percent likelihood

FIGURE 2–8

Blood cultures

To determine if there are infectious agents in the blood by promoting their growth in special medium and detecting their presence by CO_2 production

Expense: High   **In most laboratories it
is now highly automated**

Sample collection	The surface of the arm overlying the venipuncture site must be meticulously cleaned with agents that eliminate skin microorganisms before venipuncture– if not, non-pathogenic skin bacteria can contaminate the blood culture
	Blood with or without microorganisms is collected into bottles for growth in aerobic or anaerobic environments

Growth of organisms	Bottles are placed into specially equipped incubator for detection of carbon dioxide generated within individual blood culture bottles

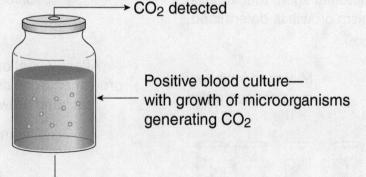

CO_2 detected

Positive blood culture— with growth of microorganisms generating CO_2

Sample from positive blood culture bottle is then processed for organism isolation, identification, and antimicrobial sensitivity

FIGURE 2–9

Antimicrobial sensitivity tests

To determine which antibiotics are likely to effectively eliminate an infectious organism by exposing the organism to different antibiotics in vitro

Expense: High

Can be highly manual, as in disc diffusion method, or semiautomated, as in dilution method

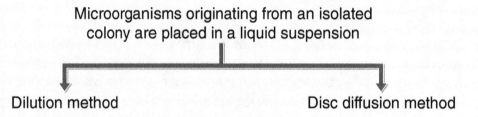

Microorganisms originating from an isolated colony are placed in a liquid suspension

Dilution method

Disc diffusion method

Organisms into multiple tubes

Organisms spread to completely cover a large agar plate which supports organism growth

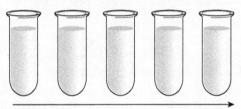

More antimicrobial agent into each sequential tube

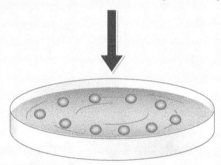

Discs with different antimicrobial agents placed onto agar surface and drug slowly diffuses from disc

After incubation, concentration of antimicrobial agent that inhibits organism growth is determined

After incubation, agents which inhibit growth of organisms are identified because bacterial growth is far from the disc

Minimum inhibitory drug concentration

Organism-free zone

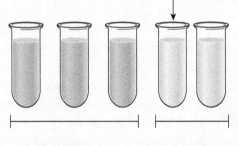

Organisms growing

Organisms not growing

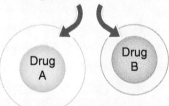

Drug A is a better antimicrobial agent than drug B

FIGURE 2–10

Direct and indirect immunofluorescence for antigen detection

To assess for a variety of specific antigens by using antibodies to the antigens with detection by fluorescence in a microscopic examination

Expense: Moderate   **Manual with microscopic evaluation**

Direct immunofluorescence   Indirect immunofluorescence

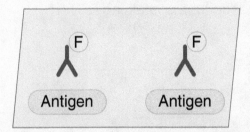

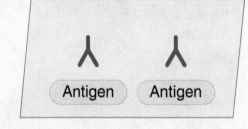

Fluorescent ⒡ labeled antibody binds to antigen of interest on a glass slide or other surface

Antibody which is *not* fluorescent-labeled binds to antigen of interest on a glass slide or other surface

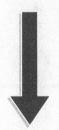

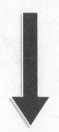

Slides read using a fluorescent microscope

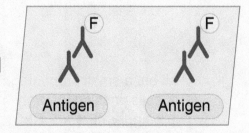

Fluorescent ⒡ labeled antibody to IgG is added and binds to antibody previously bound to antigen

FIGURE 2–11

Counting of blood cells with automated white blood cell differential count

To enumerate the number of white blood cells and the major white blood cell types; the number of red blood cells by cell counting and hemoglobin analysis, along with determination of red blood cell indices; and the number of platelets

Expense: Low   **Highly automated**

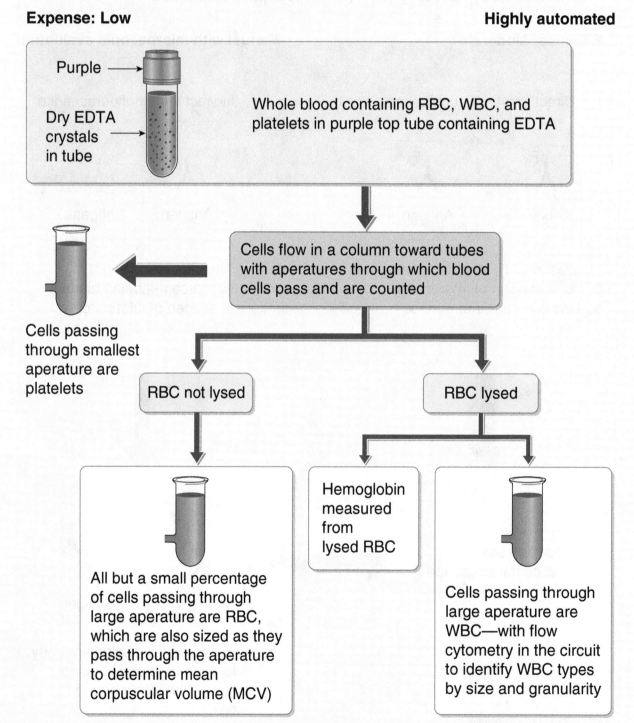

Purple

Dry EDTA crystals in tube

Whole blood containing RBC, WBC, and platelets in purple top tube containing EDTA

Cells flow in a column toward tubes with aperatures through which blood cells pass and are counted

Cells passing through smallest aperature are platelets

RBC not lysed

RBC lysed

Hemoglobin measured from lysed RBC

All but a small percentage of cells passing through large aperature are RBC, which are also sized as they pass through the aperature to determine mean corpuscular volume (MCV)

Cells passing through large aperature are WBC—with flow cytometry in the circuit to identify WBC types by size and granularity

Hematocrit or packed RBC volume is calculated from number and size of RBC

FIGURE 2–12

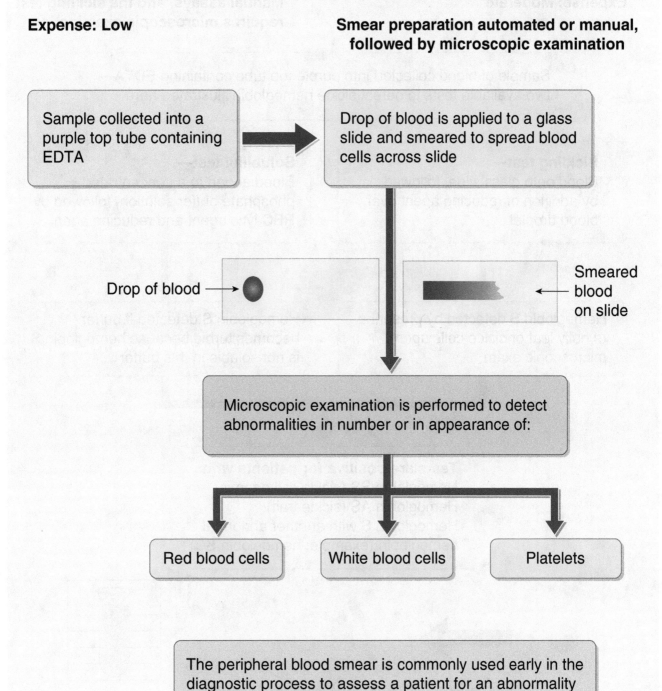

Peripheral blood smear analysis

To determine the size, shape, and any abnormal morphology of all blood cell types by examining a stained preparation of blood cells microscopically

Expense: Low

Smear preparation automated or manual, followed by microscopic examination

Sample collected into a purple top tube containing EDTA

Drop of blood is applied to a glass slide and smeared to spread blood cells across slide

Drop of blood →

Smeared blood on slide

Microscopic examination is performed to detect abnormalities in number or in appearance of:

Red blood cells

White blood cells

Platelets

The peripheral blood smear is commonly used early in the diagnostic process to assess a patient for an abnormality involving circulating blood cells

FIGURE 2–13

Sickle cell screening assay

To rapidly assess for the presence of hemoglobin S by using methods involving either predisposition of red blood cells to sickle or the limited solubility of hemoglobin S.

Expense: Moderate

Manual assays, and the sickling test requires microscopic examination

Sample of blood collected into purple top tube containing EDTA— two available tests to detect sickle hemoglobin illustrated here

Sickling test—
Blood onto glass slide, followed by addition of reducing agent over blood droplet

Solubility test—
Blood added to a concentrated phosphate buffer solution, followed by RBC lytic agent and reducing agent

Hemoglobin S detected by presence of holly leaf or sickle cells upon microscopic exam

Hemoglobin S detected if buffer becomes turbid because hemoglobin S is not soluble in this buffer

Tests are positive for patients with:
Hemoglobin SS (sickle cell anemia)
Hemoglobin AS (sickle trait)
Hemoglobin S with another abnormal hemoglobin (example: hemoglobin SC)

 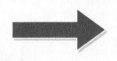

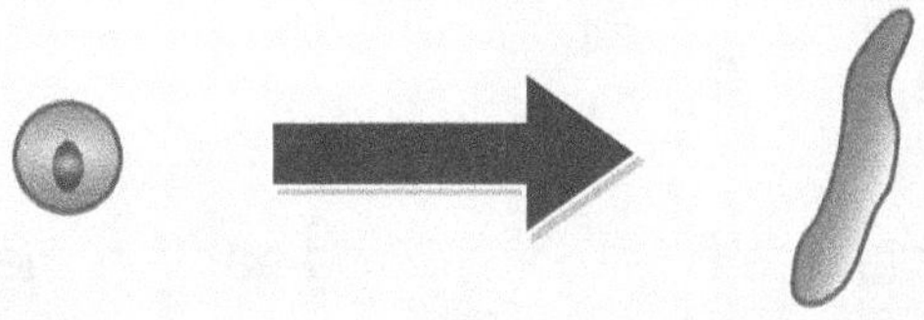

RBC with normal morphology

RBC with abnormal morphology after addition of reducing agent

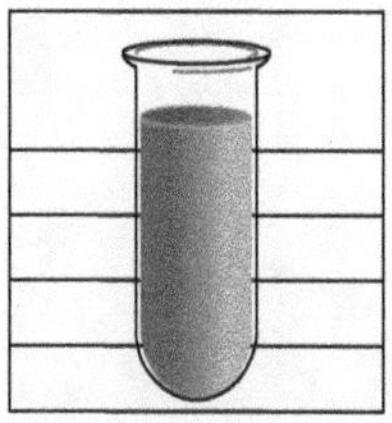

Cannot see through the specimen to visualize black lines on card behind tube if hemoglobin S is present

FIGURE 2–14

Hemoglobin analysis

To determine the different hemoglobins present by one or more methods which separate hemoglobin types

Expense: Moderate   **Semiautomated**

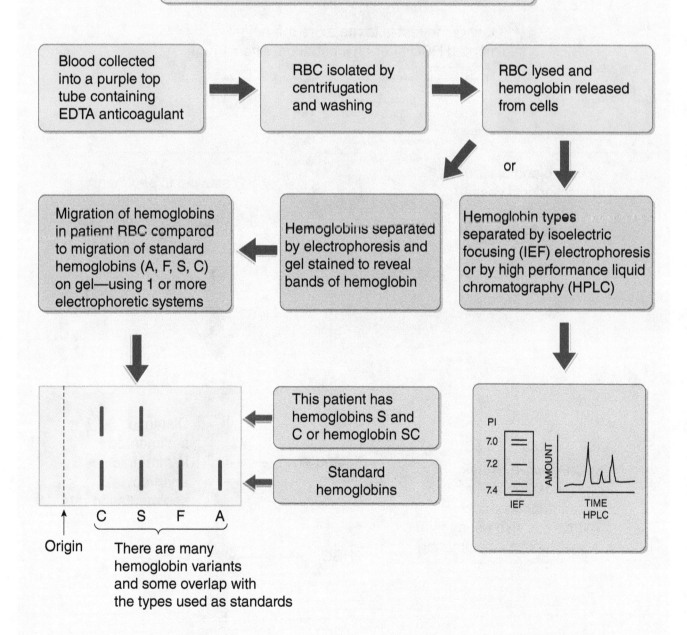

Goal of the test is to identify the hemoglobin types present in a patient's red blood cells (RBC)

Blood collected into a purple top tube containing EDTA anticoagulant

RBC isolated by centrifugation and washing

RBC lysed and hemoglobin released from cells

or

Migration of hemoglobins in patient RBC compared to migration of standard hemoglobins (A, F, S, C) on gel—using 1 or more electrophoretic systems

Hemoglobins separated by electrophoresis and gel stained to reveal bands of hemoglobin

Hemoglobin types separated by isoelectric focusing (IEF) electrophoresis or by high performance liquid chromatography (HPLC)

This patient has hemoglobins S and C or hemoglobin SC

Standard hemoglobins

C   S   F   A

Origin

There are many hemoglobin variants and some overlap with the types used as standards

PI
7.0
7.2
7.4
IEF

AMOUNT

TIME
HPLC

FIGURE 2–15

Erythrocyte sedimentation rate and C-Reactive Protein Measurement

To assess systemic inflammation by measuring the extent of red blood cell sedimentation over a fixed period of time or the amount of C-Reactive Protein in the plasma or serum

Expense: Low   **Manual or semiautomated**

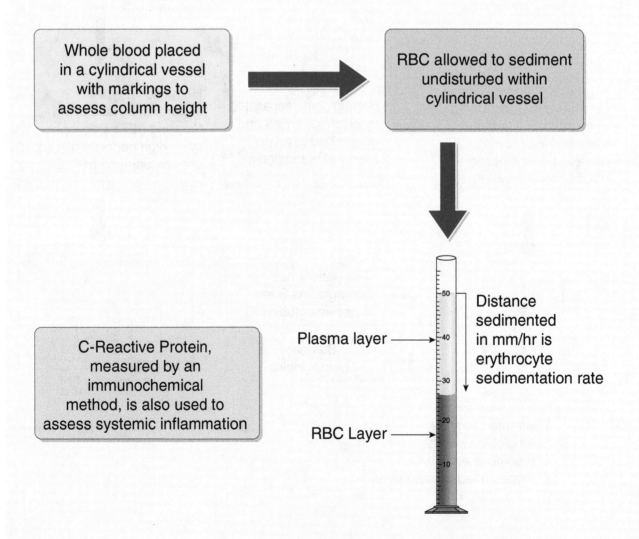

Goal of the test is to measure the height of sedimented RBC after an incubation, often 1 hour

Whole blood placed in a cylindrical vessel with markings to assess column height

RBC allowed to sediment undisturbed within cylindrical vessel

C-Reactive Protein, measured by an immunochemical method, is also used to assess systemic inflammation

Plasma layer

RBC Layer

Distance sedimented in mm/hr is erythrocyte sedimentation rate

FIGURE 2–16

The PT and PTT assays

To assess the amount of coagulation factor activity by measuring the time to clot formation after adding agents to activate the coagulation cascade

Expense: Low   **Highly automated**

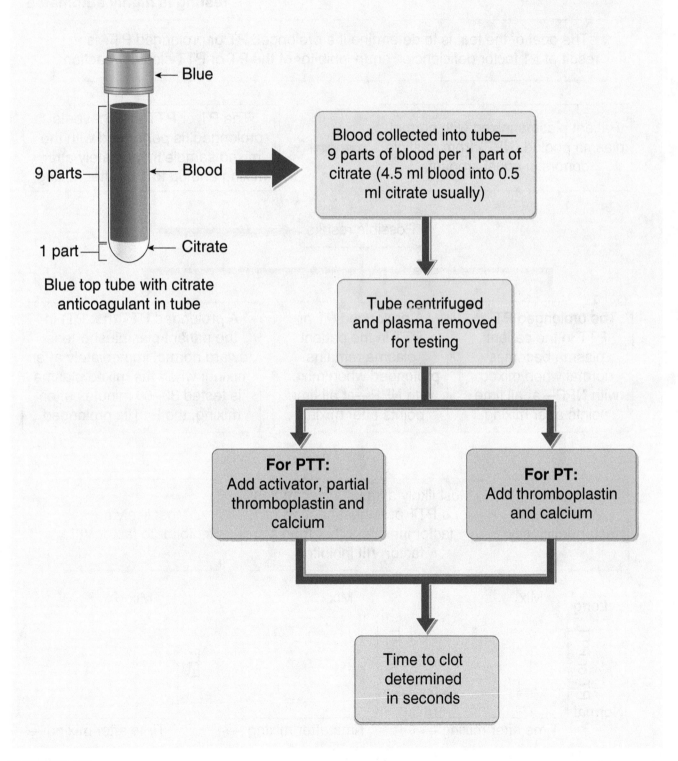

FIGURE 2–17

PT and PTT mixing studies

To determine if a prolonged PT or prolonged PTT is a result of a coagulation factor deficiency or an inhibitor that affects the coagulation cascade, by measuring the time to clot formation using the patient plasma after it is mixed in equal parts with normal plasma

Expense: Low

After samples are mixed, the testing is highly automated

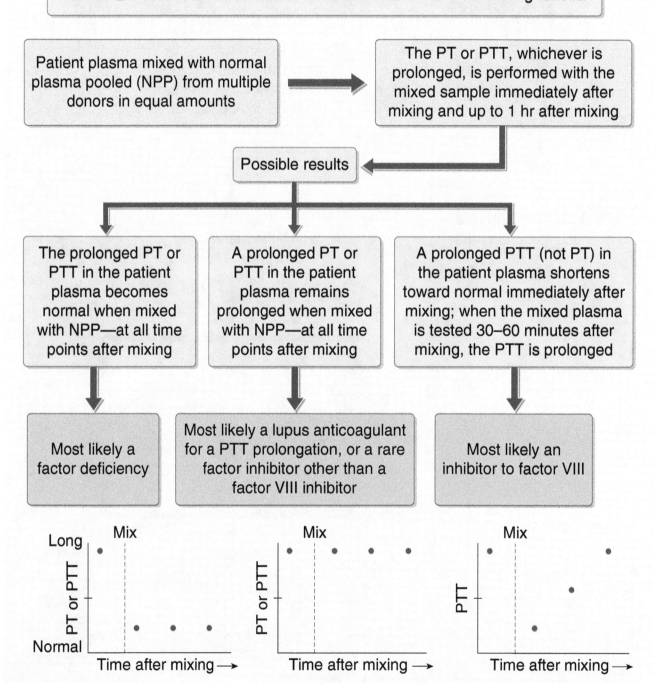

The goal of the test is to determine if a prolonged PT or prolonged PTT is a result of ≥1 factor deficiencies or an inhibitor of the PT or PTT clotting reaction

Patient plasma mixed with normal plasma pooled (NPP) from multiple donors in equal amounts

The PT or PTT, whichever is prolonged, is performed with the mixed sample immediately after mixing and up to 1 hr after mixing

Possible results

The prolonged PT or PTT in the patient plasma becomes normal when mixed with NPP—at all time points after mixing

A prolonged PT or PTT in the patient plasma remains prolonged when mixed with NPP—at all time points after mixing

A prolonged PTT (not PT) in the patient plasma shortens toward normal immediately after mixing; when the mixed plasma is tested 30–60 minutes after mixing, the PTT is prolonged

Most likely a factor deficiency

Most likely a lupus anticoagulant for a PTT prolongation, or a rare factor inhibitor other than a factor VIII inhibitor

Most likely an inhibitor to factor VIII

FIGURE 2-18

Coagulation factor assays

To quantitate the amount of a specific coagulation factor by determining the time to clot formation using the patient plasma mixed with plasma deficient only in the coagulation factor being measured

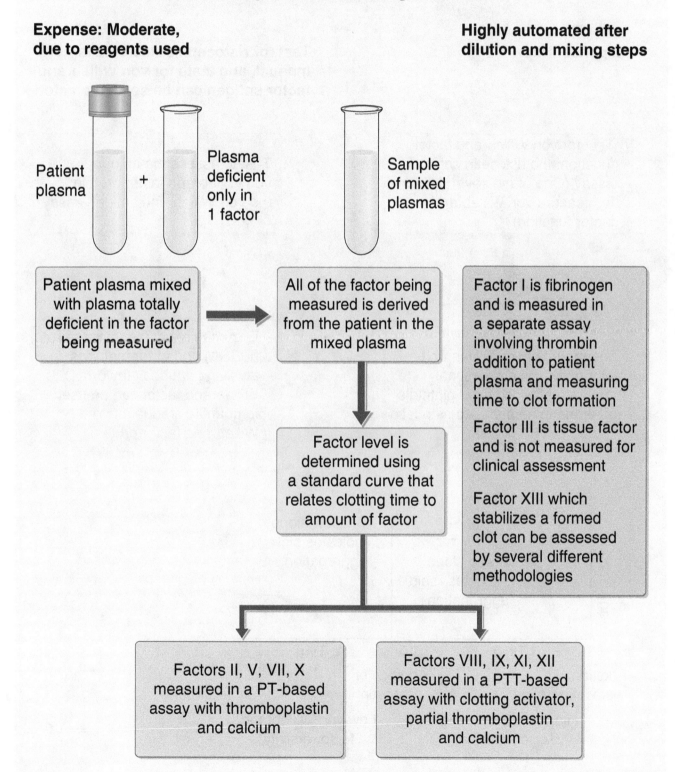

Expense: Moderate, due to reagents used

Highly automated after dilution and mixing steps

Patient plasma + Plasma deficient only in 1 factor

Sample of mixed plasmas

Patient plasma mixed with plasma totally deficient in the factor being measured

All of the factor being measured is derived from the patient in the mixed plasma

Factor level is determined using a standard curve that relates clotting time to amount of factor

Factor I is fibrinogen and is measured in a separate assay involving thrombin addition to patient plasma and measuring time to clot formation

Factor III is tissue factor and is not measured for clinical assessment

Factor XIII which stabilizes a formed clot can be assessed by several different methodologies

Factors II, V, VII, X measured in a PT-based assay with thromboplastin and calcium

Factors VIII, IX, XI, XII measured in a PTT-based assay with clotting activator, partial thromboplastin and calcium

FIGURE 2–19

von Willebrand factor assays

To measure the activity of von Willebrand factor by measuring the ability of von Willebrand factor to promote platelet aggregation; and to measure the amount of von Willebrand protein using an immunoassay.

Expense: High

Test for ristocetin cofactor is largely manual, and tests for von Willebrand factor antigen can be semiautomated

Test for von Willebrand factor function: the ristocetin cofactor assay (One of the several tests to measure von Willebrand factor function)

Test to assess the amount of von Willebrand factor protein: the von Willebrand antigen assay

The amount of von Willebrand factor activity is proportional to the rate at which fixed platelets aggregate in response to ristocetin

Enzyme-linked immunoassay (ELISA) and other methods involving antibody to von Willebrand factor can be used to quantify amount of von Willebrand factor protein

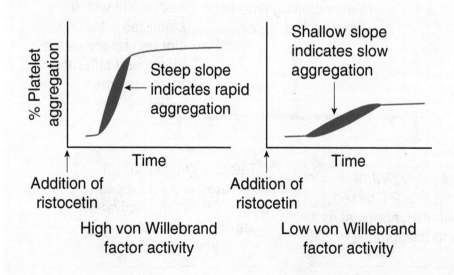

FIGURE 2–20

Platelet aggregation

To determine the function of platelets by assessing their ability to aggregate when exposed to platelet activating agents

Expense: High

Manual test requiring careful performance to generate accurate result

Goal of the test is to assess the function of circulating platelets

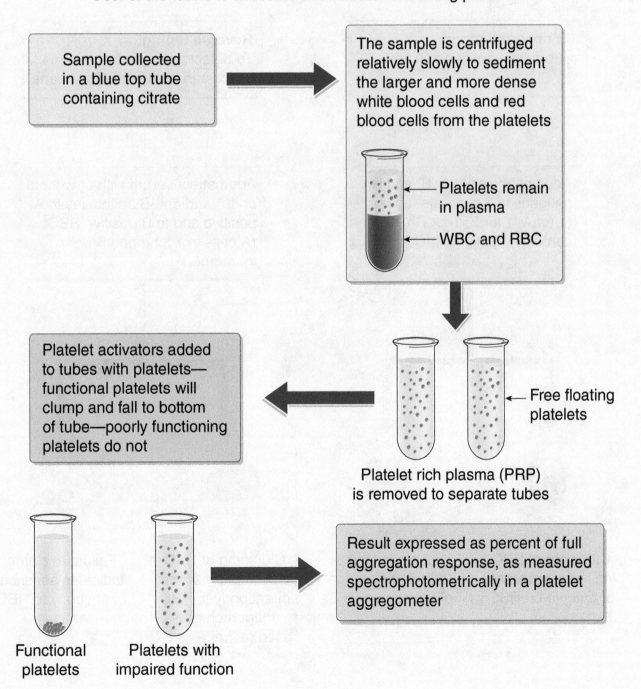

Sample collected in a blue top tube containing citrate

The sample is centrifuged relatively slowly to sediment the larger and more dense white blood cells and red blood cells from the platelets

Platelets remain in plasma

WBC and RBC

Platelet activators added to tubes with platelets— functional platelets will clump and fall to bottom of tube—poorly functioning platelets do not

Free floating platelets

Platelet rich plasma (PRP) is removed to separate tubes

Functional platelets

Platelets with impaired function

Result expressed as percent of full aggregation response, as measured spectrophotometrically in a platelet aggregometer

FIGURE 2–21

ABO/Rh typing

To determine the ABO blood type and Rh status by measuring the clumping of red blood cells after addition of antibodies to A, B, and Rh antigens; and by assessing for clumping of red blood cells known to have A or B surface antigens after addition of patient serum

Expense: Low   **Automated or manual**

| **Forward typing:** To detect antigens on RBC | **Reverse typing:** To detect antibodies in serum which can bind to RBC antigens |

| Add antibodies to A, B, and Rh antigens in 3 separate tubes (1 for A, 1 for B, 1 for Rh) containing patient RBC | Add patient serum with or without anti-A and anti-B antibodies to A positive and to B positive RBC (A cells in 1 tube and B cells in another) |

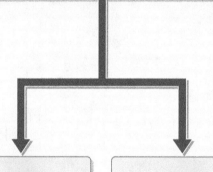

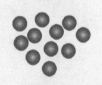

| Clumping of RBC indicates presence of antigen on RBC | Failure to clump indicates absence of antigen on RBC | Clumping of RBC indicates presence of antibody to RBC antigen on cells used (either A or B) | Failure to clump indicates absence of antibody to RBC antigen |

FIGURE 2–22

Blood component preparation

To produce packed red blood cells, fresh frozen plasma, platelet concentrates, and plasma-derived products including cryoprecipitate, immunoglobulins, albumin and coagulation factor concentrates by different centrifugation and precipitation steps

Expense: Blood products are expensive; separation of whole blood into blood components is moderately expensive

The process of component preparation is manual

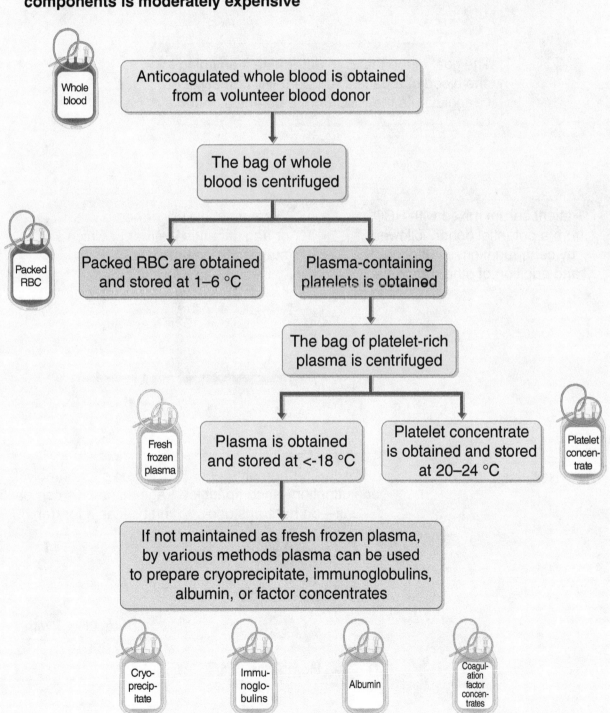

FIGURE 2–23

Blood crossmatch

To determine the suitability of a donated packed red blood cell product for a potential recipient by assessing for donor red blood cell agglutination or hemolysis when mixed with serum from the potential recipient

Expense: Low   **Process described below is manual**

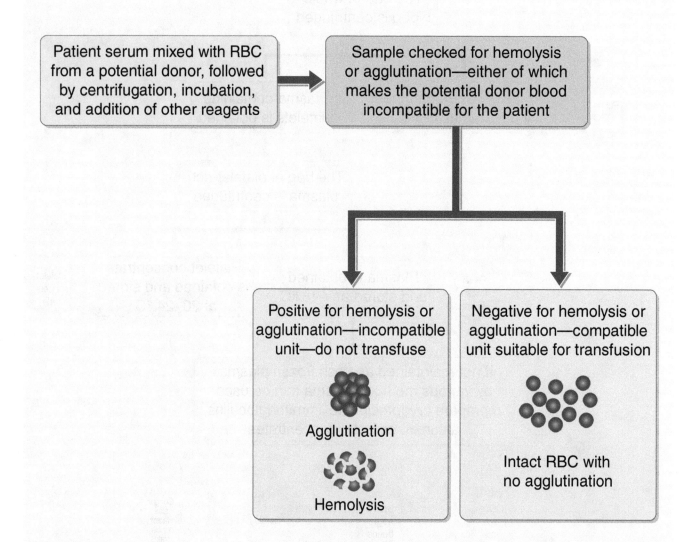

The goal of the test is to determine if anything in the blood of a patient recipient will hemolyze or agglutinate the RBC from a potential donor

Patient serum mixed with RBC from a potential donor, followed by centrifugation, incubation, and addition of other reagents

Sample checked for hemolysis or agglutination—either of which makes the potential donor blood incompatible for the patient

Positive for hemolysis or agglutination—incompatible unit—do not transfuse

Agglutination

Hemolysis

Negative for hemolysis or agglutination—compatible unit suitable for transfusion

Intact RBC with no agglutination

FIGURE 2–24

Direct antiglobulin test (DAT)

To determine if IgG or C3d is bound to the red blood cell surface by assessing for red blood cell clumping or hemolysis when the patient red cells are mixed with antibody to IgG or C3d

Expense: Moderate   **Largely manual method**

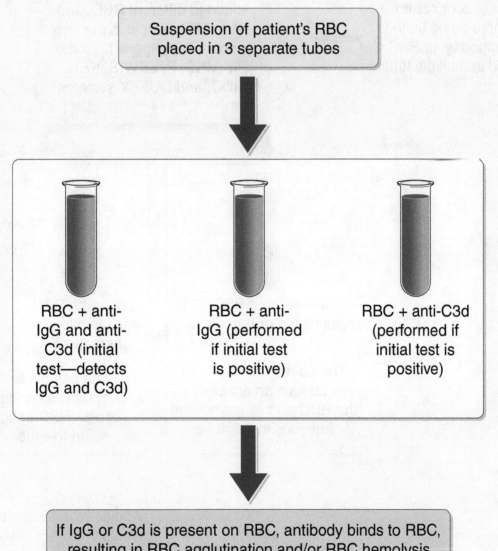

Goal of the test is to determine if IgG immunoglobin or C3d complement is bound to the surface of the patient's red blood cells

Suspension of patient's RBC placed in 3 separate tubes

RBC + anti-IgG and anti-C3d (initial test—detects IgG and C3d)

RBC + anti-IgG (performed if initial test is positive)

RBC + anti-C3d (performed if initial test is positive)

If IgG or C3d is present on RBC, antibody binds to RBC, resulting in RBC agglutination and/or RBC hemolysis

FIGURE 2–25

Indirect antiglobulin test (IAT)

To detect antibodies in the plasma or serum that can become bound to red blood cells by assessing for red blood cell clumping or hemolysis when the patient plasma or serum is mixed with red blood cells that have specific known antigens

Expense: Moderate   **Largely manual method**

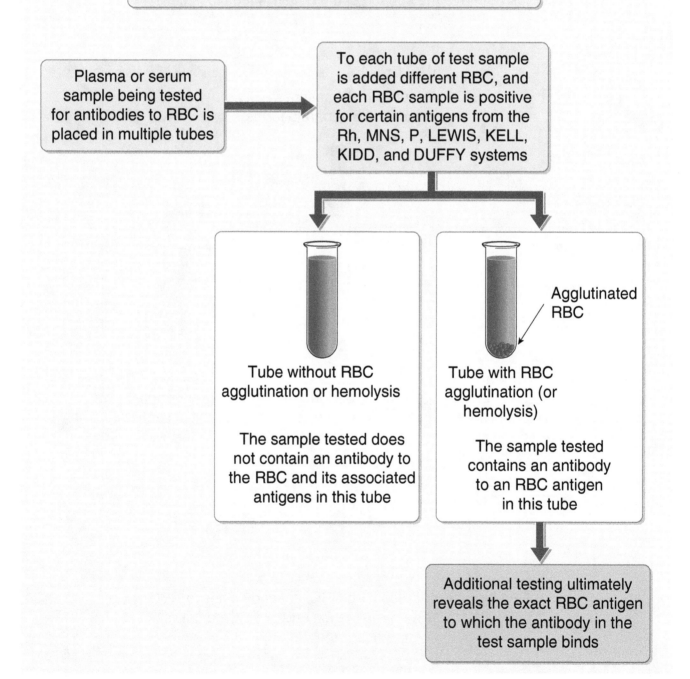

Goal of the test is to detect antibodies *not* bound to RBC present in the plasma or serum of a patient or donor that *can become* bound to RBC

Plasma or serum sample being tested for antibodies to RBC is placed in multiple tubes

To each tube of test sample is added different RBC, and each RBC sample is positive for certain antigens from the Rh, MNS, P, LEWIS, KELL, KIDD, and DUFFY systems

Tube without RBC agglutination or hemolysis

The sample tested does not contain an antibody to the RBC and its associated antigens in this tube

Agglutinated RBC

Tube with RBC agglutination (or hemolysis)

The sample tested contains an antibody to an RBC antigen in this tube

Additional testing ultimately reveals the exact RBC antigen to which the antibody in the test sample binds

FIGURE 2–26

Apheresis

To remove plasma or specific blood cells from patients for therapeutic purposes; or to remove platelets from healthy donors for transfusion of patients who will benefit from an increase in platelet count

Expense: Very high

Moderately invasive clinical procedure

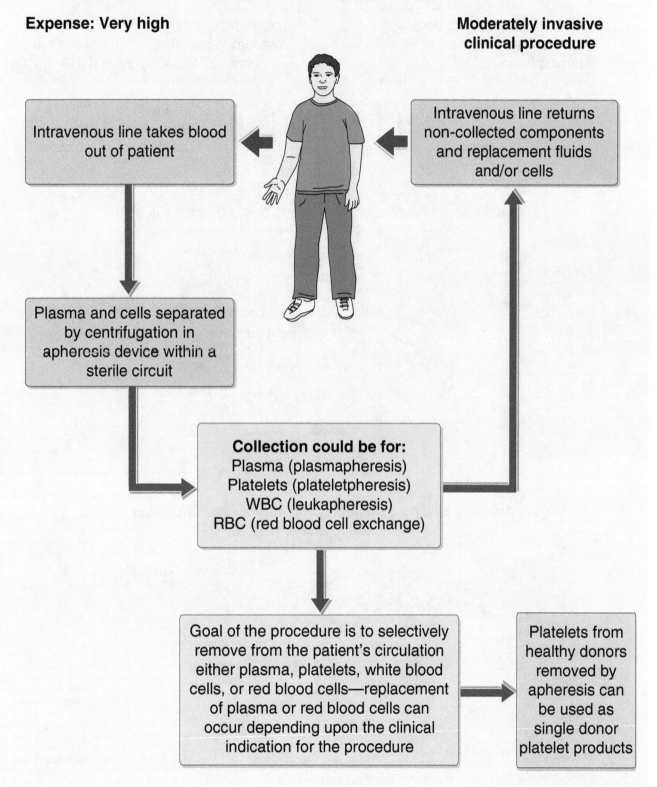

Intravenous line takes blood out of patient

Intravenous line returns non-collected components and replacement fluids and/or cells

Plasma and cells separated by centrifugation in apheresis device within a sterile circuit

Collection could be for:
Plasma (plasmapheresis)
Platelets (plateletpheresis)
WBC (leukapheresis)
RBC (red blood cell exchange)

Goal of the procedure is to selectively remove from the patient's circulation either plasma, platelets, white blood cells, or red blood cells—replacement of plasma or red blood cells can occur depending upon the clinical indication for the procedure

Platelets from healthy donors removed by apheresis can be used as single donor platelet products

FIGURE 2–27

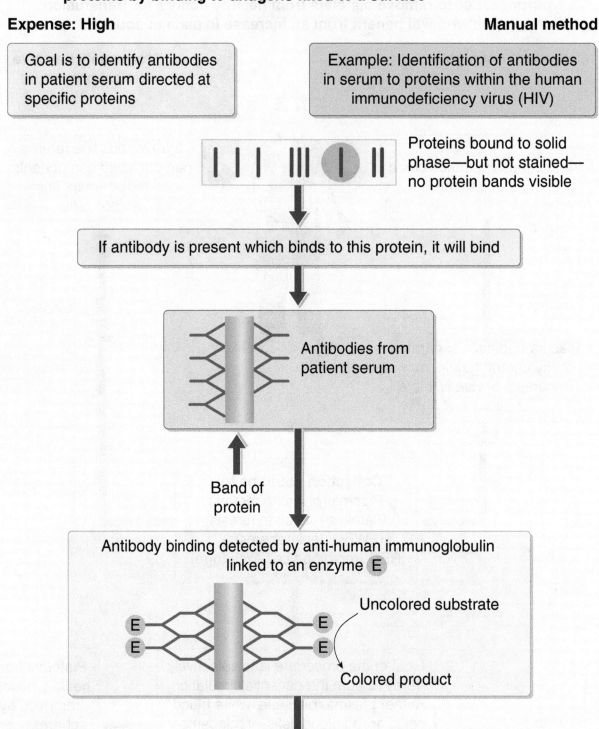

Western blot

To identify antibodies in the blood of patients directed at specific proteins by binding to antigens fixed to a surface

Expense: High   **Manual method**

Goal is to identify antibodies in patient serum directed at specific proteins

Example: Identification of antibodies in serum to proteins within the human immunodeficiency virus (HIV)

Proteins bound to solid phase—but not stained—no protein bands visible

If antibody is present which binds to this protein, it will bind

Antibodies from patient serum

Band of protein

Antibody binding detected by anti-human immunoglobulin linked to an enzyme E

Uncolored substrate

Colored product

Protein band with bound antibody becomes visible

FIGURE 2–28

Electrolyte measurements: Sodium (Na), Potassium (K), and Chloride (Cl)

To quantitate the major ions in patient plasma or serum using ion selective electrodes for each one

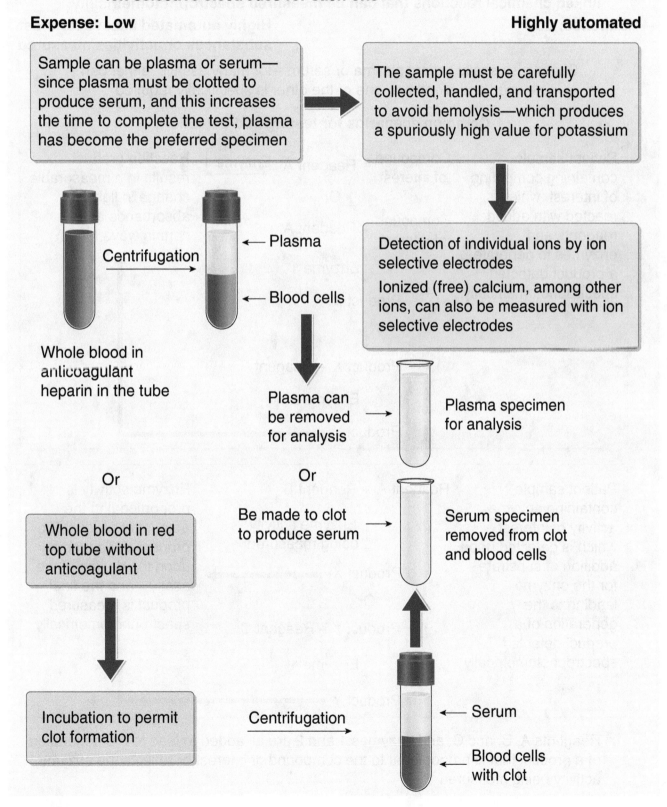

Expense: Low

Sample can be plasma or serum—since plasma must be clotted to produce serum, and this increases the time to complete the test, plasma has become the preferred specimen

Highly automated

The sample must be carefully collected, handled, and transported to avoid hemolysis—which produces a spuriously high value for potassium

Whole blood in anticoagulant heparin in the tube

Centrifugation →

← Plasma

← Blood cells

Detection of individual ions by ion selective electrodes

Ionized (free) calcium, among other ions, can also be measured with ion selective electrodes

Plasma can be removed for analysis →

Plasma specimen for analysis

Or

Whole blood in red top tube without anticoagulant

Or

Be made to clot to produce serum →

Serum specimen removed from clot and blood cells

Incubation to permit clot formation

Centrifugation →

← Serum

← Blood cells with clot

FIGURE 2–29

Assays measuring concentration of compounds or enzyme by spectrophotometry

To measure the concentration of a compound or the activity of a clinically relevant enzyme in patient plasma or serum by generating a compound in linked chemical reactions that can be measured spectrophotometrically

Expense: Low

Highly automated assays for most substances or activities measured

Sample is usually patient plasma or serum—for many assays, either can be used and for others, one or the other is specifically required

Common scenarios for testing and detection:

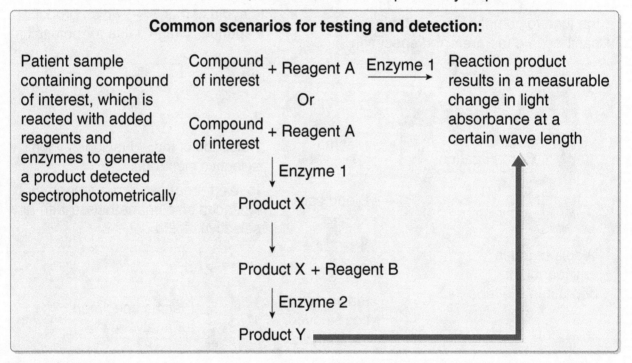

Patient sample containing compound of interest, which is reacted with added reagents and enzymes to generate a product detected spectrophotometrically

Patient sample containing enzyme activity of interest, which is detected upon addition of substrate for the enzyme leading to the generation of a product detected spectrophotometrically

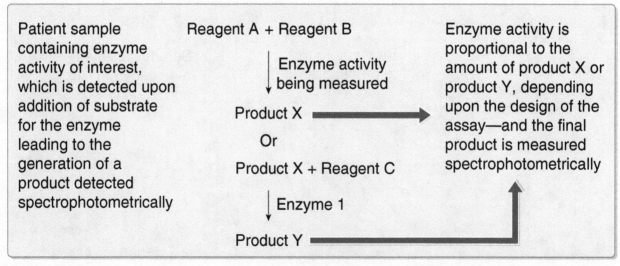

Reagents A, B, and C, and enzymes 1 and 2 are all added to lead to the generation of a product that is proportional to the compound of interest or reflects the enzyme activity being measured

FIGURE 2–30

Blood gas measurements

To quantitate the pH, pCO$_2$, and pO$_2$ in whole blood from a patient using ion selective electrodes for each one

Expense: Low

Requires injection of whole blood sample into instrument with no additional manipulation

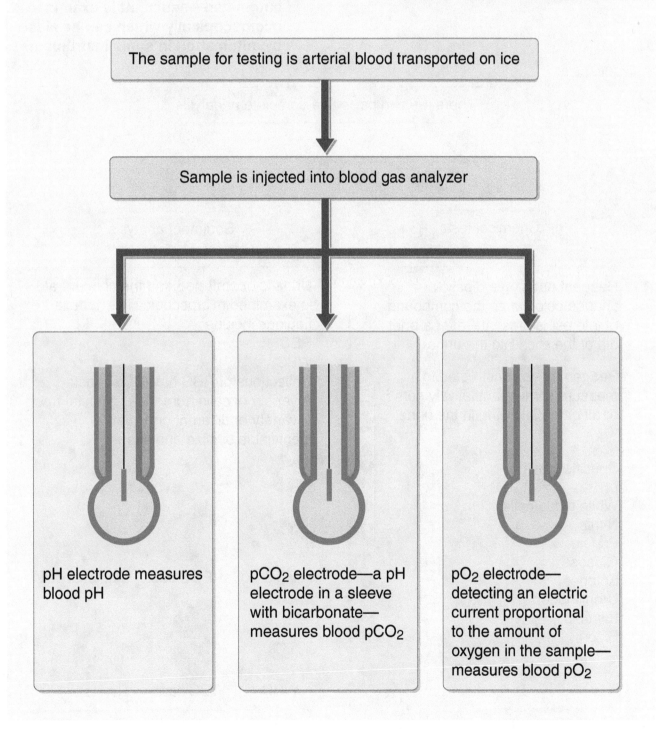

The sample for testing is arterial blood transported on ice

Sample is injected into blood gas analyzer

pH electrode measures blood pH

pCO$_2$ electrode—a pH electrode in a sleeve with bicarbonate— measures blood pCO$_2$

pO$_2$ electrode— detecting an electric current proportional to the amount of oxygen in the sample— measures blood pO$_2$

FIGURE 2–31

Urinalysis

To measure selected constituents, including red and white blood cells in the urine by semiquantitive chemical reactions on a reagent strip; and to microscopically analyze the urine sediment after centrifugation for red and white blood cells, red and white blood cell casts, epithelial cells, and crystals of various types

Expense: Low

Can be completely manual or highly automated—sediment is examined microscopically which can be aided by automation in some instruments

There are two parts to a complete urinalysis

Chemical tests

Sediment analysis

Reagent pads on a dipstick change color when the compound of interest is present—after a brief dip of the stick into the urine

Reagent pads constructed to measure semi-quantitatively some or all of the following in the urine:

Specific gravity
pH
White blood cells
Nitrite
Protein
Glucose
Ketones
Urobilinogen
Bilirubin
Blood

Urine is centrifuged and the concentrate is examined microscopically—notable findings include:
RBC
WBC
Collections of RBC or WBC in casts
A variety of cells from the urogenital tract
A variety of different crystals identifiable by size and shape

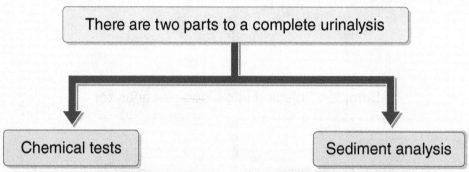

RBC   RBC cast   Epithelial cell

WBC   WBC cast   Crystals

FIGURE 2–32

Enzyme-linked immunosorbent assay (ELISA)

To detect antibodies in patient plasma or serum by binding them to a corresponding antigen fixed to a surface; or to detect an antigen in patient plasma or serum by binding the antigen to corresponding antibodies fixed to a surface

Expense: Moderate

Semiautomated to almost fully automated

To detect antibodies in the patient's serum

To detect an antigen in the patient's serum

Antibodies are detected by binding to a corresponding antigen fixed to a surface

Antigens are detected by binding to corresponding antibodies fixed to a surface

Antibody in patient serum

Antigen in patient serum

Antigen fixed to surface

Antibody fixed to surface

Detection with anti-human antibody linked to an enzyme E

Detection with antibody to antigen that has an enzyme E linked to the antibody

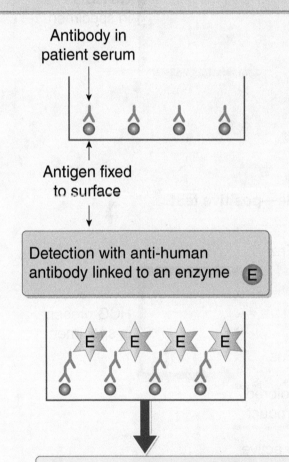
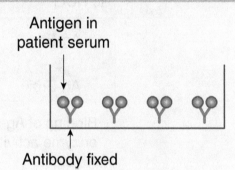
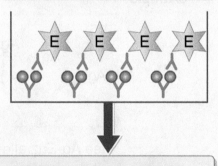

Add uncolored substrate for enzyme and enzyme converts it to a colored product—the darker the color, the more antibody or antigen in the patient serum

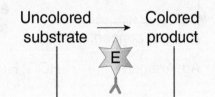

Uncolored substrate → Colored product

FIGURE 2–33

Fully automated immunoassay with all reagents in solution

To detect an antigen in any sample by using a competitive binding assay which has a linear increase in enzyme activity with increased antigen concentration

Expense: Low   **Automated**

No antigen in sample—negative test

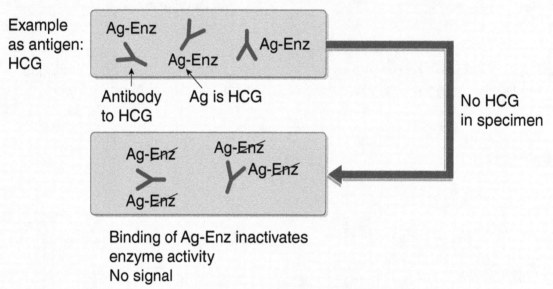

Example as antigen: HCG

Antibody to HCG   Ag is HCG

No HCG in specimen

Binding of Ag-Enz inactivates enzyme activity
No signal

Antigen in sample—positive test

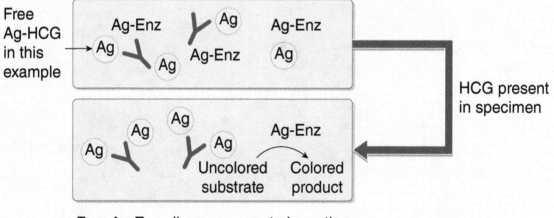

Free Ag-HCG in this example

HCG present in specimen

Uncolored substrate   Colored product

Free Ag-Enz allows enzyme to be active

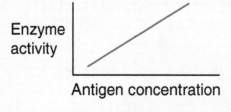

Enzyme activity

Antigen concentration

Enzyme conjugate activity is linearly proportional to antigen concentration in sample

Enz: Enzyme   Ag: Antigen   HCG: Human chorionic gonadotropin

FIGURE 2–34

Latex agglutination

To detect a compound in a liquid sample by allowing it to bind to latex particles with antibodies to the compound, which clumps the latex beads

Expense: Low   **Automated or manual**

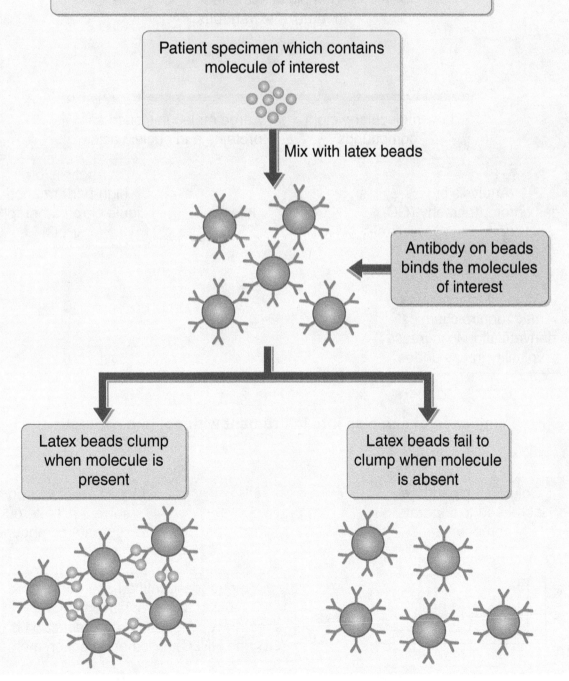

FIGURE 2–35

Chromatography for separation, identification, and quantitation of substances in biologic fluids

To separate compounds in a single sample by one of several methods, so that individual compounds can be quantitated by an appropriate assay

Expense: High

Test requires manual processing and data analysis

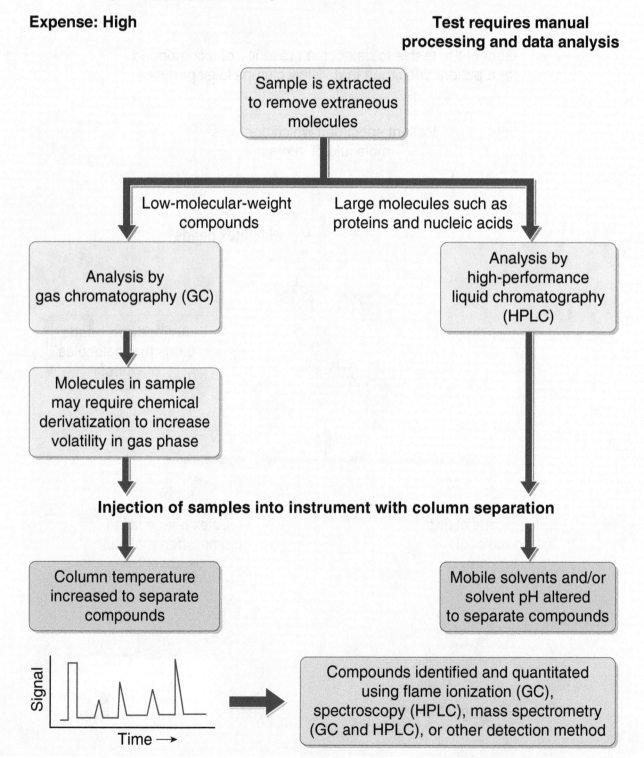

FIGURE 2–36

Mass spectrometry for molecular identification

To identify a compound in a patient sample by causing it to break into smaller pieces; the pattern of the pieces is characteristic for the compound, and it can be identified by comparison to fragment patterns from a large database of known compounds.

Expense: High

Semiautomated with high complexity of laboratory instrumentation

A patient sample is processed to render it suitable for analysis

Molecular compounds of interest are isolated from other molecules in sample by liquid chromatography or gas chromatography

In mass spectrometer, molecule is broken into different size mass fragments creating a "fingerprint" for the molecule

The fingerprint of the molecule in the patient specimen is compared to a large library of molecular fingerprints

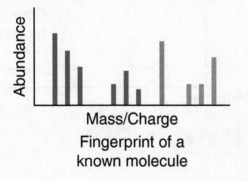

Fingerprint of a known molecule

=

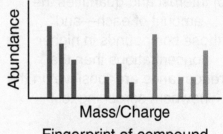

Fingerprint of compound in patient specimen

Molecule is identified because fingerprints match with very high percentage of agreement

FIGURE 2–37

Newborn screening by liquid chromatography/mass spectrometry (LC-MS)

To detect and measure substances in newborn blood which are suggestive of certain diseases using liquid chromatography combined with mass spectrometry

Expense: High for instrumentation; moderate for test performance

Semiautomated with high-complexity instrumentation

After 24 h of life, heel of neonate is punctured to obtain whole blood—which is spotted onto a special card and sent to a central laboratory

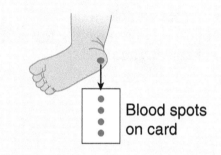

Blood spots on card

Molecular compounds of interest are extracted from a portion of the blood spot and separated by liquid chromatography

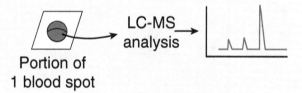

Portion of 1 blood spot

LC-MS analysis

A tandem mass spectrometer identifies the compounds of interest and quantifies the amount of each—and those compounds in higher concentrations than the reference range are "positive" in the newborn screening test

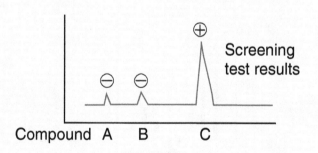

Screening test results

Compound   A   B   C

Confirmation of positive test for compound C is performed to determine if result is true-positive

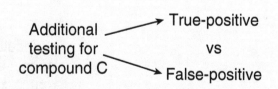

Additional testing for compound C

True-positive

vs

False-positive

FIGURE 2–38

Point-of-care glucose testing

To quantitate glucose in blood using a small handheld device

Expense: Low

After sample is added to test strip, testing is automated

Result display

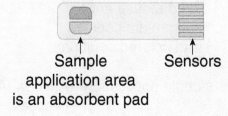

Test strip   Glucometer
with sample

Top-down view of strip

Sample   Sensors
application area
is an absorbent pad

Side view of strip

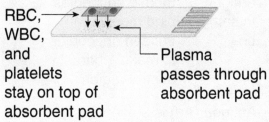

RBC,
WBC,
and
platelets
stay on top of
absorbent pad

Plasma
passes through
absorbent pad

Top-down view of strip
below absorbent pad

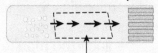

Reagents that react with
glucose embedded here as
plasma moves toward sensors

A blood sample, which is
commonly from a finger stick,
is applied to a test strip

Sample application occurs
onto an absorbent pad
that separates blood cells
from plasma

Glucose within plasma mixes
with reagents embedded on
test strip as plasma moves
toward sensors

Enzyme reactions with glucose
as substrate produce electrons
detected by sensors at the
end of the test strip
inserted into glucometer

Sensor signal is proportional
to concentration of glucose
in sample, which is shown
in the result display window
of the glucometer

FIGURE 2–39

Point-of-care immunoassay on a test strip

To identify the presence of a compound in a liquid sample using test strips with antibodies to the compound fixed to the strip; designed for point-of-care use

Cost: Moderate

Manual test requiring interpretation

Negative test

Top-down view of strip

Side view of test strip: Before application of sample

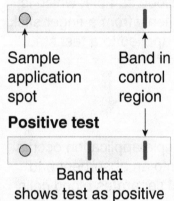

Sample application spot

Band in control region

Sample application— blood or urine

Anti-antigen antibodies fixed to strip

Goat anti- mouse antibodies fixed to strip

Area has dried mouse anti- antigen antibodies with colored conjugate

Positive test

Band that shows test as positive

Negative test

Side view of test strip after sample application—Antigen (Ag) is absent

Fluid migration with wicking action out of sample application spot

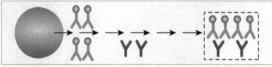

Sample added to well

Solubilizes mouse anti-antigen antibodies with colored conjugate

No antigen in sample so–

Goat anti- mouse antibodies bind mouse anti- antigen antibodies to make 1 band in control region

Positive test

Side view of test strip—Antigen (Ag) is present

Example antigen is HCG—in a pregnancy test

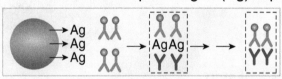

Mouse anti-antigen antibodies fixed to strip bind Ag—and the solubilized mouse anti-antigen antibodies with the colored conjugate also bind Ag to form a colored band where fixed antibodies are imbedded onto strip

Goat anti-mouse antibodies fixed to strip bind excess solubilized mouse anti-antigen antibodies to create a second colored band—bands shown within dashed lines

Ag: Antigen

FIGURE 2–40

Molecular genetic analysis overview

To detect genetic variations/mutations in tumors, to establish malignant and non-malignant diagnoses, to identify adverse drug–gene interactions, and to find infectious organisms

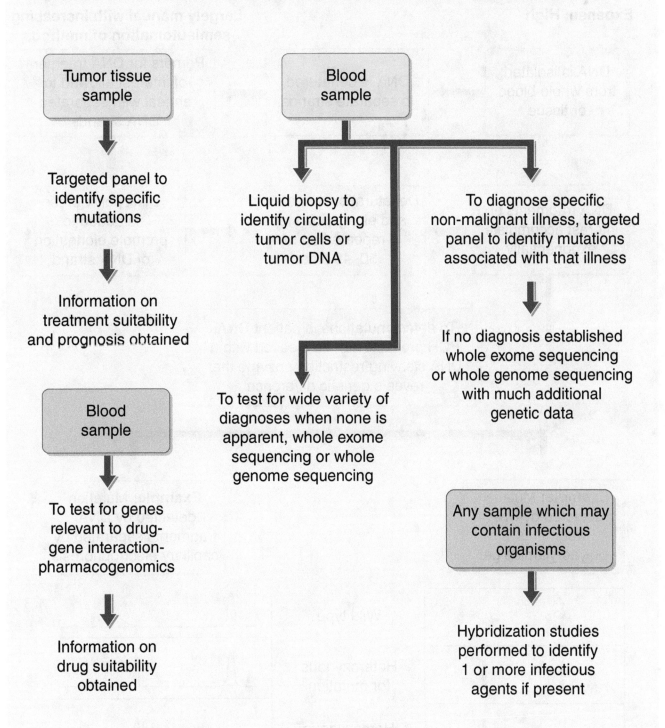

FIGURE 2–41

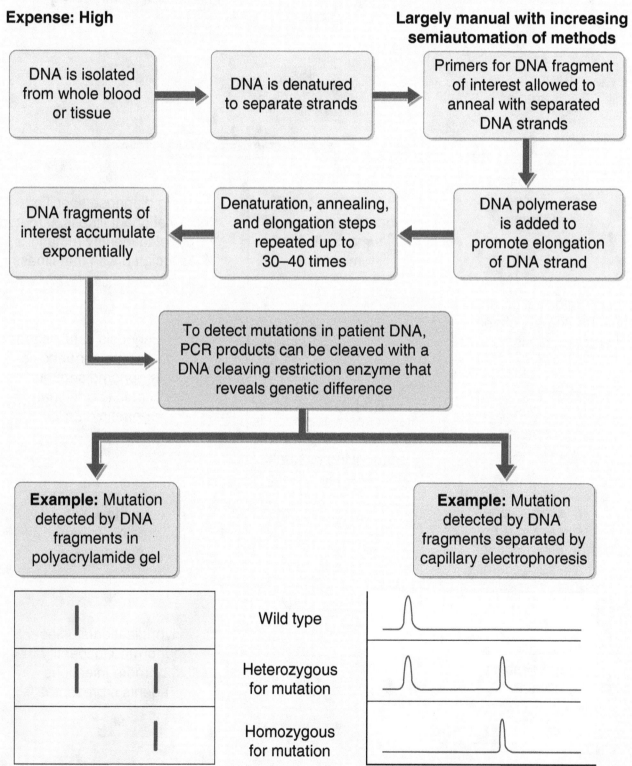

FIGURE 2–42

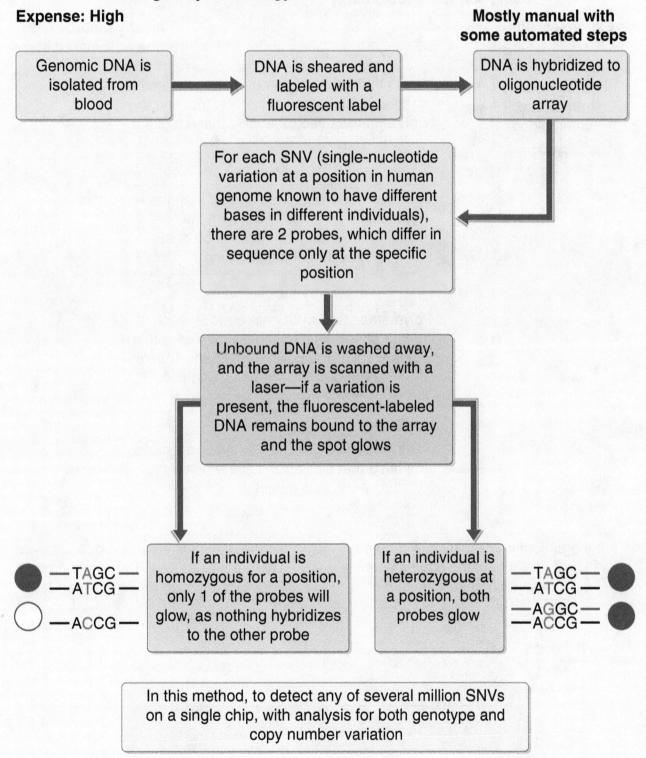

Single-nucleotide variation (SNV) identification by array analysis

To detect any of millions of single-nucleotide variations using array technology

Expense: High

Mostly manual with some automated steps

Genomic DNA is isolated from blood

DNA is sheared and labeled with a fluorescent label

DNA is hybridized to oligonucleotide array

For each SNV (single-nucleotide variation at a position in human genome known to have different bases in different individuals), there are 2 probes, which differ in sequence only at the specific position

Unbound DNA is washed away, and the array is scanned with a laser—if a variation is present, the fluorescent-labeled DNA remains bound to the array and the spot glows

If an individual is homozygous for a position, only 1 of the probes will glow, as nothing hybridizes to the other probe

If an individual is heterozygous at a position, both probes glow

—TAGC—
—ATCG—
—ACCG—

—TAGC—
—ATCG—
—AGGC—
—ACCG—

In this method, to detect any of several million SNVs on a single chip, with analysis for both genotype and copy number variation

FIGURE 2–43

Genotyping method to detect single-nucleotide variations, and insertion or deletion of nucleotides

To detect any single-nucleotide variation, and insertion or deletion using sequence technology

Expense: High

Mostly manual with some automated steps

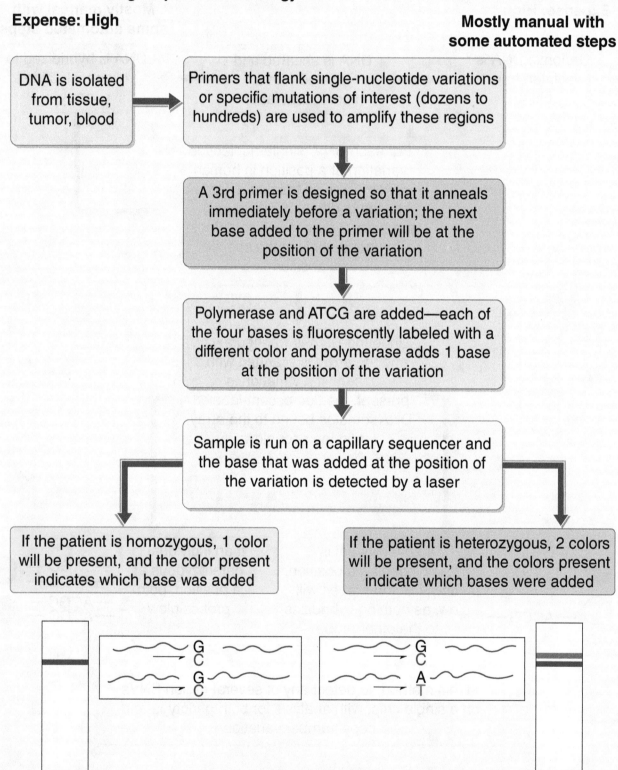

DNA is isolated from tissue, tumor, blood

→

Primers that flank single-nucleotide variations or specific mutations of interest (dozens to hundreds) are used to amplify these regions

A 3rd primer is designed so that it anneals immediately before a variation; the next base added to the primer will be at the position of the variation

Polymerase and ATCG are added—each of the four bases is fluorescently labeled with a different color and polymerase adds 1 base at the position of the variation

Sample is run on a capillary sequencer and the base that was added at the position of the variation is detected by a laser

If the patient is homozygous, 1 color will be present, and the color present indicates which base was added

If the patient is heterozygous, 2 colors will be present, and the colors present indicate which bases were added

FIGURE 2–44

Gene sequencing method

To determine the sequence of a gene to detect any genetic variation which may be present

Expense: High

Mostly manual with some automated steps

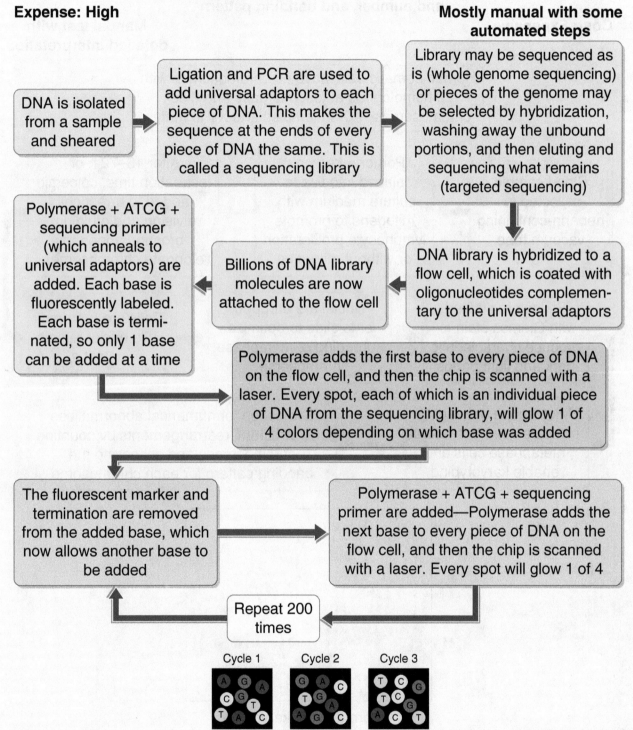

Each spot = 1 library molecule. Images are recorded in each cycle, and the color for each cycle is used to determine the base sequence. There are billions of spots on a flow cell. Thus, sequence for spot in upper left corner is A G T

FIGURE 2–45 (Reproduced, with permission, from Shendure J, Ji H. Next-generation DNA sequencing. *Nat Biotechnol.* 2008;26(10):1135-1145.)

The Karyotype

To evaluate chromosomal structure and number, and banding pattern

Cost: Expensive

Manual test with detailed interpretation

Human somatic cells have 46 chromosomes with 22 homologous autosomal pairs and 2 sex chromosomes—XX in females and XY in males

Blood sample collected in heparin-containing vacuum tube

Portion of sample placed into tissue culture medium with mitogens to promote lymphocyte proliferation or without mitogens

After 16–72 h of incubation time, colcemid added to arrest cell division and ethidium bromide added to elongate chromosomes

Slides are stained with Giemsa stain to produce characteristic dark and light bands

Nuclei are dropped onto slide to optimize spreading of metaphase chromosomes

Cells are ruptured while nuclei remain intact

Microscope or imaging software used to capture metaphase cells and enable karyotyping

Evaluation for numerical abnormalities and structural rearrangements by counting chromosomes and assessing the banding pattern for each chromosome

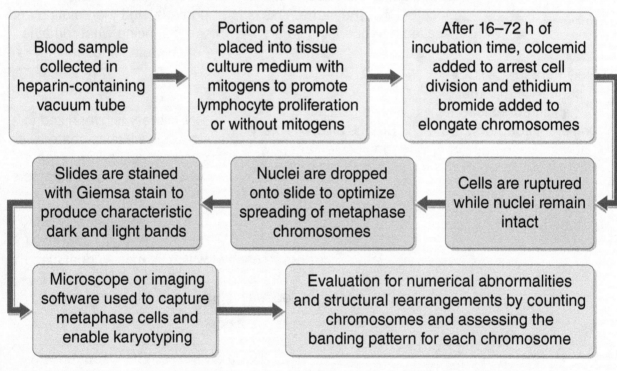

A normal male karyotype
(Courtesy of Dr Ferrin Wheeler)

Description of karyotype is total number of chromosomes, the sex chromosomes, description of any abnormality
Example: 47, XY, +21 is a male with trisomy 21.

FIGURE 2–46

Fluorescence in situ hybridization (FISH)

To detect the chromosomal location of specific genes using fluorescent single-stranded DNA probes which bind to complementary sequences of denatured, single-stranded patient DNA in metaphase chromosomes, viewed by fluorescence microscopy

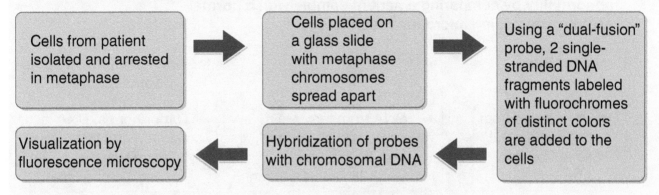

| Cells from patient isolated and arrested in metaphase | → | Cells placed on a glass slide with metaphase chromosomes spread apart | → | Using a "dual-fusion" probe, 2 single-stranded DNA fragments labeled with fluorochromes of distinct colors are added to the cells |

| Visualization by fluorescence microscopy | ← | Hybridization of probes with chromosomal DNA | ← |

Example of Results Using a
Green (G) and a Red (R) Probe

NORMAL

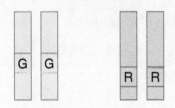

2 Different homologous chromosomes—one labeled by green DNA probe and one by red DNA probe

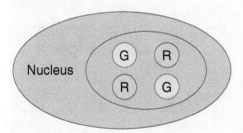

Genes located by probes- and fluorescence microscopy of chromosomes show no translocation of genes probed

ABNORMAL

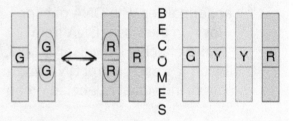

Neoplastic cell with reciprocal translocation shows split signals for both green and red probes
When chromosome fragments are exchanged, two yellow (red + green) (Y) signals are generated

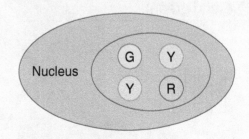

Two normal chromosomes and two "derivative" chromosomes identified by fluorescence microscopy

FIGURE 2–47

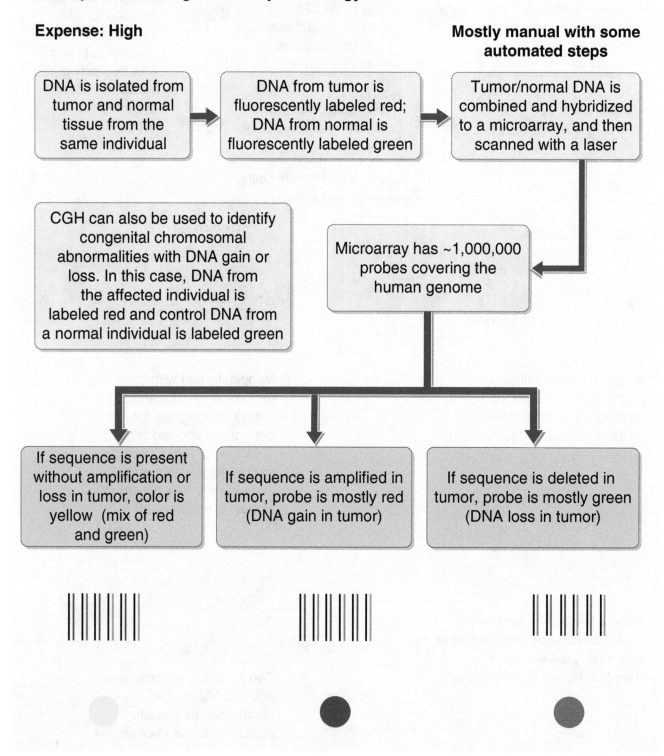

Comparative genomic hybridization (CGH)

To determine if there is a DNA gain or loss in a tumor relative to normal tissue; to determine if there is a congenital chromosomal abnormality by comparing a patient sample with a normal sample; both using microarray technology

Expense: High

Mostly manual with some automated steps

DNA is isolated from tumor and normal tissue from the same individual

DNA from tumor is fluorescently labeled red; DNA from normal is fluorescently labeled green

Tumor/normal DNA is combined and hybridized to a microarray, and then scanned with a laser

CGH can also be used to identify congenital chromosomal abnormalities with DNA gain or loss. In this case, DNA from the affected individual is labeled red and control DNA from a normal individual is labeled green

Microarray has ~1,000,000 probes covering the human genome

If sequence is present without amplification or loss in tumor, color is yellow (mix of red and green)

If sequence is amplified in tumor, probe is mostly red (DNA gain in tumor)

If sequence is deleted in tumor, probe is mostly green (DNA loss in tumor)

FIGURE 2-48

SELF-ASSESSMENT QUESTIONS

1. What is the name of the test based on the following description of the methodology?
Cells on glass slides are incubated with a patient's serum. Antibody is detected as present by adding fluorescent-labeled anti-IgG antibodies. Fluorescence staining of the nucleus of the cells on the glass slide can be homogeneous, rimmed, speckled, or nucleolar.
   A. Serum protein electrophoresis
   B. Antinuclear antibody (ANA) testing
   C. Immunofixation electrophoresis
   D. Flow cytometry

2. What is the name of the test based on the following description of the methodology?
Patient's serum or urine is added to lanes on an agarose gel and the proteins are separated by electrophoresis. Antibodies are added on top of each individual lane with specificity for the immunoglobulin heavy chains, mu, gamma, and alpha, and the immunoglobulin light chains, kappa and lambda.
   A. Serum protein electrophoresis
   B. Antinuclear antibody (ANA) testing
   C. Immunofixation electrophoresis
   D. Flow cytometry

3. What is the name of the test based on the following description of the methodology?
A sample of acellular body fluid is incubated with an antibody to the compound being measured. When the compound is present, antigen–antibody complexes form, which scatter light from a beam of light shone through the sample. The amount of scattered light is proportional to the compound being measured.
   A. Flow cytometry for identification of cell type
   B. Cryoglobulin analysis
   C. Nephelometry for quantitation of proteins
   D. Immunofixation electrophoresis

4. Which of the following compounds is commonly used in the detection of a positive blood culture?
   A. Carbon dioxide
   B. Oxygen
   C. Nitrogen
   D. Hydrogen

5. In a test for antimicrobial sensitivity of a pathogenic organism on an agar plate using a disk diffusion method, the following diameters with no growth of microorganisms were obtained for the drugs noted. Which of the following drugs is most likely to be effective against the organism identified as pathogenic?
   A. Penicillin, 2 mm
   B. Clindamycin, 5 mm
   C. Vancomycin, 10 mm
   D. Clarithromycin, 25 mm

6. In the automated blood cell counter, which of the following is a calculated value that is not measured directly by the instrument?
   A. Platelet count
   B. Hemoglobin
   C. Mean corpuscular volume (MCV)
   D. Mean corpuscular hemoglobin concentration (MCHC)

7. Which of the following hemoglobins is the least commonly detected hemoglobin by hemoglobin analysis in the US population?
   A. Hemoglobin S
   B. Hemoglobin C
   C. Hemoglobin A
   D. Hemoglobin G

8. The erythrocyte sedimentation rate has been a longstanding test to measure inflammation. Which of the following tests is also used as a marker of inflammation?
   A. Albumin
   B. Ceruloplasmin
   C. C-reactive protein (CRP)
   D. Immunoglobulin M

9. What is the unit of measurement for the PT and PTT assays?

   A. mg/dL
   B. Seconds
   C. Units/L
   D. nmol/L

10. Which set of test results is most consistent with the presence of a factor VIII inhibitor in a PTT mixing study at time points 0 hours (immediately), 30 minutes, and 1 hour after mixing?

    A. 60 seconds, 35 seconds, 58 seconds
    B. 60 seconds, 62 seconds, 58 seconds
    C. 60 seconds, 32 seconds, 30 seconds
    D. 60 seconds, 25 seconds, 28 seconds

11. Which of the statements about blood typing is true?

    A. Forward typing detects antibodies in the serum that can bind to red blood cell antigens.
    B. Reverse typing detects antigens that bound to the red blood cell.
    C. In forward typing, antibodies to A, B, and Rh antigens are added to three separate tubes containing red blood cells.
    D. The failure of red blood cells to clump upon addition of antibodies to the A antigen indicates the presence of A antigen on red blood cells.

12. Which of the following statements about storage of blood components is correct?

    A. Packed red blood cells are stored at 20–24°C
    B. Platelet concentrates are stored at 1–6°C
    C. Plasma is stored at below 18°C (i.e., at least 18° below 0°C)
    D. Whole blood is stored at below 18°C

13. What is the name of the test that determines if immunoglobulin G (IgG) or complement component C3d is bound to a patient's red blood cells?

    A. The blood crossmatch
    B. The indirect antiglobulin test
    C. Red blood cell antigen detection test to identify antibodies to red blood cells
    D. The direct antiglobulin test

14. The measurement of the electrolytes in serum or plasma is most commonly performed using a/an

    A. Ion-selective electrode
    B. Spectrophotometer
    C. Mass spectrometer
    D. Gas chromatograph

15. Linked enzyme reactions to measure a compound or an enzyme activity in plasma, which generate a color change proportional to the concentration of the compound, are most commonly which one of the following?

    A. Highly automated and relatively inexpensive to perform
    B. Manual tests and relatively inexpensive to perform
    C. Highly automated and expensive to perform
    D. Manual tests and expensive to perform

16. The sample most commonly used for blood gas testing is which one of the following?

    A. Venous plasma
    B. Serum
    C. Whole blood
    D. Arterial plasma

17. Which of the following is detected by analysis of the sediment from a centrifuged urine specimen?

    A. Specific gravity
    B. Red blood cell casts
    C. Bilirubin
    D. Urobilinogen

18. When molecular compounds are separated by liquid or gas chromatography and then the molecules are broken into different size fragments creating a "fingerprint" for each molecule, the detector is a/an

    A. Spectrophotometer
    B. Ion-selective electrode
    C. Flame ionization detector
    D. Mass spectrometer

19. Which of the following point-of-care tests is used more than the others?
    A. International normalized ratio (INR)
    B. Blood glucose
    C. Troponin
    D. Hemoglobin A1c

20. The evaluation of chromosomes by performance of a karyotype is
    A. Chromosomal analysis for structural abnormalities and abnormal number of chromosomes
    B. Total genome sequencing of an individual chromosome
    C. Identification of single-nucleotide variations
    D. Sequencing of an individual gene on a chromosome

21. Which of the following assays is a mostly automated and inexpensive test?
    A. Single-nucleotide variation identification by array
    B. Next-generation sequencing
    C. Troponin I measurement
    D. Comparative genomic hybridization

Autoimmune Disorders Involving the Connective Tissue and Immunodeficiency Diseases

Mandakolathur R. Murali

LEARNING OBJECTIVES

1. Learn the common autoimmune diseases involving primarily the connective tissue.

2. Understand the disorders associated with immune deficiencies and their underlying pathophysiology.

3. Learn the diagnostic tests required to establish a diagnosis for autoimmune disorders and for immunodeficiency disorders.

CHAPTER OUTLINE

The immune system is a tightly regulated network that incorporates both innate and adaptive pathways. The genes regulating the innate system are coded in the germ line. The innate immune system is not antigen specific. The cells and soluble factors of the innate system have **p**attern **r**ecognition **r**eceptors (PRRs, such as toll-like receptors) to common motifs on pathogens and altered self-motifs. The motifs on pathogens are called **p**athogen-**a**ssociated **m**olecular **p**atterns (PAMPs). Altered self-antigens include **d**anger-**a**ssociated **m**olecular **p**atterns (DAMPs) as found in heat shock protein, and **a**poptosis-**a**ssociated **m**olecular **p**atterns (AAMPs) as found in ds DNA, RNP, and histones. This response is rapid and there is no memory of the encounter.

The receptors on the T and B cells of the adaptive immune system are antigen or epitope specific and clonally variable, and their diversity is derived from gene recombination. The cells retain memory of the encounter and on subsequent engagement with that antigen, the cells exhibit more rapid and robust responses.

TABLE 3–1   Systemic Autoimmune Diseases: Diseases Associated with Positive Test Results for Antinuclear Antibodies (ANA)

Disease	% ANA Positive	Titer	Common Patterns
Systemic lupus erythematosus—active	95–98	High	H > S > R
Systemic lupus erythematosus—remission	90	Moderate–high	H > S
Mixed connective tissue disease	93	High	S > N
Scleroderma/CREST	85	High	S > C > N
Sjogren syndrome	48	Moderate–high	S > H
Polymyositis/dermatomyositis	61	Low–moderate	S > N
Rheumatoid arthritis	41	Low–moderate	S
Drug-induced lupus	95	Low–moderate	H>S
Pauciarticular juvenile chronic arthritis	71	Low–moderate	S

Note: ANA patterns on Hep-2 cells by indirect immunofluorescent technique (IFA). Patterns: H, homogeneous; S, speckled; R, rim; C, centromere; N, nucleolar. Titers: high = 1:1280 to 1:5120; moderate = 1:160 to 1:640; low = 1:40 to 1:80.

The immune network is tightly regulated by cells and cytokines, and a derangement in this immune homeostasis can result in immune response to self-antigens as in autoimmunity (failure of self-tolerance), or failure to recognize pathogens and eliminate them as occurs in immunodeficiency syndromes (failure of immunity). The following two groups of disorders are the focus of this chapter: the autoimmune diseases involving the connective tissue and the primary immunodeficiency diseases.

Diseases in which immune responses to self-antigens occur in the context of a genetic predisposition resulting in disease expression are called autoimmune diseases. Some involve organ-specific pathologic autoimmunity such as Hashimoto thyroiditis and celiac disease, and these are discussed in Chapters 22 and 15, respectively. The autoimmune disorders discussed in this chapter are systemic diseases with predominant involvement of the connective tissue, manifesting clinical features including inflammation of the joints, skin, muscles, and other soft tissues (see **Tables 3–1** and **3–2** and **Figure 3–1**).

The immunodeficiency diseases are subdivided into the relatively rare primary and the more common secondary immunodeficiency diseases. Primary immunodeficiency diseases are a direct consequence of either structural or functional derangement in the immune network. Secondary immune deficiency is the consequence of an alteration in the immune status resulting in the manifestation of infectious diseases, such as HIV infection, disseminated herpes simplex, and cytomegalovirus infections or a malignancy, with lymphoma and multiple myeloma as examples. Immunosuppressive therapy using monoclonal antibodies, such as rituximab (anti-CD20) or agents against TNF-α, and radiation are emerging as important causes of secondary immunodeficiency. Advances in immunotherapy for malignant diseases, such as chimeric antigen receptor therapy or **CART**, also results in some off-target responses manifesting as secondary immunodeficiency.

The following two groups of disorders are the focus of this chapter: the autoimmune diseases involving the connective tissue and the immunodeficiency diseases.

TABLE 3–2   Specific Organ Autoimmune Diseases: Diseases Associated with Positive Test Results for Antinuclear Antibodies (ANA)

Disease	% ANA Positive	Titer	Common Patterns
Graves disease	50	Low–moderate	S
Hashimoto thyroiditis	46	Low–moderate	S
Autoimmune hepatitis	63–91	Low–moderate	S
Primary biliary cirrhosis	10–40	Low–moderate	S

Patterns: S, speckled. Miscellaneous causes: low titer positive ANA patterns (mostly speckled) have been described in chronic infectious diseases such as infectious mononucleosis, hepatitis C infection, HIV, subacute bacterial endocarditis, and certain lymphoproliferative diseases.

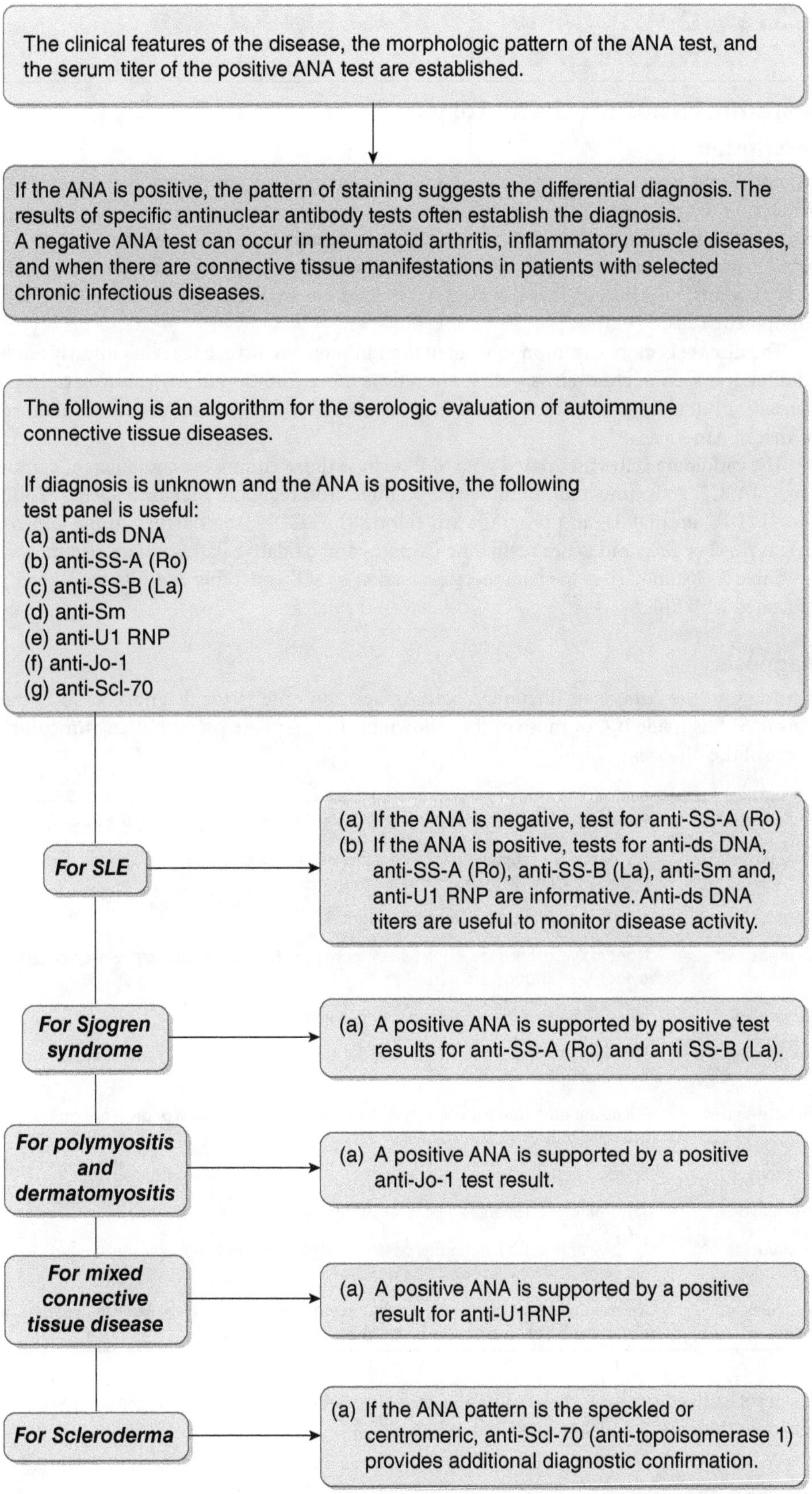

The clinical features of the disease, the morphologic pattern of the ANA test, and the serum titer of the positive ANA test are established.

If the ANA is positive, the pattern of staining suggests the differential diagnosis. The results of specific antinuclear antibody tests often establish the diagnosis.
A negative ANA test can occur in rheumatoid arthritis, inflammatory muscle diseases, and when there are connective tissue manifestations in patients with selected chronic infectious diseases.

The following is an algorithm for the serologic evaluation of autoimmune connective tissue diseases.

If diagnosis is unknown and the ANA is positive, the following test panel is useful:
(a) anti-ds DNA
(b) anti-SS-A (Ro)
(c) anti-SS-B (La)
(d) anti-Sm
(e) anti-U1 RNP
(f) anti-Jo-1
(g) anti-Scl-70

For SLE

(a) If the ANA is negative, test for anti-SS-A (Ro)
(b) If the ANA is positive, tests for anti-ds DNA, anti-SS-A (Ro), anti-SS-B (La), anti-Sm and, anti-U1 RNP are informative. Anti-ds DNA titers are useful to monitor disease activity.

For Sjogren syndrome

(a) A positive ANA is supported by positive test results for anti-SS-A (Ro) and anti SS-B (La).

For polymyositis and dermatomyositis

(a) A positive ANA is supported by a positive anti-Jo-1 test result.

For mixed connective tissue disease

(a) A positive ANA is supported by a positive result for anti-U1RNP.

For Scleroderma

(a) If the ANA pattern is the speckled or centromeric, anti-Scl-70 (anti-topoisomerase 1) provides additional diagnostic confirmation.

FIGURE 3–1 An approach to the diagnosis of autoimmune disorders involving connective tissue.

SYSTEMIC AUTOIMMUNE DISEASES INVOLVING THE CONNECTIVE TISSUE

Systemic Lupus Erythematosus

Description

Systemic lupus erythematosus (SLE) is a multisystem autoimmune disease, associated with the production of antibodies to a variety of nuclear and cytoplasmic antigens. The hallmark characteristic is the generation of antibodies to ds DNA. These antibodies complex to these self-antigens, and the ensuing immune complexes contribute to the inflammation in many organs, particularly the skin, joints, kidney, and, to a lesser extent, the cardiovascular and nervous systems, lung, and hemopoietic cells.

The disease is more common in women than in men and usually appears in early adulthood, although it is seen in children as well. It not only is more common in African Americans than in Caucasians but also has a more severe clinical phenotype with renal and vasculitic manifestations in African Americans.

The candidate genes associated with SLE include those coding for complement components C1q, C4A, C2, activating and inhibitory FcγR, interferon regulatory factor 5 (IRF5), TNF, MHC class II (DR2 and DR3), and programmed cell death (PCD). Homologues to *Bcl*-family genes, such as *Bcl-2* or *Bax*, and genes regulating caspases and oxidative pathways are also involved.

Table 3–3 summarizes the laboratory evaluation of SLE and **Table 3–4** lists the autoantibodies associated with SLE.

> Systemic lupus erythematosus (SLE) is a multisystem autoimmune disease, associated with the production of antibodies to a variety of nuclear and cytoplasmic antigens. The hallmark characteristic is the generation of antibodies to ds DNA.

Diagnosis

According to the American Rheumatologic Association criteria for diagnosis of SLE, the diagnosis of SLE is made if 4 or more of the following 11 criteria are present at any time during the course of the disease:

Malar rash	Flat or raised fixed erythema over the malar eminences and sparing the nasolabial folds
Discoid rash	Erythematous raised patches with adherent keratotic scaling and follicular plugging; scarring may occur in older lesions
Photosensitivity	Skin rash resulting from reaction to light
Arthritis	Nonerosive arthritis involving two or more peripheral joints that are swollen or tender and evidence of effusion
Oral ulcers	Mostly painless ulcers in the oral cavity and pharynx
Serositis	Pleuritis with pleural rub or effusion; pericarditis documented by rub, EKG change, or pericardial effusion
Renal diseases	Persistent proteinuria greater than 0.5 g/day or 3+ on dipstick or presence on RBC, granular, tubular, or mixed cellular casts
Neurologic	Seizures or psychosis in the absence of metabolic or drug-induced causes
Hematologic	Any immune cytopenia—RBC, WBC, or platelets
Immunologic	Positive anti-ds DNA antibody, positive antiphospholipid antibody, positive anti-Sm antibody, and false-positive serologic test for syphilis
Antinuclear antibody	An abnormal ANA titer by immunofluorescence or an equivalent assay in the absence of drugs known to be associated with "drug-induced lupus"

Tests utilized in the initial evaluation and subsequent monitoring of patients with SLE are shown in **Tables 3–3** and **3–4** and **Figure 3–1**.

Sjogren Syndrome

Description

Sjogren syndrome (SS) is a systemic connective tissue disease, more common in women than in men. Pathologically, it is an autoimmune exocrinopathy involving the lacrimal glands, salivary

TABLE 3–3   Laboratory Evaluation of Systemic Lupus Erythematosus (SLE): General Laboratory Tests

Laboratory Tests	Results/Significance
Complete blood count and erythrocyte sedimentation rate (ESR)	Decrease in RBC, WBC, and platelets either singly or in combination suggests the presence of autoimmune cytopenias; serial CBC is useful to monitor bone marrow response to immunosuppressive therapy; ESR if elevated is a useful parameter to follow with therapy
Urinalysis and BUN/creatinine	Urinalysis is useful to evaluate proteinuria and any cellular sediments and casts; 24-hour protein excretion and BUN/creatinine are useful to monitor renal function
Liver function tests and lipid profile	For evaluation of possible autoimmune hepatitis; alterations in plasma lipids either due to disease or as a sequelae of therapy are to be appropriately managed to prevent cardiovascular complications
VDRL/RPR test for syphilis	False-positive VDRL test is noted in SLE; a positive VDRL in the absence of syphilis (negative RPR) is a diagnostic criterion for SLE
Antinuclear antibody	95%–98% of patients with active SLE have a positive ANA
Complement assay	C3, C4, and factor B are useful to evaluate complement activation; CH50 to detect congenital complement deficiency especially in familial SLE; low complement values may reflect disease activity

glands, and less often the pancreas. The immune inflammation of these glands contributes to the sicca syndrome, with dry eyes (keratoconjunctivitis) and dry mouth (xerostomia) as characteristic clinical features. The disease can be primary or secondary. The primary syndrome is characterized by dry eyes, dry mouth, decreased production of tears as tested by the Schirmer test, and a lip biopsy that demonstrates inflammation of the minor salivary glands. Serologically, patients with primary Sjogren show a positive ANA, positive SS-A (Ro), positive SS-B (La), and positive rheumatoid factor (RF) in the absence of another connective tissue disease. A prospective study of 80 patients with primary SS followed for a median of 7.5 years reported the following frequencies of clinical manifestations: (a) keratoconjunctivitis sicca and/or xerostomia occurred in all patients and were the only disease manifestations in 31%; (b) extraglandular involvement occurred in 25%; and (c) non-Hodgkin lymphoma developed in 2.5%. Secondary SS is clinically similar to the primary disorder, but it is additionally associated with clinical and serologic features of another connective tissue disease, such as rheumatoid arthritis (RA) or scleroderma.

TABLE 3–4   Autoantibodies and Clinical Associations in Systemic Lupus Erythematosus (SLE)

Antigen Specificity	Prevalence (%)	Pattern on Hep-2 Cells	Clinical Associations
ds DNA	40–60	Homogeneous	Marker of active disease; titers fluctuate with disease activity; correlates best with renal disease
SS-A/Ro	40	Speckled, fine	Subacute cutaneous lupus (75%), neonatal lupus with heart block, complements deficiencies and photosensitivity
SS-B/La	10–15	Speckled, fine	Neonatal lupus
Sm	20–30	Speckled, coarse	Specific marker for SLE; may be associated with CNS disease; not useful in monitoring disease activity
RNP (U1 RNP)	30–40	Speckled, coarse	Generally coexists with Sm; RNP is a marker for MCTD
Histones	50–95	Homogeneous	50%–70% in SLE and >95% in drug-induced SLE
Phospholipids (beta-2 glycoprotein I antibodies)	30	None specific	Associated with thrombocytopenia, later trimester abortions, and hypercoagulable states
Proliferating cell nuclear antigen (PCNA)	3	Finely granular nuclear staining in rapidly dividing cells	Not sensitive but specific (>95%); not seen in RA, other connective tissue disease; antibody rapidly diminished by steroids and immunosuppressive drugs; correlates with arthritis

Sjogren syndrome is characterized by immune-mediated destruction of exocrine glands, particularly the salivary and lacrimal glands, with secondary development of keratoconjunctivitis and xerostomia. A positive ANA along with antibodies to SS-A (Ro) and/or SS-B (La) is a serologic feature. Transition from a polyclonal rheumatoid factor (RF) positive to a RF-negative oligoclonal or monoclonal process suggests a malignant lymphomatous transformation.

Diagnosis

The diagnostic features are revealed by tests that document the sicca features. The dry eyes are evaluated by the Schirmer test. This test is a measurement of tear flow over a 5-minute period. Filter paper is allowed to hang from the lateral inferior eyelid and the length of the paper that becomes wet is measured. This test is not reliable, as early in the disease there is excessive lacrimation giving a false-negative test. Demonstration of devitalized corneal epithelium due to keratoconjunctivitis is evaluated by rose Bengal or fluorescein stain. The most accurate test is the slit lamp examination of the cornea and conjunctiva. Tests for quantitating salivary secretion are not standardized and also are not specific to SS. Biopsy of the minor salivary gland in the lower lip demonstrating focal lymphocytic infiltration is a useful confirmatory test.

Table 3–5 summarizes the laboratory tests useful in diagnosis of both primary and secondary SS.

TABLE 3–5   Laboratory Evaluation for Sjogren Syndrome

	Findings in Sjogren Syndrome
Diagnostic tests for dry eyes	
Schirmer test	<5 mm wet zone on filter paper in 5 minutes
Rose Bengal dye test	Visualization of devitalized areas in cornea
Tear breakup time	Measuring breakup time and tear osmolality after installation of fluorescein; identifies those who respond to anti-inflammatory therapy
Diagnostic tests for dry mouth	
Salivary gland scintigraphy	Low uptake of radionuclide is specific for SS, but 33% of patients have a positive test; not a sensitive test
Lower lip biopsy	Presence of lymphoid infiltrate around salivary glands is consistent with disease
Magnetic resonance imaging (MRI)	MRI is superior to ultrasonography and CT studies and is equivalent to sialography; correlates well with salivary gland biopsy
General laboratory tests	
Complete blood count including differential count	Anemia, neutropenia, lymphopenia, and thrombocytopenia may suggest immune destruction. Marked lymphocytosis may suggest clonal proliferation
Serum electrolytes and liver elevated function tests	Hypokalemia if associated with renal tubular acidosis, elevated alkaline phosphatase suggests primary biliary cirrhosis
Erythrocyte sedimentation rate and C-reactive protein	Markers for chronic and acute inflammation
Urinalysis	Proteinuria, casts imply renal involvement
Quantitative immunoglobulins (IgG, IgM, IgA)	Polyclonal increase is often noted
Serum and urine protein electrophoresis (SPEP and UPEP) and serum-free light chains with altered kappa/lambda ratio	Transformation from polyclonal to monoclonal gammopathy implies evolution to a B-cell lymphoma. Presence of urine Bence-Jones protein confirms monoclonal transformation
Laboratory tests for autoimmunity	
Antinuclear antibody (ANA) titer	Commonest pattern is speckled; titer greater than 1:160; in 75% of patients
Antibodies to SS-A (Ro)	With ELISA >90% have a positive test
Antibodies to SS-B (La)	With ELISA >90% have a positive test
Rheumatoid factor	70% have positive RF
Cryoglobulins, C3, and C4	Presence of cryoglobulins and low C3 and C4 are found with multisystem disease
Anti-ds DNA antibody	In 25%–30% of patients with primary SS

Systemic sclerosis is characterized by excessive and often widespread deposition of collagen in many organ systems of the body. Pathologically, the hallmark is the deposition of altered collagen in the extracellular matrix and a proliferative and occlusive small vessel vasculopathy.

Systemic Sclerosis/Scleroderma

Description

Systemic sclerosis is characterized by excessive and widespread deposition of collagen in many organ systems of the body. The hallmark of this pathologic process is the deposition of altered collagen in the extracellular matrix. The disorder is characterized pathologically by three features: (1) tissue fibrosis; (2) a proliferative and occlusive vasculopathy of the small blood vessels; and (3) a specific autoimmune response associated with distinctive autoantibody profile.

The immunologic basis is not well understood, but an aberration in TGF-beta-mediated deposition of collagen has been observed. Antibodies to platelet-derived growth factor receptors have been incriminated in the development of fibrosis. Both the triggering event and genetic predisposition are not well defined. Although the common organ involved is the skin, the gastrointestinal tract, kidney, lung, and muscles are also affected as the disease progresses. Renal ischemia leading to hypertension escalates the complications of this disease. Preponderance in females is common.

Clinically there are four major subtypes described:

1. Diffuse cutaneous scleroderma with widespread involvement of skin and visceral organs.
2. Limited cutaneous scleroderma, in which the disease is limited to the digital extremities and face. CREST syndrome is a variant of this entity. The name is derived from its features—Calcinosis, Raynaud syndrome, Esophageal dysmotility, Sclerodactyly, and Telangiectasia.
3. Localized scleroderma that affects primarily the skin of the forearms, the fingers, and later the systemic organs.
4. Overlap syndromes with features of RA or muscle involvement.

Diagnosis

Ninety percent to 95% of all patients with scleroderma have a positive ANA test. The most common pattern is finely speckled, followed by centromeric and nucleolar patterns. The ANA activity is directed against DNA topoisomerase (also known as Scl-70). A definitive diagnosis is achieved when the characteristic clinical findings are accompanied by a positive ANA test, and often confirmed by an antibody directed to Scl-70 by ELISA.

Tables 3–6.1 and 3–6.2 summarize the laboratory evaluation for systemic sclerosis/scleroderma.

Inflammatory Muscle Diseases

Description

Inflammation of the muscle leading to injury and weakness is the basis of the three most common but distinct diseases in this category. They are dermatomyositis (DM), polymyositis (PM), and inclusion body myositis. These diseases are more common in women, and their etiology remains unknown, although immune mechanisms have been incriminated. DM may occur as a specific entity or be associated with scleroderma or mixed connective tissue disease. Rarely, it is a manifestation of a malignancy. Skin manifestations such as a heliotrope rash, the shawl sign, and Gottron papules are common in DM. Like DM, PM may also be associated with another connective tissue disease. In addition, it may be associated with viral, parasitic, or bacterial infections. DM is characterized by immune complex deposition in the vessels and is considered to be in part a complement-mediated vasculopathy. In contrast, PM appears to reflect direct T-cell-mediated muscle injury. Inclusion body myositis is a disease of older individuals and is not associated with malignancy. It is occasionally associated with another connective tissue disease.

> Inflammation of the muscle leading to injury and weakness is the basis of the three most common but distinct diseases in this category. They are dermatomyositis (DM), polymyositis (PM), and inclusion body myositis.

TABLE 3–6.1   Laboratory Evaluation for Systemic Sclerosis/Scleroderma

Laboratory Test	Scleroderma	CREST Syndrome
Pattern of ANA (Hep-2)	Speckled	Centromeric
Commonly found autoantibody	Anti-Scl-70 (greater in diffuse disease than in localized disease)	Mostly anticentromeric with a distinctive pattern on Hep-2 cells

TABLE 3–6.2   Autoantigens and Phenotypes in Systemic Sclerosis/Scleroderma

Autoantigens	Description of Phenotype
Scl-70/Topo 1 or topoisomerase 1	25%–40% of patients with diffuse scleroderma; associated with severe lung disease
ACA or centromere	55%–96% of patients with CREST syndrome. CENP-B (100%) and CENP-C (50%) are the targets. Seen in Raynaud phenomenon and in about 10% of patients with primary biliary cirrhosis
RNA polymerase I, II, and III	4%–20% of patients with diffuse skin disease and renal involvement and less lung and muscle involvement
Fibrillarin (U3 snRNP)	8%–10% of patients with cardiopulmonary and muscle involvement. Higher prevalence in blacks and Native Americans
PM-Scl	A nucleolar complex seen in association with inflammatory muscle disease in scleroderma
Th/To RNP (endoribonuclease)	10% of patients with limited scleroderma and associated with pulmonary hypertension and fibrosis
U1 snRNP (U1 RNP and polypeptides)	Associated with overlap syndrome and mixed connective tissue disease
B-23 (nucleophosmin)	A nucleolar phosphoprotein associated with pulmonary hypertension and overlap syndrome

Antisynthetase syndrome, characterized by antisynthetase antibodies that are highly specific for DM and PM, is seen in about 30% of patients with DM or PM. These patients typically experience a relatively acute onset of disease, constitutional symptoms such as fever, Raynaud phenomenon, arthritis, and interstitial lung diseases. Their hands exhibit a roughening and cracking of the radial sides of the fingers and the palm, resembling a condition found in people who labor with their hands such as mechanics, and hence called "mechanic's hands." HLA DR 52 has a strong association (90%) with antisynthetase antibody-positive myositis in people of both European and African descent. The antisynthetase antibodies include antibodies to aminoacyl-tRNA synthetase; antihistidyl-tRNA synthetase, also known as Jo-1; anti-signal recognition particle (SRP) antibodies directed against SRP; and anti-Mi-2 antibodies directed against a helicase involved in transcriptional activation.

Diagnosis

Although there are several common features between DM and PM, a characteristic feature of DM itself is the heliotrope hue around the eyes. Pulmonary interstitial fibrosis is seen in about 10% of cases in both diseases, occurring in the context of antisynthetase syndromes. There are five distinctive features described for both of these diseases. At least three of the following features are essential to fulfill the clinical diagnostic criteria for each:

1. Proximal and symmetrical muscle weakness
2. History of muscle pain and tenderness on palpation
3. Electromyographic evidence of spontaneous muscle activity and myopathic changes
4. Elevated serum or plasma concentrations of muscle enzymes such as aldolase, creatinine kinase (CK), and AST
5. Muscle biopsy demonstrating cellular inflammation

The laboratory diagnosis begins with documentation of muscle inflammation and injury as shown by elevation of serum or plasma concentrations of muscle enzymes such as aldolase, CK, and AST, together with the expected inflammatory histological features on muscle biopsy. The detection of autoantibodies is found in about one-third of the patients, and supports a diagnosis of inflammatory muscle disease. The antibodies are directed at tRNA synthetases. Anti-Jo-1 is such an antibody, with specificity to histidyl-tRNA synthetase. It is found in about 40% of

TABLE 3-7.1   Laboratory Evaluation for Inflammatory Muscle Diseases

Test	Polymyositis	Dermatomyositis	Inclusion Body Myositis (IBM)
Creatine kinase (CK)	The CK concentration is elevated >50 times and levels reflect disease activity	The CK concentration is elevated >50 times and levels reflect disease activity	CK concentrations may be normal or elevated no more than 10 times the upper limit of normal
Muscle biopsy	The inflammatory infiltrates are usually within the fascicles surrounding the healthy muscle fibers; no perifascicular atrophy; increased CD8+ cells and enhanced expression of major histocompatibility antigens by muscle fibers	The inflammatory infiltrate is usually around the fascicles. The presence of perifascicular atrophy is diagnostic; complement-mediated vasculopathy is present	The pattern of inflammation is similar to that seen in polymyositis, with the addition of basophilic-rimmed vacuoles within the muscle fiber sarcoplasm that are characteristic of IBM; the presence of all 3 of the following on muscle biopsy confirms IBM and effectively excludes other idiopathic inflammatory myopathies: (1) vacuolated muscle fibers, (2) muscle fiber inclusions with staining characteristics of beta-amyloid deposits, and (3) demonstration of paired helical fibers by electron microscopy or immunohistological staining
Anti-Jo-1 antibodies	Present in about 40% of patients	Present in about 40% of patients	Present in about 40% of patients

TABLE 3-7.2   Autoantibodies and Phenotypes in Inflammatory Myositis

Autoantibodies	Description of Phenotype
Anti-Jo-1 and other antisynthetases	Relatively acute onset of myositis, frequent interstitial lung diseases, fever, Raynaud phenomenon, mechanic's hand. Muscle disease dominates the picture in even those who meet criteria for SLE and RA
Anti-signal recognition particle (SRP)	Very acute onset of myositis with severe muscle weakness, predominantly in females and often in autumn. Rash is absent
Anti-Mi-2	Relatively acute onset of myositis with classical rashes of dermatomyositis such as V sign and shawl sign
Anti-200/100	Necrotizing myopathy with minimal muscle wasting, preceded by statin therapy, and very high CPK values
Anti-155/140	Juvenile dermatomyositis and malignancy-associated dermatomyositis
Anti-CADM-140	Clinically amyopathic dermatomyositis with interstitial lung diseases

patients with PM, and generally indicates a worse prognosis. It is also more commonly found in patients with pulmonary fibrosis. Jo-1 is more commonly detected in cases of autoimmune myositis than in those with other causes of muscle inflammation. As with many autoimmune diseases, the integration of clinical features with laboratory findings forms the basis of definitive diagnosis. Tables 3–7.1 and 3–7.2 present the laboratory evaluation for inflammatory muscle disorders.

The entity known as mixed connective tissue disorder (MCTD) has some of the features of SLE, some of systemic sclerosis, and some of polymyositis.

Mixed Connective Tissue Disease

Description

The entity known as mixed connective tissue disease (MCTD) has some of the features of SLE, some of systemic sclerosis, and some of PM. The patients have variable clinical presentations with arthralgias, myalgias or myositis, fatigue, and Raynaud phenomenon. These features are superimposed on other findings that can add in over time, including malar rash, sclerodactyly, arthritis of the hands, and Raynaud phenomenon. Pulmonary manifestations occur in over 85% of these patients and include interstitial pneumonitis, pulmonary hypertension, progressive interstitial fibrosis, and, rarely, dysfunction of diaphragm and esophagus. On rare occasion, patients with MCTD develop diffuse proliferative glomerulonephritis, psychosis, or seizures.

TABLE 3–8   Laboratory Evaluation for Mixed Connective Tissue Disorders

Laboratory Tests	Results
Antinuclear antibody	Speckled pattern on Hep-2 cells
Autoantibody to extractable nuclear antigens (ENA)	Predominantly anti-U1 RNP
Autoantibodies for SLE, SS, and polymyositis	Often positive, except for anti-Sm that is negative

The appropriate constellation of clinical findings suggests the need for laboratory testing, described in **Table 3–8**.

Diagnosis

The diagnosis of MCTD is largely made on the basis of the clinical features consistent with multiple autoimmune diseases. A high titer of anti-U1 RNP in the serum is a prerequisite for the diagnosis along with three or more clinical features, including Raynaud's phenomenon, swollen hands, synovitis, myositis or myalgia, and acrosclerosis. One of these features must include synovitis or myositis.

Rheumatoid Arthritis

Description

RA is a systemic autoimmune connective tissue disorder that primarily affects the synovial joints, often starting as a synovitis. It affects 1% to 2% of the adult population worldwide, and is predominantly a disease of young women. Susceptibility and resistance to RA is associated with HLA genotypes. The criteria for diagnosis of RA were revised in 1987 to include clinical features, laboratory values, and radiographic findings. To establish a definitive diagnosis, at least three of the following seven criteria must be present along with morning stiffness for a period of at least 6 weeks:

> RA is a systemic autoimmune connective tissue disorder that primarily affects the synovial joints, often starting as a synovitis. It affects 1% to 2% of the adult population worldwide, and is predominantly a disease of young women.

1. Arthritis in three or more small joints
2. Morning stiffness lasting >30 minutes
3. Arthritis of the small joints of the hand
4. Rheumatoid nodules
5. Symmetrical arthritis, often with synovitis
6. A positive test for RF
7. Radiographic changes of the affected joints

Diagnosis

An increased serum titer of RF has been a long-standing marker of RA, until the validation of anti-cyclic citrullinated peptide antibody (anti-CCP). This antibody not only is highly associated with RA but is also a marker for progressive and erosive joint disease. Anti-CCP is approximately 98% specific and 85% sensitive as a serum marker for RA. RF is an IgM autoantibody directed against the Fc region of IgG. While high titers of RF are associated with severe RA, it is not specific for diagnosis of RA, as it is also found in chronic infections and other connective tissue diseases. **Table 3–9** summarizes the laboratory tests useful in the evaluation of RA.

Amyloidosis

Description

Amyloidosis and cryoglobulinemia (which follows) are systemic diseases resulting from the deposition in the tissues of insoluble proteins from a soluble circulating precursor. Both represent the consequences of immune dysregulation, and their diagnosis depends on laboratory evaluation and confirmation.

Amyloidosis is a heterogeneous group of diseases resulting from the extracellular deposition of low-molecular-weight fibrils from a soluble circulating precursor giving a "waxy" or "lardaceous"

TABLE 3–9   Laboratory Evaluation for Rheumatoid Arthritis

Laboratory Test	Results and Significance
Complete blood count (CBC)	Patients with RA may have a normochromic, normocytic anemia (Hbg of about 10 g/dL), and elevated platelet count with neutrophilia; in Felty syndrome there is neutropenia; patients on immunosuppressive therapy have decreased counts of all lineages
ESR	An index of inflammation and often elevated; in RA patients, its level often parallels disease activity
C-reactive protein	This acute phase reactant is increased in RA and is an index of inflammation; useful in monitoring disease activity over time and in response to therapy
Rheumatoid factor (RF) titer	RF is detectable in 70%–80% of patients with RA; diagnostic utility is limited by its lack of specificity as it is found in almost all patients with cryoglobulinemia, in 70% of patients with Sjogren syndrome, in 20%–30% of those with SLE, and in 5%–10% of healthy individuals; its prevalence increases with age
Anti-CCP	Most useful, as its specificity is 95%–98% and sensitivity is around 85%; predicts erosive disease in RA; valuable in diagnosis of early RA; positive titers to CCP have better predictive value in diagnosis of RA in the IgM-RF-negative subgroup; negative RF in combination with negative anti-CCP is better in excluding RA than either alone in patients with polyarthritis
Anti-citrullinated α enolase	Predictor of radiographic progression
Anti-citrullinated fibrin	Detected in Felty syndrome and vasculitis
Matrix metalloproteinase (MMP) 1 and 3	Radiographic damage
Cartilage oligomeric protein (COMP)	High levels detected in early RA associated with severe disease of both large and small joints
Aggrecan cleavage fragments	Noted in slow-onset destructive disease of large and small joints
Pyridinoline cross-links	Metabolic marker of activity of bone involvement
Serum cryoglobulins	Presence correlates with extra-articular disease
Radiological studies	Periarticular osteoporosis, soft tissue swelling, joint space reduction and erosions should be determined at baseline and monitored with use of disease-modifying antirheumatic drugs; MRI is sensitive but expensive
Joint fluid analysis	If a single joint exhibits heightened inflammation in a patient with polyarticular disease, need to exclude septic arthritis or crystal-induced arthritis by cell count and differential, culture, and crystal identification

appearance to the infiltrated organs. Ultrastructurally, amyloid deposits are composed of unbranching fibrils 8 to 10 nm in width and with a molecular weight of 5 to 25 kDa. At least 25 biochemically distinct forms of human amyloid protein have been identified. The two most common forms are primary, with amyloid light chain (AL) derived from light chains of plasma cells, and secondary, with amyloid-associated protein (AA), a nonimmunoglobulin protein. Congo red staining of amyloid deposits demonstrates a characteristic apple-green birefringence on polarized microscopy, while staining with Thioflavin T produces yellow-green fluorescence.

The classification of amyloidosis is based on whether the amyloidosis is associated with a plasma cell dyscrasia such as multiple myeloma or light chain myeloma (primary amyloidosis), or the sequelae of an infectious or inflammatory disease (secondary or reactive amyloidosis). Amyloidosis may also be classified as hereditary or acquired, localized or systemic, or by the type of fibril deposited in tissues, such as transthyretin (TTR) and Alzheimer amyloid precursor protein (APP). A partial list of the chemical classification of human amyloid is given in **Table 3–10.1**.

The most common form of the disease, representing 75% to 80% of the cases, is primary amyloidosis, as an acquired disorder, with multiorgan systemic involvement. Primary amyloidosis has a male to female preponderance of 2:1. Its incidence increases with age, often starting at age 40 years.

Reactive amyloidosis or type AA amyloidosis is a serious outcome of a group of diseases called autoinflammatory syndromes. This group of diseases represents too much inflammation

The diagnosis of amyloidosis is based on the histological and immunochemical demonstration of amyloid deposits in affected organs and tissues. The preferred tissue for biopsy is obtained by fine needle aspiration of the abdominal fat pad.

TABLE 3–10.1   Chemical Classification of Amyloid

Amyloid Protein	Precursor Protein	Clinical Syndromes	Tissues Involved
AA	(Apo) serum AA	Chronic inflammation, familial Mediterranean fever (FMF), familial amyloid nephropathy (FAN) with urticaria and deafness, Muckle–Wells syndrome	Kidney, liver, and spleen
AL	Ig light chain, kappa, or lambda	Primary or myeloma associated	Kidney, heart, tongue, bone marrow, and peripheral nerves
AH	Ig heavy chain	Primary or heavy chain disease associated	Kidney, heart, tongue, bone marrow, and peripheral nerves
ATTR	Transthyretin	FAN, familial amyloidotic cardiomyopathy, senile systemic (cardiac) amyloid	Peripheral and autonomic nerves, heart, and kidney
AGel	Gelsolin	Corneal lattice dystrophy and cranial neuropathy	Cornea, cranial and peripheral nerves, kidney
ACys	Cystatin C	Hereditary cerebral hemorrhage with amyloid	Cranial vessels
Aβ	Aβ protein precursor (AβPP)	Alzheimer disease, aging	Central nervous system
Atau	Tau	Alzheimer disease, aging, other cerebral conditions	Brain
Aβ2M	β2-Microglobulin	Dialysis-related amyloid	Synovium, carpal tunnel, tongue
AApoAI	Apolipoprotein A-I	Familial amyloidotic polyneuropathy	Heart, skin, kidney, nerves, liver, larynx, and blood vessels
AApoAII	Apolipoprotein A-II	Familial nephropathy	Kidney
ACal	Procalcitonin	Medullary thyroid carcinoma	Thyroid
AANF	Atrial natriuretic factor	Atrial amyloid of aging	Cardiac atria
AprP	Prion protein	Creutzfeldt–Jakob disease, Gerstmann–Straussler–Scheinker disease, fatal familial insomnia	Central nervous system

secondary to dysregulation of the innate immune system, in the absence of high-titer autoantibodies or antigen-specific T cells. The hereditary autoinflammatory syndromes, also known as hereditary periodic fever syndromes, represent a group of genetic disorders characterized by recurrent inflammatory episodes of noninfectious origin, often starting in childhood and persisting lifelong. These syndromes are characterized by a variety of features that include fever, abdominal symptoms, arthralgias, arthritis, lymphadenopathy, ocular and skin manifestations. In disorders of the inflammasome (a component of the innate immune system which include caspases and other proteins), genetic mutations coding for proteins cause persistent or recurrent inflammation. Examples include a mutation in the gene *MEFV* coding for pyrin in familial Mediterranean fever (FMF) and a mutation in the gene *CIAS1* coding for cryopyrin in Muckle–Wells syndrome. An exuberant acute phase response with elevated C-reactive protein (CRP), serum amyloid A (SAA), and leukocytosis is associated with the inflammatory clinical presentation. The soluble SAA protein is degraded to the insoluble fibrils composed of AA, which is the hallmark of secondary amyloidosis. The mutated genes in these syndromes all code for proteins that play a role in the regulation of innate immunity.

Diagnosis

The diagnosis of amyloidosis is based on the histological and immunochemical demonstration of amyloid deposits in affected organs and tissues. The preferred tissue for biopsy is obtained by fine needle aspiration of the abdominal fat pad. Its advantages over rectal biopsy are that multiple

TABLE 3-10.2   Laboratory Evaluation for Amyloidosis

Laboratory Tests	Results/Comments
Abdominal fat pad aspiration/biopsy	Preferred site due to ease of obtaining multiple samples, better yield than rectal biopsy, and less invasive; has replaced rectal biopsy
Labial salivary gland biopsy	Better yield than abdominal pad biopsy for both AL and AA amyloidosis
Serum and urine protein electrophoresis	Primary amyloidosis is often associated with a monoclonal gammopathy; serum and urine electrophoresis followed by immunofixation studies to identify the specific monoclonal protein; assays for serum-free light chains and their ratio in serum are essential to detect light chain disease
Bone marrow biopsy	Indicated when serum electrophoresis, serum free light chain assays, and urine electrophoresis indicate a monoclonal gammopathy; flow cytometry and special stains for amyloid facilitate diagnosis
Coagulation factor X level	About 10% of patients with primary amyloidosis have factor X deficiency; about half of the patients with isolated and acquired factor X deficiency have primary amyloidosis; detection of this deficiency prior to biopsy with prothrombin time and factor X assay is essential
Protein sequencing	Useful in identifying genetic abnormalities in hereditary amyloidosis and identifying rare forms of amyloidosis
Serum amyloid P (SAP) component scanning	Scintigraphy with radiolabeled SAP used to identify and estimate total body burden of amyloid; its value is limited because SAP is obtained from blood donors and carries potential infectious risk

samples can be obtained for study, and it is less painful and invasive. Since a plasma cell dyscrasia is commonly found in patients with amyloidosis, a serum protein electrophoresis together with a determination of serum-free kappa and lambda light chains by nephelometry and a calculation of the kappa/lambda ratio is necessary to exclude a monoclonal gammopathy as the cause of the amyloidosis. Amyloid fibrils may bind to coagulation factor X causing a coagulopathy. Determination of the factor X level is important to explain bleeding tendencies in amyloidosis patients and is useful prior to biopsy of organs and tissues to identify a coagulopathy that would permit excess bleeding at the biopsy site.

To define the extent of the disease and the type of amyloidosis, the patient should be evaluated for renal, cardiac, pulmonary, neurologic, cutaneous, articular, liver, and spleen involvement. Cardiac involvement is extremely common in primary amyloidosis and much less in secondary amyloidosis. Virtually all of the familial amyloidosis manifests with nephropathic, neuropathic, or cardiopathic features. Laboratory evaluation for amyloidosis is summarized in **Table 3–10.2**.

Cryoglobulinemia

Description

Cryoglobulinemia refers to the presence in the serum of one or more immunoglobulins that precipitate at a temperature below 37°C. This precipitation is reversible, as it redissolves on warming to 37°C. The cause of cryoprecipitation remains to be determined.

Cryoglobulins are classified into three types. Type I consists of a single monoclonal immunoglobulin that does not have RF activity. It is typically IgM or IgG and less often IgA. Type I, also called simple cryoglobulinemia, is often associated with monoclonal lymphoproliferative malignancies of B cell lineage such as Waldenstrom macroglobulinemia or multiple myeloma or chronic lymphatic lymphoma (CLL). Patients with this disorder may present with features of vasculopathy involving the digits, resulting in gangrene. Type II consists of monoclonal IgM RF mixed with polyclonal IgG or IgA. The most common association for this form of cryoglobulinemia is hepatitis C infection. Type II may rarely be associated with lymphoma. Type III is also a mixed cryoglobulinemia, with polyclonal IgM RF associated with polyclonal IgG or IgA. Type III is found in patients with connective tissue disease and chronic infections. Both type II and III cryoglobulinemia patients may show fixation of complement and be associated with hypocomplementemia. Immune complex vasculitis, arthritis, neuropathy, and renal involvement may be the presenting features in patients with type II or III cryoglobulinemia.

Cryoglobulinemia refers to the presence in the serum of one or more immunoglobulins that precipitate at a temperature below 37°C. This precipitation is reversible, as it redissolves on warming to 37°C.

TABLE 3–11   Laboratory Evaluation for Cryoglobulinemia

Laboratory Test	Comment
Cryocrit	This is the (volume of the cryoprecipitate/volume of serum) × 100; necessary to keep the sample at 37°C until it reaches the laboratory and serum is separated; serum is then refrigerated at 4°C for 72 h; the cryocrit is then measured after centrifugation at 4°C; increased fibrinogen and lipids may lead to falsely elevated values
Immunofixation and immunodiffusion	Used to evaluate the constituents of the cryoglobulin and their clonality, and allow classification as type I, II, or III
Urinalysis, BUN, creatinine	To evaluate renal function
C3, C4, and RF	To assess for complement fixation by RF in the cryoglobulin
Liver enzymes	To evaluate liver function
Hepatitis serology/viral load by PCR	To evaluate hepatitis B or C infections and monitor response to therapy
Renal biopsy and immunofluorescence studies	Proteinuria, abnormal urinalysis, and altered renal function are an indication for renal biopsy with immunofluorescence for renal pathology
Lymph node and bone marrow biopsy	Indicated when a lymphoproliferative disease is suspected from the type of cryoglobulin, usually type I or II

Diagnosis

When present, the cryoglobulins are quantitated using a Wintrobe tube, and the amount of cryoglobulin present is reported as a cryocrit. It is important to remember that it is not the quantity as reported by a cryocrit that is important, but the biological inflammatory properties of the cryoglobulin. This inflammatory potential is reflected by hypocomplementemia, tissue inflammation, and organ injury. With therapy, the cryocrit decreases along with mitigation of inflammatory markers such as CRP, ESR, and complement activation. When a cryoglobulin is identified, the components comprising the cryoprotein are identified by immunodiffusion and immunofixation, using specific antisera directed at the immunoglobulin isotypes and against C3 and C4. Based on the clonality and the constituent isotypes, the cryoglobulin is then categorized as type I, II, or III. **Table 3–11** summarizes the laboratory evaluation for cryoglobulinemia.

DISEASES OF THE IMMUNE SYSTEM

X-linked Agammaglobulinemia
Description

X-linked agammaglobulinemia (XLA), also known as Bruton agammaglobulinemia, is the prototype humoral immune deficiency. It is a disease restricted to males, and is characterized by a near total absence of B lymphocytes from an arrest in B lymphocyte development. The deficiency of B cells results in pan-hypogammaglobulinemia. Patients with XLA are asymptomatic for the first several months of life. Recurrent infections manifest between 4 and 12 months after birth as the maternal antibodies wane. Lack of the opsonic antibodies results in recurrent bacterial infections due to pyogenic, encapsulated bacteria such as *Streptococcus pneumoniae*, *Haemophilus influenzae*, *Staphylococcus aureus*, and *Pseudomonas* species. Upper and lower respiratory tract infections are most common, including otitis media, sinusitis, bronchitis, and pneumonia. Skin infections and urinary tract infections also occur. The cause of XLA is due to loss of function mutations of a tyrosine kinase protein known as *btk* that is essential for B-cell development. The availability of intravenous as well as subcutaneous gammaglobulin replacement therapy has improved outcome as well as longevity for these patients.

Diagnosis

Early diagnosis is essential to prevent infections and complications of infections, such as bronchiectasis, meningitis, bacterial sepsis, septic arthritis, and even osteomyelitis. Recognizing that

X-linked agammaglobulinemia (XLA) is the prototype humoral immune deficiency and is due to a loss of function mutation in the *BTK* (Bruton tyrosine kinase) gene that is essential for B-cell development. It is a disease restricted to males, and is characterized by a near total absence of B lymphocytes from an arrest in B lymphocyte development.

TABLE 3–12.1   Laboratory Evaluation for X-Linked Agammaglobulinemia (XLA)

Laboratory Test	Result for XLA	Result for Carriers
Serum IgG	<200 mg/dL in patients greater than 6 months of age	Normal
Serum IgM and IgA	Low to absent if greater than 6 months of age	Normal
B-cell markers—CD19 and CD20	Low at birth and is diagnostic even at <6 months of age	Normal
btk gene mutation	Although not clinically needed, it is the definitive diagnostic test	Definitive test for carrier state
Antibody response to childhood vaccines	Markedly decreased to absent	Normal

B cells are CD19 and CD20 positive, a definitive diagnosis can be made at birth by enumerating B cells in cord blood by flow cytometry using monoclonal antibodies to CD19 and CD20. In children less than 6 months of age, measuring serum immunoglobulin concentration is not diagnostically useful due to the presence of transplacentally acquired maternal antibody in the blood. Thus, to establish a diagnosis in the first 6 months, it is necessary to enumerate B cells by flow cytometry. The molecular diagnosis is made by mutational analysis of the *btk* gene. This is seldom needed in clinical practice as clinical features including lack of tonsils and low numbers of CD19 or CD20 cells can establish the diagnosis. Deficient expression of *btk* protein can be detected by flow cytometry, a technique that can also be used for carrier detection. **Table 3–12.1** summarizes the laboratory approach to the diagnosis of this disorder.

Advances in the molecular basis for primary immunodeficiency syndromes are rapidly occurring, and current classification follows the system developed by World Health Organization (WHO) and the International Union of Immunological Societies (IUIS). These are summarized in the "Practice Parameters for the Diagnosis and Management of Primary Immunodeficiency," which can be found online at http://www.jcaai.org/resources/practice parameters. Gene defects causing agammaglobulinemia are depicted in **Table 3–12.2**.

Common Variable Immunodeficiency

Description

Common variable immunodeficiency (CVID) affects both males and females equally. The disease usually manifests in adult life. Unlike agammaglobulinemia, in which B cells and tonsils are absent, patients with CVID have tonsils and normal numbers of B cells in blood and lymphoid tissues. Some patients even have mediastinal and abdominal lymphadenopathy. The primary defect in CVID is that the B cells are dysfunctional, and do not differentiate into plasma cells and secrete antibody. The clinical presentation is the consequence of the hypogammaglobulinemia, namely,

TABLE 3–12.2   Gene Defects Causing Agammaglobulinemia

Defect or Disease(s)	Gene and Associated Protein
X-linked (Bruton) agammaglobulinemia	BTK (Bruton tyrosine kinase)
μ-Heavy chain deficiency	IGHM (immunoglobulin heavy constant mu)
Ig-α deficiency	CD 79A (cluster of differentiation CD79A)
Ig-β deficiency	CD 79B (cluster of differentiation CD79B)
Surrogate light chain (λ5) deficiency	CD 179B (immunoglobulin lambda like polypeptide 1 (IGLL1) or cluster of differentiation 179B)
B cell linker protein (BLINK) deficiency	BLNK (B cell linker protein)
Phosphoinositide 3-kinase kinase deficiency	PIK3R1 (phosphatidylinositol 3-kinase regulatory subunit 1)

TABLE 3–13.1   Laboratory Evaluation for Common Variable Immunodeficiency (CVID)

Laboratory Test	Result/Comments
Serum protein electrophoresis	Marked decrease in the gamma globulin fraction; rarely it may be normal in the dysfunctional variant
Serum IgM, IgG, and IgA levels	Usually low, but may be normal in dysfunctional variant
CD19 and CD20 cells	Usually normal, may be increased; rarely, low normal but never absent
IgM-CD27+ B cells	Absence of this memory B-cell marker is associated with a phenotype that is more severe and associated with granulomatous pulmonary lesions and lymphadenopathy
Response to polysaccharide and protein antigens	There is a failure to respond to these antigens; the expected fourfold rise in titer following vaccination is not observed; defines the functional defect

Common variable immunodeficiency (CVID) affects both males and females equally. The phenotypic expression of this disease is characterized by hypogammaglobulinemia, and there are many genetic defects in the B-cell maturation pathway that apparently cause this disorder.

recurrent pyogenic infections, often of the upper and lower respiratory tracts. Lack of mucosal immunity also results in enteroviral infections and giardiasis. Autoimmune diseases such as immune hemolytic anemia, neutropenia, and pernicious anemia occur. B-cell lymphomas may manifest with time. Studies of B-cell function in CVID have revealed a subset of CVID patients who have normal or low normal IgM, IgG, and IgA but fail to make functional antibody to polysaccharide and protein antigens. Long-term clinical studies have found that there is a subset of CVID patients who manifest lymphadenopathy and granulomatous nodules in the lung (also called granulomatous interstitial lung disease or GLILD). The liver and spleen do not respond to IVGG and often need immunosuppressive, such as mycophenalate mofetil, to mitigate the exuberant aberrant lymphocytic response. They have a deficiency of class switch to memory B cells which carry the marker IgM-CD 27+. On the other hand, those CVID patients that respond well to IVGG have a better prognosis and have memory B cells by flow cytometry. Thus, flow cytometry is not only necessary for diagnosis, but also for stratifying subsets of cells for a syndrome. Therapy with intravenous as well as subcutaneous gamma globulin has improved the clinical outcome for CVID patients.

Diagnosis

Table 3–13.1 describes the laboratory tests useful to establish the clinical diagnosis. The phenotypic expression of this disease is characterized by hypogammaglobulinemia, and there are many genetic defects in the B-cell maturation pathway that apparently cause this disorder. These are depicted in **Table 3–13.2**.

Hyper-IgM Syndrome

Description

Hyper-IgM syndrome (HIGM) is characterized by markedly reduced IgG and IgA, with normal to elevated IgM and normal numbers of circulating B cells. The low IgG and IgA is due to an inability of IgM-positive B cells to switch to other isotypes. The increased IgM reflects polyclonal expansion of IgM synthesis in response to infections from encapsulated bacteria. Both X-linked and autosomal recessive forms exist. The molecular causes include the X-linked loss of function mutation of the CD40 ligand (CD154) found on activated T cells, which is needed to engage with CD40 on B cells to promote the isotype switch. Other causes include loss of functional mutations of activation-induced deaminase (AID) and of uracil-DNA glycolase (UNG). These enzymes are involved in class switch recombination and in mending error-prone repair.

Selective IgA deficiency is the most common primary immunodeficiency syndrome. The defect is due to a B-cell differentiation arrest in the IgG to IgA isotype switch.

Diagnosis

The diagnosis is established by measuring serum IgM, IgG, and IgA along with enumerating CD19 and CD20 cells by flow cytometry. Normal or elevated IgM, with low IgG and IgA, with normal B cells, suggests the diagnosis, which can be confirmed by molecular studies.

TABLE 3–13.2   Gene Associations with Common Variable Immunodeficiency (CVID)-Like Disorders

Common Variable Immunodeficiency-Like Disorders	Gene and Associated Protein
Inducible costimulator	*ICOS (inducible T-cell costimulator)*
CD19	*CD19 (B cell lymphocyte antigen CD19)*
CD20	*CD20 (B cell lymphocyte antigen CD20)*
CD21	*CD21 (Epstein–Barr virus B cell attachment receptor)*
CD81, TAPA-1	*CD81 (target of antiproliferative antibody 1)*
TACI (Transmembrane activator and calcium modulator and cyclophilin ligand)	*TNFRSF13B (TNF superfamily member 13B)*
B-cell activating factor receptor (BAFF)	*TNFRSF13C (TNF superfamily member 13C)*
Phosphoinositol 3′ kinase regulatory catalytic subunit mutation	*PIK3CD (phosphatidylinositol 3-kinase catalytic subunit delta)*
Phosphoinositol 3′ kinase regulatory subunit 1 defect	*PIK3R1 (phosphatidylinositol 3-kinase regulatory subunit 1)*
LPS-responsive beige-like anchor protein deficiency	*LRBA (LPS-responsive beige-like anchor protein)*
TWEAK deficiency	*TWEAK (TNF superfamily member 12)*
NF-$_\kappa$B2 deficiency	*NFKB2 (nuclear factor kappa B2)*
Protein kinase Cδ deficiency	*PRKCD (protein kinase C delta)*
Kabuki syndrome	*KMT2D (lysine methyltransferase 2D)*

Selective IgA Deficiency

Description

Selective IgA deficiency is the most common primary immunodeficiency syndrome. Its prevalence varies from 1 in 500 in Caucasians to 1 in 10,000 to 15,000 in Asians. The clinical picture is variable, and includes asymptomatic individuals and those with allergies, autoimmune disorders, recurrent infections, and gastrointestinal diseases. The defect is due to a B-cell differentiation arrest in the IgG to IgA isotype switch. There are low numbers of IgA-bearing B cells. Anti-IgA antibodies are found in the serum of some patients, and these individuals can experience an anaphylactoid reaction to any blood or blood product containing IgA. These patients are to be given IgA-deficient blood and blood products and washed red blood cells. Patients with pure IgA deficiency and normal IgG subclasses should not receive gammaglobulin replacement therapy as these preparations do not replace IgA and any trace IgA in the gamma globulin preparations can provoke IgA antibodies and subsequent anaphylactoid reactions.

Diagnosis

The diagnosis is made by documenting an IgA level of <5 mg/dL in the presence of normal IgG and IgM. It is important to evaluate for IgG subclasses, as subjects with IgA deficiency and a low IgG2 subclass are prone to recurrent infections. This subset of patients with IgA as well as low IgG2 subclass does benefit from intravenous or subcutaneous gamma globulin therapy. The replacement is designed to correct the IgG2 deficiency, as IgG2 is an important opsonin for polysaccharide antigens.

DiGeorge Syndrome

Description

DiGeorge syndrome is due to deletion of chromosome 22q11.2 and is part of the spectrum described as "CATCH 22" (**c**ardiac anomalies, **a**bnormal facies, **t**hymic hypoplasia, **c**left palate, and **h**ypocalcemia). This deletion leads to failure of the development of third and fourth pharyngeal pouches and consequent abnormalities in the development of the thymus and parathyroid glands. Thymic dysfunction leads to T-cell abnormalities, and also B-cell dysfunction, while parathyroid abnormalities cause hypocalcaemia and tetany. Defects in the third and fourth pharyngeal pouches also result in congenital heart diseases, anomalies of the great vessels, and abnormal facies with low-set ears, fish-like mouth, and cleft palate. Patients with complete DiGeorge syndrome manifest marked defects in T-cell function and are prone to viral infections. Those with partial DiGeorge syndrome have fewer infections but have cardiac and facial abnormalities.

Diagnosis

A child with neonatal tetany and abnormal facies should be evaluated for DiGeorge syndrome by enumerating T and B cells, along with measurement of serum calcium and parathyroid hormone (PTH). The chromosome 22q11.2 deletion is documented by fluorescence in situ hybridization (FISH).

Neonatal detection of T cell disorders such as SCID and others like DiGeorge syndrome is rapidly performed by evaluating for **T** cell **r**eceptor **e**xcision **c**ircles or TREC by PCR using umbilical cord cells. Lack of a TREC signal suggests a defect in T cell maturation and possible T cell defects. This is then followed by detailed flow cytometry of the T cell compartment and functional evaluation of the T cells. Such an approach has resulted in early diagnosis and effective therapy such as stem cell or bone marrow transplantation or even gene therapy.

Severe Combined Immunodeficiency (SCID) Syndrome
Description and Diagnosis

As the name implies, SCID syndrome is characterized by profound defects in both cellular and humoral immunity. Affected neonates manifest severe and widespread viral, fungal, and bacterial infections soon after birth. The protection from maternal antibody is minimal, and the child fails to thrive. Respiratory failure often supervenes and is a cause of death. Patients with this disorder were the "bubble babies" decades earlier. Haploidentical, allogeneic bone marrow transplantation has altered the natural history of the disease. The path to recovery is often complicated by graft-versus-host (GVH) disease, and restitution of B-cell function is often incomplete. As a result, SCID patients may need intravenous gamma globulin to increase their antibody repertoire. Hematopoietic stem cell transplant with cytokine modulation to facilitate differentiation has been found to be superior, as there is less GVH disease. Early detection of SCID by TREC analyses has improved the outcome among this cohort, so much so that testing of a sample from a neonatal heel prick for TRECs is now mandatory in many states in the United States.

> SCID syndrome is characterized by profound defects in both cellular and humoral immunity. Affected neonates manifest severe and widespread viral, fungal, and bacterial infections soon after birth.

Based on T-cell, B-cell, and NK-cell enumeration, the SCID syndrome is classified according to the position of the block/defect in T-cell and B-cell development. Currently, the spectrum of primary immunodeficiency diseases includes many underlying mutations. One group of these mutations results in different combinations of T-, B-, and NK-cell alterations, to produce SCID and related cellular immunodeficiency diseases (CID). A second group of mutations alters the amount of antibody to produce primary immunodeficiency diseases. Finally, a third group of mutations is linked to syndromes involving autoimmunity and immune dysregulation. **Figure 3–2** shows 13 sites where a block in development of a T, B, or NK cell exists. The first nine are associated with SCID or CID, and the last four are linked to antibody deficiency diseases. This classification permits an insight to the molecular mechanisms of the disease and provides a framework for evaluating patients for SCID.

Figure 3–3 depicts a pathway to evaluate the causes as well as molecular basis of SCID based on flow cytometry. Such an approach is paving the way to genetic immune reconstitution and personalized therapy for the individual syndromes.

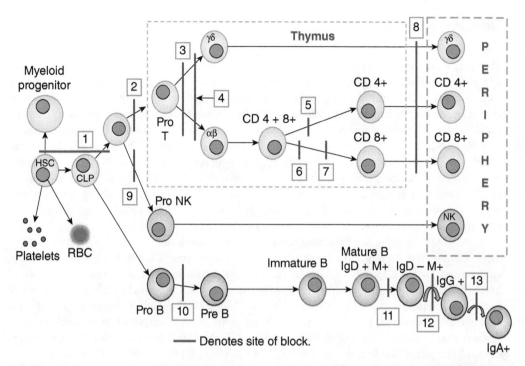

FIGURE 3–2 Primary immunodeficiency diseases and associated blocks (shown in numbered boxes) in T-cell, B-cell, and natural killer (NK)-cell development. CLP, clonal lymphoid progenitor; HSC, hematopoietic stem cell; NK, natural killer cell.

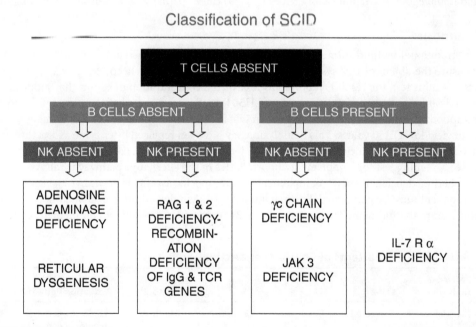

FIGURE 3–3 Classification of severe combined immunodeficiency (SCID) based upon B, T and NK cell type status.

Deficiencies of Complement Proteins

Description

The complement system of proteins and their receptors protect the host against pathogens and non-self-antigens and also abrogate the emergence of autoimmune diseases by scavenging self-antigens such as DNA so that they do not become immunogenic. Deficiencies of the complement system, therefore, result in susceptibility to infections and predispose to autoimmune diseases such as SLE. Deficiency of C3 results in increased susceptibility to infections by encapsulated, pyogenic bacteria. Deficiencies of C5, C6, C7, and C8 result in recurrent or disseminated *Neisseria* infections. Deficiencies of C1q (which scavenges DNA released from apoptotic cells), C2, and C4 predispose to SLE and other autoimmune diseases. Deficiency of C1 inhibitor due to a defect in *SERPING1* (serpin family G, member 1) gene causes hereditary angioedema (HAE). In type 1 HAE, there is deficiency of both the antigenic and functional C1 inhibitor protein. In type 2, the protein is antigenically normal and hence normal serum levels are noted when it is measured by an antigenic assay. However, in type 2 HAE, the protein is functionally abnormal and hence cannot inhibit the kinin, complement, kallikrein, and plasminogen pathways. This results in generation of bradykinin that causes angioedema. Lack of C1 inhibitor causes C4 consumption even in the basal state so that C4 is always low. In HAE patients with angioedema, C2 is also decreased. C3 is normal as this activation occurs in the fluid phase. Acquired C1 INH deficiency leads to a similar clinical phenotype and is called acquired angioedema (AAE). AAE is seen in lymphoproliferative states such as monoclonal B cell diseases that activate C1 leading to consumption of C1 INH via C1qrs activation. In autoimmune diseases, the autoantibody is directed to C1 INH leading to C1 INH–anti-C1 INH immune complexes that activate C1qrs. Activated C1 in the fluid phase contributes to the same sequence of events leading to bradykinin generation and angioedema. The important differentiating factor is that C1q is normal in HAE, but C1q is low in AAE. Factor I deficiency is associated with recurrent infections, and factor H deficiency with hemolytic uremic syndrome and age-related macular degeneration. Deficiency of membrane inhibitors such as decay accelerating factor (DAF or CD55) and homologous restriction factor (HRF or CD59) causes paroxysmal nocturnal hemoglobinuria.

Diagnosis

The traditional method to measure the functional integrity of the complement cascade was to measure the ability of this system to hemolyze antibody-coated sheep red cells in a hemolytic assay. In this test, the result is reported as titer or the concentration of serum that supports 50% hemolysis in the S-shaped titration curve (CH50 test). Serum depleted of complement due to consumption by immune complexes, and serum that is congenitally deficient in complement proteins both yield low CH50 values. This hemolysis assay has been replaced by enzyme assays that detect neoantigens exposed during the activation of terminal complement components. The hemolysis-based screening test for complement abnormalities in the alternative pathway is the AH50 assay. In inherited deficiencies of the complement system, specific assays for the individual complement component must be performed. Further, it must be shown that addition of that component alone will restore the full hemolytic activity. **Table 3–14** provides a profile of complement activation

TABLE 3–14   Patterns of Complement Activation

Pattern of Activation	CH50	C4	C3	Factor B	Conditions with Activation Pattern
Classical	Decreased	Decreased	Decreased	No change	SLE, SS, RA, and cryoglobulinemia
Alternative	Decreased	No change	Decreased	Decreased	Endotoxemia; type II MPGN and factor H mutation
Classical and alternative	Decreased	Decreased	Decreased	Decreased	SLE, shock, and immune complex diseases
Fluid phase activation—classical	Decreased	Decreased	No change	No change	Hereditary angioedema; malarial infection (*P. vivax*)

SLE, systemic lupus erythematosus; SS, Sjogren syndrome; RA, rheumatoid arthritis; MPGN, membranoproliferative glomerulonephritis.

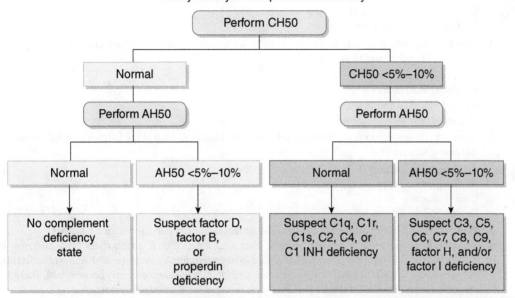

• Recurrent pyogenic infection with normal antibody function
• Disseminated neisserial infection
• Autommune diseases with normal antibody function
• Family history of complement deficiency

CH50: screening test to check any deficiencies in the complement system
AH50: screening test for complement abnormalities in the alternative pathway

FIGURE 3–4   Evaluation for inherited complement deficiency disease.

that is useful in clinical diagnosis. **Figure 3–4** provides a framework for evaluating complement deficiency diseases.

SELF-ASSESSMENT QUESTIONS

1. Which of the following diseases is not associated with positive test results for antinuclear antibodies?

    A. Systemic lupus erythematosus (SLE)
    B. Mixed connective tissue disease
    C. Scleroderma
    D. DiGeorge syndrome

2. Identify the one test below which is least relevant to establishing a diagnosis or disease severity for a patient with systemic lupus erythematosus (SLE).

    A. Antinuclear antibody test
    B. Complement assay—particularly C3 and C4
    C. Double-stranded DNA
    D. Muscle biopsy

3. Which one of the following tests is not related to establishing a diagnosis or determining the severity of Sjögren syndrome?

    A. Magnetic resonance imaging (MRI) of the salivary gland
    B. Antinuclear antibody test
    C. Antibodies to SS-A (Ro)
    D. Antibodies to cyclic citrullinated peptide (CCP)

4. Which of the following autoimmune diseases does this patient likely to have? The patient has positive tests for antinuclear antibodies with the speckled pattern; the patient is found to have an anti-Scl-70 antibody; and clinically the patient has calcinosis, Raynaud syndrome, esophageal dysmotility, sclerodactyly, and telangiectasia.

    A. Systemic sclerosis/scleroderma
    B. Rheumatoid arthritis
    C. Systemic lupus erythematosus
    D. Sjögren syndrome

5. A positive test for anti-Jo-1 is more likely to be present in a patient with which of the following autoimmune diseases?
   A. Mixed connective tissue disease
   B. Scleroderma
   C. Polymyositis and dermatomyositis
   D. Systemic lupus erythematosus

6. Which of the following tests is least likely to be informative in the laboratory evaluation of a patient known to have rheumatoid arthritis?
   A. C-reactive protein
   B. Rheumatoid factor
   C. Abdominal fat pad biopsy
   D. Anticitrullinated α-enolase

7. A patient with amyloidosis develops amyloid fibrils that bind to which of the following protein to induce a bleeding tendency?
   A. Coagulation factor VII
   B. Coagulation factor X
   C. Fibrinogen
   D. von Willebrand factor

8. Which of the following diseases of the immune system is described in the paragraph below?
   The disease is restricted to males who have near total absence of B lymphocytes from an arrest in B-lymphocyte development. The patient has a pan-hypogammaglobulinemia. Recurrent infections between 4 and 12 months after birth as maternal antibodies wane are commonly encountered. There is a loss of function mutation of the *btk* protein that is essential for B-cell development.
   A. Severe combined immunodeficiency (SCID)
   B. Common variable immunodeficiency
   C. X-linked agammaglobulinemia
   D. DiGeorge syndrome

9. A patient with recurrent pyogenic infections and normal antibody function is being evaluated for an inherited complement deficiency. The CH50 screening test for deficiencies in the complement system shows a markedly low value of <10%. The AH50 screening test for complement abnormalities in the alternative pathway is also <10%. Which of the following complement deficiencies is most likely in this patient?
   A. Factor B
   B. C2
   C. No complement deficiency state is likely
   D. C5

FURTHER READING

Alarcon Segovia D, Villareal M. Classification and diagnostic criteria for mixed connective tissue disease. In: Kasukawa R, Sharp G, eds. *Mixed Connective Tissue Disease and Anti-nuclear Antibodies.* Amsterdam: Elsevier; 1987:33.

Alspaugh MA, Tan EM. Antibodies to cellular antigens in Sjogren's syndrome. *J Clin Invest.* 1975;55:1067.

Arbuckle MR, et al. Development of autoantibodies before the clinical onset of systemic lupus erythematosus. *N Engl J Med.* 2003;349:1526.

Betteridge Z, et al. Anti-synthetase syndrome: a new auto antibody to phenylalanyl transfer RNA synthetase (anti-Zo) associated with polymyositis and interstitial pneumonia. *Rheumatology.* 2007;46:1005.

Bhat A, et al. Current concepts on the immunopathology of amyloidosis. *Clin Rev Allergy Immunol.* [Published online: July 21, 2009].

Bonilla FA, Khan DA, Ballas ZH, et al. Practice parameter for the diagnosis and management of primary immunodeficiency. *J Allergy Clin Immunol.* 2015;136:1186–1205.

Buckley RH, et al. Human severe combined immunodeficiency: genetic, phenotypic, functional diversity in one hundred eight infants. *J Pediatr.* 1997;130:378.

Castigli E, Geha RS. Molecular basis of common variable immunodeficiency. *J Allergy Clin Immunol.* 2006;117:740.

Cavazzana-Calvo M, et al. Gene therapy of human severe combined immunodeficiency (SCID)—X1 disease. *Science.* 2000;288:669.

Conley ME, et al. Genetic analysis of patients with defect in early B-cell development. *Immunol Rev.* 2005;203:216.

Cunningham-Rundles C, Ponda PP. Molecular defects in T- and B-cell primary immunodeficiency diseases. *Nat Rev Immunol.* 2005;11:880.

Dalakas MC, Hohlfeld R. Polymyositis and dermatomyositis. *Lancet.* 2003;362:971.

Davis AE3rd. The pathophysiology of hereditary angioedema. *Clin Immunol.* 2005;114:3.

Dispenzieri A, et al. International Myeloma Working Group guidelines for serum-free light analysis in multiple myeloma and related disorders. *Leukemia.* 2009;23:215.

Durand A, et al. Hyper-immunoglobulin M syndromes caused by intrinsic B-lymphocyte defects. *Immunol Rev.* 2005;203:67.

Ferri C, et al. Cryoglobulin. *J Clin Pathol.* 2002;55:4.

Glovsky MM, et al. Complement determinations in human disease. *Ann Allergy Asthma Immunol.* 2004;93:513.

Griggs RC, et al. Inclusion body myositis and myopathies. *Ann Neurol.* 1995;705:13.

Harley JB. Autoantibodies are central to the diagnosis and clinical manifestations of lupus. *J Rheumatol.* 1994;21:1183.

Heinlen LD, et al. Clinical criteria for systemic lupus erythematosus precede diagnosis, and associated autoantibodies are present before clinical symptoms. *Arthritis Rheum.* 2007;56:2344.

Hochberg MC. Updating the American College of Rheumatology revised criteria for the classification of systemic lupus erythematosus. *Arthritis Rheum.* 1997;40:1725.

Hu PQ, et al. Correlation of serum anti-DNA topoisomerase I antibody levels with disease severity and activity in systemic sclerosis. *Arthritis Rheum.* 2003;48:1363.

Kawai T, Akira S. Pathogen recognition with Toll-like receptors. *Curr Opin Immunol.* 2005;17:338.

Kissel JT, et al. Microvascular deposition of complement membrane attack complex in dermatomyositis. *N Engl J Med.* 1986;329:34.

Kwan A, Abraham RS, Currier R, et al. Newborn screening for severe combined immunodeficiency in 11 screening programs in the United States. *JAMA.* 2014;312:729–738.

Mahler M, Miller FW, Fritzler MJ. Idiopathic inflammatory myopathies and the anti-synthetase syndrome: A comprehensive review. *Autoimmun Rev.* 2014;13:367–371.

Nakamura RM, Bylund DJ. Contemporary concepts for the clinical and laboratory evaluation of systemic lupus erythematosus and "lupus-like" syndromes. *J Clin Lab Anal.* 1994;8:347.

Notarangelo LD. Primary immunodeficiencies. *J Allergy Clin Immunol.* 2010;125:S182–S194.

Oliveira JM, et al. Applications of flow cytometry for the study of primary immunodeficiencies. *Curr Opin Allergy Clin Immunol.* 2008;8:499–509.

Phan TG, et al. Autoantibodies to extractable nuclear antigens: making detection and interpretation more meaningful. *Clin Diagn Lab Immunol.* 2002;9:1.

Pratt G. The evolving use of serum free light chain assays in hematology. *Br J Haematol.* 2008;141:413.

Ramos-Casals M, et al. Primary Sjogren's syndrome: new clinical and therapeutic concepts. *Ann Rheum Dis.* 2005;64:347.

Reveille JD, Solomon DH. Evidence-based guidelines for the use of immunologic tests: anticentromere, Sci-70, and nucleolar antibodies. *Arthritis Rheum.* 2003;49:399.

Rider LG, Miller FW. Laboratory evaluation of the inflammatory myopathies. *Clin Diagn Lab Immunol.* 1995;2:1.

Rojas-Serrano J, et al. Very recent arthritis: the value of initial rheumatological evaluation and anti-cyclic citrullinated peptide antibodies in the diagnosis of rheumatoid arthritis. *Clin Rheumatol.* 2009;28:1135.

Rothfield NF. Autoantibodies in scleroderma. *Rheum Dis Clin North Am.* 1992;18:483.

Sanchez-Guerrero J, et al. Utility of Sm, anti-RNP, anti-Ro/SS-A and anti-La/SS-B (extractable nuclear antigens) detected by enzyme-linked immunosorbent assay for the diagnosis of systemic lupus erythematosus. *Arthritis Rheum.* 1996;39:1055.

Schroeder HW Jr, et al. The complex genetics of common variable immunodeficiency. *J Invest Med.* 2004;52:90.

Smeenk R, et al. Antibodies to DNA in patients with systemic lupus erythematosus. Their role in diagnosis, the follow-up and the pathogenesis of the disease. *Clin Rheumatol.* 1990;9:100.

Solomon DH, et al. Evidence-based guidelines for the use of immunologic tests: antinuclear antibody testing. *Arthritis Rheum.* 2002;47:434.

Talal N. Sjogren's syndrome: historical overview and clinical spectrum of disease. *Rheum Dis Clin North Am.* 1992;18:507.

Tedeschi A, et al. Cryoglobulinemia. *Blood Rev.* 2007;21:183.

Von Muhlen CA, Tan EM. Autoantibodies in the diagnosis of systemic rheumatic diseases. *Semin Arthritis Rheum.* 1995;24:323.

Walport MJ. Complement. First of two parts. *N Engl J Med.* 2001;344:1058.

Walport MJ. Complement. Second of two parts. *N Engl J Med.* 2001;344:1140.

Histocompatibility Testing and Transplantation

Yash P. Agrawal and Susan L. Saidman

CHAPTER OUTLINE

INTRODUCTION

An animal will generally accept an organ transplant from itself, but will reject a transplant from other animals, even if the donor animal is of the same species. Organ rejection is primarily a consequence of the interactions between the immune system of the transplant recipient and the histocompatibility antigens present on the transplanted cells. Clinical laboratories play an important role in the histocompatibility testing for solid organ as well as hematopoietic cell and bone marrow transplantation (BMT). This chapter provides a brief background to some of the issues and techniques involved in histocompatibility testing related to transplantation. Other applications of histocompatibility testing such as in the characterization of disease states (e.g., HLA-B27 in ankylosing spondylitis) or before initiation of some drug therapy (e.g., HLA-B*57:01 is a risk factor for hypersensitivity to abacavir) use similar techniques and are not discussed further.

    The histocompatibility antigens that are the primary stimulus in graft rejection are encoded by a complex of closely linked genes called the major histocompatibility complex (MHC). In mice, these genes are located on the H2 region of chromosome 17. In humans, the analogous MHC region is located in a 4000-kb region on the short arm of chromosome 6 and encodes for the HLA system (**Figure 4–1**).

HLA GENES AND GENE PRODUCTS

The HLA class I region encodes for certain glycoprotein molecules that are present on all nucleated cells. The main function of the HLA class I molecules is to bind to fragments resulting from the breakdown of intracellular pathogens, such as viruses. The HLA molecule and the bound peptide are then presented on the cell surface so that an immune response can be initiated against the pathogen. Class I molecules consist of two noncovalently linked chains. A gene in the MHC encodes the heavy chain, and a gene outside the MHC on chromosome 15 encodes the β2-microglobulin light chain. In humans, there are three important class I genes known as HLA-A, B, and C. These genes are highly polymorphic. Polymorphism refers to multiple variations of a single genetic locus and its gene product. Each variation of the gene is called an *allele*. The HLA-A, B, and C genes encode for over 100 gene products that can be defined by serology—that is, by matching antibodies against the different HLA antigens (**Table 4–1**). However, the antigens identified by serotyping are far outnumbered by the alleles that are recognized by sequencing the gene. This is because not all gene polymorphisms result in distinct antibody specificities, although they may stimulate a T-cell immune response.

The class II region encodes for the α and β chains that make up the HLA-DR, DQ, and DP molecules (**Figure 4–1**). These HLA class II molecules have a more restricted expression than the class I molecules. They are found mainly on B lymphocytes, dendritic cells, monocytes, activated T cells, and some endothelial cells. Antigen-presenting cells such as macrophages can phagocytose and engulf bacteria and other parasites via endocytosis. Once these pathogens gain entry to the cell, they can be broken down by proteases into peptides that are able to bind to the class II molecules. These peptides are then presented on the cell surface, and an immune response is initiated. The class III region contains approximately 40 genes that do not encode HLA molecules, but encode certain complement components and numerous other proteins not involved in antigen presentation.

The HLA genes are linked together—in what is called a *haplotype*—on the chromosome and inherited en bloc. Each individual inherits one haplotype from each parent, and the two

> In humans, there are three important class I genes known as HLA-A, B, and C. The class II region encodes for the α and β chains that make up the HLA-DR, DQ, and DP molecules.

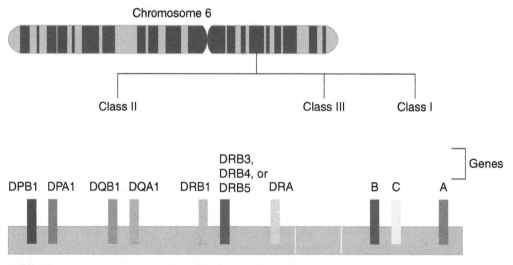

FIGURE 4–1 Genes of the human MHC system. The human major histocompatibility complex (MHC) is located on the short arm of chromosome 6. It contains over 200 genes that can be divided into different regions (class I–III). Only the major genes encoding the HLA molecules important in transplantation are shown. The class I region contains genes that encode the α chains of the classic transplantation antigens, HLA-A, B, and C. The class II region has genes that encode both the α and β chains of HLA-DP, DQ, and DR molecules. Genes encoding the α and β chains are designated as "A" or "B," and are followed by a number if there is more than one gene encoding a particular chain or a related pseudogene. For example, DRB1 is one of the genes that encodes the β chain of DR molecules. The class III region is located between regions I and II and does not encode for HLA molecules. (Adapted with permission from *Clinical Laboratory Reviews* [a newsletter publication of the Massachusetts General Hospital]. 2000;8:3.)

TABLE 4–1   Number of HLA Alleles and Serologic Specificities

HLA Gene	Number of Alleles Determined by Gene Sequencing[a]	Number of Serologic Specificities
HLA-A	>3900	28
HLA-B	>4800	63
HLA-C	>3600	10
HLA-DRB1	>2100	21
HLA-DQB1	>1100	9

[a]This number increases continually as new sequences are identified.

haplotypes represent the HLA genotype. The alleles from both of these haplotypes are expressed on an individual's cells. This is referred to as a codominant expression of the gene. Therefore, even though there are multiple HLA genes, usually only four genotypes are possible in the offspring. There is a 25% chance of any two siblings being HLA identical and a 50% chance of the siblings sharing a haplotype.

HLA antigens and alleles are named by the World Health Organization Nomenclature Committee for Factors of the HLA System. New alleles are named on an ongoing basis as they are identified, and the number of HLA alleles has grown rapidly, with over 17,500 currently listed. The DNA sequences of all recognized HLA alleles are maintained in the IPD-IMGT/HLA Database and are available online (http://www.ebi.ac.uk/ipd/imgt/hla/). Each HLA allele name follows a strict format defined by the Nomenclature Committee (**Figure 4–2**).

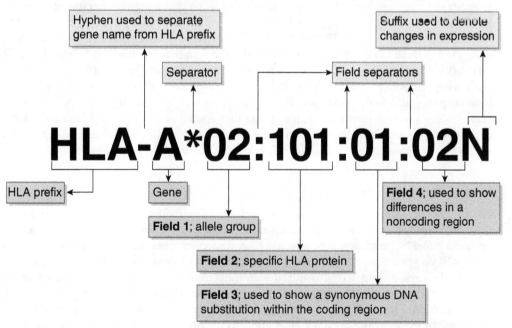

FIGURE 4–2   HLA nomenclature. The letters following the HLA prefix (e.g., HLA-A) designate the gene name in the MHC system. An asterisk (*) separates the gene name from the allele name. A *low-resolution* DNA typing is reported at the level of the allele group with only the first set of digits (e.g., HLA-A*02). This is usually the equivalent of a serologic typing result. The specific HLA protein or allele is reported by the second set of digits in a *high-resolution* typing (e.g., HLA-A*02:01). The third set of digits is used only when necessary to indicate synonymous (silent) nucleotide substitutions, and the fourth set of digits is used when necessary to denote substitutions in noncoding regions of the gene. A letter at the end may be used to denote changes in expression (e.g., N, null or not expressed). (This figure is kindly provided by Professor Steven G.E. Marsh, Anthony Nolan Research Institute, London, UK, and is from the website hla.alleles.org.)

HISTOCOMPATIBILITY TESTING ASSAYS

HLA Typing

The HLA genes are linked together—in what is called a haplotype—on the chromosome and inherited en bloc. Each individual inherits one *haplotype* from each parent, and the two haplotypes represent the HLA genotype.

The HLA type of a potential graft recipient or donor can be determined by serology using a microlymphocytotoxicity assay. T lymphocytes are used for typing class I antigens, and B lymphocytes for typing class II antigens. The assay involves mixing known HLA typing sera with the separated lymphocytes, followed by the addition of complement. Complement-mediated lysis of lymphocytes follows when the antibody in the serum binds to the appropriate HLA antigen. The extent of cell lysis is visualized under a fluorescence microscope after exposing the cells to DNA-binding dyes such as ethidium bromide. HLA typing for class I and II antigens typically involves mixing the cells with over 200 different HLA typing sera, each in a different well of a microtiter tray.

Molecular methods allow high-resolution HLA typing at the allele level, so different alleles that cannot be distinguished by serologic assays can be identified. Such techniques also have applications in typing nonlymphocytes (e.g., blasts or epithelial cells from cheek swabs) and in patients with cytopenias. One technique involves amplification of genomic DNA by polymerase chain reaction (PCR) (see Chapter 2) using primers that are *locus specific* (e.g., all DQB1 alleles) or *group specific* (e.g., all DR4 alleles). The amplified DNA is then hybridized with a panel of sequence-specific oligonucleotide probes (PCR-SSOP) specific for each allele or group of alleles. Even a single nucleotide mismatch will prevent the annealing of the probe. The bound probe is visualized using various methods, including autoradiography and color development, by blotting the DNA onto multiple membranes (dot blot hybridization). More commonly, the probes may be bound to a single membrane (reverse hybridization) or to groups of different colored beads (Luminex technology).

In a related technique, *sequence-specific* primers for an allele are used in a PCR amplification reaction (PCR-SSP). The presence or absence of PCR amplification is detected by gel electrophoresis and ethidium bromide visualization. In this technique, a positive amplification reaction signifies the presence of that specific allele.

In recent times, the PCR-SSOP and PCR-SSP methods are being replaced by sequence-based typing (SBT) methods using PCR combined with the Sanger method of DNA sequencing. The SBT methods do not always resolve sequence ambiguities that may be important in BMT, especially when the ambiguities are due to the *cis/trans* assignment of nucleotide bases in alleles of heterozygous individuals. Next-generation sequencing (NGS) holds the promise of resolving these ambiguities because the technique utilizes the creation of DNA libraries to produce clones of phase-defined sequences that are then sequenced in a massively parallel manner. The technique allows the simultaneous sequencing of multiple long DNA fragments in a single run.

HLA Antibody Screening

The patient's serum can be screened for the presence of antibodies that may have resulted from prior transfusions, pregnancies, or transplants. Serum from patients is screened for reactivity against a panel of lymphocytes or purified HLA molecules from individuals (panel cells) with known HLA types. Screening can be done using either cell-based or solid-phase assays. In the cell-based assays, patient serum is mixed with different panel cells. If the cells are lysed (in a cytotoxicity assay) or if antibody binds to them (detected using a flow cytometry assay), then it is evident that the patient's serum contains HLA antibody against the antigens expressed on that panel cell. In the solid-phase assays, HLA antigens are extracted from the panel cells. The antigens are purified and bound to a solid support, either to the wells of an ELISA plate or to colored beads that can be detected using flow cytometry or Luminex technology. Antibody binding to the molecules on the well or bead is detected using an enzyme or fluorescence conjugated anti-immunoglobulin reagent.

The number of panel cells showing lysis or antibody binding is noted, and the results are expressed as percent panel reactive antibody (PRA). Patients who have HLA antibody are referred to as "sensitized." If the patient's serum reacts with 90% of the panel cells, it is likely that the patient will have to wait longer for a compatible donor than someone who shows a PRA of 0% (i.e., no HLA antibody). Identification of the HLA antigen specificity of the antibody is an important feature of the antibody screening assays, and may reduce unnecessary crossmatches between patients who have antibodies against specific HLA antigens and donors who are positive for those antigens. Knowledge of antibody specificity can also increase opportunities for identifying compatible donors for these difficult-to-match patients. Highly sensitized (high PRA) patients may also be managed differently posttransplant since they have a higher risk of rejection. Pretransplant screening for HLA antibodies is also indicated in patients undergoing autologous stem cell transplants, since posttransplant patients with a high PRA are more likely to become refractory to platelet transfusions and may require careful observation regarding their need for HLA-matched platelets.

Crossmatching

The lymphocyte crossmatch is a critical step, especially before renal transplantation. It is also important in sensitized patients who are undergoing a heart or lung transplant. In this assay, the graft recipient's serum is mixed with donor lymphocytes (similar to that shown for red blood cells in Chapter 2 under Blood Crossmatch). If the recipient has preformed HLA antibodies against donor antigens, the cells will be lysed, the crossmatch is considered positive, and the transplant will likely not be done. The crossmatch may also be performed by measuring antibody binding to cells by flow cytometry. A "virtual crossmatch" may be done by comparing the HLA specificity of a recipient's antibodies to the HLA antigens of the donor to predict donor compatibility. In most cases a virtual crossmatch would be followed up by a lymphocyte crossmatch test either prior to or immediately posttransplant.

HISTOCOMPATIBILITY REQUIREMENTS FOR SOLID ORGAN TRANSPLANTS

In general, HLA matching is not an absolute requirement with respect to solid organ transplants (**Table 4–2**). It is usually a requirement for BMT. The application of HLA typing, crossmatching, and antibody screening in histocompatibility testing prior to transplantation of specific organs or tissues is described hereafter.

> In general, HLA matching is not an absolute requirement with respect to solid organ transplants. It is usually a requirement for bone marrow transplantation.

Kidney

Kidney transplantation from living donors, whether HLA matched or unmatched, is preferable to kidney transplantation from deceased donors. Recent national data shows that the 10-year graft failure for living donor transplants is 37% compared to 53% for deceased donors.

In a large multicenter study involving primary deceased donor renal transplants, multiple factors were shown to influence the outcome. These included the age of donor and recipient, presence of diabetes in the recipient, the cause of the donor's death, cold ischemic time of the donated kidney prior to transplant, ABO blood group compatibility, PRA, and crossmatch results between donor lymphocytes and recipient serum. A positive crossmatch is usually a contraindication

TABLE 4–2   General Requirements for HLA and ABO Blood Group Matching in Transplants

Organ	HLA	ABO
Kidney	No[a]	Yes
Cornea	No	No
Liver	No	Yes
Heart	No	Yes
Lung	No	Yes
Pancreas	No[a]	Yes
Stem cell/Bone marrow	Yes	No

[a]HLA matching preferable but not required.

to transplant. However, techniques to remove recipient circulating HLA and/or ABO antibody have been developed, allowing successful transplantation with previously incompatible kidneys, although graft survival rates are not as high as they are with compatible donors.

In the United States, approximately 30% of the kidney transplants are from living donors, including genetically unrelated donors such as spouses or friends. Patients who do not have a compatible living donor may have to wait from 3 to 5 years on the deceased donor waitlist, or even longer depending on their location, blood type, and level of HLA antibody. Patients can have a high rate of death while waiting; so rather than staying on the waitlist or undergoing treatment to remove antibody, a better alternative for patients with a potential living donor with ABO or HLA antibody incompatibilities may be kidney exchange. In kidney exchange, a person donates their kidney to another compatible recipient in exchange for their original intended recipient receiving a kidney from a different donor. HLA typing of the donors and determination of all HLA antibody in the recipient (to allow virtual crossmatching) is extremely important for such programs to optimize efficiency and allow for the most likely compatible donor to be identified.

> In the United States, nearly 35% of the kidney transplants are from living donors, including genetically unrelated donors such as spouses or friends.

Liver

HLA matching does not appear to correlate with better outcomes in liver transplantation. There are conflicting reports regarding the importance of a negative crossmatch in the pre-transplant setting, but donor-specific HLA antibodies are not a contraindication to transplantation. ABO matching, in contrast, is associated with better outcomes in both adult and pediatric populations.

Heart

The benefits of HLA matching in heart transplantation are difficult to evaluate because there are few studies that utilize prospective HLA matching. The usual priorities in cardiac transplantation are short ischemia time for the donated heart prior to transplant (<4 hours), heart size, and blood group matching. Most centers screen for HLA antibodies prior to transplant surgery and perform, when possible, a prospective crossmatch using donor cells only on sensitized patients. Alternatively, since there is often not time for a prospective crossmatch, the virtual crossmatch is an important tool. The presence of HLA-specific antibodies and a positive crossmatch against donor cells are generally accepted to be associated with an adverse outcome.

Lung

While there may be a small survival advantage with HLA-matched lung transplants, there is no consensus on the hierarchical importance of the various HLA loci. Lungs are allocated on the basis of recipient medical urgency, ABO compatibility, and size. Similar to heart transplant patients, crossmatches are usually done only on patients known to have HLA antibody and virtual crossmatch is often used.

Pancreas

Pancreata are transplanted based on ABO compatibility. HLA antibody screening is performed on transplant candidates, and a positive crossmatch is usually a contraindication to transplantation with that donor. Patients with pancreas-only transplantation have a lower survival rate than those undergoing combined pancreas and kidney transplantation. Most pancreata are transplanted in patients undergoing kidney transplants for diabetic renal failure. Evidence suggests that the kidney–pancreas transplant combination is associated with a long-term reduction in mortality, as compared with renal transplant only, in end-stage diabetic renal disease.

Cornea

The cornea is the most commonly transplanted tissue. There is no convincing evidence for the utility of HLA and ABO group matching for corneal transplants. However, the long-term

TABLE 4-3   **Examples of HLA Antigens or Alleles Associated with Adverse Reactions to Specific Drugs or Disease States**

HLA Allele	Drug Reactions
HLA-B*15:02	Increased risk of hypersensitivity to carbamazepine
HLA-B*58:01	Increased risk of hypersensitivity to allopurinol
HLA-B*57:01	Increased risk of hypersensitivity to abacavir
	Disease state
HLA-A29	Birdshot retinochoroidopathy
HLA-B27	Ankylosing spondylitis or reactive arthritis or uveitis
HLA-B51	Behcet's disease
HLA-DQ2 or DQ8	Celiac disease
HLA-DQB1*06:02	Narcolepsy

graft survival is approximately 50% and rejection remains the most common cause of graft loss. Because corneal rejection is not life-threatening, the routine use of systemic immunosuppression for prevention of rejection is not a consideration.

HEMATOPOIETIC CELL TRANSPLANTATION (HCT)

Hematopoietic cell transplantation is a therapeutic option in which normal hematopoietic stem or progenitor cells are used to replace abnormal hematopoietic cells or to reconstitute the bone marrow of patients undergoing high-dose cytotoxic therapy for malignancy. The hematopoietic cells can be harvested from the bone marrow under general anesthesia or from the peripheral blood after giving the donor multiple doses of growth factors/cytokines such as granulocyte colony-stimulating factor (G-CSF) or granulocyte–monocyte colony-stimulating factor (GM-CSF).

HLA matching is usually a requirement for allogeneic HCT. A positive crossmatch between donor and recipient is a strong predictor of graft failure, but because most patients and donors are HLA matched, this is rarely a concern. Recently, success has been obtained in cases involving partially mismatched BMT, which has increased transplantation opportunities for many patients.

In the past, serologic techniques were used extensively for HLA typing in BMT. As noted earlier, it is now known that the number of identifiable serologic specificities at any locus is far less than the number of true alleles at that locus (**Table 4–1**). Individuals who appear to be HLA matched after serologic typing may in fact have some mismatched alleles. Patients transplanted with genotypically HLA-matched marrow from siblings or unrelated individuals have a graft failure rate of approximately 2%. The risk of graft failure is much higher in the presence of a mismatch of two or more class I alleles.

The widespread availability of high-resolution allelic typing methods that allow better matching of donors with recipients has resulted in improved outcomes.

HLA TYPING AND NON-TRANSPLANTATION RELATED APPLICATIONS

Clinically HLA typing can be used to help define disease associations or to identify increased risk of drug hypersensitivity. Some of the more common HLA alleles that are tested in the United States laboratories are shown in **Table 4–3**.

A substantial portion of this chapter also appeared previously in Clinical Laboratory Reviews (a newsletter publication of the Massachusetts General Hospital, 2000;8:3).

Hematopoietic cell transplantation is a therapeutic option in which normal hematopoietic stem or progenitor cells are used to replace abnormal hematopoietic cells or to reconstitute the bone marrow of patients undergoing high-dose cytotoxic therapy for malignancy.

SELF-ASSESSMENT QUESTIONS

1. In the term, HLA-A*02:101:01:02N, which portion refers to the specific *HLA* gene?
    A. *02
    B. A
    C. 101
    D. 01

2. For which of the following organ transplants is HLA testing of least clinical value?
    A. Kidney
    B. Stem cells/bone marrow
    C. Pancreas
    D. Liver

FURTHER READING

Agrawal YP, Saidman SL. Histocompatibility testing for solid organ and bone marrow transplantation. *Clin Lab Rev* [a publication of the Massachusetts General Hospital]. 2000;8:3.

Bohmig GA, et al. Transplantation of the broadly sensitized patient: what are the options? *Curr Opin Organ Transplant*. 2011;16:588.

Cecka JM. HLA matching for organ transplantation ... Why not? *Int J Immunogenet*. 2010;37:323.

Eng HS, Leffell MS. Histocompatibility testing after fifty years of transplantation [Review]. *J Immunol Methods*. 2011;369:1.

Erlich H. HLA DNA typing: past, present, and future [Review]. *Tissue Antigens*. 2012;80:1.

Ferrari P, et al. Kidney paired donation: principles, protocols and programs [Review]. *Nephrol Dial Transplant*. 2015;30:1276.

Gebel HM, et al. Pre-transplant assessment of donor-reactive, HLA-specific antibodies in renal transplantation: contraindication vs. risk. *Am J Transplant*. 2003;3:1488.

Marsh SGE, et al. Nomenclature for factors of the HLA system, 2010. *Tissue Antigens*. 2010;75:291–455.

McCluskey J, Peh CA. The human leucocyte antigens and clinical medicine: an overview. *Rev Immunogenet*. 1999;1:3.

Morris PJ, et al. Analysis of factors that affect outcome of primary cadaveric renal transplantation in the UK. *Lancet*. 1999;354:1147.

Petersdorf EW, et al. Human leukocyte antigen matching in unrelated donor hematopoietic cell transplantation [Review]. *Semin Hematol*. 2005;42:76.

Picascia A, et al. Current concepts in histocompatibility during heart transplant [Review]. *Exp Clin Transplant*. 2012;10:209.

Reinsmoen NL, et al. Anti-HLA antibody analysis and crossmatching in heart and lung transplantation [Review]. *Transplant Immunol*. 2004;13:63.

Reisner Y, et al. Haploidentical hematopoietic transplantation: current status and future perspectives [Review]. *Blood*. 2011;118:6006.

Robinson J, et al. The IMGT/HLA database. *Nucleic Acids Res*. 2011;39(suppl 1):D1171–D1176.

Ruiz R, et al. Implications of a positive crossmatch in liver transplantation: a 20-year review. *Liver Transplant*. 2012;18:455.

Smets YFC, et al. Effect of simultaneous pancreas–kidney transplantation on mortality of patients with type-1 diabetes mellitus and end-stage renal failure. *Lancet*. 1999;353:1915.

Wolfe RA, et al. Comparison of mortality in all patients on dialysis, patients on dialysis awaiting transplantation, and recipients of a first cadaveric transplant. *N Engl J Med*. 1999;341:1725.

Infectious Diseases

Eric D. Spitzer

LEARNING OBJECTIVES

1. Determine if an organism of interest is a bacterium, fungus, parasite, or virus and learn how it is further classified among related organisms.

2. Learn the organisms that produce the commonly encountered and better characterized infectious diseases.

3. Distinguish pathogenic organisms from those found in normal flora.

4. Learn the laboratory test results associated with the individual infectious diseases and how they are used in establishing the diagnosis.

CHAPTER OUTLINE

INTRODUCTION

Humans live in a world of microbes. Many types of microbes are part of the normal human flora and rarely cause disease. Others have a greater potential for virulence and can cause disease depending on complex interactions between the host and the microbe. A small group of organisms are highly virulent and usually cause disease whenever they infect humans. This chapter on infectious diseases and clinical microbiology focuses on common pathogens and frequently encountered clinical syndromes. Infectious agents include a daunting array of viruses, bacteria, fungi, protozoans, and helminths. **Table 5–1** provides information on the basic microbiology and clinical significance of common pathogens. The organisms are grouped based on shared properties because these are often relevant to the diagnostic process. Microbial taxonomy is constantly evolving as we learn more about organisms, partly as a result of more complete knowledge of microbial genomes. These changes can be confusing to clinicians as organisms are moved from one species to another (*Streptococcus bovis* type I is now *S. gallolyticus*), species are subdivided (some organisms formerly known as *Coccidioides immitis* are now classified as *C. posadasii*), and the fungal phylum zygomycota is replaced by the subphylum mucorales [PMC4382724].

Because of the large number of potential pathogens, it is not technically possible, practical, or cost-effective to attempt to rule out all of them in each patient who may have an infection. It is therefore important for the clinician to know what organisms are most likely in a particular patient and whether routine diagnostic tests will detect them or whether specialized tests are needed. Identification of the causative agent is usually important for determining the most appropriate therapy. It can also have infection control or public health implications. The clinical findings are the first major clues in determining the site of infection and identifying a pathogenic organism. For example, a cough is usually indicative of a process in the respiratory tract while pain on urination is a clue to a urinary tract infection (UTI). Radiographic studies can further clarify the type of process and may point to specific categories of organisms.

Often, a single species of microbe can cause multiple syndromes. Conversely, a single syndrome may be caused by multiple organisms. This can lead to a large array of diagnostic possibilities. In order to determine a specific etiological diagnosis in a timely and cost-efficient manner, it is essential to take into consideration the clinical setting. For example, the organisms responsible for a community-acquired pneumonia are usually different from those that cause nosocomial pneumonia. If the patient is immunosuppressed, this further enlarges the list of potential organisms. It also matters whether the immunosuppression is due to decreased cell-mediated immunity, for example, due to HIV infection or inhibitors of tumor necrosis factor (TNF), versus neutropenia secondary to chemotherapy because each has its own associated group of opportunistic infections. Other underlying conditions such as diabetes or sickle cell disease, or the presence of prosthetic devices, are associated with specific infections. A history of travel or exposure to arthropod vectors may raise the possibility of additional organisms.

The organization of this chapter reflects the common associations between selected organisms and the site of infection. The discussion of a particular organism in a specific anatomic site in this chapter does not imply that infection by that organism is restricted to that location. Several infectious diseases, such as viral hepatitis (see Chapter 16) and *Helicobacter pylori* infections (see Chapter 15), are presented elsewhere in this book because these infections are intimately associated with a specific organ or tissue. The organisms and diseases selected for presentation

TABLE 5-1   Selected Clinically Significant Microorganisms

Aerobic Gram-Positive Cocci	**Aerobic Gram-Negative Bacilli**	***Mycoplasma* and *Ureaplasma***

Aerobic Gram-Positive Cocci

Occur singly or in pairs, tetrads, chains, or clusters
Catalase positive
  Micrococcus
  Staphylococcus aureus
  Coagulase-negative staphylococci
Catalase negative
  Aerococcus
Abiotrophia and *Granulicatella* (nutritionally
  variant streptococci)
  Enterococcus faecalis
  Enterococcus faecium
  Gemella
Leuconostoc
Streptococcus agalactiae (group B
  streptococci)
Streptococcus gallolyticus (bovis)
Streptococcus dysgalactiae (multiple species
  within group C or group G streptococci are
  classified as *S. dysgalactiae*)
Streptococcus anginosus/intermedius group
  (viridans streptococci)
Streptococcus mitis/Sanguinis group
  (viridans streptococci)
Streptococcus mutans group (viridans
  streptococci)
Streptococcus pneumoniae (pneumococcus)
Streptococcus pyogenes (group A streptococci)
Streptococcus salivarius group (viridans
  streptococci)

Aerobic gram-negative cocci

Occur singly or in pairs or clumps; catalase
positive, oxidase positive
Moraxella catarrhalis
Neisseria gonorrhoeae
Neisseria meningitidis

Aerobic gram-positive bacilli

Rod-like organisms; only *Bacillus* species
produce spores; some organisms in category
are partially acid-fast

Bacillus
Corynebacterium
Erysipelothrix
Gardnerella vaginalis (Gram variable)
Lactobacillus
Listeria
Nocardia

Mycobacteria

Rod-like organisms; acid-fast stain positive;
some stains are gram-positive; most are slow
growing

Mycobacterium tuberculosis
Mycobacterium avium complex
Mycobacterium kansasii
Mycobacterium marinum
Mycobacterium fortuitum complex (rapid grower)
Mycobacterium abscessus (rapid grower)
Mycobacterium chelonae (rapid grower)

Aerobic Gram-Negative Bacilli

Enterobacteriaceae; rod-like organisms;
oxidase-negative; ferment sugars
Citrobacter
Edwardsiella
Enterobacter
Escherichia
Ewingella
Hafnia
Klebsiella
Morganella morganii
Plesiomonas (oxidase-positive)
Proteus
Providencia
Salmonella
Serratia
Shigella
Yersinia enterocolitica
Yersinia pestis
Yersinia pseudotuberculosis

Aerobic gram-negative bacilli

Nonenterobacteriaceae, fermentative;
rod-like organisms; oxidase-positive;
ferment sugars

Aeromonas
Chromobacterium
Pasteurella
Vibrio

Aerobic gram-negative bacilli

Nonenterobacteriaceae; rod-like
organisms; catalase positive; do not
ferment sugars; oxidase variable

Acinetobacter
Alcaligenes
Burkholderia
Elizabethkingia
Empedobacter (Flavobacterium)
Pseudomonas
Shewanella
Stenotrophomonas

Aerobic fastidious gram-negative bacilli

Small, straight or curved gram-negative
bacilli or coccobacilli; may require special
conditions for adequate growth

Aggregatibacter
Afipia
Bartonella
Bordetella
Brucella
Campylobacter (microaerophilic)
Cardiobacterium
Eikenella
Francisella
Haemophilus
Helicobacter pylori
Kingella
Legionella

Mycoplasma* and *Ureaplasma

Small highly pleomorphic organisms; difficult to
observe with routine stains and require complex
medium for growth
Mycoplasma
Ureaplasma

Treponemes

Spiral organisms that may or may not stain with
routine stains and require complex medium or
animal host for growth
Borrelia
Leptospira
Spirillum
Treponema

Anaerobic gram-negative bacilli

Bacteroides
Bilophila
Fusobacterium
Prevotella
Porphyromonas

Anaerobic gram-negative cocci

Acidaminococcus
Veillonella

**Anaerobic gram-positive bacilli:
nonspore forming**

Actinomyces
Lactobacillus
Propionibacterium

Anaerobic gram-positive bacilli: spore forming

Clostridium

Anaerobic gram-positive cocci

Finegoldia
Parvimonas
Peptostreptococcus
Staphylococcus saccharolyticus

Obligate intracellular bacteria

Anaplasma
Chlamydia
Coxiella
Ehrlichia
Rickettsia

Fungi of medical significance[a]

Acremonium	*Malassezia*
Aspergillus	*Microsporum*
Blastomyces	*Mucor*
Candida	*Paracoccidioides*
Coccidioides	*Penicillium*
Cryptococcus	*Pseudallescheria (Scedosporium)*
Epidermophyton	*Rhizopus*
Fonsecaea	*Sporothrix*
	Talaromyces
Fusarium	*Trichophyton*
Geotrichum	*Trichosporon*
Histoplasma	*Wangiella*

(Continued)

TABLE 5–1   (Continued)

Virusesᵇ

Family	Representative Species Pathogenic for Humans	Family	Representative Species Pathogenic for Humans
DNA viruses		Arenaviridae	Lymphocytic choriomeningitis virus
Poxviridae	Vaccinia virus		Lassa fever virus
	Variola virus (smallpox)		Junin (Argentine hemorrhagic fever virus)
	Molluscum contagiosum virus		Machupo (Bolivian hemorrhagic fever virus)
Herpesviridae	Herpes simplex virus, type 1	Picornaviridae	*Enteroviruses*
	Herpes simplex virus, type 2		Poliovirus (3 types)
	Varicella zoster virus		Coxsackie A virus (23 types)
	Epstein–Barr virus		Coxsackie B virus (6 types)
	Cytomegalovirus		Echovirus (30 types)
	Human herpesvirus 6 (HHV 6)		Enteroviruses 68-71 (4)
	Human herpesvirus 8 (HHV 8, Kaposi sarcoma-associated herpesvirus)		Rhinovirus (common cold virus) (>115 types)
			Hepatitis A virus (enterovirus 72)
Adenoviridae	Human adenoviruses (51 serotypes)	Caliciviridae	*Noroviruses*
Papillomaviridae	Human papillomaviruses (>96 types)		Norwalk and Norwalk-like gastroenteritis viruses
Polyomaviridae	BK virus		
	JC virus	Hepeviridae	Hepatitis E virus (enterically transmitted)
Parvoviridae	B19 virus (human parvovirus)	Astroviridae	Human astroviruses
Hepadnaviridae	Hepatitis B virus	Coronaviridae	*Human coronaviruses (229E, HKU1, NL63, OC43)*
RNA viruses			MERS-CoV
Reoviridae	Orthoreoviruses	Flaviviridae	*Flaviviruses (mosquito-borne)*
Paramyxoviridae	Colorado tick fever virus		St. Louis and Japanese encephalitis viruses,
	Rotaviruses A-C		West Nile virus, yellow fever virus, dengue
Rhabdoviridae	*Respiroviruses*		virus, Zika virus
	Parainfluenza virus (types 1 and 3)		*Flaviviruses (tick-borne)*
	Morbilliviruses		Omsk hemorrhagic fever, European and Far
	Measles virus		Eastern tick-borne encephalitis viruses
	Rubulaviruses		Hepatitis C virus (parenterally transmitted)
	Mumps virus, parainfluenza virus (types 2 and 4)	Togaviridae	*Alphaviruses*
	Pneumoviruses		Western, Eastern, and Venezuelan equine
	Respiratory syncytial virus		encephalitis viruses; Ross River and Semliki
	Metapneumovirus		Forest viruses (mosquito-borne)
Filoviride	Rabies virus		*Rubivirus*
Orthomyxoviridae	Marburg and Ebola viruses		Rubella virus
	Influenza A virus	Retroviridae	Human T-cell lymphotropic virus
	Influenza B virus		HTLV 1 and 2
Bunyaviridae	*Orthobunyaviruses (mosquito-transmitted)*		Human immunodeficiency virus
	California serogroup (e.g., California encephalitis and La Crosse viruses)		HIV 1 and 2
	Hantaviruses (rodent-associated)		
	Hantaan virus (hemorrhagic fever with renal syndrome),		
	Sin Nombre virus (hantavirus pulmonary syndrome)		

Subviral agents	Endolimax	**Flagellates (blood, tissue)**
	Iodamoeba	*Leishmania*
Satellites	Blastocystis	*Trypanosoma*
Hepatitis delta (D) virus		
	Amebas (other body sites)	**Flagellates (other body sites)**
Prions	*Naegleria*	*Trichomonas vaginalis*
Kuru, Creutzfeldt–Jakob disease (CJD),	*Acanthamoeba*	
Gerstmann–Straussler–Scheinker syndrome	*Balamuthia*	**Ciliates (intestinal)**
(GSS), fatal familial insomnia (FFI)		*Balantidium*
	Flagellates (intestinal)	
Parasites of clinical significanceᶜ	*Giardia*	**Coccidia (intestinal)**
	Dientamoeba	*Cryptosporidium*
Protozoa	*Trichomonas hominis*	*Cyclospora*
Amebas (intestinal)		*Isospora*
Entamoeba histolytica		

(Continued)

TABLE 5-1   (Continued)

Coccidia (other body sites) *Toxoplasma*	*Trichostrongylus* *Trichuris*	*Hymenolepis* *Taenia solium* *Taenia saginata*
Microsporidia (intestinal and other sites) *Enterocytozoon* *Encephalitozoon*	**(Tissue)** *Trichinella* Visceral and ocular larva migrans (*Toxocara canis* or *Toxocara cati*)	**(Tissue—larval forms)** *T. solium* *Echinococcus*
Sporozoa (blood) *Plasmodium* *Babesia*	Cutaneous larva migrans (*Ancylostoma braziliense* or *Ancylostoma caninum*) *Dracunculus* *Angiostrongylus*	**Trematodes (flukes)** **(Intestinal)** *Fasciolopsis*
Fungal-like organism (formerly classified as a protozoan) *Pneumocystis*	*Gnathostoma* *Anisakis* *Capillaria*	**(Liver/lung)** *Clonorchis* *Opisthorchis* *Fasciola*
Nematodes (roundworms) **(Intestinal)** *Ascaris*	**(Blood and tissues)** *Wuchereria* *Brugia*	*Paragonimus*
Enterobius *Ancylostoma* *Necator* *Strongyloides*	*Loa* *Onchocerca*	**(Blood and tissue)** *Schistosoma mansoni* (intestine) *Schistosoma japonicum* (intestine) *Schistosoma haematobium* (bladder)
	Cestodes (tapeworms) **(Intestinal)** *Diphyllobothrium*	

[a]The fungi are listed by genus. As with the bacteria, certain species within a genus are more commonly associated with infections than other species. The list includes the fungi associated with the majority of human fungal infections. There are many more fungi in nature than are listed here. Compiled from data in McGinnis MR, Rinaldi MG. Some medically important fungi and their common synonyms and obsolete names. *Clin Infect Dis*. 1997;25:15.

[b]The viruses are grouped by family. Listed within each family are representative viral species that are pathogenic for humans. Compiled from data in Miller MJ. Viral taxonomy. *Clin Infect Dis*. 1997;25:18–20 and updated based on Knipe DM, Howley PM, eds. *Fields' Virology*. 5th ed. Philadelphia, PA: Wolters Kluwer; 2007.

[c]These organisms are listed by type of organism and most common site of infection. They are listed by genus only unless an individual species within a genus is located in one category and another species within the same genus is in a different category. Compiled from data in Garcia LS. Classification of human parasites. *Clin Infect Dis*. 1997;25:21.

in this chapter were chosen primarily by their incidence, with a preference for common infections. Many lower-incidence infections also have been included because they are often within a differential diagnosis, new information on their diagnosis and treatment is emerging, or they can be overlooked if appropriate tests are not requested. The chapter focuses on infections commonly encountered in the United States, although several travel-associated infections are discussed.

A general clinical approach to the patient with an infectious disease is diagrammed in **Figure 5–1**.

The organization of this chapter reflects the common associations between selected organisms and the site of infection.

LABORATORY TESTS FOR INFECTIOUS AGENTS

The laboratory diagnosis of infectious disease utilizes five distinct types of tests: direct examination, culture, antigen detection, nucleic acid detection, and serology. Each of these tests has strengths and weaknesses. The types of test(s) that are used in a specific case depend in large part on the organisms that are in the differential diagnosis, as well as the type of specimens that are available. See Chapter 2 for illustrations of these laboratory methods.

The laboratory diagnosis of infectious disease utilizes five distinct types of tests: direct examination, culture, antigen detection, nucleic acid detection, and serology.

Direct Stains

Direct examination involves preparing a smear of the specimen and then using an appropriate staining technique to detect the relevant microorganisms. The Gram stain is rapid and detects most types of bacterial pathogens if they are present in sufficient numbers. It provides a preliminary characterization in terms of the Gram reaction, that is, positive or negative, as well as the

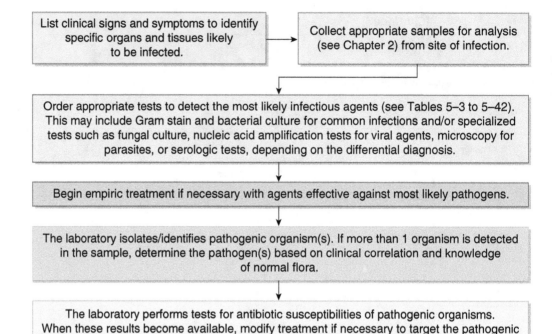

FIGURE 5–1   **A general clinical approach to the patient with an infectious disease.**

morphology (cocci, coccobacilli, or bacilli) and arrangement of the cells (individual cells, pairs, chains, or clusters). It also provides information on the host response, for example, the presence or absence of neutrophils. This stain is routinely performed on most specimen types including respiratory specimens, sterile fluids, tissue biopsies, wounds, and abscesses. It is not routinely performed on stool because of the large numbers of normal flora, urine because similar information is available from the urinalysis, and blood because of the small number of organisms typically found in cases of bacteremia. The analytic sensitivity of the Gram stain is relatively low because the observation of an average of one organism per oil immersion field corresponds to a concentration of 10^5 organisms per milliliter in the specimen. The sensitivity can be increased by concentration of the specimen through centrifugation. Other direct stains include acid-fast stains for mycobacteria and calcofluor white for fungi. Wright stains of peripheral blood are used to detect *Plasmodium* and *Babesia* infections. Routine hematoxylin and eosin stains as well as Gram, acid-fast bacteria (AFB), and Gomori methenamine silver (GMS) stains can reveal the presence of microorganisms in paraffin-embedded tissue in the surgical pathology laboratory.

Culture

Isolation of organisms in pure culture continues to be the mainstay of microbiologic diagnosis. In general, culture is very sensitive and specific and remains the "gold standard" for diagnosing many types of infection. Culture provides relatively rapid detection (within usually 1 to 3 days) of a wide array of organisms that are then available for definitive identification and antimicrobial susceptibility testing. One of the great advantages of culture assays is that microbiology laboratories routinely inoculate a combination of nonselective and selective media that support the growth of many types of pathogenic bacteria. The person ordering the test does not need to specify which organism or organisms are suspected of causing the infection. A clinician who submits a blood-culture bottle does not have to order a *Staphylococcus* culture, a *Streptococcus* culture, a gram-negative rod culture, etc. Nonetheless, it is essential to remember that routine cultures only detect typical bacteria. If other classes of agents, such as mycobacteria, fungi, parasites, or viruses, are in the differential diagnosis, then the clinician must request the appropriate tests. For example, mycobacteria and fungal cultures utilize media designed to inhibit the growth of routine bacteria and they also require prolonged incubation.

Identification of Organisms from Positive Cultures

The majority of commonly encountered bacterial pathogens can be identified by the presence of specific combinations of phenotypic traits including production of enzymes, such as catalase, coagulase, oxidase, and urease; ability to ferment or utilize different types of sugars; and additional metabolic reactions. Many of these individual tests have been combined into commercial identification kits. In contrast, slow-growing organisms, such as mycobacteria, and bacteria that are difficult to identify with traditional biochemical methods are now often identified by nucleic acid amplification and sequencing of conserved genes such as 16S ribosomal RNA or RNA polymerase. Yeasts are generally identified with biochemical tests similar to those used for bacteria. Finally, identification of molds is based on colonial and microscopic morphology.

More recently, commercial identification systems have been developed that use matrix-assisted laser desorption-ionization time-of-flight (MALDI-TOF) mass spectroscopy (MS) to generate protein spectra that can be compared with databases to identify bacteria and other microbes. The advantage of MALDI-TOF/MS is that it requires few reagents and can identify organisms in minutes as opposed to the 12- to 24-hour incubations required for most biochemical panels; this has led to its widespread adoption in clinical laboratories.

Susceptibility Testing

Once an organism has been identified in the clinical microbiology laboratory, the second major task, in most cases, is determining the organism's antibiotic susceptibility profile. Susceptibility tests involve the measurement of the minimum inhibitory concentration (MIC), the lowest concentration of antimicrobial agent that inhibits the growth of the organism. The reference method is the microbroth dilution technique. The MICs are then interpreted as sensitive, intermediate, or resistant according to tables of interpretive breakpoints that are related to therapeutically achievable serum levels for each antibiotic. Other susceptibility methods such as disk diffusion (measuring the diameter of the zone of inhibition surrounding an antibiotic-containing disk) can be correlated with the results of the broth dilution technique.

Susceptibility testing has become increasingly complex due to the widespread dissemination of increasingly resistant pathogens that include methicillin-resistant *Staphylococcus aureus* (MRSA); vancomycin-resistant enterococci (VRE); and multidrug-resistant strains of *Klebsiella pneumoniae*, *Pseudomonas aeruginosa*, and *Acinetobacter baumannii*. These organisms harbor a variety of resistance mechanisms that include altered penicillin-binding proteins, extended-spectrum beta-lactamases, carbapenemases, inducible clindamycin resistance, and multidrug efflux pumps. While molecular methods can be used for rapid detection of specific resistance genes, such as the *mecA* gene in MRSA, the *vanA* and *vanB* genes in VRE, and the *bla*$_{KPC}$ genes in *K. pneumoniae*, most susceptibility testing continues to depend on phenotypic (MIC-based) methods that require overnight incubation.

Antigen Detection

Antigen detection tests do not require the growth of microorganisms; therefore, they have the potential to provide rapid detection of infectious agents. Immunoassays that detect soluble antigens vary in speed, complexity, sensitivity, and specificity. Usually there is a trade-off between simplicity and sensitivity. Rapid immunochromatographic assays require very few procedural steps and are the basis of many point-of-care tests. These assays are less sensitive than traditional solid-phase enzyme immunoassays (EIAs) that are used for batch testing in the laboratory. Unlike culture-based assays, an immunoassay can only detect the organism that is recognized by the reagent antibodies; a separate assay must be performed for each organism. Immunoassays generally exhibit good but not perfect specificity. Furthermore, they cannot distinguish viable from nonviable organisms. Direct or indirect fluorescent immunoassays utilize microscopy to identify organisms that bind the reagent antibody. These assays often have high sensitivity and specificity compared with other types of immunoassays, but they require extensive training to ensure proper interpretation.

Nucleic Acid Amplification

The introduction of nucleic acid amplification techniques (NAATs) has led to major advances in the ability to diagnose and manage a wide variety of infectious diseases. These tests are particularly valuable for detecting difficult-to-grow or slow-growing organisms that may be present in small numbers. Examples include viral load assays for monitoring HIV and HCV infections, diagnosis of Herpes simplex virus (HSV) encephalitis, rapid assays for tuberculosis, and diagnosis of Chlamydial genital infections. NAAT tests have the potential for very high sensitivity and specificity; however, as with antigen tests, they can only be used to diagnose infections caused by organisms that the assay is designed to detect. Although current technology is not at the stage where it can eliminate the use of traditional culture methods in the routine bacteriology laboratory, commercial multiplex NAAT panels are now widely used to diagnose respiratory infections caused by influenza, RSV, and other respiratory viruses, and to diagnose gastrointestinal infections caused by a variety of bacterial, viral, and protozoan infections.

Serology

Serologic tests detect host antibodies that are produced in response to infection with a particular infectious agent. The most important limitation of these assays is that antibody is usually not detectable early in the course of infection. Even if antibody is detected, it may represent a past infection. Serologic diagnosis usually requires demonstration of seroconversion, a fourfold rise in IgG titer between sequential specimens, or a positive IgM assay. While the latter is usually thought of as a marker of acute infection, IgM can persist for 6 to 12 months. For the reasons outlined above, serologic assays are mainly used to diagnose infections, such as syphilis, that cannot be detected using more direct methods.

SEPSIS AND BLOODSTREAM INFECTIONS

Bacteremia

Description

Normally the blood is sterile. Infection in any of the organs or tissues can result in entry of bacteria into the circulation. Replication of bacteria in the blood can contribute to the signs and symptoms of sepsis (e.g., fever, tachycardia, leukocytosis, and hypotension) and may lead to dissemination of the organism to other tissues and organs; however, patients can be septic without having demonstrable bacteria in their blood. Bacteremia is often described as transient, intermittent, or continuous based on the number of positive specimens. Transient bacteremia occurs when small numbers of a commensal organism present on a mucosal surface gain access to the bloodstream. These infections are usually not clinically significant when they occur in an otherwise healthy host. Intermittent bacteremias are usually associated with a sequestered infection somewhere in the organs or tissues (e.g., an abscess). Continuous bacteremias are associated with an intravascular focus of infection. Examples include endocarditis or an infected vascular catheter. The isolation of certain species may have additional significance; for example, bacteremia caused by *S. gallolyticus* or *Clostridium septicum* is often associated with the presence of colon cancer. (See Chapter 14 for an additional discussion of sepsis.)

Diagnosis

Blood cultures are routinely collected as part of the diagnostic evaluation of patients who present with signs and symptoms of sepsis or disseminated infection. To maximize sensitivity and specificity, it is recommended that two to three sets of blood cultures be collected per septic episode. Most hospitals use continuous blood culture systems that utilize colorimetric, fluorescent, or manometric methods to detect bacterial growth. Positive bottles are then subcultured to agar plates for further evaluation of the organisms. More recently, fluorescent hybridization probes and NAAT panels have been introduced that can rapidly identify common pathogens that may be present in positive blood culture bottles.

To identify intermittent bacteremias, the timing of the blood collection is important to maximize the likelihood of finding organisms while they are in the blood (see the section on sample collection in microbiology in Chapter 2). Ideally, blood from patients with intermittent bacteremias is collected during the hour before a temperature spike, but this is not practical because the

TABLE 5–2 **Features of the Human Microbiome (i.e., "Normal Bacterial Flora")**

Anatomic Site	Bacterial Phyla (Predominant in Bold) and Common Genera (Italics)	Examples of the Significance of the Microbiome on Disease and/or Diagnostic Tests
Mouth	**Firmicutes** *Streptococcus* **Bacteriodetes** **Proteobacteria** Fusobacteria	Oral flora are common contaminants of poorly collected sputum samples; viridans group streptococci are common contaminants in blood cultures; streptococci and fastidious gram-negative rods (Proteobacteria) are important causes of endocarditis
Gut	**Bacteriodetes** **Firmicutes** Proteobacteria the gut microbiome is a complex mixture with extensive differences between individuals and across ages (e.g., young children, adults, and the elderly)*	Interaction of the gut microbiome with the host immune system is thought to play a role in inflammatory bowel diseases; disruption of fecal microbiome by antibiotics is a major risk factor for development of *Clostridium difficile* infection (CDI); fecal microbiota transplantation is used to treat recurrent CDI
Skin	**Actinobacteria** *Corynebacterium* *Propionibacterium* **Firmicutes** *Staphylococcus*	Coagulase-negative staphylococci, corynebacteria, and propionibacteria are common contaminant in blood cultures; these same organisms can cause infections of intravenous catheters and prosthetic implants
Vagina	**Firmicutes** *Lactobacillus* Bacteroidetes Actinobacteria Proteobacteria	Bacterial vaginosis results from loss of lactobacilli and overgrowth of other anaerobic organisms

*Microbiome composition is based on high throughput sequencing of 16S rRNA genes and metagenomic analysis. The main bacterial phyla are described below.

Actinobacteria—Gram-positive rods with high G+C content; examples of genera include *Corynebacterium* (aerobic) and *Propionibacterium* and *Bifidobacterium* (anaerobic).

Bacteriodetes—anaerobic gram-negative rods; examples of genera include *Bacteroides, Porphyromonas,* and *Prevotella.*

Firmicutes—Gram-positive organisms with low G+C content; examples of genera include *Staphylococcus* and *Streptococcus* (aerobic cocci), *Bacillus* and *Lactobacillus* (aerobic rods), and *Clostridium* and *Eubacterium* (anaerobic rods).

Fusobacteria—Anaerobic gram-negative rods, e.g., *Fusobacterium.*

Proteobacteria—Gram-negative rods, coccobacilli, and cocci; three major subdivisions: examples of alphaproteobacteria genera include *Bartonella, Brucella,* and *Rickettsia;* examples of betaproteobacteria genera include *Burkholderia* and *Neisseria;* examples of gammaproteobacteria genera include members of the family Enterobacteriaceae (e.g., *E. coli, Klebsiella, Proteus, and Salmonella*), *Pseudomonas,* and *Vibrio.*

febrile episodes are often not predictable. It is common practice for blood to be collected at 30- to 60-minute intervals (if possible) when a febrile patient is suspected of having an intermittent bacteremia. As one might expect, one is much more likely to detect a continuous bacteremia in the first blood culture than to detect an intermittent bacteremia.

A major problem in the interpretation of the blood culture results is incidental contamination of the specimen with the normal bacterial flora from the skin (**Table 5–2**). The clinical significance of a positive blood culture is dependent on both the number of positive specimens and the type of organism. The isolation of recognized pathogens such as *S. aureus, S. pneumoniae,* betahemolytic streptococci (*S. pyogenes* and *S. agalactiae*), enterococci, gram-negative rods (aerobic and anaerobic), or yeast from one or more blood cultures is almost always clinically significant (**Table 5–3**). In contrast, if only one of the multiple blood culture specimens is positive for an organism found on the skin (e.g., coagulase-negative staphylococci or *Corynebacterium* spp.), the result is likely to reflect contamination during specimen collection rather than true septicemia. This frequently encountered problem is one reason why at least two blood samples should be collected for blood cultures. Although skin-derived bacteria are often thought of as nonpathogenic, it is important to remember that they can cause clinically significant infections, particularly in immunosuppressed patients and in patients with intravascular catheters or prosthetic devices. The isolation of the same skin flora organism in two separately collected specimens increases the probability that it represents a clinically significant bacteremia.

To avoid the problem of contamination of the blood culture bottles with skin organisms, meticulous preparation of the skin with a bactericidal agent is necessary. The number of blood cultures required for detection of a pathogenic organism is determined by the volume of blood collected per bottle, the timing of the blood collection, the type of organism producing the infection, and previous antibiotic exposure. Three or more blood culture collections may be required to document the presence of certain organisms.

A major problem in the interpretation of the blood culture results is incidental contamination of the specimen with the normal bacterial flora from the skin.

To avoid the problem of contamination of the blood culture bottles with skin organisms, meticulous preparation of the skin with a bactericidal agent is necessary.

TABLE 5-3   Clinical Significance of Organisms that Are Frequently Isolated From Blood Cultures

Organism	Probability that the Organism Is a True Pathogen[a,b]
Gram-positive aerobic bacteria	
Staphylococcus aureus	High
Coagulase-negative staphylococci	Low/intermediate
Enterococcus spp.	Intermediate/high
Viridans group streptococci	Intermediate
Beta-hemolytic streptococci	High
Streptococcus pneumoniae	High
Bacillus spp.	Low
Corynebacterium spp.	Low
Gram-negative aerobic bacteria	
Escherichia coli	High
Klebsiella pneumoniae	High
Enterobacter cloacae	High
Pseudomonas aeruginosa	High
Acinetobacter baumanii	Intermediate/high
Anaerobic bacteria	
Clostridium spp.	Intermediate
Propionibacterium spp.	Low
Bacteroides fragilis group	High
Yeast	
Candida spp.	High
Cryptococcus neoformans	High

[a]High, 90% to 100%; intermediate, >10% to <90%; low, 0% to 10%.

[b]Based on data from Pien BC, et al. The clinical and prognostic importance of positive blood cultures in adults. *Am J Med*. 2010;123:819–828 and Weinstein MP, et al. The clinical significance of positive blood cultures in the 1990s: a prospective comprehensive evaluation of the microbiology, epidemiology, and outcome of bacteremia and fungemia in adults. *Clin Infect Dis*. 1997;24;584–602.

Infections Caused by *Rickettsia*, *Ehrlichia*, and Related Organisms

Description

Rickettsia, *Ehrlichia*, and *Anaplasma* are obligate intracellular bacteria that cannot be detected in routine bacterial cultures. These organisms are transmitted to humans by ticks; therefore, the risk of acquiring these infections depends on the geographic distribution of the tick vectors and the time of year (see **Table 5–4**).

Rickettsia rickettsii, the agent of Rocky Mountain spotted fever (RMSF), is mainly transmitted by the dog tick (*Dermacentor variabilis*) and infects endothelial cells. The resulting vascular injury elicits a widespread vasculitis, consisting of vasodilation with perivascular edema, and at times complicated by thrombosis and hemorrhage. Erythrocytes extravasating into the dermis form non-blanching petechial or purpuric lesions. The characteristic rash is often absent during the early stages of infection, and the infection can progress to a life-threatening encephalitis if not promptly treated.

Ehrlichia chafeensis is transmitted by the lone star tick (*Amblyomma americanum*) and infects monocytes. Patients present with nonspecific findings including fever, leukopenia, thrombocytopenia, and/or elevations of hepatic enzymes. Similar clinical manifestations are seen with *Anaplasma* (*formerly Ehrlichia*) *phagocytophilum* that is transmitted by deer ticks (*Ixodes* spp.) and infects granulocytes.

Diagnosis

None of these agents can be cultured on artificial media. RMSF is usually diagnosed retrospectively with serologic tests; however, this should not delay treatment that should be initiated based on clinical findings and potential history of exposure. If the rash is present, organisms can be demonstrated by immunohistochemical staining of a skin biopsy in 70% of cases. Examination of peripheral blood smears in patients with *Anaplasma* can reveal the presence of organisms within inclusions in neutrophils, but many cases are negative. *Ehrlichia* infects monocytes but is rarely observed in peripheral blood smears. NAAT-based tests of blood and/or serologic tests are the best methods for diagnosing *Anaplasma* and *Ehrlichia* infections.

TABLE 5–4   Infections Caused by Anaplasma, Ehrlichia, Rickettsia, and Related Organisms

Disease	Etiologic Agent	Mechanism of Transmission to Humans	Clinical Features	Laboratory Tests
Rocky Mountain spotted fever	*Rickettsia rickettsii*	Tick vector	Higher rate seasonally and in specific geographic areas; rash from a vasculitis, fever, and headache	Serology: increase in antibody titer after exposure; immunohistochemical tests on tissue (sensitivity approximately 70%), PCR available from CDC
Boutonneuse fever	*Rickettsia conorii*	Tick vector	Seasonal: distribution in Europe, Asia, and Africa; rash, fever, headache, and black spot at the site of tick attachment	Serology: increase in antibody titer after exposure
Rickettsial pox	*Rickettsia akari*	Bite of mouse mite	Similar to but milder than Rocky Mountain spotted fever and Boutonneuse fever; uncommon in the United States	Serology: increase in antibody titer after exposure; PCR tests on tissue available from CDC
Murine typhus	*Rickettsia typhi*	Flea feces inoculated into flea bite wound on human	Seasonal and geographic; rash, fever, and headache	Serology: increase in antibody titer after exposure
Epidemic typhus	*Rickettsia prowazekii*	Infected louse feces inoculated into human skin wounds	Associated with domestic crowding plus poor hygiene (as in refugee camps); clinically similar to Rocky Mountain spotted fever	Serology: increase in antibody titer after exposure
Scrub typhus	*Orientia tsutsugamushi*	Bite of a larval mite	Rash, fever, and headache	Serology: increase in antibody titer after exposure
Q fever	*Coxiella burnetii*	Inhalation of infected aerosols, ingestion of contaminated dairy products, or, rarely, by tick vector	Acutely, it is usually an asymptomatic or self-limited febrile pneumonia; can become chronic with damage to heart valves and bone	Serology: increase in antibody titer after exposure (most common method); PCR of blood available in reference labs
Erhlichiosis	*Ehrlichia chaffeensis*	Tick vector	From asymptomatic to a severe Rocky Mountain spotted fever-like illness	Serology: increase in antibody titer after exposure; PCR of blood; blood smears have low sensitivity
Anaplasmosis	*Anaplasma phagocytophilium*	Tick vector	Fever, headache, myalgias	Serology: increase in antibody titer after exposure; PCR of blood; blood smears have low sensitivity

Fungemia

Description

Yeast belonging to the genus *Candida* are a major cause of hospital-acquired bloodstream infections. These organisms are frequently part of the oral and gastrointestinal flora. Treatment with broad-spectrum antibiotics that disrupt the normal bacterial flora, the presence of intravenous catheters, and neutropenia all predispose to the development of candidemia.

Cryptococcus neoformans and *Histoplasma capsulatum* are important causes of fungemia in patients with markedly depressed cell-mediated immunity (*Cryptococcus* is further discussed in the section "Chronic Meningitis" and *Histoplasma* is further discussed in the section "Infections of the Lung and Pleurae"). Although molds such as *Aspergillus* spp. can cause disseminated infections in immunosuppressed patients, they are rarely detected in the bloodstream.

Diagnosis

Candidemia can usually be detected with routine blood cultures. Specialized techniques (e.g., lysis–centrifugation cultures) are usually required to detect *H. capsulatum* and may enhance the detection of *C. neoformans*. Immunoassays that detect antigens produced by *H. capsulatum* and *C. neoformans* are also used to diagnose disseminated infections caused by these organisms.

Malaria is one of the largest causes of mortality and morbidity in the world. Individuals who travel to areas where malaria is endemic and develop fever within weeks of return should be suspected of suffering from malaria.

Parasitic Infections of the Blood
Overview
Several vector-borne parasites can infect the blood. These include protozoans such as *Plasmodium* spp. (malaria), *Babesia* spp., and *Trypanosoma* spp., and nematodes such as the agents of lymphatic filariasis. *Plasmodium* infections are an important cause of nonspecific febrile illnesses in returning travelers, and *Babesia* infections are endemic in parts of the United States; these infections are discussed below. Other blood parasites are uncommon in the United States.

Malaria
Description
Malaria is one of the largest causes of mortality and morbidity in the world. Individuals who travel to areas where malaria is endemic and develop fever within weeks of return should be suspected of suffering from malaria.

There are four species of *Plasmodium* that cause most cases of human malaria. These parasites are transmitted by *Anopheles* mosquitoes that are widely distributed throughout Africa, Asia, and Latin America. The most dangerous of the four species is *Plasmodium falciparum*. This organism can achieve very high levels of parasitemia and adheres to capillary endothelium, and this can lead to severe organ damage. *P. falciparum* infection may be fatal within days. *P. vivax* and *P. ovale* are morphologically similar and generally cause less severe infection, but unlike *P. falciparum*, they can establish persistent infection and cause relapses several months after the initial infection. *P. malariae* is the least virulent species and can cause low-level infection that may cause few symptoms, but it can persist for years. *P. knowlesi*, which infects monkeys, can also cause human infections.

Diagnosis
Currently, the diagnosis of malaria and the identification of the species of *Plasmodium* responsible for malaria are usually based on the microscopic examination of stained erythrocytes in thick and thin blood films. These organisms have maturation cycles involving a variety of specific structures in the RBC, including ring trophozoites, growing trophozoites, mature schizonts, and gametocytes. The stippling of the RBCs with different dot patterns is also important in differentiating between the four species. Thus, the size and shape of the various malarial forms, their alteration of RBC morphology, and the stippling pattern in the RBCs provide the identification of the particular type of malaria. Quantitation of the level of parasitemia is also important. Marked parasitemia is a poor prognostic sign for *P. falciparum* infection. However, ill patients may have relatively low levels of parasitemia due to trapping of organisms in capillaries. PCR is starting to be used for the diagnosis of malaria and is particularly useful when low levels of parasitemia make it difficult to identify individual species. A rapid immunodiagnostic test for malaria may also be useful in settings where microscopy is not immediately available. **Table 5–5** summarizes the relevant laboratory information for the diagnosis of malaria.

Babesiosis
Description
Babesia species are protozoa that, like *Plasmodium* species, infect erythrocytes. They are delivered to the infected host by the same tick (*Ixodes*) that transmits the agent of Lyme disease and human granulocytic anaplasmosis. Babesiosis mimics malaria, in that it causes hemolysis, fever, anorexia, and hemoglobinuria. In the United States, *B. microti* is responsible for most cases of human babesiosis. In Europe, *B. bovis* and *B. bigemina* have been implicated as agents of human disease. Babesiosis occurs mainly in the Northeast and upper Midwest in the United States. It affects patients of all ages, but most cases occur during the sixth and seventh decades of life. The infection from *Babesia* tends to be self-limited. In most cases, it lasts from weeks to months, following an incubation period of 1 to 6 weeks. Mild symptoms, including malaise, fever, and headache, characterize the disease in normal hosts, but asplenic patients often develop severe infections with high levels of parasitemia. Transfusion-transmitted babesiosis is a significant concern because blood donors

Babesia are protozoa that, like *Plasmodium* species, infect erythrocytes. They are delivered to the infected host by the same tick (*Ixodes*) that transmits the agent of Lyme disease.

TABLE 5–5 **Laboratory Evaluation for Malaria**

Laboratory Test	Results/Comments
Identification of organisms within RBC in blood smears	First-line test in the diagnosis of malaria; for best results, blood should be collected from the patient during or after a febrile episode and before the administration of antiparasitic medications; to rule out malaria, it is recommended that negative results be demonstrated in blood samples collected every 6–12 h for 24 h
	Preparation of smears: thick and thin blood smears should be prepared; thick smears allow for a rapid examination of a relatively large volume of blood and have approximately a 10-fold increase in sensitivity over thin smears; thin smears allow for superior preservation of morphology and are needed for species determination; the best stain is the aqueous Giemsa stain buffered with phosphate to pH 7.2
	Reading of smears: no single criterion except for the crescentiform (banana-shaped) gametocyte of *Plasmodium falciparum* is pathognomonic; multiple morphologic criteria are used to determine the species of *Plasmodium*; it is very difficult to speciate when mixed *Plasmodium* infections occur or only small numbers of rings are present; PCR can be used to confirm identification when morphology is not definitive
Quantitation of parasitemia	Reported as percent of RBC parasitized or as number of parasites per 100 WBC; quantitation should be repeated after treatment to monitor effectiveness
Rapid immunodiagnostic test	Useful in settings where microscopy is not immediately available; detects *Plasmodium* spp. and *P. falciparum*
PCR	Mainly used for speciation rather than as a front-line test

may have subclinical/asymptomatic infections, and Babesia screening tests are still in the investigational stage. [*N Engl J Med.* 2016;375:2236–2245.]

Diagnosis

The laboratory diagnosis rests upon the identification of the *Babesia* organisms inside erythrocytes in stained thick and thin peripheral blood smears. There are a number of morphologic features that differentiate *Babesia* from *Plasmodium*. Despite its relative shortcomings, serologic testing for *B. microti* can be performed as noted in **Table 5–6**. The level of parasitemia with *Babesia* does not always correlate with the severity of symptoms.

Viral Infections of the Blood

Overview

Many viruses such as varicella zoster virus (VZV), measles, enteroviruses, and arboviruses (such as West Nile virus) exhibit a viremic phase. These viruses also exhibit organ-specific manifestations and are discussed in other sections of this chapter. Cytomegalovirus (CMV), Epstein–Barr virus (EBV), and parvovirus B19 are discussed below because they are common viruses that can have a direct effect on the blood (e.g., mononucleosis or anemia) or their presence in blood is associated with opportunistic infections in immunosuppressed patients.

Infectious Mononucleosis/Epstein–Barr Virus

Description

Most cases of mononucleosis are caused by EBV, a member of the herpesvirus family, which infects B lymphocytes and causes them to proliferate. This in turn stimulates the proliferation of cytotoxic T cells that control the active infection but do not eradicate the latent state. Although infection with EBV is extremely common, the majority of individuals have asymptomatic infections. Patients with infectious mononucleosis typically present with fever, sore throat, and enlarged cervical lymph nodes.

The diagnosis of EBV-associated infectious mononucleosis is usually confirmed by a positive serum heterophile antibody test that detects the presence of antibodies that agglutinate horse or cow erythrocytes.

TABLE 5–6   Laboratory Evaluation for *Babesia*

Laboratory Test	Results/Comments
Identification of organism in RBC on blood film	Primary method of diagnosis; differentiating features in infected RBC suggesting *Babesia* rather than *Plasmodium* include (1) a tetrad of structures that resembles a "Maltese cross" and (2) the absence of pigment granules
Indirect immunofluorescent testing for antibodies to *B. microti*	A titer of >1:64 is considered indicative of exposure to the organisms, and a titer of >1:256 is diagnostic for an acute *Babesia* infection; at titers <1:256, the result does not clearly differentiate between patients who were exposed in the past and those who are actively infected
PCR amplification	Useful for confirming identification in low-level infections or detecting very low numbers of organisms; available in reference laboratories

TABLE 5–7   Evaluation for Infectious Mononucleosis

Laboratory Tests	Comments
Heterophile antibody tests	Heterophile antibodies are IgM antibodies reactive with antigens on the cells from multiple species, and on this basis are termed heterophilic; they are detected in agglutination assays with horse or sheep RBCs or by their capacity to induce an agglutination response on antigen-coated latex particles; in infectious mononucleosis, the heterophile antibody test result is positive approximately 1 week after the symptoms first appear; the highest titers appear in the second to third week of the illness; relatively high titers persist for up to 8 weeks
Antibodies to EBV-specific antigens	Although heterophile-negative infectious mononucleosis is uncommon, it does occur, mostly in young children; in these cases, a characteristic clinical picture and the presence of IgM against the EBV viral capsid antigen (VCA-IgM) or a rising titer of VCA-IgG can confirm acute infection, whereas a negative VCA-IgM and positive VCA-IgG and positive EBNA antibodies (EBV nuclear antigen) indicate past infection
WBC differential	Patients with mononucleosis typically have a mild-to-moderate leukocytosis after the first week, with more than 60% of the WBCs as lymphocytes and 10% to 20% of all lymphocytes being atypical; the maximum percentage of atypical lymphocytes appears between days 5 and 10 after the onset of symptoms, with a decrease to normal by approximately 3 weeks in most patients

EBV, Epstein–Barr virus.

In addition to mononucleosis, EBV is associated with two types of human tumor (Burkitt lymphoma and nasopharyngeal carcinoma) and is responsible for lymphoproliferative disorders in patients with severe immunosuppression following organ transplantation or AIDS. It also causes oral hairy leukoplakia in HIV-infected patients.

Diagnosis

Large atypical lymphocytes (cytotoxic T cells) are usually present in peripheral blood smears of patients with infectious mononucleosis caused by EBV, but they are also found in many other infections. The diagnosis of EBV-associated infectious mononucleosis is usually confirmed by a positive serum heterophile antibody test that detects the presence of antibodies that agglutinate horse or cow erythrocytes. The heterophile test is often negative in young children or in patients with atypical presentations; EBV-specific serologic tests are especially important in establishing the diagnosis in these situations. Quantitation of EBV DNA in peripheral blood is important in the diagnosis and management of EBV-associated lymphoproliferative disease in solid organ and bone marrow transplant recipients.

The use of laboratory tests in the diagnosis of infectious mononucleosis is shown in **Table 5–7**.

Cytomegalovirus

Description

CMV causes several clinical syndromes. It infects leukocytes, where it remains latent in immunocompetent individuals but readily reactivates in immunosuppressed individuals. CMV is a

TABLE 5–8 **Laboratory Testing for Cytomegalovirus (CMV)**

Laboratory Test	Results/Comments
Conventional cell culture	Detection of CMV infection typically requires 7–28 days with conventional viral inoculation of cell cultures; CMV can be isolated from a variety of specimens including blood, bronchoalveolar lavage fluid, urine, and tissue
Shell vial culture	This is a modification of the conventional cell culture methodology for more rapid viral detection; viruses are detected earlier using this technique in which the specimen is inoculated onto the monolayer of cultured cells by low-speed centrifugation which enhances infectivity; infected cells are detected with fluorescently labeled antibodies; this assay often provides a positive result in 1-2 days
CMV antigen testing	The CMV "antigenemia" test detects CMV antigen in polymorphonuclear leukocytes using a monoclonal antibody; it has largely been superceded by quantitative PCR testing
Enzyme immunoassay (EIA) for IgM and IgG	Seroconversion from negative to positive or a significant rise in anti-CMV IgG titer provides evidence of infection; assays for anti-CMV IgM are available, but detection of anti-CMV IgM does not always indicate primary infection because the IgM can persist for up to 18 months; most adults are seropositive and therefore serologic tests have limited utility for diagnosis; serologic testing of donor and recipient is important for predicting risk of CMV infection in transplant recipients
Polymerase chain reaction (PCR)-based detection of CMV	DNA- and RNA-based detection is available for the detection of CMV in blood, body fluids, and tissues; quantitative assays are important for diagnosis of active infection in immunosuppressed patients; PCR is now generally preferred over culture in most situations because of increased sensitivity
Histopathology	Detecting viral inclusions or infected cells by immunohistochemistry is important in tissue such as lung or colon where it can be difficult to distinguish colonization from active infection

leading cause of opportunistic infections in transplant recipients and AIDS patients. In transplant recipients, it often presents as a nonspecific febrile illness, but it can also cause more invasive infections including esophagitis, hepatitis, colitis, pneumonitis, and retinitis, particularly in severely immunocompromised patients. CMV is also the most common congenital viral infection. It affects approximately 40,000 infants born each year in the United States. Hematogenous spread appears to be responsible for transmission of the virus to the fetus. Most congenital infections occur when the mother has a primary CMV infection during the pregnancy. Neonates can also acquire the infection from maternal breast milk. Approximately 10% of infants congenitally infected with CMV are symptomatic at birth. Common sites of involvement are liver, spleen, lungs, and central nervous system (CNS). Because specific antiviral therapy is available for treatment of these infants, rapid detection of CMV infection is necessary. Although most congenitally infected infants are asymptomatic at birth, approximately 10% to 15% will develop later problems such as hearing loss and other neurologic problems. In children and young adults, primary CMV infection can cause a mononucleosis-like illness.

> CMV is the most common congenital viral infection. It affects approximately 40,000 infants born each year in the United States.

Diagnosis

The detection of CMV in blood and tissues generally correlates with active disease, whereas detection of CMV in urine is not necessarily diagnostic of active CMV disease, even in immunocompromised patients. Quantitative PCR assays of CMV DNA in blood (viral load assays) are more useful than qualitative assays. High levels of CMV correlate with increased risk of serious opportunistic infections in a variety of organs; however, the interpretation of CMV viral loads depends on the underlying condition (e.g., solid organ transplant vs. hematopoietic stem cell transplant vs. AIDS). Congenital CMV infection is established when CMV is isolated from the urine of neonates who are less than 3 weeks of age. CMV serology is used to determine whether donors and/or recipients are latently infected with CMV. This has important implications for preventing subsequent infections. For example, a seronegative individual who receives a transplant from a seropositive donor has the highest risk of developing CMV infection. Diagnostic testing for CMV is summarized in **Table 5–8**.

Parvovirus B19

Description

Parvovirus B19 is a small single-stranded DNA virus that is transmitted by respiratory droplets. It is a common cause of infection in children in whom it causes a distinctive rash known as fifth disease. In young adults, it often causes a significant arthropathy. An unusual feature of this virus is that it replicates in erythroid precursor cells and causes a temporary cessation of RBC production until the virus is cleared by the immune system. In normal hosts this has little, if any, consequence, but in patients who have a chronic hemolytic anemia such as sickle cell disease or hereditary spherocytosis, parvovirus B19 infection causes a transient aplastic crisis in which there is a profound drop in the hematocrit. Parvovirus B19 can also cause a chronic anemia in immunocompromised patients who are unable to clear the virus. Intrauterine infection of the fetus can cause a severe anemia that leads to congestive failure and hydrops fetalis.

Diagnosis

Acute parvovirus infection can be confirmed by demonstration of IgM antibodies or detection of viral DNA by PCR. During a transient aplastic crisis, the reticulocyte count decreases to <0.1% even as the hematocrit is declining.

ENDOCARDITIS: INFECTION OF THE HEART

Description

The clinical features of infectious endocarditis, a microbial infection of the valvular or nonvalvular endothelium of the heart, depend on the type of organism, location, and type of valve. Acute infective endocarditis can present with temperatures ≥103°F, shaking chills, rapid worsening of valve function, and a variety of septic embolic complications. Subacute bacterial endocarditis is more clinically variable and is characterized by low-grade or absent fever (as a result of infection by low-virulence organisms) and a variety of nonspecific signs and symptoms such as anorexia, weight loss, and malaise. Acute bacterial endocarditis typically occurs on native heart valves. It is most often caused by virulent organisms such as *S. aureus*, beta-hemolytic streptococci, and less commonly by *S. lugdunensis*, enterococci, and *S. pneumoniae*. Subacute bacterial endocarditis is usually caused by viridans group streptococci, enterococci, and fastidious gram-negative rods from the oral cavity. Several difficult-to-grow organisms are associated with "culture-negative" endocarditis. Prosthetic valve endocarditis is often caused by coagulase-negative staphylococci but can also be caused by *S. aureus*, other skin flora, enteric gram-negative rods, and fungi.

There are a number of risk factors for endocarditis, particularly in the acute form. These include diabetes, alcoholism, intravenous drug use, malignancy, infections in other sites, and immunosuppression. Anatomic defects also predispose patients to the development of infectious endocarditis. Such defects include mitral valve prolapse, congenital or rheumatic heart disease, and calcific aortic stenosis. The worst prognosis among patients with valvular disease is associated with those who have aortic valve involvement. The mitral valve, however, is the most frequently involved. Most individuals with endocarditis are between 45 and 60 years of age.

Diagnosis

The clinical and laboratory features of bacterial endocarditis are summarized in **Table 5–9**. Laboratory confirmation of infective endocarditis usually involves isolation of the same organism from multiple blood cultures. Organisms are more likely to be isolated from blood cultures in patients who have acute bacterial endocarditis because they have a high-grade persistent bacteremia. If three sets of blood cultures are obtained, the blood cultures are positive in more than 99% of patients who have not received antibiotics. At least two sets of blood cultures should be obtained by separate venipunctures at presentation. The erythrocyte sedimentation rate is a nonspecific test that is almost always elevated in cases of endocarditis, but it is useful for monitoring the response to therapy. It is not uncommon to obtain negative blood cultures in patients who meet the clinical and echocardiographic criteria for infectious endocarditis. Many of these "culture-negative" cases are due to prior antibiotic therapy. In the past, the "HACEK" group of fastidious oral gram-negative

TABLE 5–9   Evaluation of the Patient with Infective Endocarditis (IE)

Microbiology[a]	Isolation of microorganisms consistent with IE from 2 separate blood cultures (collect 3 sets): e.g., *Staphylococcus aureus*, viridans group streptococci, community-acquired enterococci, HACEK group; serology for non-cultivatable organisms (e.g., *Coxiella*)
Echocardiography[a]	Echocardiogram positive for IE (e.g., vegetation on valve or supporting structure, abscess)
Clinical findings	Fever >38°C; vascular phenomena (e.g., arterial emboli, septic pulmonary infarcts, intracranial hemorrhage, conjunctival hemorrhages, and Janeway lesions); immunological phenomena (e.g., glomerulonephritis, Osler nodes, Roth spots)
Other potentially useful laboratory tests	Elevated WBC, markedly elevated C-reactive protein, and/or erythrocyte sedimentation ratio (can be used to monitor response to therapy).[b] Molecular methods are useful for "culture-negative" cases caused by agents such as *Bartonella* and *Tropheryma*.
Evaluation of excised valve tissue	Histopathology with H&E and special stains (Gram stain and GMS); molecular testing (broad-range or targeted PCR, available in reference labs) is more sensitive than Gram stain and culture[c]

[a]Microbiology and echocardiography results are "major" criteria in the AHA Modified Duke Criteria (*Circulation*. 2015;132:1435–1486).

[b]*Eur Heart J.* 2005;26:1873–1881.

[c]*J Clin Microbiol.* 2017;55:2599–2608.

rods was linked to culture-negative endocarditis, but these organisms are readily detected by modern blood culture systems. More recently, interest has focused on *Coxiella burnetii*, *Bartonella* spp., *Tropheryma whipplei*, and *Brucella* spp. as potential causes of "culture-negative" endocarditis. These agents can be detected by a combination of serologic and/or molecular methods.

> Laboratory confirmation of infective endocarditis usually involves isolation of the same organism from multiple blood cultures. Organisms are more likely to be isolated from blood cultures in patients who have acute bacterial endocarditis because they have a high-grade persistent bacteremia.

INFECTIONS OF THE CENTRAL NERVOUS SYSTEM

Overview

Many organisms can produce an infection within the CNS. The major sites of infection are the meninges and brain parenchyma. Most organisms gain access to the CNS by hematogenous spread or by direct extension from an adjacent site. Bacterial infections can cause acute meningitis or may lead to formation of a brain abscess. Viral infections can present as meningitis or encephalitis, but often both sites are involved and the infection is more appropriately described as meningoencephalitis. Both fungi and mycobacteria can cause chronic meningitis while several parasites can cause intracerebral mass lesions. Each of these syndromes is often associated with specific organisms, information that can be used to guide the diagnostic workup. Rational test ordering based on clinical presentation is particularly important in patients with CNS infections since diagnostic specimens are difficult to obtain and are often present in limited quantities. **Table 5–10** provides information on organisms that are frequently known to cause meningitis and/or encephalitis, and the clinical characteristics of each of these infections.

> Many organisms can produce an infection within the CNS. The major sites of infection are the meninges and brain parenchyma. Most organisms gain access to the CNS by hematogenous spread or by direct extension from an adjacent site.

Acute Bacterial Meningitis

Description

Bacterial meningitis may present as a progressive illness over several days, or as a fulminant process that develops within hours. There is no single clinical sign that is pathognomonic of meningitis. Adolescents and adults typically present with combinations of fever, headache, nuchal rigidity, and other meningeal signs, and a decreased level of consciousness that can range from lethargy to coma; however, these findings are not present in all patients. Neonates and infants often present with nonspecific signs such as irritability, while nausea and vomiting are frequent complaints in children. Confusion, often without fever, is a common presenting sign in the elderly.

In most cases, the bacteria responsible for meningitis are acquired through the upper respiratory tract and then invade the blood. From the blood, they can then seed the meninges. There are a variety of factors that increase the risk for development of meningitis. These include splenectomy, sickle cell disease, cerebrospinal fluid leak, fistula or shunt, recent neurosurgical procedure, and infection contiguous to the CNS.

TABLE 5–10   Laboratory Evaluation for Meningitis and Encephalitis

Disease/Organism	Age of Highest Incidence	Higher Incidence in	Primary Diagnostic Test(s) on CSF	Other Tests of Potential Use
Bacteria				
Group B *Streptococcus* (*Streptococcus agalactiae*)	<1 month	Neonates	Gram stain and culture	Rapid antigen detection, mainly useful for partially treated infection; commercial NAAT panel
Streptococcus pneumoniae	All ages >3 months	Hypogammaglobulinemia	Gram stain and culture	Rapid antigen detection, mainly useful for partially treated infection; commercial NAAT panel
Escherichia coli and other gram-negative bacteria (75% of *E. coli* cases are K1 strains)	<1 month and >60 years	Immunocompromised	Gram stain and culture	Rapid antigen detection for *E. coli* K1, mainly useful for partially treated infection; commercial NAAT panel
Listeria monocytogenes	<1 month and >60 years	Immunocompromised	Gram stain and culture	Commercial NAAT panel
Haemophilus influenzae (type b very rare due to vaccination, other capsule types are occasionally seen)	1 month to 5 years	Immunocompromised; unvaccinated	Gram stain and culture	Rapid antigen detection, mainly useful for partially treated infection, commercial NAAT panel
Neisseria meningitidis	1 month	Patients with complement deficiencies	Gram stain and culture	Rapid antigen detection, mainly useful for partially treated infection; commercial NAAT panel
Mycobacteria, especially *M. tuberculosis*	≥1 month	Immunocompromised	Acid-fast stain (rarely positive) and AFB culture	Nucleic acid amplification
Treponema pallidum	Adults	Tertiary syphilis patients	VDRL (relatively poor sensitivity)	Several tests for syphilis available (see the section "Syphilis")
Pseudomonas aeruginosa	All ages	Neurosurgical postoperative patients	Gram stain and culture	
Staphylococcus aureus	All ages	Neurosurgical postoperative patients	Gram stain and culture	
Coagulase-negative staphylococci	All ages	Neurosurgical postoperative patients	Gram stain and culture	
Other streptococci	All ages	Neurosurgical postoperative patients	Gram stain and culture	
Fungi				
Cryptococcus neoformans/gattii	Adults	Immunocompromised	Lateral flow assay for capsular antigen; fungal culture	Capsular antigen immunoassays are much more sensitive than India ink
Coccidioides immitis	Adults	Immunocompromised; those living in the southwestern United States, parts of Latin America	Serologic testing of serum and CSF	CSF culture lacks sensitivity; PCR
Histoplasma capsulatum	Adults	Immunocompromised; those living in the Ohio and Mississippi River Valleys, and parts of Central America	Histoplasma antigen EIA	CSF culture lacks sensitivity; serologic testing of serum and CSF
Viruses				
Enteroviruses (includes echovirus and coxsackievirus)	All ages including infants	Late summer and early fall	RT-PCR	Yes—viral culture using throat swab, and stool; CSF culture less sensitive than RT-PCR

(Continued)

TABLE 5-10   (Continued)

Disease/Organism	Age of Highest Incidence	Higher Incidence in	Primary Diagnostic Test(s) on CSF	Other Tests of Potential Use
Herpes simplex virus-1	All ages including infants	Can be primary or reactivation infections	PCR	Serologic testing (rarely performed); histochemical staining and/or culture of brain biopsy (rarely performed)
Herpes simplex virus-2	Neonates	Infant of infected mother (also recurrent aseptic meningitis in adults)	PCR	
Cytomegalovirus	All ages	Immunocompromised	PCR	Antigen detection in circulating WBCs; serum test for antibody to virus Shell vial culture of CSF or tissue
Arboviruses	Peak age group varies for the different viruses in this group	Depends on specific virus; geographic and seasonal variation linked to insect vector, usually mosquitoes or ticks	RT-PCR for early infection (<7 days) with WNV; IgM after 7 days	Serologic tests on serum and CSF for less common encephalitis viruses
Rabies virus	All ages	Individuals bitten or scratched by rabies-prone animal	Contact public health lab	Fluorescent antibody test on punch biopsy of skin from nuchal region; virus neutralization assay on serum or CSF, RT-PCR on saliva
Measles virus	Childhood	Nonvaccinated individuals recently exposed to measles infection	Not routinely performed	See section on measles
Mumps virus	Childhood	Nonvaccinated individuals recently exposed to mumps infection	Not routinely performed	See section on mumps
Varicella zoster virus	All ages	Immunocompromised	PCR	
Epstein–Barr virus	Children, adolescents, and young adults	Immunocompromised	PCR	

The organisms responsible for acute bacterial meningitis are highly dependent on the age of the patient and the clinical setting. *S. agalactiae* (group B *Streptococcus* [GBS]), *E. coli*, or *Listeria monocytogenes* are responsible for most cases of neonatal and infant meningitis. *S. pneumoniae* and *N. meningitidis* are responsible for most cases of community-acquired bacterial meningitis in children and adults (widespread vaccination for *Haemophilus influenzae* type b has nearly eliminated this previous childhood scourge). Elderly patients are at increased risk of infection with *L. monocytogenes* and aerobic gram-negative rods. In contrast, staphylococci and gram-negative rods are major causes of CNS shunt infections and postneurosurgery nosocomial infections. Knowledge of these patterns is important when deciding on empiric antibiotic therapy.

Diagnosis

Examination and culture of CSF is essential. There is usually a markedly elevated WBC count with a preponderance of neutrophils, elevated protein, and decreased glucose (relative to the blood level). Gram stain of CSF reveals the causative organism in 70% to 90% of cases of pneumococcal and meningococcal meningitis. The percentage is generally lower for other bacteria. Bacterial culture is essential in all cases because it has the greatest sensitivity and specificity. Patients who have rapidly progressive or severe disease frequently receive a dose of antibiotics before a CSF specimen can be collected. Although this may cause a false-negative culture, it should have little or no effect on the cell count and differential, protein, glucose, and Gram stain. Immunoassays that detect *S. pneumoniae* and *N. meningitidis* capsular antigens in CSF are useful in these patients with partially treated meningitis, but they are *not* more sensitive than a Gram stain. The diagnosis of acute meningitis is likely to benefit from the recent introduction of commercial NAAT panels.

Acute Viral Meningitis

Description

Viral meningitis (often described as aseptic meningitis due to the absence of bacteria) presents with fever, headache, and meningeal signs. There may be a mildly decreased level of consciousness. At least 75% of these infections are caused by members of the enterovirus family that includes the coxsackieviruses and echoviruses. Arboviruses (arthropod-borne viruses), HSV-2, HIV, and many other viruses can also cause this syndrome. Both enterovirus and arbovirus infections exhibit seasonal variation; most cases occur in the summer and early fall. Viral meningitis is usually a self-limited illness with a generally good prognosis. This is fortunate since there are currently no clinically useful antiviral drugs that are active against the enteroviruses and arboviruses. The clinical diagnosis of viral meningitis is often not clear-cut because there can be parenchymal involvement leading to varying degrees of encephalitis (see below). In addition, several other conditions can cause a similar clinical syndrome. These include partially treated bacterial meningitis, neoplastic diseases that have spread to the meninges, and immune-mediated diseases. It is important to identify these conditions because each of them is treatable and requires specific therapy.

Diagnosis

Acute bacterial meningitis must be differentiated from viral and fungal meningitis. There is a significant difference in the CSF findings between viral and bacterial meningitis (**Table 5–11**).

In viral meningitis, CSF analysis usually reveals an elevated WBC count with a preponderance of mononuclear cells, elevated protein, and a normal glucose. Identification of the causative agent is best achieved through the use of specific nucleic acid amplification tests and/or immunoassays, depending on the specific virus; viral culture has a relatively poor yield in most cases and is not routinely used for diagnosis. Many clinical or reference laboratories offer NAAT assays for enteroviruses, HSV and other herpesviruses, and West Nile virus. Immunoassays for detection of virus-specific IgM and IgG are often used to detect other viruses. Bacterial culture and cytopathology examination may be indicated if the diagnosis is unclear.

Chronic Meningitis

Description

Patients suffering from chronic meningitis usually present with a variety of signs including low-grade fever, headache, lethargy, confusion, nausea, vomiting, and stiff neck that develop over a period of 1 to 4 weeks. Fungi and mycobacteria are responsible for many cases of chronic meningitis. The encapsulated yeast, *C. neoformans*, is one of the most common causes, particularly in patients with depressed cell-mediated immunity due to HIV infection or immunosuppressive therapy. *C. neoformans* is acquired by inhalation that usually causes an asymptomatic pulmonary infection. These organisms then spread to the CNS by the hematogenous route. *C. gattii*, previously classified as a subspecies of *C. neoformans*, often causes meningitis in patients who are not infected with HIV. *C. immitis* and *C. posadasii*, dimorphic fungi that are prevalent in the

> Viral meningitis (often described as aseptic meningitis due to the absence of bacteria) presents with fever, headache, and meningeal signs. At least 75% of these infections are caused by members of the enterovirus family that includes the coxsackieviruses and echoviruses.

TABLE 5–11   Typical Cerebrospinal Fluid (CSF) Findings in Meningitis[a]

	Normal	Bacterial	Viral	Fungal or Tuberculous
WBC (count/mL)	0–5	>100–5000	100–1000	50–500
Neutrophils (% of total WBC)	0–15	>80	<50[b]	<50
Glucose (mg/dL)	45–65	<40	45–65	30–45
CSF/blood glucose ratio	0.6	<0.4	0.6	<0.4
Protein (mg/dL)	20–45	>150	50–100	100–500

[a]Data from Segretti J, Harris AA. Acute bacterial meningitis. *Infect Dis Clin North Am*. 1996;10:797–809 and Derber CJ, Troy SB. Head and neck emergencies: bacterial meningitis, encephalitis, brain abscess, upper airway obstruction, and jugular septic thrombophlebitis. *Med Clin North Am*. 2012;96:1107–1126.

[b]The percentage of neutrophils can be elevated during early stages of infection.

southwestern United States, are also acquired by inhalation and have a predilection for infecting the meninges and CNS. Immunosuppressed patients who harbor *Mycobacterium tuberculosis* are at increased risk of CNS tuberculosis (TB). Neoplastic and immune-mediated diseases can also cause chronic meningeal symptoms; it is important to distinguish between these conditions and infection.

Diagnosis

The diagnosis of chronic meningitis requires evaluation of the CSF. Typically there are an increased number of mononuclear cells, mildly elevated protein, and normal glucose (except in TB). Immunoassays for *C. neoformans*/*C. gattii* capsular polysaccharide can be performed in less than an hour, have a very high sensitivity and specificity, and are superior to visual examination of India ink preparations (the antigen test does not distinguish between *C. neoformans* and *C. gattii*). Fungal culture should also be performed. If the patient is at increased risk of disseminated TB (i.e., purified protein derivative [PPD]-positive or a history of pulmonary TB), then the CSF should be tested for mycobacteria. AFB smears of CSF are quite insensitive. PCR of CSF can provide early confirmation of *M. tuberculosis* infection in many cases; however, culture should still be performed to obtain an isolate for susceptibility testing.

Encephalitis

Description

Viral encephalitis is an infection of the brain parenchyma that can produce permanent neurologic damage or death in persons of all ages. A higher incidence of viral encephalitis is found in young children, the elderly, and persons with impaired immunity. For some viruses, there is a seasonal variation for infection. Most of the viruses that produce encephalitis enter the CNS via the hematogenous route. In its mildest form, viral encephalitis can present with fever and headache, and in its most severe form as an acute fulminating disorder with seizures and death. Prominent clinical findings include altered level of consciousness, altered mental status, headache, seizures, and other signs of neurologic dysfunction. The most important cause of sporadic encephalitis is HSV-1 that often causes permanent neurologic damage or death. Fortunately, there is effective antiviral therapy for HSV encephalitis that can prevent most of these complications if given early in the infection. Arboviruses transmitted by mosquitoes are responsible for periodic epidemics of encephalitis. A dramatic example of this phenomenon was the appearance of West Nile virus in the eastern United States in the summer of 1999 and its subsequent spread across the country during the next 4 years. Arboviral encephalitis is usually a self-limited infection. Most patients recover, but a significant number have persistent neurologic symptoms. Amebas such as *Naegleria* should also be considered in the differential diagnosis of encephalitis since they require specific therapy. Autoimmune disorders, such as production of antibodies against the NMDA receptor, can also present with symptoms and signs suggestive of encephalitis.

> Viral encephalitis is an infection of the brain parenchyma that can produce permanent neurologic damage or death in persons of all ages. The most important cause of sporadic encephalitis is HSV-1 that often causes permanent neurologic damage or death.

Diagnosis

The diagnosis of viral encephalitis includes evaluation of CSF. In patients with viral encephalitis, there is a predominantly lymphocytic pleocytosis, with a slight to moderate elevation of CSF protein, and no change in glucose content from normal. However, there are variations, depending on the virus that produces the encephalitis. Some of the agents can produce CSF findings that mimic those of bacterial meningitis (e.g., pleocytosis with an increased number of neutrophils), particularly during the early stages of infection. The diagnosis of HSV encephalitis should be confirmed with a PCR assay of CSF that detects HSV DNA. This test is very sensitive and specific. Because of the severity of HSV infections and the availability of effective treatment, it should be performed on any patient with suspected encephalitis. Viral culture of CSF is insensitive and should not be routinely performed. Encephalitis caused by other viruses is often diagnosed by detection of viral nucleic acid or virus-specific IgM and IgG in serum or CSF.

Table 5–10 presents the laboratory evaluation for meningitis and encephalitis by disease and/or organism. Organisms not listed in the table also may cause CNS infections. Chapter 2 provides descriptions of many of the tests mentioned in the table.

Brain Abscess

Description

A brain abscess is a focal lesion and therefore presents differently from meningitis and encephalitis. The most common clinical presentation is persistent, worsening headache. More than half of patients will have focal neurologic deficits, but only half have fever. Bacterial abscesses can result from hematogenous dissemination or extension from an adjacent site. The most common organisms are viridans group streptococci such as *S. anginosus*, *Haemophilus/Aggregatibacter* spp., and anaerobic gram-negative rods. If the patient is immunosuppressed, then the abscess could be caused by *Aspergillus* or other fungi, *Nocardia* spp. or *Mycobacterium* spp., or *Toxoplasma gondii*. Neurocysticercosis, a mass lesion that results from infection with the pork tapeworm *Taenia solium*, often presents as new-onset seizures in an adult.

Diagnosis

Unlike other CNS infections, examination of CSF is unlikely to yield useful information and even performing a lumbar puncture may be contraindicated. The initial diagnosis is usually based on CT and MRI findings. Identification of the causative agent is important for guiding therapy. This usually requires stereotactic biopsy of the abscess to obtain material for microscopic examination and culture. Serologic assays performed on serum may be helpful in the diagnosis of *Toxoplasma* infections and neurocysticercosis.

BONE INFECTIONS/OSTEOMYELITIS

Description

Osteomyelitis is an infection of the bone characterized by progressive, inflammatory destruction of the bone tissue. It can be classified by the route of infection (hematogenous, contiguous spread, direct traumatic, or surgical inoculation), the site of infection, the type of patient, or duration of infection (acute or chronic). Hematogenous osteomyelitis is most common in prepubertal children, where it usually involves the long bones, and older adults where it usually involves the vertebrae. Less common sites of osteomyelitis include the sternoclavicular and sacroiliac joints, and symphysis pubis. Children with acute osteomyelitis appear ill with fever, chills, localized pain, and leukocytosis. In contrast, adults with vertebral osteomyelitis often have a subacute course with slowly worsening back pain and little or no fever or leukocytosis. Hematogenous osteomyelitis is usually caused by a single organism. *S. aureus* accounts for half of cases. Other frequently encountered organisms are streptococci and enterobacteriaceae in neonates, gram-negative rods in the elderly, *Salmonella* spp. in patients with sickle cell disease, *P. aeruginosa* in intravenous drug users, and *Candida* spp. in patients with intravascular catheters. TB and brucellosis can cause vertebral osteomyelitis in patients who have been exposed to these organisms.

> Osteomyelitis caused by a contiguous focus of infection often results from an injury associated with an open fracture or following surgery for reconstruction of bone.

Osteomyelitis caused by a contiguous focus of infection often results from an injury associated with an open fracture or following surgery for reconstruction of bone. It is also common in patients with poorly controlled diabetes mellitus due to peripheral neuropathy and vascular insufficiency. This form of osteomyelitis is found almost exclusively in the foot and starts insidiously in areas of traumatized skin. The infection of the skin may be easily overlooked as the organism makes its way to the bones in the toes, metatarsal heads, and tarsal bones. Unlike hematogenous osteomyelitis, these contiguous focus infections are usually polymicrobial involving combinations of staphylococci, streptococci, enterococci, and gram-negative rods. Additional classes of organisms may be present in the wound if the injury site was contaminated with soil. With between 500,000 and 1,000,000 hip replacements per year worldwide, infections associated with prosthetic joints are also common (see the section "Infections of the Joints").

Diagnosis

Imaging techniques can be used to detect osteomyelitis in the early phase and reveal the extent of damage to bones and joints. Definitive diagnosis requires biopsy and culture of the infected tissue in most cases. This permits an accurate identification of the organisms responsible for the osteomyelitis. In some situations, the organisms suspected of causing osteomyelitis may be identified

TABLE 5–12 Organisms Associated with Osteomyelitis and Populations at Risk

Organism	Population with Highest Incidence or Predisposing Condition
Staphylococcus aureus	All ages, including infants and children; most frequent organism causing hematogenous osteomyelitis
Salmonella spp.	Sickle cell disease patients; immunocompromised individuals
Pseudomonas aeruginosa	Intravenous drug abusers; those with a puncture wound to the foot; patients with urinary catheters
Aerobic gram-negative rods (e.g., *Enterobacter* and *Proteus*)	Urinary tract infections, diabetic foot infections, or vascular insufficiency
Aerobic streptococci	Patients with bites, diabetic foot lesions, or vascular insufficiency
Anaerobic streptococci	Patients with foreign body-associated infections such as those induced by prosthetic joints (chronic infection), bites, diabetic foot lesions, or decubitus ulcers
Mycobacterium tuberculosis	Patients with a history of pulmonary tuberculosis; immunocompromised individuals
Fungal species (includes *Candida* and *Aspergillus*)	Patients with catheter-related fungemia; intravenous drug abusers; immunocompromised individuals

from the culture of synovial fluid, blood, or biopsy of contiguous lesions. Microbiologic culture of blood or contiguous tissue does not definitively identify the organism in the bone, but it may provide a strong indication of the organisms responsible for the osteomyelitis.

Table 5–12 lists the organisms most likely to cause osteomyelitis and identifies the populations at risk for infection by the named organisms.

INFECTIONS OF THE JOINTS

Description

Acute pain and swelling in the joint can be produced by infectious agents, crystals of monosodium urate or other compounds, and a variety of less common causes. Because some organisms can destroy cartilage in a matter of days, the diagnosis of infectious arthritis must be made quickly. Organisms can seed the joint through the hematogenous route (from intravenous drug abuse, indwelling catheters, or endocarditis), through direct inoculation from intra-articular injections or arthroscopy, or from a contiguous site of infection, especially the bones and bursae. Septic arthritis can resemble a variety of noninfectious processes, but an acutely inflamed joint should be considered septic until proved otherwise. Septic arthritis is most often monoarticular with polyarticular involvement in less than 20% of the cases.

> The mainstays of the laboratory investigation for a joint infection are synovial fluid Gram stain and culture to identify infecting organisms, and polarized microscopy of the synovial fluid to identify crystals in crystal-induced arthritis.

Diagnosis

The mainstays of the laboratory investigation for a joint infection are synovial fluid Gram stain and culture to identify infecting organisms, and polarized microscopy of the synovial fluid to identify crystals in crystal-induced arthritis. It should be noted, however, that crystal-induced and infectious arthritis can coexist. Synovial fluid WBC counts consistent with infection are ≥50,000/µL, with more than 90% as neutrophils. **Table 5–13** summarizes the organisms associated with joint infection and the relevant clinical features for each infection.

INFECTIONS OF THE SKIN AND ADJACENT SOFT TISSUE

Overview

Many different organisms can produce infections of the skin and soft tissue. Clinical manifestations and severity vary widely and include aggressive, fast-moving infections such as necrotizing fasciitis, abscesses that require incision and drainage, chronic superficial fungal infections, and rashes that can be caused by local or systemic viral infections. A brief description of infections associated with

> Abscesses, infected wounds, and cellulitis are common acute infections of the skin. The most common organisms are *S. aureus*, group A beta-hemolytic streptococci, other streptococci and staphylococci, and several gram-negative rods.

TABLE 5–13   Evaluation for Organisms Associated with Infections of the Joints

Organism	Population with Highest Incidence and/or Predisposing Conditions	Clinical Features	Laboratory Tests
Staphylococcus aureus	Damaged joint; cutaneous abscess; intravenous drug abuse; prosthetic joint	Most common cause of septic arthritis; can produce rapid destruction of the joint	Gram stain of synovial fluid is positive in majority of cases
Selected streptococcal species (excluding *Streptococcus pneumoniae*)	Diabetes mellitus	Second most common cause of septic joint after *S. aureus*; from benign to severe, depending on the specific organism and predisposing conditions	Gram stain and culture of synovial fluid and blood cultures reveal infecting organism in majority of cases
Coagulase-negative staphylococci	Prosthetic joint	Inflammation and tenderness around a prosthetic joint	Gram stain and culture of synovial fluid, with blood cultures, may reveal organism
Cutibacterium (Propionibacterium) acnes	Prosthetic joint	Commonly affects prosthetic shoulder joints; pain and stiffness	Prolonged incubation (10–14 days) improves recovery of organism; sonication of prosthetic material may increase yield of culture
Neisseria gonorrhoeae	Young adults	May have genitourinary findings of gonococcal infection; dermatitis and synovitis not uncommon	Gram stain of synovial fluid is positive in 25%–30% of cases; synovial fluid culture is positive in 25%–50% of cases; blood culture is positive in 10%–15% of cases
Gram-negative bacilli (pathogens include *Pseudomonas aeruginosa, Serratia, Klebsiella,* and *Enterobacter,* which may be specific for certain joints)	Immunocompromised patients; urinary or biliary tract infection; intravenous drug abusers (especially for *Pseudomonas*); prosthetic joint; SLE and sickle cell disease (especially for *Salmonella*)	Up to 20% of septic arthritis cases are caused by gram-negative organisms	Gram stain of synovial fluid reveals organisms in about 50% of cases; culture of synovial fluid and blood also may lead to organism identification
S. pneumoniae	Splenic dysfunction	Accounts for <5% of septic arthritis cases	Gram stain and culture of synovial fluid and blood cultures reveal infecting organism in majority of cases
Mycobacterial species (includes *M. tuberculosis* and *M. marinum*)	Earlier tuberculous infection reactivated by age or immunosuppression	Up to 50% of patients with *M. tuberculosis* joint involvement also have pulmonary tuberculosis	Culture of synovial fluid or synovial tissue may reveal organism
Fungal species (pathogens include *Sporothrix, Cryptococcus, Blastomyces, Coccidioides,* and *Candida*)	Alcoholism; myeloproliferative disorders	*Sporothrix* is the most common cause of fungal arthritis; *Cryptococcus* and *Blastomyces* infections may be associated with adjacent osteomyelitis; blastomycosis arthritis may be associated with pulmonary infection	Repeated cultures of synovial fluid and tissue are often required for identification of the organism; a calcofluor fungal smear of synovial fluid may be helpful
Borrelia burgdorferi (Lyme disease agent)	Patients with Lyme disease or history of tick exposure	Intermittent attacks of swelling in a large joint	One of several tests for Lyme disease (see the section "Lyme Disease")

SLE, systemic lupus erythematosus.

particular organisms is provided in **Table 5–14**. The diagnostic information to identify infecting organisms is also included in the table. Lyme disease and *Bartonella* infections are discussed in **Tables 5–15** and **5–16**. A number of other infectious diseases, such as syphilis and herpes simplex infections, also have skin manifestations and are more fully described elsewhere in this chapter.

Acute Bacterial Infections

Abscesses, infected wounds, and cellulitis are common acute infections of the skin. The most common organisms are *S. aureus*, group A beta-hemolytic streptococci, other streptococci and

TABLE 5-14   Selected Skin and Soft Tissue Infections Caused by Bacteria

Skin/Soft Tissue Infection	Description	Predisposing Condition(s)	Etiologic Agent(s)	Clinical Findings	Laboratory Diagnosis
Superficial folliculitis	Infection of hair follicles of the skin	Poor hygiene, occupational exposure to oils and solvents	*Staphylococcus aureus* most common	Single or multiple superficial, dome-shaped, pruritic pustules at the ostium of hair follicles on the scalp, back, and/or extremities	Diagnosis usually made clinically; Gram stain and bacterial cultures support the clinical diagnosis
Hot tub folliculitis	Infection of hair follicles of the skin	Whirlpools and hot tubs with low chlorine, high pH, and high water temperatures	*Pseudomonas aeruginosa*	Small erythematous pruritic papules topped by pustules in areas submerged in hot water	Clinical diagnosis supported by bacterial culture and Gram stain of infected pustule or water source
Furuncle	Acute bacterial infection of perifollicular skin, usually from preexisting folliculitis	Skin areas subject to friction and perspiration, poor hygiene, occupational exposure to grease or oil, malnutrition, alcoholism, and immunosuppression	*S. aureus*	Indurated, dull red, tender nodule with central purulent core on the face, buttocks, perineum, breast, and/or axilla	Diagnosis usually made clinically; Gram stain and culture of suppurative lesion support the clinical diagnosis
Carbuncle	Coalescence of interconnected furuncles; involves subcutaneous tissue with drainage at multiple sites	For untreated furuncles, complications include bacteremia, endocarditis, and osteomyelitis	*S. aureus*	Multiple abscess formations separating connective tissue septae with drainage to surface along hair follicles	Diagnosis usually made clinically; Gram stain and culture of suppurative lesion support the clinical diagnosis
Paronychia	Infection of the nail folds	Minor trauma causing break in the skin, as produced by splinters Chronic: frequent immersion of hands in water	Acute: staphylococci, beta-hemolytic streptococci, gram-negative enteric bacteria Chronic: *Candida albicans*	Tender, red, swollen areas extending around the nail fold with or without pus	Clinical diagnosis supported by bacterial and/or fungal cultures of infected areas
Impetigo contagiosa (nonbullous)	Localized purulent infection of the skin	Children (2–5 years old) living in warm, humid climates; poor hygiene; preexisting superficial abrasions from insect bites, trauma, and other causes	Group A beta-hemolytic streptococci and *S. aureus*	Small superficial vesicles that form pustules rupture, forming characteristic yellow-brown, "honey-colored" crusted lesions	Clinical diagnosis supported by culture/Gram stain of base of early lesion positive for staphylococci and/or streptococci; anti-DNase B and antihyaluronidase titers may be elevated
Bullous impetigo	Localized purulent infection of the skin causing bullous lesions	Occurs in newborns and younger children on nontraumatized skin of the buttocks, perineum, trunk, and/or face	Usually due to *S. aureus* producing exfoliative toxins	Begins as small vesicles that quickly enlarge to form bullae with clear fluid that rupture and leave a brownish black crust	Clinical diagnosis supported by culture/Gram stain of base of lesion or clear fluid from bullae showing staphylococci
Staphylococcal scalded skin syndrome (SSSS)	Widespread bullae and exfoliation as a severe manifestation of an infection by *S. aureus* strains producing exfoliative exotoxins	Higher incidence in newborns and younger children	*S. aureus* producing exfoliative exotoxins	Scarlatiniform rash with widespread tender bullae with clear fluid; bullae rupture, resulting in separation of skin; exfoliation exposes large areas of red skin	Diagnosis usually made clinically

(Continued)

TABLE 5–14   (Continued)

Skin/Soft Tissue Infection	Description	Predisposing Condition(s)	Etiologic Agent(s)	Clinical Findings	Laboratory Diagnosis
Ecthyma	A variant of impetigo on the lower extremities causing punched-out ulcerative lesions	May occur de novo or secondary to preexisting superficial abrasions such as insect bites; occurs in children and elderly most often	Usually group A beta-hemolytic streptococci	"Punched-out" ulcers with yellow crust extending into dermis, typically on lower extremities	Clinical diagnosis supported by culture and Gram stain of base of lesion that is positive for streptococci
Erythrasma	Superficial chronic bacterial infection of the skin	More common in males, obese patients, and patients with diabetes mellitus	*Corynebacterium minutissimum/C. amycolatum*	Slowly spreading pruritic, red brown macules with scales—affecting axillae, groin, and toes	Gram-stained imprints of skin lesions reveal gram-positive bacilli; examination of skin under Wood's lamp reveals distinctive red coral fluorescence
Erysipelas	Acute inflammation of superficial layers of the skin with lymphatic involvement	Occurs most often in infants, young children, and elderly; those with skin ulcers, local trauma/abrasion, and eczematous lesions; increased susceptibility in sites with impaired lymphatic drainage	Group A beta-hemolytic streptococci; rarely, group B, C, G streptococci and *S. aureus*	5%–20% facial, 70%–80% lower extremity; painful, bright red, edematous, indurated lesions with raised border, well demarcated from uninvolved skin; regional lymphadenopathy common	Difficult to culture group A streptococci from lesion; up to 20% of throat cultures positive for group A streptococci; blood culture positive in 5% of cases
Cellulitis	Diffuse suppurative inflammation of skin and subcutaneous tissues	Occurs in sites of previous tissue damage such as operative wounds, ulcers, and focal trauma; increased incidence in intravenous drug abusers	Nonimmunosuppressed hosts: commonly group A beta-hemolytic streptococci; less commonly *S. aureus*; group B and G streptococci in patients with lower extremity edema; gram-negative rods in immunosuppressed patients; *Pasteurella* in cat and dog bites; *Vibrio vulnificus* when wounds are exposed to marine environment	Localized, painful, erythematous, warm lesions, poorly demarcated from uninvolved skin; regional lymphadenopathy may be present; bacteremia and gangrene may occur if untreated	Gram stain/culture of purulent exudate from advancing edge may reveal etiologic agent; blood cultures positive in 25% of cases
Synergistic necrotizing cellulitis (nonclostridial anaerobic cellulitis)	A variant of necrotizing fasciitis (see following entities) involving skin, muscle, subcutaneous tissue, and fascia	Diabetes mellitus, obesity, advancing age, cardiac, and renal disease	Mixture of anaerobes (anaerobic streptococci and *Bacteroides* most commonly) and facultative bacteria (*Klebsiella, E. coli, Proteus*)	Acute onset of tender skin ulcers in lower extremity draining foul-smelling, red-brown ("dishwater") pus, with underlying gangrene of subcutaneous tissue and muscle; tissue gas in 25% of patients; systemic toxicity is significant	Culture/Gram stain of exudate aspirated from lesion

(Continued)

TABLE 5–14 (Continued)

Skin/Soft Tissue Infection	Description	Predisposing Condition(s)	Etiologic Agent(s)	Clinical Findings	Laboratory Diagnosis
Necrotizing fasciitis (Type I)	A deep-seated, severe necrotizing infection of the subcutaneous tissue, resulting in progressive destruction of superficial and, in some cases, deep fascia and fat	Diabetes mellitus, alcoholism, parenteral drug abuse; occurs at sites of trauma such as an insect bite, and following laparotomy performed in the presence of perineal soiling, decubitus ulcers, and perirectal abscesses	At least one anaerobic species (most commonly *Bacteroides* or *Peptostreptococcus*) along with a facultative anaerobic species such as streptococci or gram-negative enteric bacilli such as *E. coli, Enterobacter, Klebsiella,* and *Proteus*	Sudden onset of tender, warm, erythematous, well-demarcated cellulitis, usually involving the lower extremity, abdominal wall, perianal, and/or groin areas; sequential skin color changes from red-purple to patchy blue-gray over several days; within 3–5 days, skin breakdown occurs with bullae, a seropurulent exudate, frank cutaneous gangrene, and skin anesthesia; high fevers and systemic toxicity with early shock and organ failure common	Surgical exploration required to distinguish from cellulitis; leukocytosis, thrombocytopenia, azotemia, and increased serum levels of creatine kinase (CK) may be present; Gram-stained smears of exudates reveal a mixture of organisms; blood cultures are frequently positive; subcutaneous gas and soft tissue swelling detectable on radiographs
Necrotizing fasciitis (Type II) (also known as hemolytic streptococcal gangrene)	A deep-seated, severe, necrotizing infection of the subcutaneous tissue, resulting in progressive destruction of superficial and, in some cases, deep fascia and fat	Occurs in 50% of patients with streptococcal toxic shock syndrome; predisposing factors also include diabetes mellitus, long-term steroid therapy, cirrhosis, peripheral vascular disease, a recent history of minor trauma, stab wounds, and surgical procedures	Group A streptococci, either alone or in combination with other species, most commonly *S. aureus*	Sudden onset of tender, warm, erythematous, well-demarcated cellulitis, usually involving the lower extremity, abdominal wall, perianal, and groin areas; sequential skin color changes from red-purple to patchy blue-gray over several days; within 3–5 days, bullae develop with seropurulent exudate, frank cutaneous gangrene, and skin anesthesia; high fevers and systemic toxicity with early shock and organ failure	Surgical exploration required to distinguish from cellulitis; leukocytosis, thrombocytopenia, azotemia, and increased serum levels of CK may be present; Gram-stained smears of exudate reveal gram-positive cocci in chains; surgical debridement provides tissue for culture and Gram stain; subcutaneous gas and soft tissue swelling present on radiograph
Clostridial anaerobic cellulitis	A necrotizing clostridial infection of devitalized subcutaneous tissue with rare involvement of deep fascia or muscle	Dirty or inadequately debrided traumatic wounds; preexisting localized infection; contamination of surgical wounds	Clostridial species, usually *Clostridium perfringens*	Localized edema of wound site; thin, foul-smelling drainage of wound with minimal pain, extensive gas formation in tissues, and frank crepitant cellulites	Gram stain of drainage shows numerous blunt-ended, thick, gram-positive bacilli and variable numbers of neutrophils; soft tissue radiographic films show abundant gas

(Continued)

TABLE 5–14 **(Continued)**

Skin/Soft Tissue Infection	Description	Predisposing Condition(s)	Etiologic Agent(s)	Clinical Findings	Laboratory Diagnosis
Clostridial myonecrosis (gas gangrene)	Rapidly progressive infection characterized by muscle necrosis and systemic toxicity caused by potent clostridial exotoxins	Wounds associated with trauma and open fractures such as gunshot wounds; intestinal and biliary tract surgery	*C. perfringens* accounts for 80% of cases; other species include *C. septicum*, *C. novyi*, and *C. sordelli*; the toxins released by these organisms are responsible for much of the morbidity and mortality associated with these infections	Sudden onset of severe pain at the site of a wound with rapid progression to localized tense edema and pallor; crepitance is a late finding and is neither a sensitive nor a specific feature; as the lesion progresses, the skin progresses to magenta or brown discoloration with brown serosanguinous discharge and "mousey" odor	Surgical exploration critical in demonstrating devitalized muscle tissue; CT scan shows gas in the muscle and in fascial planes with soft tissue swelling; Gram stain of exudate shows typical gram-positive or gram-variable rods with spores and lysed or absent neutrophils; with *C. perfringens*, organism shows typical boxcar appearance without spores on Gram stain, "double-zone hemolysis" on anaerobic blood plate, and lecithinase activity (alpha-toxin); elevated CK, LDH, and myoglobin due to myonecrosis
Spontaneous or nontraumatic gas gangrene	Rapidly progressive infection characterized by muscle necrosis and systemic toxicity caused by clostridial infection	Hematologic malignancies, colon cancer, diabetes mellitus, peripheral vascular disease; commonly with no obvious portal of entry; not associated with traumatic or surgical wounds	Most cases due to *C. septicum*	Sudden onset of pain and localized swelling of extremity, followed by discoloration, blister formation, and crepitance; associated fever, abdominal pain, vomiting, and diarrhea	Surgical exploration critical in demonstrating myonecrosis; CT scan shows gas in the muscle and fascial planes with soft tissue swelling; Gram stain of exudate shows typical gram-positive or gram-variable rods with spores and lysed or absent neutrophils; elevated CK, LDH, and myoglobin due to myonecrosis

CT, computed tomography; LDH, lactate dehydrogenase.

staphylococci, and several gram-negative rods. Certain underlying conditions, such as diabetes and peripheral vascular disease, predispose to polymicrobial infections involving gram-positive cocci and gram-negative rods.

Cat/dog and human bite wounds are commonly infected with the above organisms, but they are also associated with specific organisms (*Pasteurella multocida* and *Eikenella corrodens*, respectively).

Necrotizing fasciitis (usually caused by *S. pyogenes*) and clostridial myonecrosis (also known as gas gangrene) are uncommon, but they are life-threatening infections that require prompt surgical and medical intervention. Traumatic gas gangrene is usually caused by contamination of wounds by *Clostridium perfringens* (an anaerobic spore-forming gram-positive rod). Spontaneous gas gangrene is usually caused by *C. septicum*, often in patients with underlying gastrointestinal malignancies or neutropenia.

Lyme Disease
Description

The causative agent of Lyme disease is *Borrelia burgdorferi*, which is spread by the bite of a tick of the genus *Ixodes*. Lyme disease is the most common vector-borne infection in North America and in Europe. It can go unnoticed in some patients because the associated "flu-like" symptoms are not specific for the disease. Within days to weeks of infection, a distinctive skin rash, known as erythema migrans, appears. It is important to treat the patient at the time that this rash appears to prevent subsequent potential neurologic, cardiac, or musculoskeletal complications.

The causative agent of Lyme disease is *Borrelia burgdorferi*, which is spread by the bite of a tick of the genus *Ixodes*. Lyme disease is the most common vector-borne infection in North America and in Europe.

TABLE 5–15 Laboratory Evaluation for Lyme Disease

Laboratory Test	Results/Comments
Enzyme-linked immunoassay (ELISA)—total antibodies	Detects serum IgM and IgG that react with a sonicated extract of *B. burgdorferi*; used as a screening test; because of the potential for false-positive reactions a positive EIA is followed by Western blot in the CDC-recommended 2-step algorithm; EIA can also be used to determine CSF/serum indices
Indirect immunofluorescence assay (IFA)	This assay also detects serum antibodies against *B. burgdorferi*; it has been replaced by EIAs in most laboratories
Western blot analysis	This assay detects serum antibodies to specific antigens of *B. burgdorferi* as a qualitative yes/no answer; the results should be interpreted according to CDC guidelines: a positive IgG blot is defined as the presence of antibodies that react with at least 5 out of 10 specific proteins; a positive IgM blot is defined as the presence of antibodies that react with at least 2 out of 3 specific proteins; Western blots can also be performed on CSF
Anti-C6 ELISA	A recently developed ELISA that detects antibodies against a highly immunogenic, highly conserved epitope of *B. burgdorferi*; more sensitive than the 2-step algorithm (because of low sensitivity of the Western blot in early Lyme disease) but slightly less specific than the 2-step algorithm
PCR analysis	May be useful for testing CSF or joint fluid in selected cases

CSF, cerebrospinal fluid; PCR, polymerase chain reaction.

Diagnosis

Unlike many infections, this laboratory diagnosis is rarely based on culture of *B. burgdorferi*. This is because there are few organisms in clinical specimens, and these organisms require specialized media for growth with prolonged incubation. Therefore, the diagnosis rests upon a characteristic clinical findings picture supported by positive serologic tests for *B. burgdorferi*. In patients who present with erythema migrans, the diagnosis is straightforward. However, for many patients with less specific symptoms and equivocal serologic test results, it is difficult to make a definitive diagnosis. The traditional approach for serologic testing for Lyme disease consists of a screening EIA utilizing a whole cell sonicate, followed by a confirmatory Western blot immunoassay which requires the presence of specific diagnostic bands (see Chapter 2 for a description of these assays). There are several important issues regarding the use serologic assays to diagnose Lyme disease:

- The serologic tests are not entirely specific for Lyme disease.
- Serum samples collected in the early stage of the disease may not contain antibodies to the organism because there is little or no antibody production in many patients until 3 to 4 weeks after the onset of the illness.
- The immune response is variable, and treatment with antibiotics can reduce the magnitude of the response.

Cross-reactivity between the antigens from *B. burgdorferi* and antigens from other organisms may occur. For example, false-positive serologic reactions for Lyme disease have been reported in patients with RMSF, leptospirosis, and syphilis. False-positive reactions can also occur in some patients with autoimmune diseases. The development of newer serologic assays such as those based on the C6 peptide may replace parts of the standard algorithm.

PCR-based assays for detection of *B. burgdorferi* DNA may be useful for testing joint fluid or CSF. Only properly validated assays should be used since in a low-prevalence population (i.e., patients with nonspecific symptoms and no history of a tick bite) the positive predictive value can be very low. A summary of the different assays currently available for diagnosis of Lyme disease is provided in **Table 5–15**.

Cat-Scratch Disease and Bacillary Angiomatosis

Descriptions

Several organisms of the genus *Bartonella* were found to be associated with human disease in the 1990s when they were identified as the etiologic agents in cat-scratch disease and bacillary angiomatosis. Most cases of cat-scratch disease are caused by *B. henselae* (other *Bartonella* spp. and *Afipia felis* may account for a small percentage of these cases). Initially a papule or pustule forms at the site of the scratch, but most individuals seek medical attention several weeks later because of the development of a regional lymphadenopathy (mainly in the neck or upper extremity). In most cases, it resolves spontaneously, although in rare cases severe complications can occur, including encephalitis, conjunctivitis, and neuroretinitis. Bacillary angiomatosis is a disorder in which there are distinctive and potentially lethal vascular proliferative responses in the skin, the bones, and other organs. Bacillary angiomatosis is most commonly diagnosed in individuals infected with HIV.

> Several organisms of the genus *Bartonella* were found to be the etiologic agents in cat-scratch disease and bacillary angiomatosis.

Diagnosis

A further description of cat-scratch disease and bacillary angiomatosis and recommendations for their diagnosis are included in **Table 5–16**. Serologic tests and PCR-based tests may be useful to support the histopathologic findings from lymph node biopsies in cat-scratch disease and from skin biopsies in bacillary angiomatosis. *Bartonella* spp. are difficult to culture.

Fungal Infections

Fungal infections of the skin can be characterized as superficial, cutaneous, and subcutaneous. Infections caused by fungi such as *Malassezia* spp. are limited to the superficial layers of the skin and can result in patchy alteration of pigmentation. The more invasive cutaneous infections caused by dermatophytes and subcutaneous infections are discussed in the following sections.

Descriptions

The dermatomycoses (also known as ringworm) are skin infections caused by dermatophytes. These organisms are closely related fungi that invade keratinous tissues such as skin, hair, and the fur of animals. The dermatophytes are classified into three genera, *Epidermophyton*, *Microsporum*, and *Trichophyton*. Dermatophyte infections are named according to the anatomic location (in Latin) for the body site, following the word "tinea." For example, tinea pedis is a dermatophyte infection of the foot. The diagnosis of a dermatophyte infection is made by microscopic examination of a scraping of the lesion and by culturing the specimen on selective agar that inhibits the growth of commensal bacteria and other fungi. When organisms are successfully grown in culture, they are identified to the species level by colony and microscopic morphology.

TABLE 5–16   Evaluation for Cat-Scratch Disease and Bacillary Angiomatosis

Infection	Description/ Clinical Findings	Predisposing Conditions	Etiologic Agents	Laboratory Diagnosis
Cat-scratch disease	Regional lymphadenopathy that develops 2–3 weeks after contact with a cat in the presence of a scratch or eye lesion; usually persists for 2–4 months	History of contact with cat	Most cases are caused by *Bartonella henselae* (rare causes include other *Bartonella* spp. and *Afipia felis*)	Lymph node biopsy with characteristic appearance (stellate necrotizing granulomas); Warthin–Starry silver stain may reveal bacilli, but only in a small percentage of specimens; diagnosis is supported by detection of antibodies to *B. henselae* in serum; PCR for *B. henselae* DNA useful in atypical cases
Bacillary angiomatosis	A disease with proliferative vascular lesions caused by infection with small gram-negative organisms of the genus *Bartonella*; cutaneous lesions: papular red nodules; bacillary angiomatosis lesions also can occur in bones, liver, spleen, CNS, and other sites	AIDS patients, especially those with low CD4 cell counts; history of contact with cat or exposure to lice	*B. henselae* (from cats) and *B. quintana* (transmitted by lice)	Skin biopsy with a characteristic vascular proliferation and numerous bacilli detected on Warthin–Starry stain; organisms can be isolated from blood using special isolator tubes and grown in culture

CNS, central nervous system; PCR, polymerase chain reaction.

Sporotrichosis is a chronic infection characterized by nodular lesions in cutaneous and subcutaneous tissues and adjacent lymphatics. This infection is caused by *Sporothrix schenckii*, a dimorphic fungus that is typically introduced by traumatic implantation into the skin (e.g., during gardening). Sporotrichosis commonly displays a lymphocutaneous pattern as it tracks up the lymphatic system in the hand and arm. Rare manifestations include pulmonary and disseminated infections. Histologic examination of a specimen will often reveal granulomatous inflammation, but organisms are rarely seen. Therefore, diagnosis usually depends on culturing the specimen to permit microbiologic isolation of the *S. schenckii* organisms.

Mycetoma is a chronic infectious disease that involves cutaneous and subcutaneous tissues, fascia, and bone, and remains localized. It is characterized by draining sinuses, with aggregates of the etiologic agent in the pus draining from the sinuses. The fungi that produce the mycetoma are associated with woody plants and soil. The organisms are usually introduced by traumatic inoculation into the skin. A tumor-like deforming disease can develop during subsequent years if untreated. Dozens of fungal organisms have been documented as causes of mycetoma. In the United States, the most common agent is *Pseudoallescheria boydii*. The asexual form of this organism is known as *Scedosporium apiospermum*. Other fungi predominate in tropical and subtropical areas. The fungal elements are most often found in the center of a suppurative and granulomatous lesion that develops in a deep site and extends out to the skin for drainage. Draining sinuses appear in essentially all patients within 1 year of the initial trauma. Identification of the causative agent is made by fungal smear and culture of the material draining from the sinus tracts. Clinically similar infections are caused by filamentous gram-positive bacteria in the genus *Nocardia*. It is important to identify the infecting agent because the therapy for fungi is very different from that used for bacteria.

Chromomycosis is a subcutaneous infection by organisms originating in the soil, with only rare cases of dissemination. It is most often seen in tropical or subtropical environments and is rare in the United States. The lesions typically appear on the lower extremities. They are pink, scaly papules that expand to form a superficial nodule, and their presence suggests the diagnosis. Examination of the lesions microscopically in potassium hydroxide (KOH) or calcofluor white preparations can be diagnostic. Without therapy, which is usually surgical, the scaly papules grow to form nodules with a verrucous and friable surface.

Diagnosis

A further description of the infections and the tests used to identify the associated organisms are included in **Table 5–17**.

Viral Infections with Prominent Skin Manifestations
Overview

Systemic viral infections can cause a variety of macular, papular, or vesicular rashes. Many of these typically occur in the pediatric age range and may be associated with systemic signs and symptoms. Enteroviruses and parvovirus B19 are discussed in other sections.

Varicella Zoster Viral Infection
Description

Primary infection with VZV causes chickenpox, a vesicular rash that occurs predominantly on the trunk, scalp, and face. This disease is usually self-limited, with the symptoms resolving after 7 days. Varicella can also produce pneumonia, with pulmonary symptoms manifested approximately 4 days after the varicella rash. After primary infection, the virus enters the latent phase and remains in sensory ganglia. On reactivation, which occurs in a minority of adults, it produces herpes zoster, a vesicular rash that occurs along a dermatome distribution. The incidence of varicella has been declining since the introduction of a live virus vaccine.

Diagnosis

Chickenpox and herpes zoster are diagnosed clinically in most cases because of the characteristic presentation of the diseases. Laboratory tests for the VZV virus, although they represent the gold

Primary infection with varicella zoster virus causes chickenpox, a vesicular rash that occurs predominantly on the trunk, scalp, and face. This disease is usually self-limited, with the symptoms resolving after 7 days.

TABLE 5-17   Evaluation for Superficial, Cutaneous, and Subcutaneous Fungal and Mycobacterial Infections

Disease/ Dermatomycosis	Etiologic Agent(s)	Clinical Findings	Anatomic Pathology	Microbiology
Tinea versicolor (pityriasis)	*Malassezia furfur*	Hypopigmented or hyperpigmented macules on trunk or proximal limbs	Skin biopsies may demonstrate yeast forms with short hyphae	Round yeast forms and short hyphae visible by direct microscopy of lesion scrapings
Tinea capitis (scalp ring worm)	*Trichophyton, Microsporum*	Pruritic, scaly, erythematous lesions associated with alopecia on the scalp	Skin biopsies usually not necessary; if performed, hyphae may be visible in biopsy material	Wet hair or skin smears treated with KOH or calcofluor white reveal hyphae; culture on selective agar that contains cycloheximide
Tinea barbae	*Trichophyton verrucosum*	Pustular lesions in bearded areas	Skin biopsies usually not necessary; if performed, hyphae may be visible in biopsy material	Wet hair or skin smears treated with KOH or calcofluor white reveal hyphae; culture on selective agar that contains cycloheximide
Tinea corporis (body ring worm)	*Epidermophyton, Microsporum,* or *Trichophyton*	Sharply demarcated skin lesions on trunk and/or legs that contain pustules or papules and have prominent edges	Skin biopsies usually not necessary; if performed, hyphae may be visible in biopsy material	Wet hair or skin smears treated with KOH or calcofluor white reveal hyphae; culture on selective agar that contains cycloheximide
Tinea cruris ("jock itch")	*Trichophyton rubrum* or *Epidermophyton floccosum*	Localized rash with scaly lesions that involve anterior aspect of thighs; pustules and papules may be present	Skin biopsies usually not necessary; if performed, hyphae may be visible in biopsy material	Wet hair or skin smears treated with KOH or calcofluor white reveal hyphae; culture on selective agar that contains cycloheximide
Tinea manum	*Trichophyton rubrum*	Dry infection of the palmar surface of the hand	Skin biopsies usually not necessary; if performed, hyphae may be visible in biopsy material	Wet hair or skin smears treated with KOH or calcofluor white reveal hyphae; culture on selective agar that contains cycloheximide
Tinea pedis (athlete's foot)	*T. rubrum, Trichophyton mentagrophytes,* or *E. floccosum*	Pruritic foot lesions that may peel and crack and form vesicles or pustules	Skin biopsies usually not necessary; if performed, hyphae may be visible in biopsy material	Wet hair or skin smears treated with KOH or calcofluor white reveal hyphae; culture on selective agar that contains cycloheximide
Chronic mucocutaneous candidiasis	*Candida albicans* most common	Uncommon disorder caused by selective inability of T lymphocytes to respond to *Candida* antigens (linked to defects in IL-17 signaling); plaque-like patches with erythematous borders	Persistent circumscribed hyperkeratotic skin lesions, crumbling dystrophic nails; yeast and pseudohyphae	Demonstration of yeast and pseudohyphae on KOH smear with confirmation by culture; identification of *Candida* species requires biochemical tests
Sporotrichosis (usually involves cutaneous and subcutaneous tissues and adjacent lymphatics)	*Sporothrix schenkii*	Papulonodular, erythematous lesions in distal extremities; secondary lesions along lymphatic channels	Skin biopsies of involved lesions reveal a granulomatous response and, in some cases, cigar-shaped yeast forms	Skin lesions may be cultured; blood cultures may be positive if sporotrichosis is multifocal
Mycetoma (madura foot)	*Madurella, Pseudallescheria boydii,* other species	Foot or hand infection that extends from skin into deeper tissue; indurated swelling and multiple sinus tracts draining pus that contains aggregates of the fungus causing the disease; mainly limited to rural areas in tropical/subtropical countries	Hyphae may be visible in tissue or drainage using various stains; deep biopsies are preferred	Causative species inferred from organisms in sinus tract drainage
Chromomycosis (also known as chromoblasto-mycosis and many other names)	*Fonsecaea pedrosoi;* other species	Verrucous, cauliflower-like skin lesions, often pruritic; may result in secondary infection or lymphedema; mainly limited to rural areas in tropical/subtropical countries	Sclerotic bodies may be visible in stained tissue	Sclerotic bodies may be visible in exudates; culture confirmation recommended with Sabouraud agar
Skin infections caused by rapidly growing mycobacteria	*Mycobacterium fortuitum* complex and *M. abscessus* are the most common	Furunculosis, wound infections, injection site abscesses; failure to respond to commonly used antibiotics	Granulomatous inflammation; AFB stains are often negative	Isolation of organism usually requires procedures and growth media specific for mycobacteria
Mycobacterium marinum infection	*M. marinum*	Chronic cutaneous lesions, usually on hands, secondary to exposure to marine environments or fish tanks	Granulomatous inflammation; AFB stains are often negative	Isolation of *M. marinum* requires incubation of mycobacterial media at 30°C

AFB, acid-fast bacilli; KOH, potassium hydroxide.

TABLE 5-18   Evaluation for Varicella Zoster Virus (VZV) Infection

Laboratory Tests	Results/Comments
PCR analysis	Most sensitive method for detection of VZV in vesicular lesions and CSF (for suspected VZV encephalitis)
Direct immunofluorescence assay (DFA)	Used to detect VZV in vesicular rashes; cells at the base of a vesicular lesion are scraped from the skin and applied to a slide for direct immunofluorescent staining for VZV; more sensitive than culture but less sensitive than PCR
Antibody detection assays (mainly for IgG, include enzyme immunoassay and fluorescent anti-membrane antibody assay)	These tests are used to confirm immunity to VZV; often used to screen health care workers; may be important to know before and during pregnancy because a number of fetal anomalies are associated with primary VZV infection during pregnancy; commercial assays may not detect serological responses to VZV vaccine
Viral culture	Can be performed on vesicle fluid but considerably less sensitive than PCR or DFA; results are typically available within 7–21 days

CSF, cerebrospinal fluid; PCR, polymerase chain reaction.

standard for diagnosis, are typically unnecessary. Cutaneous lesions may be evaluated for the presence of VZV by direct immunofluorescence or PCR-based tests. Serologic testing is often important to determine whether an individual (e.g., a health care worker) has ever been infected with VZV and is therefore presumed to have immunity. Assays for VZV infection are summarized in **Table 5–18**.

Measles (Rubeola) and Rubella

Description

Rubeola and rubella infections are often confused because of the similarity in their names and similar clinical manifestations. Measles (or rubeola) is a highly contagious childhood disease characterized primarily by fever and a rash. The primary portal of entry for the rubeola virus is the upper respiratory tract. Approximately 14 days after exposure to the rubeola virus, a characteristic measles rash appears, and within 1 to 2 additional days there is a measurable amount of antibody to rubeola virus in the bloodstream. The leading cause of death in patients with measles is secondary bacterial pneumonia. Rubella, also known as German measles, is most often a mild illness in children and young adults. It is primarily of concern because infection of the fetus in early pregnancy can cause serious congenital abnormalities. Rubella is characterized by a rash and an enlargement of lymph nodes. Like the rubeola virus, the portal of entry of rubella virus is most often the respiratory tract. The availability of vaccines against measles and rubella has greatly decreased the incidence of these infections in the United States.

Rubeola and rubella infections are often confused because of the similarity in their names and similar clinical manifestations. Measles (or rubeola) is a highly contagious childhood disease characterized primarily by fever and a rash. Rubella, also known as German measles, is most often a mild illness in children and young adults.

Diagnosis

The laboratory diagnosis of measles or rubella can be important for epidemiologic surveillance purposes and to limit its transmission to susceptible individuals. The laboratory diagnosis is usually based on detecting virus-specific IgM in serum or isolation of the virus from urine or respiratory specimens. PCR-based assays are also available in selected public health laboratories.

Within 24 to 48 hours of the development of a rash, antibodies to rubella become detectable. Primary infection stimulates production of antibodies that confer lifelong immunity. It is for this reason that the presence of antibodies to rubella is desirable before initiating pregnancy. The antibodies can be demonstrated in a serologic test that indicates exposure to the rubella virus. Serologic testing is an important component of the evaluation of a pregnant woman with the clinical signs and symptoms of rubella. **Table 5–19** summarizes the laboratory evaluation for rubeola and rubella.

TABLE 5-19   Laboratory Evaluation for Measles and Rubella (German Measles)

Laboratory Tests	Results/Comments
Serology	Virus-specific IgM is detectable in serum a few days after appearance of rash; seroconversion or fourfold rise in IgG in convalescent serum also supports the diagnosis; presence of IgG provides evidence of immunity
RT-PCR and viral culture	Preferred specimen types are nasopharyngeal secretions and urine (these tests are available in specialized reference laboratories and public health laboratories)

EYE INFECTIONS

Description and Diagnosis

Infectious agents play a prominent role in many diseases of the eye. **Table 5–20** describes the infections of the eye according to anatomic site of infection within the eye. Many organisms that produce eye infections are described in detail in other sections of this chapter. The microbiologic tests for the detection and identification of the organisms listed in **Table 5–20** are presented in other sections of this chapter.

TABLE 5-20   Infections of the Eye and Causative Organisms

Infection	Clinical Features/Definition	Causative Organisms
Eyelid infections		
Hordeolum	An acute infection of either a meibomian gland or a gland of Zeis, also known as a sty	*Staphylococcus aureus*
Chalazion	A chronic granulomatous lesion on a meibomian gland	May arise from a hordeolum
Marginal blepharitis	Diffuse inflammation of the eyelid margins	*S. aureus* has been implicated
Infections of the lacrimal system		
Dacryoadenitis	Inflammation of the lacrimal gland	*S. aureus* most common; next most common is *Chlamydia trachomatis*, and rarely *Neisseria gonorrhoeae*
Canaliculitis	An inflammation of the canaliculi	*Actinomyces israelii*
Dacryocystitis	An infection of the lacrimal system occurring as a result of outflow obstruction in the nasolacrimal duct	Acute: *S. aureus*, *Streptococcus pyogenes*, *Streptococcus pneumoniae* in infants, *Haemophilus* spp. in children. Chronic: *Actinomyces*, *Aspergillus*, and *Candida*
Conjunctivitis	Infection of the conjunctiva; a very common ocular infection	
Viral	More common than bacterial conjunctivitis in developed countries	Adenovirus is the most common virus, with herpes simplex virus, influenza A virus, enterovirus 70, and coxsackievirus as other causative agents
Bacterial (nonchlamydial)	Hyperacute bacterial conjunctivitis is the most severe form of conjunctivitis	Hyperacute: *N. gonorrhoeae* common, but also *N. meningitidis* and *Corynebacterium diphtheriae*. Acute: *S. aureus*, *S. pneumoniae*, *Haemophilus influenzae* in children, *S. pyogenes*, and "*Haemophilus aegyptius*"; gram-negative bacillary infections are rare. Chronic: *S. aureus* is the most common agent with *Moraxella lacunata* and *Moraxella catarrhalis* also causative
Chlamydial	Two distinct presentations exist—trachoma is a leading cause of blindness in endemic areas of the world (repeated episodes of conjunctivitis lead to scarring and inward turning of lid, lashes cause corneal scarring); *Chlamydia*-induced inclusion conjunctivitis is usually much less severe	See the section "Chlamydial Infections"

(Continued)

TABLE 5–20   (Continued)

Infection	Clinical Features/Definition	Causative Organisms
Infectious keratitis	Infection of the cornea; can lead to loss of vision because of corneal scarring or because of progression to perforation and endophthalmitis	
Viral	Keratitis is almost always unilateral and may affect any age group	Herpes simplex virus is the most common cause of corneal ulcers in the United States
Bacterial	Bacteria causing conjunctivitis may invade the cornea following minor trauma to the corneal epithelium; contact lens wear is a predisposing factor for bacterial keratitis	Coagulase-negative staphylococci, *S. aureus*, *Pseudomonas aeruginosa*, *S. pneumoniae*, and viridans streptococci
Fungal	This is a rare entity accounting for less than 2% of infectious keratitis cases	*Aspergillus*, *Candida*, and *Fusarium* are the most common, with geographic variation
Parasitic	Most cases are in contact lens wearers	*Acanthamoeba* is the most common cause of parasitic keratitis in industrialized countries
Endophthalmitis	Infection of the vitreous; a severe ocular infection with significant permanent impairment of vision as a result of the infection	
Postoperative	This occurs in most patients 1–3 days after cataract surgery	Coagulase-negative staphylococci, *S. aureus*, gram-negative bacilli, streptococci, and *H. influenzae*
Posttraumatic	The onset is rapid for virulent bacteria; onset is over weeks to months for fungal organisms	Coagulase-negative staphylococci, *Bacillus*, gram-negative bacilli, and fungi
Endogenous	This form of endophthalmitis does not follow surgery or trauma; usually a complication of bacteremia or fungemia	*S. aureus*, streptococci, gram-negative bacilli, *Candida*
Uveitis	Infection of the iris, ciliary body, and choroid (often with retinal involvement)	
Anterior	Presents with redness, eye pain, photophobia; most cases of anterior uveitis have a noninfectious immune-mediated etiology	
Viral		Herpes simplex 1 virus, varicella zoster virus, cytomegalovirus
Bacterial	Usually bilateral when associated with secondary syphilis	*Treponema pallidum* (syphilis)
Posterior	Visual impairment is main symptom	
Viral		Herpes simplex virus and the varicella zoster virus can cause acute retinal necrosis; cytomegalovirus retinitis mainly occurs in patients with AIDS
Bacterial		*T. pallidum* (syphilis) is rare; perform serologic tests for syphilis; also test CSF; *Mycobacterium tuberculosis* also rare
Fungal		*Candida*, *Cryptococcus*, *Histoplasma*
Parasitic		*Toxoplasma gondii* is a common cause; *Toxocara canis* mainly affects children

INFECTIONS OF THE LARYNX, PHARYNX, MOUTH, EAR, ORBIT, AND SINUSES

Description and Diagnosis

Upper respiratory infections are very common and are responsible for many visits to health care providers. The majority of the infections are caused by a number of viral and bacterial agents. **Table 5–21** describes the infections of the pharynx, larynx, mouth, ear, orbit, and sinuses. The table contains a brief description of the infections and their associated organisms as well laboratory studies that are useful for establishing a diagnosis.

TABLE 5–21   Infections of the Larynx, Pharynx, Mouth, Ear, Orbit, and Sinuses

Disease or Pathogen	Clinical Findings	Histopathology/ Radiology	Microbiology Testing	Common Pathogens
Laryngeal infections				
Laryngitis, acute	Hoarseness and occasional aphonia are associated with upper respiratory infections	Histopathologic and radiographic studies are not useful for routine diagnosis	Diagnosis usually on clinical features	Influenza viruses, rhinoviruses, adenovirus, parainfluenza viruses, *Streptococcus pneumoniae*, *Haemophilus influenzae*, and *Streptococcus pyogenes*
Laryngitis, tuberculous (laryngeal tuberculosis) (also see the section "Tuberculosis")	Cough, wheezing, hemoptysis, dysphagia, odynophagia; laryngeal lesions vary from ulcers to exophytic masses	Granulomatous changes and acid-fast organisms may be observed in laryngeal biopsy material; chest radiographs may reveal pulmonary tuberculosis	Laryngeal biopsy may be submitted for mycobacterial smears and culture	*Mycobacterium tuberculosis* (highly infectious)
Pharyngeal and oral infections				
Herpes gingivostomatitis	Painful, ulcerating vesicles in oral mucosa; fever, fetid breath, cervical adenopathy, drooling; usually in children less than 5 years old	Rapid diagnosis with Giemsa- or Wright-stained smears from lesion by identifying multinucleated giant cells (less sensitive than culture); Tzanck preparation; less sensitive than DFA or culture	DFA stain of moist lesion scrapings may be positive; can provide rapid diagnosis; less sensitive than culture; lesions may be cultured, usually for 24–48 h; PCR available in some labs (more sensitive than culture); serologic tests of acute and convalescent sera may aid in diagnosis	Herpes simplex virus is the agent of primary infection
Herpes labialis, recurrent	Painful, ulcerating vesicles beginning on the outer lip (usually lower lip); fever usually absent	Rapid diagnosis with Giemsa- or Wright-stained smears from lesion by identifying multinucleated giant cells (Tzanck preparation); less sensitive than DFA or culture	DFA stain of moist lesion scrapings may be positive; can provide rapid diagnosis; less sensitive than culture; lesions may be cultured, usually for 24–48 h; PCR available in some labs (more sensitive than culture); serologic tests generally not useful	Herpes simplex virus is the agent of recurrent disease
Oral thrush (oral candidiasis)	Creamy white patches on the tongue and oral mucosa that bleed easily when scraped	Histopathologic studies are not useful for routine diagnosis	KOH or Gram-stained smears of oral lesions reveal pseudohyphae and yeast forms	*Candida albicans*
Streptococcal pharyngitis ("strep throat")	Pharyngeal pain, odynophagia, fever, chills, headache; anterior cervical adenopathy; purulent exudates, edema, and erythema in posterior pharynx	Histopathologic studies are not useful for routine diagnosis	Rapid antigen detection test (RADT) on throat swab (less sensitive than culture); culture of throat (posterior pharynx) swab is traditional gold standard; PCR-based tests provide a sensitive and rapid alternative	*S. pyogenes* (group A streptococci); groups C and G streptococci cause milder pharyngitis; infections of the throat by respiratory viruses may mimic strep throat clinically
Neisseria gonorrhoeae infection of the pharynx (see the section "Gonorrhea")				
Diphtheria	In its mildest form, asymptomatic carriage of organisms; formation of tough membrane over pharyngeal surface; also can cause skin lesions and damage to multiple organs	Histopathologic studies are not useful for routine diagnosis	Organisms from lesion can be grown in culture (specialized agar improves sensitivity)	*Corynebacterium diphtheriae*
The "common cold"	Nasal discharge and sinus congestion; often with pharyngeal and sinus pain; may be febrile with chills and headache	Not useful	Testing to rule out a bacterial infection, usually by culture of a throat swab specimen, is often performed when pharyngeal pain is present; multiplex nucleic acid amplification tests may be useful in patients with underlying risk factors	Rhinovirus, coronavirus, and adenovirus, among others

(Continued)

TABLE 5–21 **(Continued)**

Disease or Pathogen	Clinical Findings	Histopathology/ Radiology	Microbiology Testing	Common Pathogens
Ear, orbit, and sinus infections				
Otitis externa	Pruritic and painful outer ear, with an edematous and erythematous ear canal	If invasive otitis externa present, CT or MRI of head is useful for monitoring bone or tissue infection	Wound or external auditory canal specimens for Gram stain and culture	*Pseudomonas aeruginosa* (swimmer's ear), *Staphylococcus aureus*, and *S. pyogenes*
Otitis media	Ear pain, otorrhea, hearing loss with fever, irritability, headache, lethargy, anorexia, and vomiting	Histopathologic and radiographic studies are not useful for routine diagnosis	Diagnosis usually on clinical features; tympanic fluid obtained by tympanocentesis may be cultured	*S. pneumoniae*, *H. influenzae*, *Moraxella catarrhalis*, *S. pyogenes*, *S. aureus*, and selected viruses
Orbital cellulitis	Proptosis and eye pain; eyelid swelling, redness, warmth, tenderness	Cranial CT scan of sinuses and orbit may identify abscesses	Blood, conjunctival, and wound specimens for Gram stain and culture	*S. aureus*, *S. pyogenes*, *H. influenzae*, and *S. pneumoniae*
Periorbital cellulitis	Eyelid pain, swelling, and erythema with low-grade fever	Sinus radiographs or CT scan may exclude sinus disease	Blood, conjunctival, and wound specimens for Gram stain and culture	*S. pneumoniae*, *H. influenzae*, and anaerobic bacteria
Sinusitis (acute)	Persistent upper respiratory symptoms; purulent nasal discharge, fever, facial pressure or pain, facial erythema or swelling, and nasal obstruction	For complicated cases, CT scanning of paranasal sinuses is method of choice—presence of an air-fluid level correlates with bacterial infection	Usually a clinical diagnosis; sinus puncture aspirates are specimen of choice for Gram stain and culture; endoscopic sampling of exudates less likely to identify pathogens	*S. pneumoniae*, *H. influenzae*, and rhinoviruses

CT, computed tomography; KOH, potassium hydroxide; MRI, magnetic resonance imaging.

INFECTIONS OF THE LUNG AND PLEURAE

Overview

Many categories of organisms can cause pneumonia and other types of pulmonary infections. It is important to consider the clinical setting when evaluating and managing a patient with pneumonia because the types of organisms that are responsible depend on whether or not specific risk factors are present.

Community-acquired pneumonia is commonly caused by a few common bacterial agents including *S. pneumoniae*, *Mycoplasma pneumoniae*, *H. influenzae*, and *Legionella* spp. Although respiratory viruses, such as influenza, typically involve the upper airway, they often lead to subsequent bacterial infections in the lungs. In contrast to community-acquired pneumonia, hospital-associated and ventilator infections are likely to be caused by multidrug-resistant organisms including *K. pneumoniae*, *P. aeruginosa*, *A. baumanii* complex, and MRSA. *P. aeruginosa*, *Burkholderia cepacia*, and MRSA are also important causes of lung infections in patients with cystic fibrosis. In recent years there has been an increase in the number of *Bordetella pertussis* infections that has been attributed to waning immunity following the introduction of acellular pertussis vaccines.

Travel and/or exposure history can be an important clue in patients with persistent pulmonary signs and symptoms, as they may have TB or dimorphic fungal infections (described below). Patients with depressed cell-mediated immunity (e.g., transplant recipients or HIV infection) are at increased risk of *Pneumocystis* and CMV infections. Patients who have prolonged neutropenia from chemotherapy, for example, are at increased risk of invasive infections caused by *Aspergillus* spp. and other fungi.

Table 5–22 describes the infections of the lung and pleurae. The many different lung infections are grouped into bacterial, fungal, parasitic, and viral diseases. There are two major challenges in the laboratory diagnosis of pulmonary infections. First, it can be difficult to obtain respiratory specimens that are not contaminated with oropharyngeal flora. This is particularly true of expectorated sputum. It is one of the reasons why this type of specimen is routinely

It is very important to consider the clinical setting when evaluating and managing a patient with pneumonia because the types of organisms that are responsible depend on whether or not specific risk factors are present.

TABLE 5-22 **Infections of the Lung and Respiratory Tract**

Pathogen	Clinical Findings	Histopathology and Radiology	Microbiology Testing	Other Tests
Bacterial infections				
Bordetella pertussis (whooping cough)	Paroxysmal, nonproductive cough; low-grade fever, rhinorrhea; vomiting may follow cough	CXR may show pneumonia with consolidation	Cultures and/or PCR from nasopharyngeal specimens	Peripheral blood lymphocytosis often present; serology may be useful but requires acute and convalescent specimens
Burkholderia cepacia	Causes respiratory distress or progressive respiratory failure with high fever in cystic fibrosis patients (especially females)	CXR may show widespread infiltrates	Sputum from lower respiratory tract for Gram stain and culture with special media	
Moraxella catarrhalis	Tracheitis, bronchitis, sinusitis, and otitis media can all occur	In most cases, CXR findings are not prominent	Gram stain and culture from respiratory specimens	Serologic tests not useful
Chlamydia pneumoniae	Pharyngitis, hoarseness, fever, mild pneumonitis; atypical pneumonia, especially in the elderly	CXR usually reveals single subsegmental lesion; pleural effusion may be evident	PCR is preferred test for acute *C. pneumoniae* infection	IgM and IgG serologic tests can be useful; culture requires specialized cell lines, rarely performed
Chlamydia psittaci	Symptoms can include fever and chills, headache, myalgia, and nonproductive cough	CXR may show lobar or interstitial infiltrates	IgM and IgG serologic tests for antibody to the organism are the most common method (cross reactions occur with *C. pneumoniae*)	Culture is technically difficult (only available in a small number of laboratories), PCR is available in some public health laboratories
Coxiella burnetii (Q fever)	Causes atypical pneumonia with fever, severe headache, chills, sweats, myalgias; associated with exposure to livestock	CXR often shows multiple rounded opacities	Culture and PCR only performed in specialized or reference laboratories	IgM and IgG serologic tests for antibody to the organism most useful for initial diagnosis; normal WBC count; elevated smooth muscle autoantibodies often present
Klebsiella pneumoniae	Bronchitis, bronchopneumonia, or lobar pneumonia; "currant jelly" sputum; frequent complications such as abscess and empyema	CXR may reveal pattern of pneumonia and identify complications, if they arise	Sputum from lower respiratory tract for Gram stain and culture	
Haemophilus influenzae (nontypeable)	Pneumonia with fever, productive cough; often exacerbates chronic bronchitis	CXR may show interstitial or bronchopneumonia, or pneumonia with consolidation	Sputum or other lower respiratory tract specimen for Gram stain and culture	
Legionella pneumophila (also see the section "*Legionella* Infections")	Atypical pneumonia with slightly productive cough, fever, and chest pain; diarrhea often present	CXR typically shows alveolar infiltrates; pleural effusions common	Respiratory specimens cultured on selective media; urinary antigen test is rapid and sensitive for serogroup 1	Hyponatremia often present; PCR and serologic tests may be useful for diagnosis
Mycobacterium avium complex (and other nontuberculous mycobacteria)	In the non-HIV-infected patient, pulmonary disease with productive cough, fever, weight loss, and occasionally hemoptysis	CXR mimics reactivation tuberculosis with cavitation	Sputum from lower respiratory tract specimen for acid-fast stain and culture (must distinguish active disease from colonization)	In HIV-infected population, must distinguish atypical mycobacteria from *Mycobacterium tuberculosis* infection
M. tuberculosis (see the section "Tuberculosis")				
Mycoplasma pneumoniae	Often causes an upper respiratory tract infection with fever, malaise, headache, and nonproductive cough; may cause atypical pneumonia	CXR may show extensive infiltrates, out of proportion with symptoms	Commercial PCR and other NAAT tests are available for diagnosis of acute infection	IgM and IgG tests may be useful (require acute and convalescent serum); culture requires specialized techniques, not used for routine diagnosis

(Continued)

TABLE 5–22   (Continued)

Pathogen	Clinical Findings	Histopathology and Radiology	Microbiology Testing	Other Tests
Pseudomonas aeruginosa	Causes pneumonia in elderly, hospitalized, and cystic fibrosis patients; may be fulminant with chills, fever, dyspnea, excessive purulent sputum, and cyanosis	CXR may reveal diffuse bronchopneumonia; in bacteremic pneumonia, alveolar and interstitial infiltrates with cavitation may be seen	Sputum from lower respiratory tract for Gram stain and culture; blood cultures may be positive	Mucoid isolates often obtained from cystic fibrosis patients
Staphylococcus aureus	Pneumonia with fever, purulent sputum	CXR shows infiltrates, consolidation, abscesses, pleural effusions, and/or loculations	Sputum from lower respiratory tract for Gram stain and culture; pleural fluid or empyema if present should be cultured; blood cultures may be positive	Empyema is a frequent complication that requires drainage; pleural fluid very purulent with many neutrophils
Streptococcus agalactiae (group B streptococci)	Causes pneumonia in neonates and elderly; fever present; apnea, tachypnea, grunting, and cyanosis in neonates	CXR in neonates may show pulmonary infiltrates, often similar to hyaline membrane disease	Sputum from lower respiratory tract for Gram stain and culture	Pregnant carrier females may be screened by culture of vaginal and rectal swab specimens; nucleic acid amplification tests are an alternative
Streptococcus pneumoniae	Productive cough with rust-tinged sputum, fever, shaking chills, and pleuritic chest pain	CXR may show subsegmental infiltrations; segmental or lobar consolidation may be present; empyema is an uncommon complication	Sputum from lower respiratory tract for Gram stain and culture; blood cultures are often positive	Peripheral blood leukocytosis frequent; urine antigen test can provide rapid diagnosis (higher sensitivity in pneumonia with bacteremia)
Streptococcus pyogenes (group A streptococci)	Abrupt onset of pneumonia with fever, chills, dyspnea, pleurisy, and blood-tinged sputum	CXR reveals bronchopneumonia with consolidation	Sputum from lower respiratory tract for Gram stain and culture; blood cultures may be positive	Empyema is a frequent complication
Fungal infections (see the section "Dimorphic Fungi and Other Fungal Infections")				
Pneumocystis (see the section "*Pneumocystis jirovecii* Pneumonia")				
Viral infections				
Adenovirus	Pharyngitis or tracheitis with cough, fever, sore throat, and rhinorrhea; interstitial pneumonia may develop; diarrhea also may be present	Adenoviral eosinophilic inclusions may be visible in lung biopsies if they are obtained	Adenoviral culture from respiratory specimens; rapid viral antigen detection by DFA can be useful; nucleic acid amplification is useful	With serologic testing, a fourfold rise in titer is consistent with new infection
Coronaviruses	Human coronaviruses (229E, HKU1, NL63, OC43) generally cause self-limited upper respiratory symptoms, may be associated with fever; MERS-CoV (present in camels) can cause severe respiratory disease in humans	Patchy infiltrates or consolidations, ground-glass opacities seen in MERS (overlaps with other viral pneumonias)	RT-PCR for human coronaviruses available in commercial panels	RT-PCR for MERS available from public health labs
Cytomegalovirus (CMV)	Interstitial pneumonitis with nonproductive cough, fever, dyspnea, and hypoxia	CXR shows interstitial pneumonia; nodules or cavities may be seen; lung biopsies reveal CMV inclusions ("owl's eye" cells)	Viral cultures from respiratory specimens (bronchoalveolar lavage fluid or tissue); can also use PCR	Quantitative PCR assays using blood are preferred for diagnosis of disseminated disease
Hantavirus	Fever, severe myalgias, headache, tachypnea, and shortness of breath; rapidly progressive to hypotension, respiratory failure, and shock	CXR shows rapid progression to bilateral interstitial edema and diffuse alveolar disease; pleural effusions often present	Immunohistochemistry or PCR using blood or lung biopsy may confirm infection	IgM serologic tests by capture enzyme immunoassay or Western blot are diagnostic methods of choice

(Continued)

TABLE 5–22 **(Continued)**

Pathogen	Clinical Findings	Histopathology and Radiology	Microbiology Testing	Other Tests
Influenza A or B virus	Fever, chills, myalgias, headaches, dry cough; primary viral pneumonia may occur	CXR may show bilateral infiltrates	Nucleic acid amplification (RT-PCR) performed on nasopharyngeal specimens is most sensitive method; DFA plus viral culture is also useful	Rapid antigen detection tests have poor sensitivity, often less than 50%
Human metapneumovirus	Bronchiolitis and pneumonia similar to respiratory syncytial virus infections	CXR may show interstitial infiltrates or hyperinflation	Nucleic acid amplification (RT-PCR) performed on nasopharyngeal specimens is most sensitive method; DFA test is less sensitive; grows poorly in culture	
Parainfluenza viruses 1, 2, 3, and 4	Upper respiratory tract infections, otitis media, conjunctivitis, and pharyngitis; may cause croup or bronchiolitis	CXR is negative in cases with no pulmonary involvement	Nucleic acid amplification (RT-PCR) performed on nasopharyngeal specimens is most sensitive method; DFA plus viral culture is also useful	
Respiratory syncytial virus (usually infants and young children)	Pneumonia or bronchiolitis; fever, paroxysmal cough, dyspnea	CXR may show interstitial infiltrates or hyperinflation	Nucleic acid amplification (RT-PCR) performed on nasopharyngeal specimens is most sensitive method; DFA plus viral culture is also useful	Rapid antigen detection tests have moderate sensitivity (50%–80%)
Pleural empyema: most common organisms found are *S. pneumoniae*, *S. aureus*, *H. influenzae*, *S. pyogenes*, *P. aeruginosa*, *K. pneumoniae*, and *Bacteroides*	Chest pain, chills, persistent fever, right sweats	Thoracic CT scan usually permits definitive diagnosis; ultrasound distinguishes solid lesions from pleural fluid collections; CXR may show pleural fluid accumulations in lateral decubitus views	Pleural or empyema fluid should be cultured for aerobic and anaerobic organisms	Peripheral blood leukocytosis usually present; pleural fluid values often show fluid pH below 7, glucose below 40 mg/dL, and LDH exceeding 1000 IU/L

CXR, chest radiograph; LDH, lactate dehydrogenase; PCR, polymerase chain reaction; CT, computed tomography.

screened microscopically for the presence of squamous epithelial cells to determine whether it is a true lower respiratory specimen. The other problem is that there is no single test that detects all of the potential respiratory pathogens. While routine Gram stain and sputum culture readily detects *S. pneumoniae*, common gram-negative rods, and *S. aureus*, separate cultures and/or test methods are required to detect *Legionella*, mycobacteria, fungi, respiratory viruses, CMV, and *Pneumocystis*. These are discussed in more detail in the following sections.

Tuberculosis

Description

TB is a major cause of morbidity and mortality around the world and remains a major challenge for public health officials. Approximately one-fourth of the world's population is estimated to be infected with the causative agent, *M. tuberculosis*. This slow-growing AFB continues to be an important concern in industrialized countries because of the development of drug-resistant strains and a growing population of immunosuppressed patients who are at increased risk of TB. Although it can infect a variety of organs, *M. tuberculosis* primarily causes pulmonary disease. It is usually acquired by inhalation of infectious aerosolized droplets. The majority of primary infections are asymptomatic; however, the organisms are not completely eliminated. This leads to a quiescent phase known as latent tuberculosis infection (LTBI). Otherwise healthy individuals with LTBI have an approximately 10% lifetime risk of developing secondary or reactivation pulmonary TB. Prophylaxis of asymptomatic-infected individuals reduces the risk of subsequent reactivation TB.

Approximately one-fourth of the world's population is estimated to be infected with the causative agent, *M. tuberculosis*. Early identification of patients with active pulmonary TB is crucial for preventing transmission of this serious infection to other patients and to health care workers.

Clinical features of active pulmonary TB include fever, night sweats, weight loss, productive cough, and hemoptysis in later stages of the disease. Radiographic studies often show cavitary lung lesions, usually in the lung apices. It is important to realize that immunosuppressed patients who develop active TB often have atypical clinical presentations and can have nonspecific radiographic changes. Before the epidemic of HIV infection in the United States, approximately 85% of newly diagnosed infections with TB were limited to the lung, with 15% involving nonpulmonary sites or both pulmonary and nonpulmonary sites. With advanced HIV infection, less than half the cases are limited to pulmonary involvement. Extrapulmonary TB commonly involves the lymph nodes, pleura, genitourinary tract, bones and joints, meninges, peritoneum, and pericardium.

Early identification of patients with active pulmonary TB is crucial for preventing transmission of this serious infection to other patients and health care workers. Treatment of active TB caused by sensitive strains requires combination therapy for 6 months. Multidrug-resistant and extremely resistant *M. tuberculosis* (MDR-TB and XDR-TB, respectively) are more difficult to treat and have a poorer outcome.

Diagnosis

There are two categories of laboratory tests for TB: those that detect latent infection and those that detect active disease. Skin testing with PPD detects previous exposure to *M. tuberculosis*. A delayed-type hypersensitivity response to the *M. tuberculosis* antigens (mediated by T cells) leads to induration at the site of injection. One problem with the PPD test is that individuals who have been vaccinated with bacille Calmette–Guerin (BCG) can also have a positive reaction. BCG is derived from *M. bovis*, a member of the *M. tuberculosis* complex, and is widely used outside the United States. Recent advances in immunology and genomics have led to the development of alternatives to the PPD test, such as interferon-gamma release assays (IGRAs). Peripheral blood or purified mononuclear cells are incubated with antigenic peptides that are unique to *M. tuberculosis* (i.e., they are not present in BCG) and then an immunoassay is performed to measure production of interferon-gamma. The IGRAs are at least as sensitive as the PPD and are more specific since BCG vaccination does not produce a false-positive result.

The diagnosis of secondary/active TB depends on detection of *M. tuberculosis* in clinical samples. This testing is particularly important since the PPD and IGRAs can be negative in patients with active TB. Acid-fast staining of sputum specimens (using either a fuchsin [red] stain or a fluorescent stain) enables visualization of the mycobacteria in ~70% of cases of pulmonary TB. Detection of mycobacteria in sputum using an AFB stain provides only presumptive evidence of pulmonary TB in the presence of characteristic radiologic findings. The presence of *M. tuberculosis* must be confirmed by culturing the organism in liquid and/or solid media or by using NAATs. Modern automated liquid culture systems routinely detect growth of *M. tuberculosis* in 1 to 2 weeks versus 4 to 6 weeks with traditional cultures on solid media. These systems also make it possible to perform rapid susceptibility testing in liquid culture for first-line anti-tuberculous drugs. The NAATs make possible same-day confirmation of smear-positive specimens, which contain relatively large numbers of organisms. Culture remains the gold standard for detecting *M. tuberculosis* in smear-negative specimens, although NAAT tests, some of which can also detect resistance genes, continue to improve.

Table 5–23 includes the clinical and laboratory information relevant to the diagnosis of pulmonary and extrapulmonary TB.

Other nontuberculous mycobacteria, including slow-growing organisms such as *M. avium* complex and *M. kansasii*, and rapid growers, such as *M. abscessus*, can cause chronic pulmonary disease in both normal and immunocompromised hosts.

Legionella Infections

Description

Legionella pneumophila is a fastidious, slow-growing gram-negative rod. *Legionella* species are widespread in the environment and are a cause of community-acquired pneumonia. They are usually found in surface or potable water and are associated with moist environments. Approximately 6000 cases of *Legionella* pneumonia occur each year in the United States, although many additional cases are probably not diagnosed. Most cases occur sporadically, but outbreaks have

TABLE 5–23   Evaluation for Tuberculosis (TB)

	Pulmonary Tuberculosis	CNS Tuberculosis	Genitourinary Tuberculosis	Disseminated Tuberculosis
Clinical findings	Symptoms range from none to fever with productive cough and dyspnea; hemoptysis indicates presence of advanced disease	Fever, unremitting headache, nausea, and malaise; in the United States, elderly are frequently affected; where TB is common, it primarily affects children aged 1–5 years	Most common site for extrapulmonary TB is the kidney; dysuria, frequency, and hematuria are common; women may present with a chronic pelvic inflammatory process, menstrual irregularities, or sterility; men may present with an enlarging scrotal mass	More likely to occur in HIV-positive individuals; may be present without miliary pattern in chest radiographs; patient may present with fever, weight loss, and anorexia
Tests				
PPD or interferon-gamma release assay (IGRA for TB)	In the presence of compatible radiologic and clinical findings, a positive PPD in an unvaccinated patient, or a positive IGRA, suggests TB; a negative result does not exclude active infection	In the presence of compatible radiologic and clinical findings, a positive PPD in an unvaccinated patient, or a positive IGRA, suggests TB; a negative result does not exclude active infection	In the presence of compatible radiologic and clinical findings, a positive PPD in an unvaccinated patient, or a positive IGRA, suggests TB; a negative result does not exclude active infection	In the presence of compatible radiologic and clinical findings, a positive PPD in an unvaccinated patient, or a positive IGRA, suggests TB; a negative result does not exclude active infection
Microscopy	Acid-fast bacilli in sputum smears permit rapid diagnosis; sensitivity is variable, approximately 70% if 3 specimens are tested	Acid-fast bacilli in smears of CSF have relatively low sensitivity (10%–30%); sputum samples also should be tested	Both urine and sputum samples should be examined; acid-fast bacilli in smears of urine have relatively low sensitivity (14%–39%)	Urine, lymph node, liver, bone marrow, and sputum smears have low sensitivity for organism detection
Mycobacterial culture	Culture from sputum specimen on liquid and solid media is the most sensitive method; for pediatric cases, multiple gastric lavage specimens can be used; liquid culture with DNA probe hybridization enables rapid TB confirmation	Culture of CSF has a sensitivity of 45%–70%	Urine specimens for mycobacterial culture are positive in 60%–80% of cases, although it is more likely to be positive in men than in women	Culture may be performed using bone marrow, liver, urine, and sputum specimens
Nucleic acid amplification	Very useful for rapid detection of TB but does not replace culture; sensitivity higher in smear-positive specimens; several FDA-approved assays are available; can detect some resistance mutations by NAAT	May provide a rapid diagnosis but cannot replace culture; no FDA-approved assays	Utility not well defined	Sputum specimens may be used for amplification
Other findings	Pleural fluid, if present, is an exudate (not a transudate) with mononuclear cells	With lumbar puncture, there may be an increased opening pressure and 100–1000 cells/μL of CSF (mostly mononuclear cells) and elevated CSF protein	In the appropriate clinical setting, TB may be considered if negative routine urine cultures show WBCs in acid urine	Impaired function of infected organs may be noted in routine laboratory tests of those organ systems
Radiology	Chest radiograph may detect adenopathy, effusion, cavitation, or nodule; in HIV-infected patients, the chest radiograph is less likely to show typical changes	If TB is established in the brain, it may produce a mass, or "tuberculoma," visible by CT scan	40%–75% of cases have a positive chest radiograph; other radiologic studies are not very useful	Chest radiograph may be normal and repeat testing may prove useful; CT scan or MRI may be useful to detect TB in extrapulmonary sites such as the brain or vertebrae
Anatomic pathology	Caseating granulomas may be observed in biopsies of enlarged lymph nodes	Biopsy may be diagnostic	Renal biopsy may be helpful to identify genitourinary lesions	If bronchial washings do not provide diagnosis, granulomas in bone marrow or liver biopsy may be diagnostic

CNS, central nervous system; CSF, cerebrospinal fluid; CT, computed tomography; MRI, magnetic resonance imaging; PPD, purified protein derivative.

been associated with aerosolized transmission from cooling towers, evaporative condensers, potable hot water lines, showers, respiratory therapy equipment, decorative fountains, and whirlpool spas. Outbreaks in health care facilities are especially worrisome because of the large population of patients with compromised immunity or impaired pulmonary function who are at increased risk of severe *Legionella* infections.

Legionella infections can present as subclinical infections, pneumonia, and extrapulmonary infections including endocarditis. Patients with *Legionella* pneumonia can present with a broad spectrum of symptoms, ranging from mild cough to widespread pulmonary infiltrates and multisystem failure. Patients with *Legionella* pneumonia may also experience hemoptysis, diarrhea, and a change in mental status.

Diagnosis

The diagnosis of legionellosis can be easily missed because the organisms are not detected on routine Gram stain (*Legionella* stains very poorly) and growth of the organism in culture requires special types of agar. A sputum Gram stain showing mostly neutrophils, without associated bacteria, should raise suspicion of Legionnaires disease or other atypical pneumonia. *L. pneumophila* serogroup 1 infections, which account for most community-acquired legionellosis, can be readily diagnosed using rapid immunoassays that detect a *Legionella* antigen that is excreted in urine. These tests detect 80% to 90% of cases and have good specificity. Another advantage is that they remain positive for several weeks, even after the patient has been started on antibiotics. Bacterial culture is the gold standard for the diagnosis of *Legionella* infection. Cultures from sputum, bronchoalveolar lavage (BAL), and/or lung tissue may require 4 to 5 days of growth for isolation of *Legionella* colonies. The sensitivity for organism detection is greater with a BAL specimen than with an expectorated sputum specimen. Isolation of *Legionella* from specimens requires the use of a charcoal-based bacteriologic medium, with the addition of antibiotics if the specimens are from nonsterile sites. The isolation and identification of *Legionella*, in association with pneumonia, is diagnostic for *Legionella* pneumonia; however, the sensitivity of culture can be laboratory-dependent. PCR-based tests are routinely available in reference laboratories and have good sensitivity and specificity. Serologic assays can also be used for diagnosis *Legionella* infections but interpretation of a single titer is difficult. Direct fluorescent antibody tests of respiratory specimens are no longer recommended because of limited sensitivity and specificity.

Table 5–24 summarizes the laboratory tests relevant to diagnosis of the *Legionella* infections.

Nocardiosis

Description

Nocardia spp. are aerobic gram-positive actinomycetes that are found worldwide in soil and decaying organic matter. Nocardiosis is chiefly an opportunistic infection, particularly in patients with impaired cell-mediated immunity such as hematopoietic malignancies, HIV/AIDS, those

TABLE 5–24 **Evaluation of Patients for Legionnaires Disease**

Laboratory Test	Result
Bacteriologic culture	This is the "gold standard" test, requires special media for growth and isolation of the *Legionella* organisms; sensitivity tends to be laboratory dependent
Urinary antigen	Detects only *Legionella pneumophila* serogroup 1; overall sensitivity is 60%–80% because serogroup 1 represents 60%–80% of *Legionella* pneumonia cases; within serogroup 1, the sensitivity compared with culture is ≥95%
PCR analysis	Amplification of *Legionella* DNA from respiratory specimens; good sensitivity and specificity; can detect *L. pneumophila* and other Legionella species, depending on the assay
Serology	Rising titers of antibody to *Legionella* may be useful in documentation of disease in culture-negative cases; requires acute and convalescent specimens
Direct fluorescent antibody test	Infrequently used for direct testing of clinical specimens; relatively poor sensitivity, interpretation requires expertise

PCR, polymerase chain reaction.

TABLE 5–25   Evaluation for Nocardiosis

	Pulmonary Nocardiosis	Cutaneous/Subcutaneous Nocardiosis	CNS Nocardiosis	Systemic Nocardiosis
Microbiology	Gram stain, modified acid-fast stain, or aerobic culture may generate a positive result from sputum and bronchial specimens; selective agar and prolonged incubation periods used for fungal and/or mycobacterial culture increases yield	Gram stain, modified acid-fast stain, or aerobic culture may generate a positive result from specimens obtained from fistulas, abscesses, or skin biopsies; fungal and/or mycobacterial culture also useful	Aerobic culture may generate a positive test in CSF specimens or aspirates of cerebral masses, fungal and/or mycobacterial culture increases yield; Gram stain or modified acid-fast stain may reveal filamentous bacteria	Testing is most useful for cases involving CNS and lungs; blood culture may be positive if processed to maximize organism recovery; specimens from sites of suspected involvement may be used for smears and cultures
Anatomic pathology	Biopsies of large cavitary lesions in the lung may reveal organisms	Biopsies of skin lesions may reveal organisms	Fine needle aspirate of cerebral mass may reveal organisms	Biopsies of affected organs or tissues may reveal organisms

CNS, central nervous system; CSF, cerebrospinal fluid.

receiving immunosuppressive therapy, and transplant recipients. Pulmonary nocardiosis is the most common presentation. It can exhibit the full spectrum of acute or chronic pulmonary infection, including pneumonia and abscess formation. Other clinical manifestations include anorexia, productive cough, pleurisy, dyspnea, hemoptysis, and weight loss.

Primary *Nocardia* infection in the lung, skin, or soft tissue may erode into blood vessels and spread hematogenously to a variety of different organs. *Nocardia* have a well-recognized predilection for invasion into the CNS.

Diagnosis

Detection of the organism can be accomplished by microscopic examination of specimens combined with culture. Gram staining may reveal filamentous gram-positive rods with or without branching. They are also partially acid-fast; that is, they are positive on a modified acid-fast stain (which uses a less stringent decolorizer) but are negative on a regular acid-fast stain. *Nocardia* spp. are slowly growing organisms and may be difficult to recover. In the past, these organisms were identified based on biochemical reactions; however, DNA-based methods reveal that many of organisms that would previously have been identified as *Nocardia asteroides* are separate species with distinct antibiotic susceptibility profiles.

The laboratory information for diagnosis of nocardiosis in different anatomic sites is provided in **Table 5–25**.

Pneumocystis jirovecii Pneumonia

Description

Pneumocystis spp. are single-cell organisms that were originally described as protozoans, but phylogenetic analysis indicates that they are more appropriately classified with the fungi. These organisms are a well-recognized cause of pulmonary infection in patients with profoundly impaired cell-mediated immunity. These infections were originally attributed to *P. carinii* (which is found in rats), but it is now known that human infections are caused by the morphologically similar *P. jirovecii*. From the beginning of the HIV epidemic in the early 1980s until 1993, *P. jirovecii* was the indicator infection for more than 20,000 newly diagnosed cases of AIDS in the United States reported to the Centers for Disease Control and Prevention. It has become much less common since the introduction of highly active antiretroviral therapy. In a small number of cases, *Pneumocystis* can also cause extrapulmonary infections.

Diagnosis

Pneumocystis spp. cannot be cultured in vitro. Laboratory diagnosis depends on identification of the organism in stained preparations of clinical specimens, most often induced sputum or BAL fluid. These are concentrated onto a slide by cytocentrifugation. Other specimens include

TABLE 5–26 Evaluation for *Pneumocystis jirovecii*[a]

Type of Infection	Specimen	Laboratory Tests	Results/Comments
Pneumocystis pneumonia	BAL fluid, induced sputum, or lung biopsy	Microscopy using special stains is the standard method for diagnosis of *Pneumocystis* pneumonia; PCR-based assays (performed in reference labs) are more sensitive	Fluorescently labeled monoclonal antibodies can detect cysts and trophic forms; Gomori methenamine silver (GMS) stain and calcofluor only detect cyst walls; Giemsa stain only detects trophic forms Serum beta 1-3-D-glucan assay can detect pneumocystis in addition to invasive fungal infections due to Candida, Aspergillus, and related fungi
Extrapulmonary *Pneumocystis* infection	Lymph node, spleen, bone marrow, or liver	Microscopy using special stains	Organisms can be detected with GMS or fluorescent antibodies; they do not stain with hematoxylin and eosin

[a]In older literature, this organism is referred to as *P. carinii* (see Stringer JR, Beard CB, Miller RF. Spelling *Pneumocystis jirovecii*. *Emerg Infect Dis*. 2009;15:506).

transbronchial or open lung biopsies. The *Pneumocystis* life cycle includes trophozoite and cyst stages. The most sensitive method for detecting these forms is staining the preparation with fluorescently labeled monoclonal antibodies. Other frequently used stains are GMS (stains cyst walls) and Giemsa (stains trophozoites and intracystic stages). Alternative methods for diagnosis include detection of 1-3-β-D-glucan (which is used to detect other invasive fungal infections) as well as PCR-based tests that are available in reference laboratories. [*Clin Microbiol Rev*. 2014;27:490–526.]

Table 5–26 summarizes the laboratory information that supports a diagnosis of *P. jirovecii* infection.

The dimorphic fungi grow as filamentous molds in the environment but transform into yeast (or related forms) in infected tissue.

Dimorphic Fungi and Other Fungal Infections

Description

The dimorphic fungi grow as filamentous molds in the environment but transform into yeast (or related forms) in infected tissue. The most important members of this group are *H. capsulatum* and *Coccidioides* spp. These organisms are usually acquired by inhalation, but they can disseminate and cause life-threatening systemic infections.

H. capsulatum is endemic along the Mississippi and Ohio River Valleys, as well as in parts of Central America and the Caribbean region. Most infections are asymptomatic or subclinical; however, inhalation of large quantities of spores or hyphal fragments can cause symptomatic lung infection that requires antifungal therapy. As with TB, primary infection with *H. capsulatum* is contained by the cell-mediated immune response. However, the organism may not be eradicated. *H. capsulatum* infection in patients with underlying lung disease can lead to chronic progressive pulmonary histoplasmosis that must be treated to prevent further lung damage. Patients who have depressed cell-mediated immunity (due to underlying disease or immunosuppressive therapy) are at a risk of developing disseminated histoplasmosis. This form of the disease may present with nonspecific findings such as fever, weight loss, and hepatosplenomegaly, and can be fatal if untreated. Patients who harbor *H. capsulatum* and receive drugs that inhibit TNF or its receptor are also at a high risk of developing disseminated infection.

Coccidioides spp. are endemic in the southwestern United States (*C. immitis* in the central valley of California and *C. posadasii* in Arizona). The life cycle of *Coccidioides* is similar to *H. capsulatum* except that it forms spherules in infected tissue. Immunosuppressed patients and certain ethnic groups are at increased risk of disseminated coccidioidomycosis and CNS infections. Other dimorphic fungi are described in **Table 5–27**. [For Taloromyces, see Limper AH, Adenis A, Le T, Harrison TS. Fungal infections in HIV/AIDS. *Lancet Infect Dis*. July 31, 2017.]

Immunosuppressed patients are susceptible to a variety of other fungal lung infections, including *Aspergillus* spp. and other septate molds, nonseptate molds such as *Mucor* and *Rhizopus*, and the encapsulated yeast *C. neoformans*.

Diagnosis

Diagnostic tests for *H. capsulatum* include fungal culture, immunoassays that detect a fungal cell wall antigen, and serology. Culture is the gold standard, but fungal growth is usually not detected for 1 to 2 weeks. Serology is useful for patients with chronic pulmonary histoplasmosis, but it is

TABLE 5-27   Evaluation for Systemic and/or Invasive Mycotic Infections

Pathogen	Clinical Findings	Microbiology	Histopathology
Dimorphic fungi[a]			
Blastomyces dermatitidis (occurs in parts of the central and eastern United States [Ohio and Mississippi River Valleys, Great Lakes] and St. Lawrence river)	Chronic pneumonia with productive cough, hemoptysis, weight loss, and pleurisy; may be associated with verrucous or ulcerative skin lesions, subcutaneous nodules, osteolytic bone lesions, arthritis, prostatitis, and epididymitis	Broad-based budding yeasts may be visible in calcofluor stains of wet mounts of sputum or exudates; organism forms branching septate hyphae with microconidia in culture at 30°C, identification is usually confirmed by DNA hybridization; antibody and antigen detection tests have limited utility (can cross-react with other dimorphic fungi)	Broad-based budding yeasts in tissues; microabscesses and pyogranulomas may be present in tissue
Coccidioides spp. (common in the southwestern United States)	Influenza-like syndrome or pneumonia; also may cause erythema nodosum or erythema multiforme, meningitis, and disseminated disease	Endospores or spherules may be visible in calcofluor stains of wet mounts of sputum or exudates; organism forms arthroconidia in culture at 30°C, identification is usually confirmed by DNA hybridization; serologic tests are useful in both pulmonary and disseminated diseases; Coccidioides antigen is useful in meningitis cases	Spherules with endospores may be visible within tissue; pyogenic and granulomatous (may be caseous) responses can be found in tissue
Histoplasma capsulatum (common in the Ohio and Mississippi River Valleys in the United States, and parts of Central America)	Influenza-like syndrome or pneumonia; chronic progressive pulmonary infection in patients with underlying lung disease; and disseminated disease in immunosuppressed patients	Calcofluor or Giemsa stains may reveal budding yeast or intracellular forms within macrophages in respiratory specimens or bone marrow; organism forms branching septate hyphae with tuberculate macroconidia in culture at 30°C, identification is usually confirmed by DNA hybridization; serologic tests are useful in pulmonary disease; antigen detection in serum and urine is particularly useful in disseminated disease	Yeasts may be seen intracellularly within macrophages and/or extracellularly as budding forms; epithelioid granulomas may be present
Paracoccidioides brasiliensis (restricted to Central and South America)	Respiratory symptoms such as productive cough and chest pain; fever, weight loss, ulcerative granulomas of buccal, nasal, or gastrointestinal mucosa may occur	Calcofluor stains of wet preps of sputum or pus may reveal multiple budding yeast; organism forms branching septate hyphae in culture at 30°C, identification usually confirmed by exoantigen tests or DNA-based assays	Multiple budding yeasts detectable in tissues; microabscesses and granulomas also may be present in tissue
Taloromyces (Penicillium) marneffei (restricted to Southeast Asia)	Disseminated disease in immunosuppressed patients	Grows as a septate mold at 30°C, often produces diffusible red pigment; identification confirmed by conversion to yeast form at 37°C	Yeast-like cells often contain cross-walls (divide by fission rather than budding)
Filamentous fungi			
Aspergillus spp. (*A. fumigatus* is most common pathogen)	Aspergilloma (fungus ball) in preexisting cavity; invasive pulmonary aspergillosis with fever, dyspnea, and chest pain in patients with neutropenia and/or organ and bone marrow transplantation; can progress to disseminated disease	Calcofluor white stains of respiratory or biopsy material may reveal septate hyphae; culture isolates are usually identified by colonial and microscopic morphology; the serum galactomannan assay is useful for early detection of invasive pulmonary aspergillosis; commercially available PCR-based tests can aid in the diagnosis of invasive pulmonary aspergillosis	Septate hyphae with 45° branching are visible in tissues (similar structures are seen in other invasive fungal infections, as those caused by *Fusarium* or *Pseudoallescheria*)
Mucor/Rhizopus	Invasive pulmonary disease similar to aspergillosis; rhinocerebral mucormycosis begins with facial pain and headache, can progress to invasion of the orbit and CNS	Calcofluor white stains of nasal or respiratory specimens may reveal broad nonseptate hyphae; organisms generally grow rapidly in culture but can be difficult to isolate from tissue	Broad, nonseptate hyphae with right-angle branching can be seen in tissue; often associated with necrosis
Yeasts			
Candida spp.	Invasive mucosal infections such as esophagitis; disseminated disease in immunosuppressed or neutropenic patients	KOH/calcofluor preps of mucosal scrapings may reveal budding yeast, pseudohyphae, or hyphae; *Candida* grows well on routinely used agar and blood culture media; PCR-based detection from blood may be useful in patients at risk for invasive candidiasis	Yeast, pseudohyphae, or hyphae can be seen in infected tissue
Cryptococcus neoformans/ Cryptococcus gattii	Meningitis, pneumonia, skin lesions (in disseminated disease)	Antigen detection by lateral flow immunoassay or latex agglutination of CSF is the most sensitive of the available tests; India ink smear may detect yeasts; confirmatory culture using CSF is recommended	Narrow-based budding yeasts may be visible in tissue (capsule stains with mucicarmine)

[a]The dimorphic fungi can undergo reversible transition between mold forms and yeast forms. They grow as molds in the environment but replicate as yeast (or spherules) in infected tissue.

relatively insensitive for diagnosis of disseminated histoplasmosis. The antigen test performed on serum or urine is particularly useful for diagnosing disseminated disease. Coccidioidomycosis is diagnosed by serology and/or culture depending on the clinical presentation. The diagnosis of dimorphic fungal infections can also be confirmed by demonstration of characteristic structures in biopsy specimens. Currently the diagnosis of other fungal lung infections relies on culturing respiratory secretions and/or histopathologic examination of biopsy specimens. A serum assay that detects a galactomannan antigen produced by *Aspergillus* spp. is useful in the diagnosis of invasive pulmonary aspergillosis. Serum assays for circulating β-D-glucan may also be useful for detecting invasive fungal infections.

The clinical findings associated with systemic mycotic infections are shown in **Table 5–27** along with the microbiologic evaluation and histopathology findings.

Respiratory Virus Infections

Description

Many different viruses can cause upper and lower respiratory infections. Respiratory syncytial virus (RSV) and influenza viruses cause large numbers of infections in the winter months. RSV is the major cause of bronchiolitis in infants, but it can also cause serious infections in the elderly. Influenza is often thought of as an infection of adults (in whom it causes a syndrome characterized by rapid onset of fever, headache, and myalgias followed by upper respiratory symptoms); however, it also commonly infects children and may resemble RSV. Primary influenza pneumonia is a rare but dangerous form of the infection. More commonly, the typical influenza syndrome described above is followed several days later by a secondary bacterial pneumonia. Parainfluenza viruses classically cause croup (tracheobronchitis), the clinical manifestations of which often overlap those caused by RSV and influenza. Other important respiratory viruses include adenoviruses, metapneumovirus, and coronaviruses. Because of the availability of antiviral agents that target influenza viruses, it has become important to establish a specific viral etiology in patients with "flu-like" symptoms, particularly in severely ill patients and those with underlying cardiac and pulmonary diseases. Identification of the cause of severe respiratory infections may also be needed to guide infection control activities. Immunosuppressed patients are susceptible to all of the viruses described above. They are also at increased risk of developing CMV pneumonitis.

> Nucleic acid amplification tests are the most sensitive method for detecting influenza and other common respiratory viruses in nasopharyngeal specimens (aspirates, washes, or swabs). Multiplex panels can be performed in 1 to 8 hours. A new generation of rapid antigen tests for influenza can provide an answer in 20 minutes with a sensitivity 80%.

Diagnosis

Nucleic acid amplification tests are the most sensitive method for detecting influenza virus, RSV, and other common respiratory viruses, and have replaced viral culture in most clinical laboratories. Commercial molecular assays range from large multiplexed panels that detect influenza A and B, RSV, parainfluenza virus, metapneumovirus, coronavirus, adenovirus, and rhinovirus/enterovirus, to rapid point-of-care instruments that detect influenza and RSV. These tests are generally performed on nasopharyngeal specimens (aspirates, washes, or swabs). Large multiplex panels require 1 to 8 hours, depending on the methodology whereas rapid molecular point-of-care tests require <30 minutes. Rapid influenza antigen detection tests (such as those that utilize a lateral flow immunochromatographic format) are still used in many outpatient settings since they require little or no equipment, and it is easy to set up multiple specimens in parallel. In the past, these assays had a sensitivity of only 50% to 70% compared to molecular methods and therefore produced many false-negative results. New FDA regulations now require that rapid tests now achieve a minimum sensitivity of 80%. Direct immunofluorescent assays are now rarely performed because they are labor intensive and require experienced observers, while viral culture typically requires 3 to 10 days which is not a clinically useful timeframe.

Laboratory methods for detecting respiratory viruses are summarized in **Table 5–22**.

INFECTIONS OF THE GASTROINTESTINAL TRACT

Overview

Although many organisms can cause infectious gastroenteritis, the clinical setting usually makes it possible to focus on a small group of likely pathogens. Key factors to consider are whether the infection was acquired in the community or in a health care facility, duration of symptoms, travel

TABLE 5–28   Evaluation for Viral Infections of the Gastrointestinal Tract

Pathogen	Clinical Findings	Microbiology
Rotavirus	Watery diarrhea, fever, vomiting (mostly in infants and young children in winter)	Direct antigen detection in stool specimens by immunoassay; commercial multiplex PCR-based gastrointestinal panels can detect rotavirus
Adenovirus types 40/41	Watery diarrhea in infants; fever	Direct antigen detection in stool specimens by immunoassay (gastrointestinal adenoviruses are not culturable)
Cytomegalovirus (CMV) (in immunosuppressed patients)	May have explosive diarrhea (can be watery or bloody); fever	CMV may be cultured from colonic biopsies; histopathology may reveal viral inclusions and inflammation (colitis)
Noroviruses	Nonbloody diarrhea, vomiting, myalgias, and low-grade fever	PCR-based is the method of choice for detecting noroviruses in clinical specimens (available as individual tests and in multiplex panels)

history, and whether the patient is immunosuppressed. In the past, the detection of these different classes of organisms (bacteria, viruses, and parasites) required multiple methods (bacterial culture, antigen detection, and microscopy). This situation is changing due to the introduction of commercial multiplex molecular panels that can detect a wide array of pathogens.

Viruses Inducing Gastroenteritis

Description

In immunocompetent hosts, the majority of cases of community-acquired self-limited nausea, vomiting, and/or diarrhea are caused by viruses (primarily noroviruses, rotaviruses, and enteric adenoviruses [types 40 and 41]). There has been a substantial decrease in rotavirus infections in the United States since the introduction of a pediatric vaccine in 2006. Laboratory tests for noroviruses, based on nucleic acid amplification, are generally not performed unless there are large outbreaks that have epidemiologic significance, for example, outbreaks on cruise ships or in health care facilities. Antigen detection assays are commonly used to diagnose rotavirus and adenovirus infections. Although enteroviruses are usually acquired by fecal–oral transmission, they generally cause systemic infections; gastroenteritis is not a prominent clinical manifestation. CMV, especially in immunocompromised patients, can produce an explosive, watery diarrhea.

> Community-acquired diarrhea accompanied by abdominal pain or systemic symptoms should be evaluated for a select group of bacterial pathogens, consisting of *Salmonella* spp., *Shigella* spp., *Campylobacter* spp., Shiga toxin-producing *E. coli*, and *Yersinia* spp.

Diagnosis

Table 5–28 summarizes the clinical, radiologic, histopathologic, and laboratory findings associated with the gastrointestinal illnesses produced by rotavirus, adenovirus, CMV, and noroviruses.

Aerobic Bacterial Infections

Description and Diagnosis

Community-acquired diarrhea accompanied by abdominal pain or systemic symptoms should be evaluated for a select group of bacterial pathogens, consisting of *Salmonella* spp., *Shigella* spp., *Campylobacter* spp., Shiga toxin-producing *E. coli*, and *Yersinia* spp. Recent travel or consumption of raw shellfish would raise the possibility of *Vibrio* spp. All of these organisms are very unlikely to be the cause of gastroenteritis in a patient who has been hospitalized for more than 3 days. Mycobacterial infections would need to be considered in profoundly immunosuppressed patients. **Table 5–29** describes some of the more common bacterial infections of the gastrointestinal tract. Many of these organisms also can produce infections outside of the gastrointestinal tract.

Clostridium difficile Infections

Description

C. difficile infection is frequently implicated in antibiotic-associated diarrhea and is responsible for most cases of pseudomembranous colitis, a potentially life-threatening condition that requires combined medical and surgical intervention. Antibiotics frequently implicated include ampicillin,

TABLE 5–29   Evaluation for Bacterial Infections of the Gastrointestinal Tract and for Peritonitis

Pathogen	Clinical Findings	Microbiology	Additional Diagnostic Information
Bacterial infections			
Campylobacter jejuni	Acute enteritis with diarrhea (may be watery or bloody), fever, and abdominal pain; Guillain–Barre syndrome is an uncommon complication that may occur 2–3 weeks following diarrhea	Fecal wet mounts may reveal darting motility of organisms; Gram-stained fecal smears have a sensitivity of 50%–75%; stool cultures for *C. jejuni* must be incubated under microaerophilic condition; commercial multiplex PCR panels detect several *Campylobacter* species	Leukocytes and erythrocytes often present in fecal smears; anti-GM1 ganglioside antibodies may be detected in post-*Campylobacter* Guillain–Barre syndrome
Escherichia coli (pathogenic strains include ETEC, EPEC, EIEC, and STEC)	Depends on type of *E. coli*, e.g., watery/traveler's diarrhea caused by ETEC; or bloody diarrhea and hemolytic uremic syndrome (HUS) associated with *E. coli* O157 or other Shiga toxin-producing isolates	Routine stool cultures are useful for suspected O157:H7 isolates (requires differential agar); other STEC can be detected by Shiga toxin immunoassay; STEC and EIEC included in some commercial PCR panels	Culture of Shiga toxin producing stains (STEC) is important for epidemiologic tracking
Mycobacterium avium complex (disseminated infection in AIDS patients)	Watery diarrhea, abdominal pain, nausea, vomiting, weight loss, and night sweats	Blood cultures are the most likely to yield organisms; positive stool culture by itself can represent localized or disseminated infection	Gastrointestinal symptoms precede disseminated mycobacterial disease in AIDS patients; lymph node, liver, or bone marrow biopsies may reveal acid-fast organisms; bowel biopsies not routinely performed
Salmonella enteritidis and other nontyphoidal strains of *Salmonella*	Nonbloody diarrhea, fever, nausea, vomiting, and abdominal cramping	Routine stool cultures are useful; blood cultures rarely positive (less than 5%); *Salmonella* is detected by several commercial PCR panels	Serotyping of culture isolates is important for epidemiologic tracking; fecal smears usually have neutrophils
Salmonella typhi or *paratyphi* (enteric or typhoid fever)	Fever, abdominal pain, hepatosplenomegaly, diarrhea, "rose spots," weakness, and weight loss	Routine stool cultures are useful; blood cultures are 50%–70% sensitive; bone marrow cultures are 90% sensitive; duodenal fluid collected by intestinal string rarely performed	Serologic tests are generally not useful
Shigella (shigellosis; bacillary dysentery)	Dysentery with abdominal pain and bloody diarrhea	Routine stool cultures used to detect organism; *Shigella* is detected by several commercial PCR panels	Direct fecal smears often contain abundant neutrophils; serologic tests are not useful
Vibrio cholerae and other *Vibrio* spp.	Mild or explosive watery diarrhea; dehydration may be severe	Motile vibrios may be visible in fresh fecal smears; stool cultures should include selective media (e.g., TCBS agar); *Vibrio* spp. are detected by some commercial PCR panels	Serotyping of organisms may be performed
Yersinia enterocolitica	Enterocolitis with diarrhea, abdominal pain, and fever; reactive polyarthritis and erythema nodosum may occur after diarrhea	Stool cultures on selective media are necessary to permit growth of organisms for identification	Serologic tests for arthritis may be useful for assessing patients with polyarthritis
Clostridium difficile (antibiotic-associated colitis) and *Clostridium perfringens* (food poisoning)	See **Table 5–30**		
Peritonitis			
Primary peritonitis (usually in children or patients with cirrhosis)	Fever, abdominal pain, nausea, vomiting, and diarrhea	Gram stain and culture of peritoneal (ascitic) fluid is most likely to identify (in order of likelihood)—*E. coli*, *Klebsiella pneumoniae*, *Streptococcus pneumoniae*, enterococci	Typically, peritoneal fluid protein is low (<3.5 g/L) and peritoneal fluid leukocyte count is elevated (usually >1000/μL) with neutrophils >250/μL and pH <7.35
Secondary peritonitis (due to perforation, appendicitis, cholecystitis)	Signs of sepsis with fever, tachycardia, tachypnea, and hypotension	Gram stain and culture of peritoneal fluid or aspirated abscess material usually reveals mixed aerobic and anaerobic flora; *E. coli*, *Bacteroides fragilis*, and *Candida albicans* commonly found	Peritoneal fluid studies less definitive in this setting; peripheral blood leukocytosis often present; abdominal ultrasound or CT scan may be useful for evaluation and identification of suspected intra-abdominal abscesses

CT, computed tomography.

TABLE 5–30   Evaluation for Clostridial Infections of the Gastrointestinal Tract

Diagnostic Test	*Clostridium difficile* Colitis	Food Poisoning with *Clostridium perfringens*, Type A	Neutropenic Enterocolitis Caused by *Clostridium septicum* and Other Organisms
Endoscopy with biopsy of suspicious lesions	Invasive and expensive; usually reserved for more severe cases	Not useful	Endoscopy is typically not performed, but if a sample of the bowel is removed, it will show the characteristic inflammation and/or necrosis
Tests for toxins	The presence of toxins A or B in diarrheal stools establishes the diagnosis of *C. difficile* colitis; the tissue culture test for toxin B detects a cytopathic effect from filtrates of the diarrheal stool with sensitivities of ~80% but requires 24–48 h and is technically complex; rapid immunoassays for toxins A and B are less sensitive (50%–60%); nucleic acid amplification of the toxin genes provides rapid detection as well as high sensitivity (~95%); tests for *C. difficile* should only be performed on unformed diarrheal stool, unless ileus is suspected; the clinical significance of PCR-positive/toxin-negative specimens can be difficult to determine	Various tests are available to detect the enterotoxin responsible for the toxic effect of *C. perfringens* in food poisoning; these tests are performed in public health laboratories	Not routinely performed
Stool cultures	Most sensitive method; requires special media and must confirm that isolates produce toxin; patients may be asymptomatically colonized	Routine cultures of stool samples are not useful; specialized culture methods are performed in public health laboratories; 10^6 spores per gram of stool or 10^5 organisms per gram of suspected food source supports the diagnosis of food poisoning with *C. perfringens*	Not typically performed; because bacteremia may be produced in this illness, blood cultures for the clostridial organisms can be collected

C. difficile infection is frequently implicated in antibiotic-associated diarrhea. *C. difficile* elaborates toxins A and B that induce fluid secretion, mucosal damage, and intestinal inflammation and produces heat-resistant spores that persist for months in the environment.

amoxicillin, cephalosporins, and clindamycin. The pathogenesis of *C. difficile* infection is a multistep process that involves antibiotic-mediated disruption of the normal intestinal flora, acquisition of toxigenic *C. difficile*, and "third factor," which may be a particularly virulent strain or an inadequate host immune response to *C. difficile* toxins. Colonization of the gastrointestinal tract occurs by the oral–fecal route. *C. difficile* elaborates toxins A and B that induce fluid secretion, mucosal damage, and intestinal inflammation. The organism also produces heat-resistant spores that persist for months in the environment. Organisms can be cultured from floors, toilets, bed pans, bedding, and all sites where patients with diarrhea from *C. difficile* infection have recently been treated. Although the majority of infections occur in hospitalized patients, *C. difficile* disease is also a concern in long-term care facilities and can also present as a community-acquired infection in individuals with appropriate risk factors.

C. difficile infection can affect children and adults. (Young infants exhibit asymptomatic colonization and appear to be resistant to the toxic effects of *C. difficile* infection.) Adults can also be asymptomatically colonized. Symptomatic *C. difficile* infection usually presents with mild-to-moderate diarrhea and lower abdominal cramping. Symptoms often begin shortly after antibiotic therapy, but may be delayed for several weeks after antibiotic therapy is initiated. Patients who go on to develop pseudomembranous colitis experience more severe diarrhea, abdominal tenderness, and systemic symptoms. Patients with advanced disease may present with a fulminant life-threatening colitis that must be treated promptly to avoid perforation of the bowel wall.

Diagnosis

Since patients can be asymptomatically colonized with *C. difficile*, stool tests for toxigenic *C. difficile* should only be performed on patients with a compatible clinical presentation, such as those with three or more loose stools in 24 hours. The main tests for diagnosing *C. difficile* from stool specimens are PCR-based amplification assays that detect the toxin B gene and immunoassays that detect toxins A and B ("toxin assays"). There is ongoing disagreement about the best diagnostic algorithm because it is often difficult to determine whether a PCR-positive/toxin-negative specimen represents asymptomatic colonization or clinically significant infection. **Table 5–30** summarizes the evaluation of patients for *C. difficile* infection.

Protozoal Infections

Description

Protozoa are a very diverse group of unicellular eukaryotic organisms that can be free-living or parasitic. Many have two morphologic stages—trophozoites and cysts. Trophozoites, which are metabolically active feeding forms of the organism, may encyst within a protective coating to tolerate harsh environments. The cyst is a dormant form of the protozoan, and can reemerge as a trophozoite (for asexually reproducing organisms) when exposed to favorable conditions. For protozoa that multiply by sexual reproduction, a zygote is formed from the fusion of two gametes. Encystation of a zygote produces an oocyst that may contain two or more sporocysts, each with its own cyst wall. Sporocysts contain sporozoites, infective forms of the organism.

The intestinal protozoa are divided into five main groups that differ in terms of epidemiology and clinical presentation. Several of the groups contain pathogenic as well as nonpathogenic species. Although the latter do not require treatment, their presence indicates that the individual has been exposed to oral–fecal contamination.

> The intestinal protozoa are divided into five main groups that differ in terms of epidemiology and clinical presentation. Most intestinal protozoa are detected by examination of stained stool specimens.

- **Flagellates:** Pathogenic species include *Giardia lamblia* and *Dientamoeba fragilis*. *Giardia* is the most common intestinal parasite in the United States. Sources of infection include ingestion of contaminated water and person-to-person transmission in day care centers. *Giardia* can cause diarrhea, abdominal cramps, bloating, and flatulence. Symptoms often persist for more than 1 week.
- **Amebas:** *Entamoeba histolytica* is a major cause of intestinal infections worldwide, particularly in tropical areas with limited sanitation facilities. Most infections in the United States are acquired elsewhere. Clinical manifestations range from asymptomatic colonization to diarrhea, amebic colitis/dysentery, or extraintestinal abscess formation (usually in the liver). The diagnosis of amebiasis is complicated by the fact that *E. histolytica* is morphologically indistinguishable from the nonpathogenic *E. dispar*. Other nonpathogenic amebas include *E. coli* and *Endolimax nana*.
- **Coccidia:** Human pathogens include *Cryptosporidium* spp., *Cyclospora* spp., and *Isospora belli*. These organisms are members of the apicomplexans family and are related to the tissue parasites *T. gondii* and *Plasmodium* spp. *Cryptosporidium* spp. are a relatively common cause of infection in the United States. Outbreaks have been caused by contamination of drinking water or recreational water such as pools or water parks. *Cryptosporidium* usually causes a self-limited diarrhea in immunocompetent hosts, but it can cause severe persistent diarrhea in AIDS patients. *Cyclospora* spp. have caused outbreaks linked to imported food, such as raspberries. *Isospora* infections are usually only diagnosed in immunosuppressed patients.
- **Ciliates:** *Balantidium coli* is the only pathogenic ciliate.
- **Microsporidia:** Although these organisms are included in the section on protozoans, recent phylogenetic analysis indicates that they are more closely related to the fungi. *Enterocytozoon bienusi* causes self-limited diarrhea in normal hosts and chronic diarrhea in AIDS patients in whom it can also spread to the biliary tract. *Encephalitozoon* spp. can cause diarrhea and a variety of extraintestinal infections in immunosuppressed hosts.

Diagnosis

Most intestinal protozoa are usually detected by examination of stained stool specimens. Sensitive immunoassays are available for detecting antigens produced by *Giardia* and *Cryptosporidium*. *Cryptosporidium*, *E. histolytica*, and *Giardia* are also included in recently introduced multiplex molecular panels for gastrointestinal pathogens. Serology can be useful for diagnosing invasive *E. histolytica* since *E. dispar* does not trigger an antibody response. **Table 5–31** describes infections produced by selected pathogenic protozoa. Protozoal infections are commonly found within the gastrointestinal tract, but, as noted in the table, many other organs and tissues can be infected.

Intestinal Helminth Infections

Description

Helminth (worm) infections in humans constitute a significant percentage of the global burden of illness caused by infectious diseases. The helminths are multicellular organisms that are divided into three groups: tapeworms (cestodes), roundworms (nematodes), and flukes (trematodes).

TABLE 5–31   Evaluation for Protozoal Infections

Pathogen	Clinical Findings	Histopathology/Cytology	Testing	Comments
Microsporidia				
Encephalitozoon and *Enterocytozoon* (note: phylogenetic analysis indicates that microsporidia are more closely related to fungi)	Chronic, watery diarrhea; dehydration, weight loss, fever, abdominal pain, and vomiting	Spores are visible in duodenal or biliary aspirates, or within enterocytes in small intestinal biopsies; electron microscopy may be helpful	Chromotrope-based staining of stool specimens may be used to detect organisms; PCR-based detection is more sensitive than microscopy (available in reference labs)	D-Xylose and fat malabsorption are common; serologic tests are not useful
Amebas				
Entamoeba histolytica	Infection may be asymptomatic or present as acute amebic or fulminant colitis with bloody diarrhea; hepatic abscess can be a late complication	Cysts or trophozoites may be demonstrated in colonic scrapings or biopsies; if amebic liver abscess is suspected, abdominal imaging by ultrasound or CT scan should be performed	Cysts and/or trophozoites can be detected with routine stains used in ova and parasite preparations of stool specimens; antigen detection and PCR assays are also commercially available	Serologic tests may be used in detection of an amebic liver abscess or intestinal amebiasis
Naegleria fowleri	Causes primary meningoencephalitis with abrupt onset of headaches, fever, nausea, vomiting, and pharyngitis; associated with swimming in warm freshwater lakes; can be rapidly progressive	Brain biopsy not routinely recommended because CSF yields organisms, even though brain biopsy also may reveal organisms	Fresh CSF examination (wet mount) for motile trophozoites, may also be Giemsa-stained; brain biopsies may be cultured; PCR testing available in reference and public health labs	Purulent CSF with no bacteria is common; children or young adults exposed to fresh water are at risk
Acanthamoeba	Causes keratitis with ocular pain and corneal ulceration; also causes granulomatous amebic encephalitis (GAE)	Corneal biopsies may reveal organisms in patients with keratitis; brain or skin biopsy of nodules or ulcers required for diagnosis of GAE	Giemsa, Gram, or calcofluor-stained smears of corneal scrapings may reveal amebas; culture of organisms from corneal scrapings or brain tissue is possible	Keratitis can be subacute or chronic and is often associated with soft contact lens use
Ciliates				
Balantidium coli	Infection may be asymptomatic or may cause severe diarrhea or dysentery; diarrhea may persist for weeks to months prior to development of dysentery	*B. coli* can invade the colonic mucosa, with consequent ulcer formation; in such cases, the organism is visible on histologic section	Wet preparation examination of fresh concentrated stool will demonstrate the trophozoite and cyst forms; the organisms are large and frequently can be seen under low magnification	These organisms do not stain well, making recognition and identification on a permanent stained smear difficult
Flagellates				
Giardia lamblia	Acute or chronic watery diarrhea; nausea, anorexia, low-grade fever, and chills	Trophozoites may be identified by endoscopic brush cytology, mucosal smears, or histopathologic examination of small intestinal biopsy	Cysts or trophozoites may be visible in stool specimens; direct antigen detection is a sensitive alternative; *Giardia* is detected by several commercial PCR panels	
Trichomonas vaginalis	Vaginitis with excessive discharge, dysuria, and dyspareunia	Visible on Pap smear	Trichomonads may be observed in wet mounts of vaginal secretions (60% sensitivity); endocervical or urethral cultures are more sensitive; commercial NAAT assay offers high sensitivity	Abundant neutrophils are present in vaginal wet mounts
Coccidia				
Cryptosporidium parvum and *C. hominis*	Watery, cholera-like diarrhea, abdominal pain, nausea, fever, and fatigue	Organisms may be visible in small intestine biopsies, although many infections may be missed due to sampling variation	Oocysts may be detected in concentrated specimens with acid-fast stain or DFA; direct fecal antigen tests are a sensitive alternative; *Cryptosporidium* is detected by several commercial PCR panels	Serologic tests are not useful

(Continued)

TABLE 5–31 (Continued)

Pathogen	Clinical Findings	Histopathology/Cytology	Testing	Comments
Cyclospora cayetanensis	Watery diarrhea and constipation, nausea, anorexia, abdominal cramping, and weight loss; outbreaks have been associated with imported produce	Jejunal biopsy may show inflammation, villous atrophy, or crypt hyperplasia; organisms may be detected with acid-fast stain	Oocysts are visible in fresh stool; variable appearance with acid-fast stain of stool specimen; oocysts show blue-green autofluorescence when excited at 365 nm	Serologic tests are not available
Isospora belli	Profuse, watery diarrhea; abdominal pain, cramping, weight loss, and low-grade fever; may be especially severe in HIV-infected patients	Intestinal biopsies may reveal organisms in sections	Oocysts are visible in wet smears of fresh or preserved stool; oocysts stain red with acid-fast stain	Serologic tests are not available
Toxoplasma gondii	Lymphadenopathy or mononucleosis-like syndrome in immunocompetent adults; encephalitis, pneumonitis, or chorioretinitis in immunosuppressed individuals; chorioretinitis and/or neurologic findings in congenital infections	Tachyzoites often visible in endomyocardial biopsies of heart transplant recipients; lymph node pathology is characteristic; brain biopsies lack sensitivity	Tachyzoites often visible in CSF, amniotic fluid, or bronchoalveolar lavage fluid; antigens from the organism may be detectable in the serum; PCR may identify *T. gondii* DNA in respiratory or amniotic specimens	Serologic tests remain the standard for diagnosis to determine recent versus chronic infection; however, serologic studies lack sensitivity in immunocompromised patients
Kinetoplastids (Not intestinal)				
Leishmania: cutaneous and mucosal leishmaniasis	Erythematous papules, nodules, or ulcers; regional lymphadenopathy and fever	Identification of organisms in touch preparations and sections of skin biopsy specimens	Organisms from skin biopsy specimens may be cultured in liquid media	Serum antibody titers are not useful
Leishmania: visceral leishmaniasis (kala-azar)	Fever, malaise, weight loss, hepatomegaly, splenomegaly	Fine needle aspiration of the spleen for touch preparation and culture is >96% sensitive; organisms may be visible in bone marrow aspirates	Specimens obtained by fine needle aspiration of spleen, liver, and bone marrow may be cultured	High serum antibody titers are present in immunocompetent persons with visceral leishmaniasis
Trypanosomiasis, African (sleeping sickness caused by *Trypanosoma brucei*)	Chancre, intermittent fevers, lymphadenopathy, pruritic rash, and meningoencephalitis	Histopathologic evaluation lacks sensitivity	Trypomastigotes visible in peripheral blood smears, chancre fluid, lymph node or bone marrow aspirates	WBCs in CSF and an elevated CSF IgM titer are useful for diagnosis of meningoencephalitis
Trypanosomiasis, American (Chagas disease caused by *Trypanosoma cruzi*)	Chronic illness highlighted by cardiac disease (cardiomyopathy) and embolic phenomena; lymphadenopathy and chagoma occur in acute disease	Histopathologic evaluation of heart or other tissues lacks sensitivity	In acute disease, parasites may be detected in peripheral blood or buffy coat smears; lymph node, bone marrow aspirates, pericardial fluid, or CSF also may be examined	IgG serologic tests are used to diagnose chronic Chagas disease; PCR-based detection available at the CDC

CSF, cerebrospinal fluid; CT, computed tomography; PCR, polymerase chain reaction; DFA, direct fluorescent antibody; CDC, Centers for Disease Control and Prevention.

Helminths are typically enclosed by a protective coat, inside of which may be differentiated organ systems for digestion, neuromuscular control, and reproduction. Many helminths have complex life cycles that involve two or more hosts. Helminths develop into adult worms and/or undergo sexual reproduction in the definitive host, whereas they do not develop past the larval stage in intermediate hosts. When humans are the definitive host, the parasite often causes intestinal symptoms, whereas when humans are an intermediate host, the parasite causes extraintestinal symptoms. Infections in humans usually result from ingestion of eggs, penetration of intact skin by infective larvae, or bites by insect vectors, depending on the specific helminth. Many helminth life cycles involve a stage in which the larvae migrate through tissue. This migration can be relatively asymptomatic but can also have serious clinical consequences depending on the type of helminth. These principles are illustrated by the following two examples.

The definitive host for *Echinococcus granulosis* (a tapeworm) is the dog, which harbors the adult tapeworm in its intestinal tract and excretes eggs in the feces. When an intermediate host, such as sheep or humans, ingests these eggs, the eggs hatch in the intestinal tract and larvae penetrate the intestinal wall and eventually form slowly expanding cysts in visceral organs such as the liver or lungs.

Strongyloides stercoralis is one of the several nematodes that are acquired when infective larvae present in warm moist soil penetrate human skin. The larvae migrate through tissue into the venous circulation and are transported to the lungs where they invade the alveoli, are coughed up and swallowed, and then develop into mature worms in the intestinal tract. The adult worms produce larva that are shed in feces into the environment where they can complete their life cycle. Unlike other nematodes, however, *S. stercoralis* larvae can also penetrate the gut wall or perianal skin and initiate an autoinfective cycle that results in persistent low-level infection even after the host has left an endemic area. If an infected patient subsequently receives immunosuppressive therapy, particularly with corticosteroids, the patient can develop life-threatening *Strongyloides* hyperinfection syndrome in which large numbers of nematode larvae migrate into the lungs and extraintestinal tissues.

Diagnosis

Infections with intestinal helminths are usually diagnosed by detection of eggs or larvae in feces. For many of the helminths, the identification of the organism is based on the morphologic characteristics of the organism and/or the eggs. These characteristics include size, shape, and thickness of the egg wall, special structures such as knobs and spines, and the developmental stage of the egg contents (e.g., undeveloped, developing, or embryonated).

Important information in the evaluation of a patient infected with helminths includes a history of possible exposure to the organism. Eosinophilia is commonly observed in patients with helminth infections due to larval migration through tissues. The clinical findings, mode of transmission to humans, aspects of microbiologic and serologic testing, and relevant radiologic findings for selected helminth infections are presented in **Table 5–32**.

Food Poisoning

Nausea and vomiting that occurs 1 to 8 hours after eating can be caused by ingestion of bacterial toxins that are already present in the food rather than by infection of the intestinal tract. The most common causes are enterotoxins produced by *S. aureus* (found in dairy and bakery products) and *Bacillus cereus* (found in reheated fried rice). The condition is self-limited. *C. perfringens* food poisoning results from the ingestion of food containing at least 10^8 enterotoxin-producing organisms. Often these are foods that have become grossly contaminated from storage over long periods at ambient temperature. This is particularly true of animal protein foods, such as cooked meats and gravies. Most individuals experience watery diarrhea with abdominal cramps (*B. cereus* can cause a similar syndrome). Fatalities are rare, with spontaneous resolution of symptoms within 6 to 24 hours.

Botulism
Description

Botulism is a neuroparalytic disease produced by potent toxins derived from *Clostridium botulinum*. The toxins block the release of the neurotransmitter acetylcholine at peripheral cholinergic synapses. The most common cause of botulism in humans is ingestion of preformed toxins in food contaminated with *C. botulinum*. Food products identified as sources of outbreaks include home-canned vegetable products, fish products preserved by a variety of methods, and sausage and ham preserved by salting rather than heating and then consumed without cooking. Infant botulism, which affects children up to 35 weeks of age only, is a result of colonization of the intestinal tract by *C. botulinum* after the ingestion of viable spores. Wound botulism can occur when *C. botulinum* contaminates deep wounds and secretes the toxin.

Patients suffering from botulism typically present with muscle weakness, difficulty in speaking and swallowing, and blurred vision. Such patients can progress to symmetric descending

Nausea and vomiting that occurs 1 to 8 hours after eating can be caused by ingestion of bacterial toxins that are already present in the food rather than by infection of the intestinal tract. The most common causes are enterotoxins produced by *S. aureus* (found in dairy and bakery products) and *Bacillus cereus* (found in reheated fried rice).

TABLE 5-32   Evaluation for Helminth Infections of the Gastrointestinal Tract

Pathogen	Clinical Findings	Mode of Transmission to Humans	Microbiology and Serology Testing
Tapeworms (*Cestodes*)			
Diphyllobothrium latum (fish tapeworm)	Diarrhea and abdominal pain; intestinal obstruction; can cause vitamin B_{12} deficiency and pernicious anemia	Ingestion of cysts in freshwater fish	Characteristic operculate eggs or proglottids (segments of the organism) may be present in examination of feces
Echinococcus granulosus and *Echinococcus multilocularis* (restricted to high northern latitudes)	Abdominal pain with hepatomegaly; confusion and headaches if CNS is involved; cysts in tissue, primarily liver, also lung and brain; often discovered incidentally on imaging	Ingestion of eggs; due to environmental contamination from infected canines	Serologic tests available to assess exposure; microscopy of cyst fluid reveals proglottids; however, cyst rupture can cause severe allergic reactions
Taenia saginata (beef tapeworm)	Abdominal discomfort, diarrhea, and intestinal obstruction	Ingestion of the organisms in contaminated beef	Spherical eggs or gravid proglottids (segments of the organism) often present in feces
Taenia solium (pork tapeworm)	Intestinal infection is often asymptomatic; neurocysticercosis can present with new onset seizures, focal neurologic defects, or increased intracranial pressure; CNS cystic lesions detected by CT or MRI	Ingestion of cysts in infected pork leads to intestinal infection (taeniasis) or ingestion of eggs (shed by human carrier) leads to invasive cysticercosis	Proglottids (segments of the organism) or eggs are present in stool of patients with taeniasis; serology useful in conjunction with imaging for diagnosis of neurocysticercosis
Roundworms (*nematodes*)			
Ascaris lumbricoides	Often asymptomatic or mild abdominal discomfort; can cause intestinal obstruction or obstructive jaundice; may have Loeffler syndrome (pulmonary eosinophilia) in lungs with dyspnea, cough, and rales; eosinophilia in blood	Ingestion of embryonated eggs; often hand-to-mouth transmission after contact with contaminated soil or surface	Ovoid eggs usually present in examination of feces; developing or adult worms may be present in feces
Enterobius vermicularis (pinworm)	Usually children are infected; perianal and perineal pruritus due to deposition of eggs in perianal region	Ingestion of eggs; often hand-to-mouth transmission after scratching perianal area or contact with contaminated surface; infection also may occur by inhalation of airborne eggs in dust	Cellulose tape test performed in which tape adheres to eggs in perianal folds; eggs transferred to slide for microscopy; anal swabs also useful
Filariae (*Wuchereria bancrofti* for elephantiasis and *Onchocerca volvulus* for onchocerciasis)	Elephantiasis (lymphatic filariasis)—lower extremity swelling and fevers; onchocerciasis (river blindness)—cutaneous nodules and blindness	Injection of larvae—during mosquito bite for *W. bancrofti* and during black fly bite for *O. volvulus*	*Wuchereria* microfilariae may be visible in peripheral blood smears; skin snips or core biopsy of nodules may reveal *Onchocerca* microfilariae
Hookworms (*Ancylostoma duodenale* and *Necator americanus*)	Can cause pruritus, rash, Loeffler-like syndrome, abdominal pain; primary concern is iron deficiency anemia and protein malnutrition due to chronic blood loss	Skin penetration by larvae, often through the feet in contact with contaminated soil	Partially embryonated eggs present in feces; larvae may be present in feces
Strongyloides stercoralis	Chronic infection—abnormal pain, intermittent urticarial rash, peripheral blood eosinophilia; hyperinfection (immunosuppressed patient)—colitis, abdominal distention, respiratory distress, shock	Larvae penetration of skin or colon; organism persists due to autoinfective cycle	First-stage (rhabditiform) larvae are often visible in feces; larvae may be present in sputum or duodenal aspirates; serologic tests can be useful if organisms are not seen by microscopy
Trichinella spiralis	Gastroenteritis, fever, eosinophilia, myositis, and circumorbital edema following ingestion of raw pork or raw bear meat (trichinosis)	Ingestion of larvae in contaminated meat products	Larvae may be detected in sediment from digested muscle tissue; antibodies to organism may be detected with serologic tests
Trichuris trichiura (whipworm)	Diarrhea, dysentery, and abdominal cramping; rectal prolapse may occur	Ingestion of embryonated eggs through hands, food, or drink contaminated by contact with infected soil or surfaces	Barrel-shaped eggs visible in feces

(Continued)

TABLE 5–32   (Continued)

Pathogen	Clinical Findings	Mode of Transmission to Humans	Microbiology and Serology Testing
Flukes (trematodes)			
Fasciolopsis buski (intestinal fluke)	Abdominal discomfort; travel or residence in Asia	Ingestion of metacercariae (larval form of organism) in aquatic plants	Ellipsoidal eggs in feces or bile
Liver flukes (*Fasciola hepatica* and *Clonorchis sinensis*)	Hepatomegaly, cholangitis, hepatitis; *F. hepatica* is worldwide; *C. sinensis* more common in Southeast Asian immigrants; with *F. hepatica*, hepatic nodules or linear tracks	Ingestion of metacercariae (larval form of organism) in aquatic plants (for *F. hepatica*) and in freshwater fish (for *C. sinensis*)	Ellipsoid or ovoid eggs present in feces
Paragonimus westermani (lung fluke)	Cough with brownish sputum, intermittent hemoptysis, pleuritic chest pain, and eosinophilia	Ingestion of metacercariae (larval form of organism) in crayfish or freshwater crabs	Ovoid eggs are present in feces and, less commonly, in sputum
Schistosoma haematobium (blood fluke)	Hematuria, granulomatous disease of the bladder, bladder carcinoma, and secondary bacterial urinary tract infections; obstruction, hydronephrosis, or filling defects may be observed by renal ultrasonography or intravenous pyelography	Penetration of intact human skin by cercariae (larval form of organism), often during bathing, swimming, or washing clothes in contaminated water	Eggs often visible in microscopic examination of the urine
Schistosoma japonicum (blood fluke)	Nausea, vomiting, hemoptysis, melena, hepatosplenomegaly, portal hypertension, and esophageal varices	Penetration of intact human skin by cercariae (larval form of organism) often during bathing, swimming, or washing clothes in contaminated water	Round to ovoid eggs in feces
Schistosoma mansoni (blood fluke)	Nausea, vomiting, hemoptysis, melena, hepatosplenomegaly, portal hypertension, and esophageal varices	Penetration of intact human skin by cercariae (larval form of organism) often during bathing, swimming, or washing clothes in contaminated water	Lateral-spined eggs in feces that may be bloody or mucus-laden

CNS, central nervous system; CT, computed tomography; MRI, magnetic resonance imaging.

weakness and paralysis that can affect the diaphragm. Constipation, nausea and vomiting, and abdominal cramping are also common presentations. Botulism toxin can be neutralized by antisera raised against it, but the use of antitoxin may not reverse existing neuroparalysis. Recently there has been concern about the potential use of botulinum toxin as a bioweapon.

Diagnosis

The laboratory confirmation of human botulism is established by detection of the toxin in the serum or stool of an affected patient or in a sample of food consumed prior to onset of the illness. These assays are only available in public health laboratories. Animal assays are still used because they can detect very low levels of toxin. Isolation of *C. botulinum* from stools, gastric samples, or wound specimens, in combination with the appropriate clinical signs and symptoms for botulism, also establishes the diagnosis. For wound botulism, both serum and wound specimens should be tested for the presence of toxin and organisms. For infant botulism, stool samples are required for analysis.

The laboratory diagnosis is described in **Table 5–33**.

PYELONEPHRITIS AND URINARY TRACT INFECTIONS

Description

UTIs can be divided into three categories:

- Uncomplicated infections of the lower urinary tract involving the bladder and/or urethra
- Uncomplicated infections of the upper urinary tract, or pyelonephritis, involving the ureters, renal pelvis, and kidney
- Complicated UTIs involving various sites within the urinary tract

TABLE 5–33 **Laboratory Evaluation for Botulism**

Laboratory Test	Positive Result
Mouse bioassay	This is the reference method for the detection of botulinum toxin; aliquots of serum, feces, food extract, gastric fluid, or culture supernatant are injected intraperitoneally into mice; control mice are injected with aliquots of the various samples containing botulinum antitoxin; the mice are observed for the toxic effects of the botulism toxin; if the mice receiving the botulinum antitoxin do not develop signs of botulism and the mice not receiving the antitoxin do develop signs, the diagnosis is established
Bacterial culture	The organism can be cultured anaerobically; the isolates must be shown to contain toxins by the bioassay
Antigen detection assays	Sensitive enzyme immunoassays and mass spectroscopy methods are in development

Acute symptomatic uncomplicated lower UTIs are very common in women. The typical symptoms are painful urination (dysuria), urgency, and frequency. Approximately 80% of these infections are caused by *E. coli*. Uropathogenic *E. coli* are genetically distinct from other intestinal strains and possess virulence factors that facilitate colonization of the urinary tract epithelium. Other enteric gram-negative rods, such as *Proteus* spp. and *Klebsiella* spp., and gram-positive cocci including *Staphylococcus saprophyticus* and enterococci can cause uncomplicated UTIs. The high incidence of UTIs in women is probably due to the relatively short length of the urethra and its proximity to the anus and the genital tract. Risk factors for uncomplicated lower UTI in young, sexually active women include intercourse and diaphragm and spermicide use. UTIs are uncommon in men until after the age of 50 years. UTIs in children are also more common in females. They can be associated with constipation, incomplete or infrequent voiding, sexual abuse, and anatomic defects within the urinary tract.

Acute uncomplicated pyelonephritis (upper UTI) is usually due to an ascending infection that begins in the bladder. The main clinical features are fever and chills, nausea, vomiting, and abdominal pain. Costovertebral angle tenderness is usually present. Risk factors for pyelonephritis include the presence of renal stones, obstruction of urine outflow, vesicoureteral reflux, pregnancy, anatomic abnormalities of the kidney and urinary tract, and urinary catheterization. Intrarenal infections are often the result of hematogenous dissemination of *S. aureus* or *Candida* spp.

Complicated UTI refers to infections in patients with a variety of underlying conditions such as anatomic or functional urologic abnormalities, stones, or obstruction. Imaging studies are often useful for identifying the underlying problem. Other predisposing factors are indwelling catheters or urologic instrumentation, immunosuppression, renal disease, and diabetes. These infections are typically caused by hospital-acquired bacteria including *Klebsiella* spp., *Proteus* spp., *Morganella morganii*, *P. aeruginosa*, enterococci, staphylococci, and yeast.

Asymptomatic bacteriuria occurs in 3% of women; of these, 10% will develop UTIs. A higher incidence of UTIs is found in the elderly population where 10% to 15% of women older than 60 years suffer from recurrent UTIs.

Diagnosis

The laboratory diagnosis of a UTI involves tests to detect WBCs in the urine (pyuria) and tests to detect bacteria in the urine (bacteriuria).

Rapid detection of WBCs and bacteria in the urine can be performed using a urine dipstick. The WBCs are detected with a dipstick pad containing leukocyte esterase reagents and some bacteria can be detected by their ability to convert nitrate to nitrite (see Chapter 18 for a discussion of urinalysis). WBCs and bacteria also can be identified and counted in a microscopic analysis of the urine. A urine WBC count of >5 leukocytes per high-power field is defined by most authors as significant pyuria. The level of bacteriuria in the three categories of UTIs varies.

Urine culture is the gold standard for the diagnosis of UTIs, although it may not be necessary for uncomplicated outpatient UTIs. Unlike most other specimen types, urine is always cultured using a quantitative procedure because interpretation of the results depends on both

Acute symptomatic uncomplicated lower UTIs are very common in women. The typical symptoms are painful urination (dysuria), urgency, and frequency. Approximately 80% of these infections are caused by *E. coli*.

The laboratory diagnosis of a UTI involves tests to detect WBCs in the urine (pyuria) and tests to detect bacteria in the urine (bacteriuria).

TABLE 5-34   Evaluation for Urinary Tract Infection (UTI)

Laboratory Test/ Clinical Feature	Uncomplicated Lower Urinary Tract Infection	Uncomplicated Pyelonephritis	Complicated Urinary Tract Infection
Site of infection	Bladder and urethra	Ureters, renal pelvis, and kidney	Varies
Risk factors	Intercourse and diaphragm/spermicide use	Include risk factors for both uncomplicated lower UTI and complicated UTI	Structural or functional abnormalities in the urinary tract
Symptoms	Frequency, urgency, and dysuria	Frequency, urgency, dysuria, flank pain, and fever	Depend on the site of infection
Level of pyuria	>5 WBC per high-power field using a fresh urine specimen or a positive leukocyte esterase dipstick test result	>5 WBC per high-power field using a fresh urine specimen or a positive leukocyte esterase dipstick test result	>5 WBC per high-power field using a fresh urine specimen or a positive leukocyte esterase dipstick test result
Level of bacteriuria (CFU)	For women without symptoms, >10^5 CFU/mL on 2 consecutive specimens; for women with symptoms, >10^2 CFU/mL; for men with symptoms, >10^3 CFU/mL	>10^4 CFU/mL	Same as for uncomplicated lower UTI

CFU, colony-forming unit.

the type and the number of organisms in the specimen. Because urine passes through the distal urethra, which is colonized with a variety of gram-negative rods and other organisms, isolation of bacteria from a midstream clean catch urine specimen does not automatically establish the presence of infection. Significant bacteriuria is often defined as the presence of $\geq 10^5$ colony-forming units (CFU)/mL; however, many patients with a urethral syndrome can have lower counts. The presence of three or more organisms with none predominating indicates contamination, and a new specimen should be collected. Rapid specimen transport and refrigeration of stored specimens is important because bacteria can replicate in urine that is left at room temperature, unless a preservative is used, leading to overgrowth of contaminants and inaccurate colony counts. A summary of the laboratory evaluation for UTI is presented in **Table 5–34**.

INFECTIONS OF THE MALE GENITAL TRACT

Description and Diagnosis

Epididymitis is most often caused by a sexually transmitted disease such as gonorrhea or *Chlamydia* infection (discussed in a later section). However, it can also be caused by enteric gram-negative rods or *Pseudomonas* in patients with underlying urinary tract disease.

Acute bacterial prostatitis presents with urinary tract symptoms, a tender prostate, and is often accompanied by systemic findings such as fever. Chronic infection of the prostate due to gram-negative rods or gram-positive cocci is often asymptomatic, but it can serve as a source of recurrent symptomatic bacteriuria. Chronic pelvic pain syndromes have also been attributed to chronic prostatitis, but often the etiology is unclear. Granulomatous prostatitis caused by extrapulmonary TB or systemic fungal infections produces nodular lesions that can mimic prostatic carcinoma. Histologic examination of a biopsy specimen would distinguish these possibilities. **Table 5-35** provides an association between site of infection in the male genital tract and common causative organisms.

The most common infection of the testicle is viral orchitis that is usually caused by mumps or coxsackieviruses. Mumps is an acute viral disease that causes painful enlargement of the salivary glands, particularly the parotid glands. The virus is transmitted via respiratory droplets. Orchitis in postpubertal males is often due to mumps, although the incidence is low due to vaccination. Laboratory diagnosis is important for epidemiologic investigations. The laboratory tests for mumps are summarized in **Table 5-36**.

The most common infection of the testicle is viral orchitis that is usually caused by mumps or coxsackieviruses.

TABLE 5–35   Infections of the Male Genital Tract

Site of Infection	Common Causative Organisms
Seminal vesicles	Gram-negative bacilli and *Neisseria gonorrhoeae*
Epididymis	*Chlamydia*, gram-negative bacilli, *N. gonorrhoeae*, *Mycobacterium tuberculosis*
Prostate gland	Gram-negative bacilli, enterococci (and staphylococci), and *N. gonorrhoeae*

TABLE 5–36   Laboratory Evaluation for Mumps

Laboratory Tests	Results/Comments
Serology	A positive mumps IgM assay is useful for diagnosis of acute mumps infection; measurement of a mumps IgG seroconversion (from negative to positive) in acute and convalescent specimens or a fourfold rise in mumps IgG titer also supports the diagnosis
PCR	RT-PCR is useful for detecting viral RNA; oral or buccal swab from parotid gland area is preferred specimen, urine is less useful; CSF can be tested in CNS infections
Culture	Mumps virus grows slowly; oral or buccal swab from parotid gland area is preferred specimen, urine is less useful; CSF can be tested in CNS infections; typing of viral isolates is important for epidemiologic studies

INFECTIONS OF THE FEMALE GENITAL TRACT

Description and Diagnosis

Infections of the female genital tract include vaginitis, vaginosis, and cervicitis/pelvic inflammatory disease (infection of the uterus, fallopian tubes, and adjacent structures). As with infections of the male genital tract, many of these infections are due to sexually transmitted diseases that are discussed in a later section.

The primary symptom of vaginitis is pruritus that can be accompanied by a discharge. The most common cause is the yeast *Candida albicans*. *Trichomonas vaginalis* (a protozoan) can cause a similar syndrome. The chief complaint in bacterial vaginosis is vaginal odor. In the past this condition was ascribed to overgrowth of *Gardnerella vaginalis*, but the current view is that it results from a disruption of the normal vaginal flora in which lactobacilli (gram-positive rods) are largely replaced by a mixture of gram-negative coccobacilli.

Table 5–37 briefly describes the etiologic agents, clinical features, and laboratory diagnosis of vaginitis, vaginosis, and pelvic inflammatory disease. Genital herpes and other sexually transmitted diseases are discussed in a subsequent section.

Organisms that infect or colonize the female genital tract can also cause infections of the newborn. Beta-hemolytic streptococci belonging to Lancefield group B (GBS) are also known as *S. agalactiae*. These organisms often asymptomatically colonize the gastrointestinal and female genital tracts; however, they are also an important cause of neonatal sepsis and meningitis (*E. coli* capular type K1 is another common cause of this type of infection). Risk factors associated with early onset neonatal infection include maternal colonization with GBS, premature rupture of membranes, chorioamnionitis, and previous delivery of an infected infant. Pregnant women are routinely screened during the third trimester at 35 to 37 weeks for colonization with GBS. This can be done by culture of vaginal and rectal swabs or nucleic acid amplification. Women who are colonized (or have the risk factors listed above) are given antibiotics during delivery to prevent neonatal infections. *Chlamydia trachomatis*, *Neisseria gonorrhoeae*, and *Herpes simplex* can also be transmitted to the newborn during delivery and cause serious infections.

The primary symptom of vaginitis is pruritus that can be accompanied by a discharge. The most common cause is the yeast *Candida albicans*. *Trichomonas vaginalis* (a protozoan) can cause a similar syndrome.

TABLE 5–37   Infections of the Female Genital Tract

Disease/Condition	Common Etiologic Agent(s)	Clinical Features	Laboratory Diagnosis
Vulvovaginitis	*Candida albicans, Trichomonas vaginalis*	Pruritus, irritation, external dysuria, vaginal discharge (especially with *T. vaginalis*)	Candidiasis: microscopy after treating specimen with 10% KOH to reveal yeast and hyphal forms, culture; trichomoniasis: NAAT, culture, nucleic acid hybridization, antigen detection, wet mount to detect motile trichomonads
Vaginosis	Polymicrobial (multiple anaerobes and *Gardnerella vaginalis*)	Vaginal odor, vaginal discharge	Vaginal discharge pH >4.5; "fishy" odor after addition of 10% KOH; "clue cells" (vaginal epithelial cells coated with coccobacilli) on wet mount; or Gram stain with decreased gram-positive rods and increased gram-negative or variable coccobacilli
Cervicitis, pelvic inflammatory disease (PID)	*Chlamydia trachomatis, Neisseria gonorrhoeae*	Cervicitis is often asymptomatic; PID is associated with lower abdominal pain, vaginal discharge, dysuria, and dyspareunia; long-term sequelae can include infertility and ectopic pregnancy	Nucleic acid amplification of *N. gonorrhoeae* and *C. trachomatis* from urogenital specimens is the preferred method in most situations (see **Tables 5–40** and **5–41**)

SEXUALLY TRANSMITTED DISEASES

Syphilis

Description

Syphilis is a multisystem infectious disease that has prominent dermatologic and neurologic manifestations. It is caused by *Treponema pallidum*, a thin elongated bacterium known as a spirochete. *T. pallidum* is typically spread through contact with infectious lesions during sexual activity. Transmission occurs in about one-third of patients exposed to early syphilis. Primary skin lesions, also known as chancres, usually develop within 3 weeks after initial exposure. Primary syphilis is the stage defined by the presence of lesions at the site of inoculation. Secondary syphilis is the stage of hematogenous dissemination of *T. pallidum*, with widespread physical findings and constitutional signs and symptoms. The signs and symptoms include rash, alopecia, condylomata lata, and shallow painless ulcerations of mucous membranes known as "mucous patches." Even in the absence of treatment, the signs of primary and secondary syphilis spontaneously resolve, and patients enter a latent stage of infection. Manifestations of tertiary syphilis develop in approximately 30% of untreated patients after a variable period of latency. The manifestations of tertiary syphilis involve cardiovascular and/or neurologic and ophthalmic abnormalities. Neurologic involvement, however, is not limited to patients in the tertiary stage of the disease. The clinical manifestations of neurosyphilis include meningitis, general paresis, and tabes dorsalis. Congenital syphilis can occur in newborns whose mothers have syphilis.

> *T. pallidum* cannot be cultured on microbiologic media. As a result, serologic testing is the most widely used approach for the diagnosis of syphilis. Nontreponemal screening tests for syphilis include the venereal disease research laboratory (VDRL) and rapid plasma reagin (RPR) tests. Positive screening test results are routinely confirmed with more specific tests that detect antibodies that react with *T. pallidum* antigens.

The number of cases of primary and secondary syphilis in the United States was relatively stable from the early 1960s to the mid-1980s with 20,000 to 30,000 cases per year. With the appearance of AIDS and the decline of public health programs, the number of cases of primary and secondary syphilis in the United States increased to more than 50,000 by 1990; however, by 2000 it had declined by 80%. More recently there has been a gradual increase in the number of cases.

Diagnosis

T. pallidum organisms are too narrow to be visualized by standard light microscopy, but they can be seen by dark-field microscopy. This technique requires considerable expertise to distinguish *T. pallidum* from nonpathogenic treponemes and other artifacts, and currently it is rarely available.

T. pallidum cannot be cultured on microbiologic media. As a result, serologic testing is the most widely used approach for the diagnosis of syphilis. Two types of tests are routinely used. Nontreponemal screening tests for syphilis include the venereal disease research laboratory (VDRL) and rapid plasma reagin (RPR) tests. These assays detect antibodies that react with an antigen composed of cardiolipin and other lipids. A single reactive test requires supplemental historical, clinical, or laboratory information to provide a diagnosis of syphilis, as there are many biologic causes of a false-positive VDRL or RPR.

Positive results on nontreponemal screening tests are routinely confirmed with more specific tests that detect antibodies that react with *T. pallidum* antigens (i.e., treponemal tests). The fluorescent treponemal antibody absorption test (FTA-ABS) uses indirect immunofluorescence to detect the binding of the patient's antibodies to *T. pallidum* organisms fixed onto a microscopic slide (the patient's serum is first preabsorbed with a nonpathogenic treponeme to increase the specificity of the test). The *T. pallidum* particle agglutination test (TP-PA) measures the ability of serum antibodies to agglutinate gelatin particles that are coated with surface antigens extracted from *T. pallidum*. Because these assays are more expensive and/or technically demanding than the nontreponemal screening tests, they have traditionally been used to confirm a positive nontreponemal test rather than being used for initial evaluation. The introduction of high-throughput, sensitive, EIAs utilizing specific *T. pallidum* antigens has led to the development of the "reverse algorithm": the patient's serum is initially tested with a *T. pallidum* EIA. If it is positive, an RPR is performed to determine if the patient has active infection. If the serum is EIA-positive/RPR-negative, a TP-PA is performed to distinguish a false-positive EIA from past or early infection.

The treponemal tests are specific and sensitive, but they do not distinguish current infection from past infection. Although the nontreponemal tests are less specific, they are still useful because changes in the antibody titer are used to monitor the response to therapy.

Diagnosis of syphilis in newborns is complicated by the fact that they can have substantial quantities of antitreponemal IgG as a result of transfer of this IgG from the maternal circulation to the fetus. A serologic diagnosis of congenital syphilis in the neonate can be confirmed if antitreponemal IgM, made by the fetus, is found in the neonatal circulation. An infant RPR titer greater than the maternal RPR titer also supports a diagnosis of congenital syphilis.

The laboratory tests used in the diagnosis of primary, secondary, latent and tertiary, and congenital syphilis are shown in **Table 5–38**.

Gonorrhea

Description

Gonorrhea, an infection with the organism *N. gonorrhoeae*, is a major cause of morbidity as a sexually transmitted disease, primarily because of complications of the initial infection. These complications include ascending pelvic infections in women, epididymo-orchitis in men, and disseminated gonococcal infections in women and men. Infants born to untreated mothers can also develop ophthalmia neonatorum. The clinical symptoms of gonorrhea include dysuria, urethral and/or vaginal discharge, and pelvic pain. Gonorrhea is generally more symptomatic in men than in women. Clinical features include urethral discharge and mucopurulent cervicitis, respectively. Untreated asymptomatic individuals serve as a reservoir for *N. gonorrhoeae*. Transmission from males to females is more efficient than in the reverse direction. Pharyngeal infections of *N. gonorrhoeae* are typically asymptomatic.

The incidence of gonorrhea in the United States peaked in 1978 and declined approximately 75% through the late 1990s. Since then it has leveled off. Most cases are reported in men because they are more symptomatic than women. Individuals with gonorrhea have a high rate of other sexually transmitted diseases and therefore require complete screening. Ascending pelvic infections that occur in 10% to 20% of acutely infected women can result in infertility and ectopic pregnancy.

Diagnosis

Isolation of *N. gonorrhoeae* in culture requires a nutrient-rich selective agar and an incubation period of up to 48 hours for colony formation. Due to the fastidious nature of the organism, false-negative results frequently occur as a result of poor specimen handling and delayed transport. As a result of these limitations, NAAT assays are now widely used to detect *N. gonorrhoeae* in urogenital specimens (cervical, urethral, and urine). These assays have high specificity, but caution must be used when interpreting positive results in a low-prevalence population. Other anatomic sites, for example, rectal and pharyngeal, are often tested by culture. A NAAT test can only be used for these specimens only if it has been verified that resident flora at these locations does not

N. gonorrhoeae requires a nutrient-rich selective agar for successful culture and an incubation period of up to 48 hours for colony formation. Due to the fastidious nature of the organism, false-negative results frequently occur as a result of poor specimen handling and delayed transport.

TABLE 5-38   Evaluation of Syphilis

Laboratory Test	Primary Syphilis	Secondary Syphilis	Latent and Tertiary Syphilis	Congenital Syphilis
Direct Detection Tests[a]				
Dark-field microscopy (from wet prep of exudate obtained directly from chancre or lesion); requires specialized microscope and extensive training; subject to artifacts; not widely available	In early primary stage, when other tests are less sensitive, this test is useful	If exudative secondary stage lesions are present, this test is useful	Exudative lesions are absent, so this test cannot be performed	Organisms may be present in nasal secretions
Non-Treponemal Tests				
Rapid plasma reagin (RPR) test; agglutination reaction that uses charcoal particles coated with lecithin-cardiolipin-cholesterol mixture	Lag in nonspecific serologic response results in markedly reduced sensitivity in primary syphilis	Rapid, inexpensive screening test; incidence of biologic false-positivity ranges from 0.3% to 1%; positive results must be confirmed by other anti-treponemal serology tests; important for treatment follow-up by assessing titer of antibody	Screening test for both latent and tertiary stages; VDRL recommended over RPR to diagnose neurosyphilis when using a CSF specimen	Maternal IgG antibodies cross placenta and complicate interpretation; need to compare infant and maternal titers
Venereal Disease Research Laboratory (VDRL) test; flocculation test that uses same antigen as RPR; primarily used to test CSF specimens	Lag in nonspecific serologic response results in markedly reduced sensitivity in primary syphilis	Rapid, inexpensive screening test; incidence of biologic false-positivity ranges from 0.3% to 1%; positive results must be confirmed by anti-treponemal serologies; useful for treatment follow-up by assessing titer of antibody	Screening test for both latent and tertiary stages; positive CSF VDRL is sufficient to diagnose neurosyphilis but sensitivity is only 30%–70%), a negative CSF VDRL does not exclude the diagnosis	Maternal IgG antibodies cross placenta and complicate interpretation; need to compare infant and maternal titers
Treponemal tests[b]				
Fluorescent treponemal antibody test with absorptions (FTA-ABS); indirect fluorescent antibody test utilizing *T. pallidum* organisms fixed on a slide	Used as a confirmatory diagnostic test or in lieu of RPR or VDRL; sensitivity of 80%–85% in primary syphilis	Useful as a confirmatory diagnostic test in RPR-positive or VDRL-positive patients; overall sensitivity is approximately 98%; specificity >98% (but does not distinguish syphilis from yaws or pinta); not useful for monitoring therapy	Useful as a confirmatory diagnostic test in RPR-positive or VDRL-positive patients; overall sensitivity is approximately 98%, but it is reduced in late latent phase	A modification of the standard test that detects IgM has been used for neonatal infections (only neonatal)
Immunoassays utilizing recombinant antigens for specific detection of anti-*T. pallidum* IgG (some assays detect IgG + IgM); includes enzyme immunoassay (ELISA/EIA), chemiluminescent immunoassay (CIA), and multi-bead assay formats	Useful as confirmatory diagnostic test; also more sensitive than non-treponemal tests in primary syphilis	Useful as confirmatory diagnostic test, with sensitivity and specificity approaching >99%; also used in "reverse algorithm"[c]	Useful as confirmatory diagnostic test, with sensitivity and specificity approaching 100%; also used in "reverse algorithm"[a] (despite high specificity, positive predictive value can be 70% in a low prevalence population)	Maternal anti-treponemal IgG antibodies cross placenta and complicate interpretation
T. pallidum particle agglutination assay (TP-PA); utilizes gel particles coated with *T. pallidum* antigens	Useful as confirmatory diagnostic test; not as sensitive as FT-ABS in primary infection	Used as a confirmation test if FTA-ABS is inconclusive or when a *T. pallidum* EIA assay is positive but the RPR is negative as part of the "reverse algorithm"	Used as a confirmation test if FTA-ABS is inconclusive or when a *T. pallidum* EIA assay is positive but the RPR is negative as part of the "reverse algorithm"	Maternal anti-treponemal IgG antibodies cross placenta and complicate interpretation

[a]PCR-based detection utilizing laboratory developed tests (i.e., non-FDA-approved) appear to be useful for detecting *T. pallidum* in primary lesions and in CSF but are only available in a limited number of reference labs and CDC.

[b]Other treponemal tests: (i) Western blot assays that detect anti-*T. pallidum* IgG and IgM are not performed in routine clinical laboratories; (ii) microhemagglutination assay for *T. pallidum* (MHA-TP) has largely been replaced by the TP-PA assay.

[c]See Loeffelholz MJ, Binnicker MJ. It is time to use treponema-specific antibody screening tests for diagnosis of syphilis. *J Clin Microbiol.* 2012;50:2–6.

TABLE 5-39 Sample Collection Site by Patient Type for *Neisseria gonorrhoeae*

Specimen	Patient
Urine[a]	Symptomatic (or at-risk) male or female
Urethral exudate	Symptomatic male
Urethral swab if no exudate can be expressed	Symptomatic male
Anorectal and pharyngeal swab	Male or female with rectal or pharyngeal exposure
Conjunctival swab	Infant with conjunctivitis
Blood and synovial fluid	Male or female patient presenting with arthritis and/or dermatitis and suspected of prior gonococcal infection
Swab from endocervical canal	Female suspected of infection

[a]For nucleic acid amplification, not culture.

TABLE 5-40 Evaluation for *Neisseria gonorrhoeae* Infection[a]

Laboratory Test[b]	Results/Comments
Nucleic acid amplification tests (NAAT) (methods include PCR, strand displacement amplification [SDA], and transcription-mediated amplification [TMA])	This is the preferred test for diagnosis of genitourinary tract *N. gonorrhoeae* infections; endocervical or self-collected vaginal swabs in women and urethral swabs in men have the highest yield; the yield for male urine is equivalent to urethral specimens, whereas female urine is slightly less sensitive than endocervical/vaginal swabs
	NAAT assays are also recommended for rectal and pharyngeal infections, but these are not FDA-approved indications and test performance must be validated by individual labs
Gram stain and culture	*N. gonorrhoeae* appears as gram-negative kidney-bean-shaped diplococci (within neutrophils and extracellularly) in clinical specimens; a Gram stain has high sensitivity and specificity for male urethral specimens, but it is much lower for female specimens and is not routinely performed
	Culture is sensitive and inexpensive, but improper specimen collection and handling can easily lead to loss of viability and false-negative cultures; culture and susceptibility testing is particularly important for patients who have not responded to appropriate antibiotic therapy; culture is also used for ocular specimens and other body fluids

[a]Based on Recommendations for the Laboratory-Based Detection of *Chlamydia trachomatis* and *Neisseria gonorrhoeae*—2014. *MMWR Recomm Rep*. March 14, 2014;63(RR02):1-19.

[b]Other methods such as non-amplified DNA hybridization lack sensitivity and are no longer recommended.

cause false-positive results. The samples collected for analysis depend on the site most likely to be infected and the sex of the patient (**Tables 5–39** and **5–40**).

Chlamydial Infections

Description

Chlamydiae are gram-negative, nonmotile, obligate intracellular bacteria. *C. trachomatis* is the most common cause of sexually transmitted disease in North America. It is also the agent of trachoma, a major cause of preventable blindness worldwide. *Chlamydophila pneumoniae* causes a respiratory infection that is similar to *Mycoplasma* infection. *C. psittaci*, which is common in certain birds and can be spread to humans via aerosolized feces, causes psittacosis, a respiratory and/or systemic infection.

C. trachomatis produces up to 4,000,000 infections each year in the United States as a sexually transmitted disease. Groups at increased risk for *C. trachomatis* infection include men or women who have had a new sexual partner or more than one sexual partner in the last year

TABLE 5–41   Evaluation for *Chlamydia trachomatis* Infection[a]

Laboratory Test	Results/Comments
Nucleic acid amplification tests (NAAT) (methods include PCR, strand displacement amplification [SDA], and transcription-mediated amplification [TMA])	This is the preferred test for diagnosis of *Chlamydia trachomatis* infections of the urogenital tract; endocervical or self-collected vaginal swabs in women and urethral swabs in men have the highest yield; the yield for male urine is equivalent to urethral specimens, whereas female urine is slightly less sensitive than endocervical/vaginal swabs
	NAAT methods are also recommended for rectal and pharyngeal infections but these are not FDA-approved indications and test performance must be validated by individual labs
Chlamydia culture	*Chlamydia trachomatis* is an obligate intracellular organism that is grown by inoculating a clinical specimen onto a monolayer cell culture (e.g., McCoy cells); *Chlamydia* culture is much less sensitive than NAAT assays; it is primarily used for cases of potential sexual abuse in children and for specimen types for which NAAT tests have not been validated
Other tests[b]	Serology can be used to aid in the diagnosis of lymphogranuloma venereum (LGV); NAAT assays can detect LGV strains but cannot distinguish them from non-LGV strains; a direct fluorescent antibody (DFA) test can be used to detect *C. trachomatis* in ocular specimens

[a]Based on Recommendations for the Laboratory-Based Detection of *Chlamydia trachomatis* and *Neisseria gonorrhoeae*—2014. *MMWR Recomm Rep*. March 14, 2014;63(RR02):1–19.
[b]Methods such as non-amplified DNA hybridization lack sensitivity and are no longer recommended.

and sexually active women using barrier contraceptive methods. Approximately one-third of infected males and half of infected females may have asymptomatic or mild infections. Subclinical infection and scarring of the fallopian tubes with subsequent infertility is one of the major complications of *Chlamydia* infections. *C. trachomatis* can also infect newborns during delivery and cause conjunctivitis and pneumonia. Lymphogranuloma venereum (LGV), a disease characterized by tender inguinal lymphadenopathy and often proctitis, is caused by specific serovars of *C. trachomatis*.

Diagnosis

Detection of chlamydial DNA using NAAT assays is now the preferred method for diagnosing genital *C. trachomatis* infections due to the high sensitivity and specificity of these assays. These tests use PCR, strand displacement amplification (SDA), or transcription-mediated amplification (TMA) to amplify *C. trachomatis* genes. They have largely replaced other nonculture methods such as antigen detection.

Diagnosis of a chlamydial infection also can be made on the basis of a positive culture of the organism from infected sites. This requires cells in which the organism proliferates and is a labor-intensive procedure. Careful sample collection and specimen transport are important in the maintenance of viable organisms for culture. Although culture is less sensitive than NAAT assays, it is still used in medicolegal situations. Commercial NAAT assays can detect LGV (lymphogranuloma venereum) serovars of *C. trachomatis* but cannot distinguish them from non-LGV serovars. Serologic tests for anti-*Chlamydia* antibodies involving complement fixation or immunofluorescence detect antichlamydial IgG or IgM in the serum and are sometimes used to support the diagnosis of LGV.

Table 5–41 summarizes the tests available to diagnose *Chlamydia* infections.

Herpes Simplex Virus Infections
Description

HSV is a double-stranded DNA virus surrounded by a lipid envelope and is usually transmitted by person-to-person contact. The virus initially causes a productive infection of epithelial cells and then establishes a latent infection in sensory ganglia for the lifetime of the host. It can subsequently reactivate and produce active infections. The classic pattern of infection is a group of recurring vesicles on an erythematous base; however, HSV infection is often asymptomatic, and lesions occur in a minority of infected patients. Individuals infected with HSV are potentially contagious, whether or not lesions are visible. HSV is subdivided into HSV type 1 and type 2. Oral herpes infections, which are typically present as cold sores, are primarily caused by HSV-1.

TABLE 5–42 **Evaluation for Herpes Simplex Viral Infection**

Laboratory Test	Positive Result
Nucleic acid amplification tests (NAAT)	PCR is the gold standard for the diagnosis of HSV encephalitis and meningitis because it is vastly more sensitive than culture for detection of virus in CSF
	PCR is also the most sensitive method for diagnosis of neonatal HSV infections; the test can be performed on CSF, blood, and mucocutaneous vesicular lesions
	PCR and other NAAT methods are more sensitive than culture for the detection of HSV in symptomatic genital infections; it may also detect asymptomatic shedding of the virus
Viral culture	Viral culture is useful for the diagnosis of mucocutaneous HSV infection; however, it is less sensitive than NAAT methods; the greatest likelihood for recovery of virus from culture is when a vesicular or pustular lesion is sampled within 72 h of its appearance; a negative result for a culture does not rule out HSV infection
Serologic tests for antibodies to HSV	HSV-2 infection can be detected with type-specific enzyme immunoassays or immunoblots that detect antibodies to glycoprotein G and can distinguish infection with HSV-2 from HSV-1; other serologic assays cannot distinguish antibodies directed against HSV-1 and HSV-2; antibody assays are useful for detecting HSV-2 genital infection when mucocutaneous lesions are not present; a negative result does not exclude HSV, particularly during a primary infection
Other tests	Direct fluorescent antibody (DFA) staining of cells from mucocutaneous lesions, when positive, can provide rapid confirmation of active HSV infection; however, this method is less sensitive than PCR or culture, a negative result does not rule out infection
	The presence of intranuclear inclusions and multinucleated giant cells in a Tzanck preparation (Wright–Giemsa stain) from a mucocutaneous lesion supports a diagnosis of a herpesvirus infection; however, it is less sensitive than DFA, culture, or PCR, and it cannot distinguish between HSV and VZV

HSV, herpes simplex virus; PCR, polymerase chain reaction; DFA, direct fluorescent antibody, VZV, varicella zoster virus.

Genital herpes infections are primarily caused by HSV-2. It is estimated that 50,000,000 individuals in the United States have genital HSV infection. Transmission of genital herpes occurs during sexual contact, which is not limited to intercourse. Genital HSV-2 infection is much more likely to recur and have asymptomatic virus shedding than HSV-1 infection. Neonatal herpes may be acquired when the infant comes into contact with HSV, typically through an infected birth canal (it can also be acquired from caregivers infected with HSV). Neonatal herpes can present as a severe disseminated infection predominantly affecting the liver and lungs, as a localized CNS infection, or as a skin and mucous membrane infection.

Herpes simplex viruses can be subdivided into HSV type 1 and type 2. Oral herpes infections, which are typically present as cold sores, are primarily caused by HSV-1. Genital herpes infections are primarily caused by HSV-2.

Diagnosis

The laboratory diagnosis of HSV depends on the type of infection and specimen (see **Table 5–42**). PCR-based tests are more sensitive than viral culture for detecting HSV in vesicle fluid from patients who present with genital lesions. The presence of HSV-2 infection between recurrences can be confirmed by performing type-specific serologic tests that detect antibodies to glycoprotein G. PCR testing of CSF is superior to all other methods for the diagnosis of CNS HSV infections.

SELF-ASSESSMENT QUESTIONS

1. Which one of the following general methods is unlikely to be used as a laboratory test to identify an infectious agent?
   - A. Culture of the organism
   - B. Nucleic acid amplification for selected pathogens
   - C. Susceptibility testing of organisms to different antibiotics
   - D. Karyotyping of isolated organisms that are pathogenic

2. Susceptibility tests are most widely used for which of the following types of organisms?
   - A. Bacterial infections
   - B. Fungal infections
   - C. Viral infections
   - D. Parasitic infections

3. Which of the following organisms is most likely to be an incidental contaminant of the specimen because of its presence within the normal bacterial flora of the skin?

   A. *Bacteroides*
   B. *Neisseria*
   C. Coagulase-negative staphylococci
   D. *Haemophilus*

4. Which of the following is not normally sterile?

   A. Blood
   B. Peritoneal fluid
   C. Joint fluid
   D. Sputum

5. Which of the bacteria listed below is an obligate intracellular bacterium and, as a result, cannot be detected by routine bacterial culture?

   A. *Cryptococcus*
   B. *Pseudomonas*
   C. *Rickettsia*
   D. *Candida*

6. Malaria is one of the largest causes of morbidity and mortality in the world. It is caused by protozoa of the *Plasmodium* species. Which of the four species of *Plasmodium*, transmitted by the *Anopheles* mosquito, is the most dangerous?

   A. *P. falciparum*
   B. *P. vivax*
   C. *P. ovale*
   D. *P. malariae*

7. Which one of the following tests is of less value than the others in the diagnosis of infectious mononucleosis?

   A. Heterophile antibody test
   B. Tests for antibodies to Epstein–Barr virus-specific antigens
   C. White blood cell differential with peripheral blood smear
   D. Tests for antibodies to parvovirus B19

8. Which of the below statements about the diagnosis of infectious endocarditis is not true?

   A. Endocarditis specifically affects the valvular endothelium in the heart.
   B. Laboratory confirmation of infective endocarditis commonly involves the isolation of the same organisms from multiple blood cultures.
   C. Acute bacterial endocarditis has a more persistent high-grade bacteremia than subacute bacterial endocarditis and is therefore more likely to be detected.
   D. The presence of hematuria and bacteriuria is common in patients with infective endocarditis.

9. Which of the following types of microorganisms is *least* likely to produce meningitis?

   A. Bacteria
   B. Parasites
   C. Fungi
   D. Viruses

10. A patient suspected to have meningitis has the following laboratory test results from a cerebrospinal fluid sample collected by lumbar puncture.
    White blood cell (WBC) count: 4500/μL; neutrophils 88% of total WBC; glucose 32 mg/dL; and protein 220 mg/dL. Which of the below causative reagents for meningitis is most likely?

    A. Virus
    B. Bacteria
    C. Fungus
    D. Mycobacterium—tuberculous meningitis

11. The tests useful for a synovial fluid analysis collected from a painful joint include all except which one of the following choices?

    A. Protein concentration of the synovial fluid
    B. Gram stain and culture of the synovial fluid
    C. Polarized light microscopy of the synovial fluid for crystal detection
    D. White blood cell count of the synovial fluid

12. Which of the following is not a skin or a soft tissue infection caused by a bacterium?

    A. Osteomyelitis
    B. Folliculitis

    C. Furuncle

    D. Carbuncle

13. Which of the following diseases is associated with a distinctive skin rash known as erythema migrans and requires early treatment to prevent potential subsequent complications that can be neurologic, cardiac, or musculoskeletal?

    A. Cat scratch disease

    B. Bacillary angiomatosis

    C. Lyme disease

    D. Necrotizing fasciitis

14. Which of the following viruses produces chickenpox?

    A. Rubeola

    B. Varicella zoster

    C. Herpes simplex

    D. Rubella

15. Which of the following association between the name of a superficial fungal infection and its anatomic location on the body is incorrect?

    A. Tinea pedis—Hand

    B. Tinea barbae—Beard

    C. Tinea capitis—Scalp

    D. Tinea cruris—Anterior aspect of the thighs

16. Which of the following eye infections is associated with *Chlamydia trachomatis* as a leading cause of blindness?

    A. Endophthalmitis

    B. Infections of the lacrimal system in the eye

    C. Conjunctivitis

    D. Infections of the retina

17. Three of the following are major challenges to laboratory diagnosis of pulmonary infection. Which one is not?

    A. Collection of an adequate sputum specimen that originates in the lung

    B. Contamination of the respiratory sample with oropharyngeal flora

    C. A single test that detects all the respiratory pathogens

    D. The difficulty of respiratory pathogens to be evaluated for sensitivity to antibiotics

18. Which of the following agents has been the indicator infection for more than 20,000 cases of AIDS?

    A. *Pseudomonas aeruginosa*

    B. *Pneumocystis jirovecii*

    C. *Klebsiella* species

    D. Pulmonary tuberculosis

19. Which one of the following organisms is not associated with systemic mycotic infections?

    A. *Blastomyces dermatitidis*

    B. *Histoplasma capsulatum*

    C. *Aspergillus fumigatus*

    D. *Trichophyton tonsurans*

20. Testing to identify one of the agents below is of more value than the other three when investigating a case of nosomial diarrhea. Which one is it?

    A. *Clostridium difficile*

    B. *Salmonella* species

    C. *Campylobacter* species

    D. *Shigella* species

21. What is the appropriate sample for *C. difficile* testing for toxins A and B?

    A. Formed stool

    B. Whole blood

    C. Watery diarrheal stool

    D. Plasma

22. The intestinal protozoa are divided into five main groups that differ in epidemiology and clinical presentation. Which one of the following is not an intestinal protozoon?

    A. *Giardia lamblia*

    B. *Entamoeba histolytica*

    C. *Cyelospora cayetensis*

    D. *Taenia solium*

23. Tapeworms, roundworms, and flukes are all members of what category of agents producing infections in the gastrointestinal tract?

    A. Bacteria
    B. Protozoa
    C. Helminths
    D. Yeasts

24. Ingestion of bacterial toxins already present in food can cause food poisoning. The enterotoxins from which of the following organisms are a common cause of food poisoning?

    A. *Streptococcus pneumonia*
    B. *Pseudomonas aeruginosa*
    C. *Bacillus cereus*
    D. *Enterococcus faecalis*

25. *Clostridium botulinum* produces potent toxins that primarily affect which one of the following organ systems?

    A. Nervous system
    B. Vascular system
    C. Endocrine system
    D. Genitourinary system

26. An evaluation of a patient with a possible urinary tract infection involves all but one of the following tests. Which test is least likely to be informative in such a patient?

    A. White blood cells in urine
    B. Glucose concentration in urine
    C. Bacteria in urine
    D. Urine culture

27. An infection of which one of the following anatomic sites is not considered a urinary tract infection?

    A. Bladder
    B. Kidney
    C. Ureter
    D. Prostate

28. Which of the following is not a test for a syphilis infection?

    A. Rapid plasma reagin (RPR) test
    B. Microscopy after treatment of a vaginal specimen with 10% KOH
    C. Venereal disease research laboratory (VDRL) test
    D. Fluorescent treponemal antibody test with absorptions (FTA-ABS)

29. Which of the following is not commonly considered to be a sexually transmitted disease?

    A. Gonorrhea
    B. Herpes simplex infection
    C. Chlamydial infection
    D. *Escherichia coli* infection

30. The choices below show a sample collection site on the left and a patient type on the right. Which of the following is not correct for a patient being evaluated for a *Neisseria gonorrhea* infection?

    A. Urethral exudate—Symptomatic male
    B. Conjunctival swab—Infant with conjunctivitis
    C. Swab from endocervical canal—Female suspected of infection
    D. Urethral swab—Symptomatic female

FURTHER READING

Achermann Y, Goldstein EJ, Coenye T, Shirtliff ME. Propionibacterium acnes: from commensal to opportunistic biofilm-associated implant pathogen. *Clin Microbiol Rev*. 2014;27:419–440.

Aliabadi N, Tate JE, Haynes AK, Parashar UD; Centers for Disease Control and Prevention (CDC). Sustained decrease in laboratory detection of rotavirus after implementation of routine vaccination—United States, 2000-2014. *MMWR Morb Mortal Wkly Rep*. 2015 Apr 10;64(13):337–342. PMID: 25856253.

Allos BM. *Campylobacter jejuni* infections: update on emerging issues and trends. *Clin Infect Dis*. 2001;32:1201–1206.

Arvanitis M, Anagnostou T, Fuchs BB, Caliendo AM, Mylonakis E. Molecular and nonmolecular diagnostic methods for invasive fungal infections. *Clin Microbiol Rev*. 2014;27:490–526.

Ashley RL. Performance and use of HSV type-specific serology test kits. *Herpes*. 2002;9:38–45.

Assi MA, et al. Systemic histoplasmosis: a 15-year retrospective institutional review of 111 patients. *Medicine (Baltimore)*. 2007;86:162–169.

Baron EJ, et al. Prolonged incubation and extensive subculturing do not increase recovery of clinically significant microorganisms from standard automated blood cultures. *Clin Infect Dis*. 2005;41:1677–1680.

Bauer TM, et al. Derivation and validation of guidelines for stool cultures for enteropathogenic bacteria other than *Clostridium difficile* in hospitalized adults. *JAMA*. 2001;285:313–319.

Biggs HM, Behravesh CB, Bradley KK, et al. Diagnosis and management of tickborne rickettsial diseases: Rocky Mountain spotted fever and other spotted fever group rickettsioses, ehrlichioses, and anaplasmosis—United States. *MMWR Recomm Rep*. 2016;65(No. RR-2):1–44. doi:http://dx.doi.org/10.15585/mmwr.rr6502a1.

Bortolussi R. Listeriosis: a primer. *CMAJ*. 2008;179:795–797.

Boulware DR, et al. Maltreatment of *Strongyloides* infection: case series and worldwide physicians-in-training survey. *Am J Med*. 2007;120:545.e1–545.e8.

Bryant RE, Salmon CJ. Pleural empyema. *Clin Infect Dis*. 1996;22:747–762.

Chatterjee S, Nutman TB. Filarial nematodes. In: Jorgensen JH, Pfaller MA, Carroll KC, et al., eds. *Manual of Clinical Microbiology*. 11th ed. Washington, DC: ASM Press; 2015:2461–2470.

Cho I, Blaser MJ. The human microbiome: at the interface of health and disease. *Nat Rev Genet*. 2012;13:260–270.

Chon CH, et al. Pediatric urinary tract infections. *Pediatr Clin North Am*. 2001;48:1441–1459.

Clark AE, Kaleta EJ, Arora A, Wolk DM. Matrix-assisted laser desorption ionization-time of flight mass spectrometry: a fundamental shift in the routine practice of clinical microbiology. *Clin Microbiol Rev*. 2013;26:547–603.

Couturier MR, Graf EH, Griffin AT. Urine antigen tests for the diagnosis of respiratory infections: legionellosis, histoplasmosis, pneumococcal pneumonia. *Clin Lab Med*. 2014;34:219–36.

Derber CJ, Troy SB. Head and neck emergencies: bacterial meningitis, encephalitis, brain abscess, upper airway obstruction, and jugular septic thrombophlebitis. *Med Clin North Am*. 2012;96:1107–1126.

Didier ES, Weiss LM. Microsporidiosis: current status. *Curr Opin Infect Dis*. 2006;19:485–492.

Dimaio MA, et al. Performance of BinaxNOW for diagnosis of malaria in a U.S. hospital. *J Clin Microbiol*. 2012;50:2877–2880.

Duff P. Maternal and perinatal infection. In: Gabbe SG, Niebyl JR, Simpson JL, eds. *Obstetrics: Normal & Problem Pregnancies*. 5th ed. New York, NY: Churchill Livingstone; 2007:1233–1248.

Durand ML. Eye infections. In: Betts RF, Chapman SW, Penn RL, eds. *Reese and Betts' a Practical Approach to Infectious Diseases*. Philadelphia, PA: Lippincott Williams & Wilkins; 2003:222–250.

Edelstein PH, Roy CR. Legionnaires' disease and pontiac fever. In: Bennett JE, Dolin R, Blaser MJ, eds. *Mandell, Douglas, and Bennett's Principles and Practice of Infectious Diseases*. 8th ed. New York, NY: Elsevier/Saunders; 2015:2633–2644.

Edwards MS, Baker CJ. *Streptococcus agalactiae* (group B *Streptococcus*). In: Bennett JE, Dolin R, Blaser MJ, eds. *Mandell, Douglas, and Bennett's Principles and Practice of Infectious Diseases*. 8th ed. New York, NY: Elsevier/Saunders; 2015:2340–2348.

Enright AM, Prober CG. *Herpesviridae* infections in newborns: varicella zoster virus, herpes simplex virus, and cytomegalovirus. *Pediatr Clin North Am*. 2004;51:889–908.

Eron LJ. Cellulitis and soft-tissue infections. *Ann Intern Med*. 2009;150:ITC1-1.

Espy MJ, et al. Real-time PCR in clinical microbiology: applications for routine laboratory testing. *Clin Microbiol Rev*. 2006;19:165–256.

Fang FC, Polage CR, Wilcox MH. Point-counterpoint: what is the optimal approach for detection of *Clostridium difficile* infection? *J Clin Microbiol*. 2017;55:670–680.

Fishman JA. Infection in solid-organ transplant recipients. *N Engl J Med*. 2007;357:2601–2614.

Fleming RV, et al. Emerging and less common fungal pathogens. *Infect Dis Clin North Am*. 2002;16:915–933.

Florin TA, et al. Beyond cat scratch disease: widening spectrum of *Bartonella henselae* infection. *Pediatrics*. 2008;121:e1413–e1425.

Fredricks DN, et al. Molecular identification of bacteria associated with bacterial vaginosis. *N Engl J Med*. 2005;353:1899–1911.

Freedman DO, et al. Spectrum of disease and relation to place of exposure among ill returned travelers. *N Engl J Med*. 2006;354:119–130.

Garcia HH, Jimenez JA, Escalante H. Cestodes. In: Jorgensen JH, Pfaller MA, Carroll KC, et al., eds. *Manual of Clinical Microbiology*. 11th ed. Washington, DC: ASM Press; 2015:2471–2478.

García-Arias M, et al. Septic arthritis. *Best Pract Res Clin Rheumatol*. 2011;25:407–421.

Gaydos C, Essig A. Chlamydiaceae. In: Jorgensen JH, Pfaller MA, Carroll KC, et al., eds. *Manual of Clinical Microbiology*. 11th ed. Washington, DC: ASM Press; 2015:1106–1121.

Gea-Banacloche J, et al. West Nile virus: pathogenesis and therapeutic options. *Ann Intern Med*. 2004;140:545–553.

Glaser CA, et al. Beyond viruses: clinical profiles and etiologies associated with encephalitis. *Clin Infect Dis*. 2006;43:1565–1577.

Grice EA, Segre JA. The human microbiome: our second genome. *Annu Rev Genomics Hum Genet*. 2012;13:151–70.

Gupta R, et al. Genital herpes. *Lancet*. 2007;370:2127–2137.

Gwaltney JM. Clinical significance and pathogenesis of viral respiratory infections. *Am J Med*. 2002;112:13–18.

Hall CB. Respiratory syncytial virus and parainfluenza virus. *N Engl J Med*. 2001;344:1917–1928.

Hay RJ. Dermatophytosis (ringworm) and other superficial mycoses. In: Bennett JE, Dolin R, Blaser MJ, eds. *Mandell, Douglas, and Bennett's Principles and Practice of Infectious Diseases*. 8th ed. New York, NY: Elsevier/Saunders; 2015:2985–2994.

Heiro M, Helenius H, Sundell J, et al. Utility of serum C-reactive protein in assessing the outcome of infective endocarditis. *Eur Heart J*. 2005;26:1873–81.

Ho M. The history of cytomegalovirus and its diseases. *Med Microbiol Immunol*. 2008;197:65–73.

Hurt C, Tammaro D. Diagnostic evaluation of mononucleosis-like illnesses. *Am J Med*. 2007;120: 911.e1–911.e8.

Ison MG. Adenovirus infections in transplant recipients. *Clin Infect Dis*. 2006;43:331–339.

Iverson SA, et al. Recognition and diagnosis of *Cryptococcus gattii* infections in the United States. *Emerg Infect Dis*. 2012;18:1012–1015.

Jarzembowski JA, Young MB. Nontuberculous mycobacterial infections. *Arch Pathol Lab Med*. 2008;132:1333–1341.

Johnson CC, et al. Peritonitis: update on pathophysiology, clinical manifestations, and management. *Clin Infect Dis*. 1997;24:1035–1045.

Jones MK, Keiser J, McManus DP. Trematodes. In: Jorgensen JH, Pfaller MA, Carroll KC, et al., eds. *Manual of Clinical Microbiology*. 11th ed. Washington, DC: ASM Press; 2015:2479–2492.

Kauffman C, et al. Clinical practice guidelines for the management of sporotrichosis: 2007 update by the Infectious Diseases Society of America. *Clin Infect Dis*. 2007;45:1255–1265.

Lederman ER, Crum NF. A case series and focused review of nocardiosis: clinical and microbiologic aspects. *Medicine (Baltimore)*. 2004;83:300–313.

Lednicky JA. Hantaviruses. A short review. *Arch Pathol Lab Med*. 2003;127:30–35.

Lee BE, Davies HD. Aseptic meningitis. *Curr Opin Infect Dis*. 2007;20:272–277.

Lewinsohn DM, Leonard MK, LoBue PA, et al. Official American Thoracic Society/Infectious Diseases Society of America/Centers for Disease Control and Prevention Clinical Practice Guidelines: diagnosis of tuberculosis in adults and children. *Clin Infect Dis*. 2017;64:e1–e33.

Liesman RM, Pritt BS, Maleszewski JJ, Patel R. Laboratory diagnosis of infective endocarditis. *J Clin Microbiol*. 2017;55:2599–2608.

Limper AH, Adenis A, Le T, Harrison TS. Fungal infections in HIV/AIDS. *Lancet Infect Dis*. Jul 31, 2017. doi:10.1016/S1473-3099(17)30303-1.

Lindström M, Korkeala H. Laboratory diagnostics of botulism. *Clin Microbiol Rev*. 2006;19:298–314.

Loeffelholz MJ, Binnicker MJ. It is time to use treponema-specific antibody screening tests for diagnosis of syphilis. *J Clin Microbiol*. 2012;50:2–6.

Mandell LA, et al; Infectious Diseases Society of America; American Thoracic Society. Infectious Diseases Society of America/American Thoracic Society consensus guidelines on the management of community-acquired pneumonia in adults. *Clin Infect Dis*. 2007;44(suppl 2):S27–S72.

Mazuski JE, Solomkin JS. Intra-abdominal infections. *Surg Clin North Am*. 2009;89:421–437.

McDonald LC, Gerding DN, Johnson S, et al. Clinical practice guidelines for *Clostridium difficile* infection in adults and children: 2017 update by the Infectious Diseases Society of America (IDSA) and Society for Healthcare Epidemiology of America (SHEA). *Clin Infect Dis*. Feb 15, 2018. doi:10.1093/cid/cix1085.

McGowan CC, Krieger JN. Prostatitis, epididymitis, and orchitis. In: Bennett JE, Dolin R, Blaser MJ, eds. *Mandell, Douglas, and Bennett's Principles and Practice of Infectious Diseases*. 8th ed. New York, NY: Elsevier/Saunders; 2015:1381–1387.

Moore A, Nelson CA, Molins C, Mead PS, Schriefer M. Current guidelines, common clinical pitfalls, and future directions for laboratory diagnosis of Lyme disease, United States. *Emerg Infect Dis*. 2016;22:1169–1177.

Moran GJ, et al. Methicillin-resistant *S. aureus* infections among patients in the emergency department. *N Engl J Med*. 2006;355:666–674.

Morbidity and Mortality Weekly Report (MMWR). Recommendations for the laboratory-based detection of *Chlamydia trachomatis* and *Neisseria gonorrhoeae*—2014. *MMWR Recomm Rep*. 2014;63(RR02):1–19.

Morshed MG, Singh AE. Recent trends in the serologic diagnosis of syphilis. *Clin Vaccine Immunol*. 2015;22:137–147.

Murdoch DR, et al. Clinical presentation, etiology, and outcome of infective endocarditis in the 21st century: The International Collaboration on Endocarditis—prospective cohort study. *Arch Intern Med.* 2009;169:463–473.

Murray HW, et al. Advances in leishmaniasis. *Lancet.* 2005;366:1561–1577.

Naktin J, Beavis KG. *Yersinia enterocolitica* and *Yersinia pseudotuberculosis. Clin Lab Med.* 1999;19:523–536.

Nørskov-Lauritsen N. Classification, identification, and clinical significance of *Haemophilus* and *Aggregatibacter* species with host specificity for humans. *Clin Microbiol Rev.* 2014;27:214–240.

Pai M, et al. Systematic review: T-cell-based assays for the diagnosis of latent tuberculosis infection: an update. *Ann Intern Med.* 2008;149:177–184.

Pasternack MS, Swarts MN. Cellulitis, necrotizing fasciitis, and subcutaneous tissue infections. In: Bennett JE, Dolin R, Blaser MJ, eds. *Mandell, Douglas, and Bennett's Principles and Practice of Infectious Diseases.* 8th ed. New York, NY: Elsevier/Saunders; 2015:1194–1215.

Patel R. New developments in clinical bacteriology laboratories. *Mayo Clin Proc.* 2016;91:1448–1459.

Pawlowski SW, et al. Diagnosis and treatment of acute or persistent diarrhea. *Gastroenterology.* 2009;136:1874–1886.

Pfaller MA, Diekema DJ. Epidemiology of invasive mycoses in North America. *Crit Rev Microbiol.* 2010;36:1–53.

Pichichero ME. Otitis media. *Pediatr Clin North Am.* 2013;60:391–407.

Pien BC, Sundaram P, Raoof N, et al. The clinical and prognostic importance of positive blood cultures in adults. *Am J Med.* 2010;123:819–828.

Polage CR, Cohen SH. State-of-the-art microbiologic testing for community-acquired meningitis and encephalitis. *J Clin Microbiol.* 2016;54:1197–202.

Pritt BS. *Plasmodium* and *Babesia.* In: Jorgensen JH, Pfaller MA, Carroll KC, et al., eds. *Manual of Clinical Microbiology.* 11th ed. Washington, DC: ASM Press; 2015:2338–2356.

Queiroz-Telles F, McGinnis MR, Salkin I, Graybill JR. Subcutaneous mycoses. *Infect Dis Clin North Am.* 2003;17:59–85.

Ramanan P, Bryson AL, Binnicker MJ, Pritt BS, Patel R. Syndromic panel-based testing in clinical microbiology. *Clin Microbiol Rev.* Nov 15, 2017;31. pii: e00024-17.

Ribes JA, et al. Zygomycetes in human disease. *Clin Microbiol Rev.* 2000;13:236–301.

Sande MA, Gwaltney JM. Acute community-acquired bacterial sinusitis: continuing challenges and current management. *Clin Infect Dis.* 2004;39(suppl 3):S151–S158.

Saubolle MA, et al. Epidemiologic, clinical, and diagnostic aspects of coccidioidomycosis. *J Clin Microbiol.* 2007;45:26–30.

Schmid DS, Jumaan AO. Impact of varicella vaccine on varicella-zoster virus dynamics. *Clin Microbiol Rev.* 2010;23:202–17.

Sheorey H, Biggs B-A, Ryan N. Nematodes. In: Jorgensen JH, Pfaller MA, Carroll KC, et al., eds. *Manual of Clinical Microbiology.* 11th ed. Washington, DC: ASM Press; 2015:2448–2460.

Sia IG, Berbari EF. Infection and musculoskeletal conditions: osteomyelitis. *Best Pract Res Clin Rheumatol.* 2006;20:1065–1081.

Sobel JD. What's new in bacterial vaginosis and trichomoniasis? *Infect Dis Clin North Am.* 2005;19:387–406.

Sobel JD. Vulvovaginal candidosis. *Lancet.* 2007;369:1961–1971.

Stanley SL Jr. Amoebiasis. *Lancet.* 2003;361(9362):1025–1034.

Stevens DL. The flesh-eating bacterium: what's next? *J Infect Dis.* 1999;179 (suppl 2):S366–S374.

Stevens DL, et al. Life-threatening clostridial infections. *Anaerobe.* 2012;18:254–259.

Storch GA. Diagnostic virology. In: Knipe DM, Howley PM, eds. *Fields' Virology.* 5th ed. Philadelphia, PA: Wolters Kluwer; 2007:565–604.

Strockbine NA, Bopp CA, Fields PI, Kaper JB, Nataro JP. *Escherichia, Shigella,* and *Salmonella.* In: Jorgensen JH, Pfaller MA, Carroll KC, et al., eds. *Manual of Clinical Microbiology.* 11th ed. Washington, DC: ASM Press; 2015:685–713.

Tan KE, et al. Prospective evaluation of a matrix-assisted laser desorption ionization-time of flight mass spectrometry system in a hospital clinical microbiology laboratory for identification of bacteria and yeasts: a bench-by-bench study for assessing the impact on time to identification and cost-effectiveness. *J Clin Microbiol.* 2012;50:3301–3308.

Thielman NM, Guerrant RL. Clinical practice. Acute infectious diarrhea. *N Engl J Med.* 2004;350:38–47.

Thomson RB Jr, Bertram H. Laboratory diagnosis of central nervous system infections. *Infect Dis Clin North Am.* 2001;15:1047–1071.

Tipple C, Taylor GP. Syphilis testing, typing, and treatment follow-up: a new era for an old disease. *Curr Opin Infect Dis.* 2015;28:53–60.

Vannier E, et al. Human babesiosis. *Infect Dis Clin North Am.* 2008;22:469–488.

Waites KB, et al. Molecular methods for the detection of mycoplasma and ureaplasma infections in humans: a paper from the 2011 William Beaumont Hospital Symposium on molecular pathology. *J Mol Diagn.* 2012;14:437–450.

Weinstock GM. Genomic approaches to studying the human microbiota. *Nature.* 2012;489(7415):250–256.

Whitley RJ. Herpes simplex encephalitis: adolescents and adults. *Antiviral Res.* 2006;71:141–148.

Wilson ML, Gaido L. Laboratory diagnosis of urinary tract infections in adult patients. *Clin Infect Dis.* 2004;38:1150–1158.

Wolf J, Daley AJ. Microbiological aspects of bacterial lower respiratory tract illness in children: atypical pathogens. *Paediatr Respir Rev.* 2007;8:212–219.

Wong CL. Does this patient had bacterial peritonitis or portal hypertension? How do I perform a paracentesis and analyze the results? *JAMA.* 2008;299:1166–1178.

Workowski KA, Bolan GA; Centers for Disease Control and Prevention. Sexually transmitted diseases treatment guidelines, 2015. *MMWR Recomm Rep.* 2015;64(RR-03):1–137.

Young NS, Brown KE. Parvovirus B19. *N Engl J Med.* 2004;350:586–597. Available at: https://www.aphl.org/programs/infectious_disease/tuberculosis/TBCore/2-Overview-of-Syphilis-Diagnostics-Assays-and-Algorithms.pdf. Accessed February 15, 2018.

Toxicology

James H. Nichols, Nicola J. Rutherford,
and Michael Laposata

LEARNING OBJECTIVES

1. Define therapeutic drug monitoring, and learn when it is necessary and how it is performed for commonly monitored drugs.

2. Describe basic pharmacokinetic principles as they relate to therapeutic drug monitoring.

3. Identify the common drugs of abuse and how they are detected in blood, serum, urine, and other body fluids.

4. Understand the association between occupations, industries, and exposure to specific environmental toxins.

CHAPTER OUTLINE

INTRODUCTION

Toxicology comprises several medical applications. The analysis of drugs in human specimens can be conducted for clinical or legal/forensic purposes. Clinical applications include the acute management of overdose and therapeutic monitoring of drug concentrations to achieve maximum efficacy while limiting the toxicity and side effects of medications. Forensic applications of toxicology include analysis of drugs to provide evidence for civil and criminal court cases, to investigate the cause of death, to deter the use of performance-enhancing drugs in athletic competitions, and to determine operator impairment related to traffic citations and vehicle collisions. Workplace drug testing assesses preemployment drug abuse and on-the-job impairment. Given the number of therapeutic drugs, drugs of abuse, and environmental toxins, as well as the variety of diseases, signs, and symptoms associated with drug exposure and overdose, there is an array of laboratory testing strategies. For this reason, the discussion of toxicology in this chapter will be divided into three broad sections—therapeutic drug monitoring (TDM), drugs of abuse, and environmental toxins (**Figure 6–1**).

Therapeutic drug monitoring

> TDM is the practice of measuring the concentration of a drug or its metabolites in order to optimize the dosing of that drug to an individual patient and/or to assess patient compliance with a dosing schedule.

> TDM may be required for drugs with a narrow therapeutic index, significant side effects, or low margin of safety. Monitoring is useful when the therapeutic range for a drug significantly overlaps the toxic range, when a drug cannot be dosed based on clinical observation, or when patients have compliance problems.

> Not all drugs require monitoring.

Detection of drugs of abuse

> An abused drug is any compound that is consumed in greater amounts or in a manner that is neither approved nor supervised by medical staff. Drugs of abuse are agents used recreationally for euphoria, stimulant, sedative, or other effects. Analysis is intended to detect past use by the patient.

Detection of environmental toxins

> Environmental toxins are potentially hazardous substances that contaminate the air, water, or soil. Exposure to environmental toxins may be monitored by specific tests for clinical diagnosis and treatment.

FIGURE 6–1   **Considerations in therapeutic drug monitoring, drugs of abuse detection, and detection of environmental toxins.**

THERAPEUTIC DRUG MONITORING

Overview of Therapeutic Drug Monitoring

The goal of therapeutic drug monitoring is to increase the likelihood of a therapeutic effect and avoid or minimize adverse effects. Patients do not require monitoring for most drugs.

TDM is the practice of measuring the concentration of a drug or its metabolite in order to optimize the dosing of that drug to an individual patient and/or to assess patient compliance with a dosing schedule. The goal of TDM is to improve drug efficacy—the likelihood of a therapeutic effect while avoiding or minimizing adverse effects. **Table 6–1** lists some commonly monitored drugs. Patients do not require monitoring for most drugs. However, for a limited group of agents or for patients with certain conditions (for instance, limited renal function, pregnancy, newborn or geriatric age groups), TDM plays an essential role in establishing the appropriate therapeutic dosing regimen.

Prior to the 1960s, drug dosing was entirely empirical. For certain agents, this trial-and-error approach gave wide variations in patient response and a significant incidence of toxicity. Since then, physicians have learned to optimize drug dosages and delivery while avoiding many of the drug's adverse effects. This has been achieved through the development of sensitive and rapid laboratory assays and the establishment of therapeutic ranges for common medications.

Indications for Therapeutic Drug Monitoring

TDM is performed to optimize the dose of a drug to an individual patient. Drugs with a narrow therapeutic index or margin of safety (the difference between the effective dose and the toxic dose) are potential candidates for therapeutic monitoring (**Table 6–2**). TDM is useful for drugs

TABLE 6–1   Commonly Monitored Drugs

Methotrexate

Immunosuppressants
- Tacrolimus (FK-506)
- Cyclosporin
- Sirolimus (rapamycin)

Antibiotics
- Gentamicin
- Tobramycin
- Vancomycin

Antiepileptics (first generation)
- Phenytoin
- Phenobarbital
- Carbamazepine
- Valproic acid
- Clonazepam

Antiepileptics (second generation)
- Lamotrigine
- Levetiracetam
- Oxcarbazepine

Tricyclic antidepressants
- Amitriptyline
- Desipramine
- Doxepin
- Imipramine
- Nortriptyline

Lithium

Cardiac agents
- Digoxin

Pain management
- Buprenorphine
- Methadone

TABLE 6–2   Indications for Therapeutic Drug Monitoring

The prescribed drug has a low margin of safety; that is, toxic blood drug concentrations or dosages are only slightly greater than therapeutic ones (a narrow therapeutic index)

Patient compliance with their prescribed drug regimen is uncertain

The drug does not act via irreversible inhibition ("hit and run" effect)

Symptoms of underlying disease are difficult to distinguish from drug toxicity

The treatment goal is not an objectively measured end point (such as blood pressure)

The prescribed drug has significant pharmacokinetic variability as a result of:
- Interindividual metabolic capacity
- Nonlinear (zero-order) drug kinetics
- Frequent drug–drug interactions
- Physiologic conditions (e.g., aging, pregnancy)
- Underlying disease state (e.g., liver or renal impairment)

that display significant pharmacokinetic variability that may be caused by drug interactions, genetic variation in drug metabolism, nonlinear kinetics, physiologic conditions such as pregnancy and aging, and underlying diseases that alter the effective amount of drug delivered to or metabolized by the body. When patient compliance is in question, drug monitoring may be used to demonstrate the presence or absence of the prescribed agent. TDM requires a suitable laboratory assay and the establishment of a therapeutic reference range that correlates with efficacy and/or toxicity.

TDM is performed by measuring the concentration of a drug and metabolite(s). Blood or serum/plasma is the usual sample for TDM, but in some cases, urine or oral fluid samples are used to evaluate drug concentration. The most common examples of urine and oral fluid sampling are monitoring of buprenorphine, methadone, and oxycodone for patient compliance. By using blood levels to guide drug therapy, a proportional relationship is assumed between the plasma/serum concentration, the concentration of drug at the organ cellular level, and pharmacologic effect. For practical reasons, only blood levels of the drug are measured, because tissue concentrations cannot be easily sampled or analyzed. This pharmacokinetic principle of homogeneity defines the timing of sampling for TDM, since the concentrations of drug in blood at the moment of sample collection must reflect a proportional and constant (steady-state) concentration at the end organ and be reflective of drug effects at the cellular level. Most TDM samples are collected as trough concentrations, the lowest level just prior to the next dose, or as peak concentrations, 30 to 60 minutes after the dose, when blood levels are most reflective of the tissue concentration and drug efficacy or toxicity.

Pharmacokinetic Principles

Pharmacokinetics is the study of drug interaction (absorption, metabolism, and clearance) within the body. Drug behavior in the body can be described by the LADME mnemonic. The "L" stands for liberation or release of the drug from its dosage form. The "A" is absorption that describes the movement of drug from the administration site into circulation. Distribution is the "D" and describes the reversible movement of drug through the circulatory system and body tissues. Metabolism or "M" is the chemical conversion of drug to active and inactive compounds. Finally, the "E" indicates how the body eliminates the drug.

Drugs behave in the body based on their chemical characteristics at the molecular level. Drugs can be acidic, basic, neutral, or polar (**Table 6–3**). The charge and dissociation constant (pK) of the drug influences its absorption, distribution, and elimination characteristics. The dissociation constant of the drug also affects how the drug can be extracted from patient samples and analyzed in the laboratory.

Liberation and Routes of Drug Administration

Drugs can be delivered to the body in a variety of ways. Patients may take a drug orally (PO) by pill (e.g., aspirin) or dissolve a powder in a liquid drink (e.g., laxatives). Drugs can be delivered intravascularly (IV) through a needle directly into circulation (antibiotics, like vancomycin). Some medications are delivered under the tongue, sublingual (SL), like nitroglycerin for cardiac pain or angina. Others may be injected under the skin, subcutaneous (SC), like compounds in a

---

TABLE 6–3　Characteristics of Chemical Groups on Drugs

Acidic drugs

$$\text{R–C=O} \underset{}{\overset{pK}{\longleftrightarrow}} \text{R–C=O} + \text{H}^+$$
$$\mid \qquad\qquad\quad \mid$$
$$\text{OH} \qquad\qquad\; \text{O}^-$$

Unionized　　　　　Ionized

Basic drugs

$$\text{H}^+ + \text{R–NH}_2 \overset{pK}{\longleftrightarrow} \text{R–NH}_3^+$$

Unionized　　　　　　　　　Ionized

Neutral Drugs	Polar Drugs
R–CH$_3$	R–OH
(Oil-like)	(Water-like)

The chemical groups on a drug determine the drug's characteristics and behavior in the body

Acidic and basic chemical groups on drugs are in equilibrium between the unionized (uncharged) and ionized (charged) forms of the molecule

Unionized forms can passively diffuse while charged forms require active transport and bind to proteins and other counterions

Neutral drugs carry no charge and can be hydrophobic, oil-like, or polar, hydrophilic, and attract water

tuberculosis test, or intramuscularly (IM), such as vaccinations. Rectal (suppositories) and transdermal (e.g., fentanyl pain patches) applications are other methods of delivering a drug. The route of administration will affect absorption and bioavailability of the drug to the body.

Drug Absorption

The route of drug administration and the formulation of the drug affect the rate and extent of drug absorption. For example, oral drug absorption is affected by many factors including drug solubility in enteral fluid, the acid–base characteristics of the drug, the lipid solubility of the drug, interferences with absorption by food, destruction of the drug by gastrointestinal flora, coadministration of other drugs—especially antacids, cholestyramine, and other resin-binding agents—blood flow to the gastrointestinal tract, and gastrointestinal transit time. Some orally delivered drugs are also subject to a significant "first-pass effect," whereby they are largely metabolized by the liver to inactive compounds before reaching the systemic circulation. IV administration delivers drug directly into circulation bypassing "first-pass metabolism," and the amount of drug delivered IV is often compared with other delivery options for determining the extent or amount of drug that is absorbed from a specific formulation. Significant variability in drug absorption is thus a common indication for TDM.

The chemical characteristics of a drug also affect the rate and extent of drug absorption. Acidic drugs carry a carboxyl group, $R-COOH$ (**Table 6–3**). This acidic group is unionized or uncharged at pH levels below the drug's dissociation constant and is ionized or charged ($R-COO^-$) at pH levels above the drug's dissociation constant. Drugs that act as strong acids have dissociation constants with a pK <5, such as salicylate, penicillin, and analgesics. Strongly acidic drugs are unionized and do not carry a charge at the acidic pH of the stomach while they carry a charge at the more basic pH of the intestines. So, drugs like salicylate are passively absorbed in the stomach, but require active transport for absorption across the intestines. Weak acids (barbiturates, sulfonamides, and thiazide diuretics) have dissociation constants in the range 5 to 11, and are preferentially absorbed in the intestines compared with the stomach. Strongly acidic drugs tend to be fully dissociated or charged at blood pH of 7.4 while weak acids may have significant amounts of the unionized form present in the blood. Due to the acidic pH of urine, weak acids that are ionized at blood pH may become unionized in urine and prone to greater reabsorption. Basic drugs contain an amine group ($R-NH_3$). Basic groups are ionized ($R-NH_2^+$) below and unionized (uncharged) above their dissociation constant. Basic drugs can act as weak bases (e.g., anesthetics, opiates, and antidepressants) with pK <10 or strong bases (e.g., amphetamines and bronchodilators). Basic drugs tend to be significantly ionized (charged) at blood pH. Drugs can also be neutral and carry no charge across the range of physiologic pH. Neutral drugs can be lipophilic and act like fats (e.g., corticosteroids) or polar and hydrophilic and attract water molecules (e.g., digoxin).

Distribution

After absorption, drugs distribute throughout the body through the circulatory system, lymphatic system, and tissue fluids. The amount of free drug available to act at organ receptors is affected by both protein and tissue binding. Protein binding is another consideration in TDM. Binding to plasma proteins occurs to some extent for most drugs, with bound and free (unbound) drugs existing in equilibrium. Although it is only the free drug fraction that is biologically active, most laboratory assays measure the total drug concentration, that is, the sum of the bound and the unbound drug. Several factors can cause changes in plasma proteins and, consequently, affect free drug levels. Acid/neutral drugs tend to bind albumin while basic/neutral drugs bind α_1-acid glycoprotein. Some drugs have specific binding proteins such as cortisol and corticosteroid-binding globulin, also known as transcortin. These proteins serve as transport proteins for drugs from the site of absorption to the tissue where the drug can act, and as delivery mechanisms to the liver for metabolism or the kidney for elimination. Disease alterations in protein concentration can, therefore, affect the concentration of free drug. For example, hypoalbuminemia, which occurs in the elderly and in patients with cirrhosis, may cause an increased free drug fraction in the setting of normal total drug levels. α_1-Acid glycoprotein is an acute-phase reactant and levels of this protein increase in acute and chronic diseases. Increases in α_1-acid glycoprotein create more binding sites for drug, so less free drug will be available in light of the same total drug concentration in a sample. The presence of uremia in disease results in compounds binding to albumin, displacing drug from the protein and elevating the free drug fraction. TDM can determine the proportion of free and total drugs in the setting of disease and individualize the dosage to the patient's condition.

Drug Metabolism

Drug metabolism typically renders nonpolar, lipophilic drugs into more polar, water-soluble compounds for elimination. The liver is the primary site for drug metabolism. Genetic variants, age, cirrhosis, and other hepatic conditions may adversely affect drug metabolism, and thus predispose a patient to toxicity. Many drugs are hepatic enzyme inducers or inhibitors and thus can influence the rate of their own metabolism, as well as the metabolism of many other drugs.

Pharmacogenetics

Pharmacogenetics is the study of drug action and metabolism based on genetics. Common gene variants can alter drug metabolism, the transport of drug in the body, the affinity of the drug receptor, and the signaling induced by the drug. Together, these genetic variants produce an individualized response to a drug. Testing for certain genetic variants can help clinicians predict how the patient will respond to a specific drug and/or dose of drug. This can guide clinicians to the best treatment option for their patient, avoiding a trial and error approach, to achieve therapeutic drug levels while minimizing unwanted side effects and drug toxicity.

Pharmacokinetics is the study of drug interaction (absorption, metabolism, and clearance) within the body. Pharmacogenetics is the study of how a patient will respond to a drug based on his/her own genetics.

An example of pharmacogenetics in patient care is the determination of warfarin dose, a blood thinner used to treat and prevent blood clots. One gene of interest is CYP2C9, a member of the cytochrome P450 family of enzymes, involved in the metabolism of warfarin. Depending on the genotype, an individual can be a "normal metabolizer," a "fast metabolizer," or a "slow metabolizer." Fast metabolizers will catalyze the oxidation of warfarin to hydroxywarfarin at a greater rate than normal and slow metabolizers, and will require a higher dose of the drug. On the other hand, slow metabolizers will metabolize warfarin at a slower rate and may require a lower dose of drug as they will be more prone to toxicity if prescribed the same dose of drug.

Drug Elimination

Elimination is the removal of drug and metabolites from the body. Drugs can be eliminated through the kidneys, the liver, the lungs, the skin, the feces, and by other means. Elimination of many polar, nonlipophilic drugs is achieved primarily through renal excretion, which is dependent on adequate kidney function and renal blood flow. Other parameters relevant to elimination through the kidneys include urine pH and the properties of the drug itself, such as the dissociation constant, pK, and molecular size. Drug clearance is the theoretical volume of serum/plasma that is completely cleared of a drug per unit time. Importantly, clearance is the sum of all elimination mechanisms—hepatic, renal, lung, and any other—for a particular drug. Patients with impaired drug clearance may need more frequent monitoring.

In TDM, drug levels are most often determined only after steady state has been achieved. Steady state is the condition that occurs when the amount of drug entering the system equals the amount being eliminated. Steady-state concentration is compared in relation to a target range to determine changes in dosing. The target range is established from experimental dosing studies to determine the optimum drug concentration where a drug is most effective while causing the least undesirable side effects and toxicity. The target range is a generalized range that fits most patients, but that range may need to be adjusted or altered in certain disease states and physiologic conditions. TDM allows physicians to optimize drug dosage to a patient's individual situation.

Most but not all drugs are eliminated by first-order (or linear) kinetics. This means that a constant *fraction* of drug is eliminated per unit time. Other drugs are eliminated by zero-order (or nonlinear) kinetics, such that a constant *amount* of drug is eliminated per unit time.

Most but not all drugs are eliminated by first-order (or linear) kinetics. This means that a constant fraction of total drug is eliminated per unit time. All drugs have a biological half-life. For drugs that follow first-order elimination kinetics, changes in dose will generally cause predictable changes in blood levels. Increases in drug concentration lead to increases in the rate of drug elimination. Some drugs, however, are eliminated by zero-order (or nonlinear) kinetics, such that a constant amount of drug is eliminated per unit time. Typically, metabolism by zero-order kinetics occurs when elimination pathways for that drug have been saturated. Under these circumstances, the biological half-life is not constant but depends on drug concentration. As a result, small increments in dose may cause disproportionately large increments in blood levels. Due to their lack of a predictable dose–response relationship, drugs that follow zero-order kinetics often require monitoring.

Assuming first-order kinetics, five half-lives are required after initiation of drug therapy to reach nearly complete (97%) steady state (five half-life rule). Five half-lives are also required for nearly complete clearance of a drug after the termination of therapy, and for attaining a new steady state whenever a dosing regimen has been changed.

Drug Interactions and Dose Adjustments

Many patients may take more than one medication, and those drugs can interact in the patient's body. Drug interactions may cause displacement of bound drug from proteins. The clinical significance of the interaction is likely to be increased when both drugs are highly protein bound (80% or more), when one of the drugs has a higher binding affinity, or when one of the drugs is present in higher concentration than the other. Dosing adjustments may be required in these instances. Displacement of bound drug does not inevitably lead to an increased free drug level, because free drug is subject to increased metabolism and elimination. Increases in plasma proteins and drug binding may also occur as an acute-phase response or during pregnancy, and, consequently, higher dosing may be necessary. Caution must be used when interpreting total drug levels in patients with possible protein disturbances or drug interactions, and free drug levels may be more useful in these situations.

Laboratory Methods

Currently, most clinical laboratories utilize immunoassays for the rapid and quantitative measurement of therapeutic drugs. In an immunoassay, drug in the patient's sample competes with a drug conjugate (drug attached to an enzyme or microparticle) for the binding of specific antibodies. Antibody binding results in blocking enzyme activity or in turbidity from the cross-linking of microparticles. By direct measurement of enzyme activity or indirect measurement of the inhibition of turbidity from microparticle complexes in solution, the amount of drug in the patient sample is quantitated. Chemiluminescent immunoassays offering superior sensitivity are also available for drug analysis. Other immunoassay methods such as ELISA and radioimmunoassay are less commonly used. More complex laboratory techniques, such as chromatography with ultraviolet or mass spectral detection, are also commonly utilized for drug measurements. (See Chapter 2.) Immunoassays offer advantages over chromatographic methods, because immunoassays can be automated and analyze a greater number of samples more rapidly with less labor and cost. Only the *total* drug concentrations are routinely measured. Free drug levels require a more time-consuming and expensive ultracentrifugation or dialysis equilibrium steps to separate the protein-bound drug from the free drug. Free drug concentrations are typically lower than total drug concentrations by a factor of two- to 20-fold, so more sensitive assays are required.

Specimen Collection

The appropriate specimen for therapeutic drug measurements is usually serum or plasma. Most laboratories do not accept gel separator tubes as the gel can bind drugs and interfere with drug recovery. Immunosuppressant levels are measured using whole blood due to the distribution and concentration of drug in RBCs, which are removed in the preparation of serum/plasma. EDTA-anticoagulated whole blood is the appropriate sample for these immunosuppressant drug measurements. Urine samples are frequently used to evaluate patient compliance in cases of therapeutic administration of buprenorphine, methadone, and several opiates (including oxycodone). Saliva or oral fluid may be appropriate for monitoring some medications, such as theophylline, in pediatric patients or in those for whom phlebotomy is difficult. Oral fluid is also not subject to adulteration or substitution, which can be an issue with monitoring for pain management compliance in patients prone to drug abuse. In general, trough levels are drawn just prior to the next dose and are used to evaluate the likelihood of a therapeutic effect. Peak levels are drawn at varying times, depending on the particular drug, and are used typically to assess toxicity risk.

In general, *trough* levels are drawn just prior to the next dose and are used to evaluate the likelihood of a *therapeutic* effect. *Peak* levels are drawn at varying times, depending on the particular drug, and are used typically to assess *toxicity* risk.

Selected Commonly Monitored Drugs

Selected individual drugs and considerations for TDM are presented in **Table 6–4**. The required specimen volume and preservative will vary by analytical methodology, so the described collection

TABLE 6–4   Therapeutic Drug Monitoring for Commonly Monitored Drugs

Drug	Monitoring Recommendations	Specimen Collection Tube and Instructions	Suggested Therapeutic Range	Special Considerations
Methotrexate	24, 48, 72 h after bolus; then daily until below cytotoxic levels	5 mL red top; wrap in foil to protect from light; indicate time past bolus	<10 μmol/L at 24 h <1 μmol/L at 48 h <0.4 μmol/L at 72 h	Monitoring guidelines are for high-dose therapy (>20 mg/kg) only
Tacrolimus (FK-506)	Trough levels, 12 h post dose	3 mL purple top	5–20 ng/mL	Cross-reactivity with its metabolites in immunoassays

Cyclosporin	Trough levels, 12 or 24 h post dose	3 mL purple top; avoid drawing from line of administration	Transplant of:
			(1) Liver: 400–800 ng/mL
			(2) Heart: 150–300 ng/mL
			(3) Kidney:
			   (a) <3 months: 150–250 ng/mL
			   (b) >3 months: 100–200 ng/mL
				Ranges depend on organ transplanted and time since transplant

Aminoglycosides	Peak: (1) IV: 30–60 min post dose (2) IM: 60–90 min post dose Trough: 30 min prior to next dose	5 mL red top	Gentamicin—peak: 5–10 μg/mL, trough: <2.0 μg/mL Tobramycin—peak: 4–8 μg/mL, trough: <2.0 μg/mL	Guidelines for conventional dosing only (not low-dose therapy or pulse therapy)
Vancomycin	Either peak or trough, once per day	5 mL red top	Peak: 30–40 μg/mL, trough: 5–10 μg/mL	Frequency of monitoring dependent on clinical situation
Phenytoin	Peak for toxicity is 4–5 h after dose; trough for monitoring	5 mL red top	10–20 μg/mL	Pertains to assay that measures total drug (free + bound)
Phenobarbital	Trough	5 mL red top	15–50 μg/mL	Steady state attained in 2–3 weeks
Carbamazepine	Peak level for toxicity is 2–4 h after dose; trough for monitoring	5 mL red top	4–12 μg/mL	Not helpful for idiosyncratic toxicities
Clonazepam	Peak for toxicity is 4 h after dose; trough for monitoring	1 mL red or green top	20–60 μg/mL	
Lamotrigine	Peak for toxicity is 2–4 h after dose; trough for monitoring	1 mL red or green top	3–14 μg/mL	
Levetiracetam	Peak for toxicity is 1 h after dose; trough for monitoring	1 mL red or green top	5–30 μg/mL	
Oxcarbazepine	Peak MHD for toxicity is 4–6 h after dose; trough for monitoring	1 mL red or green top	15–35 μg/mL MHD	
Valproic acid	Trough is not well defined	5 mL red top	50–100 μg/mL	Upper limit of therapeutic range
Tricyclic antidepressants	Steady state occurs in about 5 days; 10–14 h after once per day dosing; 4–6 h after twice per day dosing	5 mL red top	Amitriptyline[a]: 120–250 μg/L Desipramine: 150–300 μg/L Doxepin[a]: 150–250 μg/L Imipramine[a]: 150–250 μg/L Nortriptyline: 50–150 μg/L	Measure sum of parent and active metabolite for drugs noted with "a" in box at left
Lithium	10–14 h after dose; then biweekly or weekly until steady state; then every 1–3 months	5 mL red top	0.5–1.5 mmol/L (avoid green-top tubes)	Toxicity may occur at <1.5 mmol/L, especially in patients who show chronic toxicity
Digoxin	8 h after PO dose; 12 h after IV dose; and at steady state (1 week after initiation)	5 mL red top	0.9–2.0 ng/mL	Specimen collection time is crucial to avoid falsely high levels; STAT levels occasionally necessary

IM, intramuscular; IV, intravenous; PO, oral; MHD, monohydroxy carbazepine.
[a]Measure the sum of parent and active metabolite, that is, (amitriptyline + nortriptyline), (imipramine + desipramine), and (doxepin + desmethyldoxepin).

instructions are only a guide. The reader should refer to specific instructions from the laboratory. The general monitoring recommendations will depend on the motivation for monitoring the drug, possible drug interactions, and whether the patient is stable or showing signs of toxicity. Therapeutic ranges are only suggestions and will vary by patient, condition, and the presence of other medications.

Methotrexate

Methotrexate is a folate antagonist used in the treatment of a wide variety of neoplasms. Dose-related toxicity is common with high-dose methotrexate therapy (defined as >1 g/m^2 or 20 mg/kg). Adverse effects include immunosuppression, and diverse organ damage including renal failure, myelosuppression, hepatic toxicity, neurotoxicity, gastrointestinal toxicity, and death. Toxicity correlates with serum methotrexate concentration and duration of exposure. Patients with poor hydration, renal insufficiency, pleural effusion, ascites, or gastrointestinal obstruction are at increased risk for toxicity. Adverse effects of methotrexate are ameliorated by administration of leucovorin, a reduced folate. Serial methotrexate levels are used to guide the appropriate dosing and duration of leucovorin rescue following high-dose methotrexate administration.

Immunosuppressants

The immunosuppressant drugs, tacrolimus (FK-506), cyclosporin, and sirolimus (rapamycin), are drugs used to prevent rejection in organ transplantation. Cyclosporin is also utilized to treat psoriasis, chronic autoimmune urticaria, and rheumatoid arthritis. These drugs were originally discovered in bacteria (tacrolimus and sirolimus) and fungus (cyclosporin) from soil samples. Monitoring is indicated because these drugs have a narrow therapeutic index and highly variable pharmacokinetics. Adverse effects include nephrotoxicity, hepatotoxicity, pulmonary toxicity, neurotoxicity (light sensitivity, tingling in the palms, and tinnitus), tremor, and hypertension.

Whole blood is the preferred specimen for TDM, as the immunosuppressant drugs concentrate into erythrocytes more than the plasma/serum portion of blood. Low trough concentrations may indicate subtherapeutic immunosuppression and can be associated with increased risk of rejection. High trough concentrations cause increased toxicity including nephrotoxicity that can be particularly challenging to diagnose in renal transplant patients. Drug levels must be interpreted in conjunction with other laboratory test results and clinical findings to discriminate between toxicity and rejection. For renal transplant patients on cyclosporin therapy, the only definitive method for differentiating graft rejection from drug-induced nephrotoxicity is renal biopsy. These drugs are sometimes used in combination, and with mycophenolic acid, to enhance the immunosuppressant effects and decrease the dose and side effects.

The immunosuppressants are extensively metabolized by the liver to a number of metabolites, some of which have immunosuppressant activity. These metabolites can cross-react in laboratory immunoassays, thus overestimating parent drug concentrations in situations where elimination is impaired and when metabolites accumulate, as in cholestasis. Patients who have received mouse monoclonal antibody therapies may also have inaccurate immunoassay results from human anti-mouse heterophilic antibody (HAMA) interference. This interference occurs through nonspecific linkage of the capture antibody with the detection antibody without the presence of antigen. HAMA interference can cause both false-positive as well as false-negative results depending on the immunoassay format. HPLC with tandem mass spectrometry is increasingly being used for laboratory analysis to circumvent cross-reactivity with the immunoassays.

Antibiotics

Aminoglycosides

Gentamicin, tobramycin, and amikacin are aminoglycoside antibiotics. Ototoxicity and nephrotoxicity from aminoglycosides are related to dose and duration of exposure. Numerous factors, such as renal and cardiac function, age, liver disease, and obesity, affect the pharmacokinetic properties of aminoglycosides. Because of the many patient factors, as well as the low margin of safety and high incidence of dose-related toxicity, aminoglycoside levels are usually indicated in conjunction with renal function monitoring to minimize toxicity. In patients with normal renal function and without underlying disease, the indication for drug monitoring is less well defined.

Vancomycin

Vancomycin is a tricyclic glycopeptide antibiotic with significant dose-related nephrotoxicity and ototoxicity. The practice of measuring vancomycin levels emerged from the guidelines for aminoglycoside monitoring. However, the necessity for vancomycin monitoring is controversial, because the correlation between serum vancomycin levels and efficacy or toxicity has yet to be definitively demonstrated. Adult patients with normal renal function may not require routine monitoring. Indications for monitoring include impaired or changing renal function, concomitant use of nephrotoxic drugs, altered volume of distribution (as in a burn injury victim), prolonged vancomycin use, higher than usual doses, and use in neonates, children, pregnant women, and patients with malignancy.

Antiepileptics

Antiepileptics are frequently monitored to establish the dose necessary to reduce the frequency and magnitude of seizures. Trough levels are used to establish minimum effective dose. When toxicity is suspected, peak or random levels may be obtained. Too low a level will lead to breakthrough seizures, while too high a dose can induce seizures. A therapeutic level maintains seizure control and avoids side effects. The concentration of drug in the blood also may be used to evaluate patient compliance, and explain seizures that are refractory to drug treatment.

Phenytoin (Dilantin®)

Phenytoin (or its prodrug phosphenytoin) is a widely used anticonvulsant with nonlinear kinetics and wide interindividual variability in dose requirement. Phenytoin toxicity includes ataxia, tremor, lethargy, seizure exacerbation, and neuropsychiatric changes. Phenytoin use in certain populations requires special consideration. Neonates and the elderly have decreased clearance. On the other hand, children metabolize phenytoin more rapidly than adults, and, therefore, dose adjustment is necessary at various ages. Careful monitoring in pregnancy is required due to metabolic and volume changes that occur during pregnancy. Phenytoin is highly protein bound, and conditions such as renal failure, liver disease, burn injury, and age will affect the amount of free drug by altering the amount of plasma protein.

Extensive protein binding also predisposes phenytoin to significant interactions with other protein-bound drugs, such as valproic acid. Coadministration of valproic acid and phenytoin is common and may cause a decrease in total phenytoin. Valproic acid displaces phenytoin from albumin, which causes a transient increase in free phenytoin, but this free phenytoin is readily metabolized and cleared. The overall effect is usually a decrease in total phenytoin with an unchanged level of free phenytoin. Monitoring of total phenytoin levels is sufficient for patient management, and free phenytoin levels are not usually necessary except in renal or hepatic disease, conditions that would affect total protein or body clearance.

Phenobarbital and Primidone (Mysoline®)

Phenobarbital and primidone are used to treat all types of seizures except absence (petit mal) seizures. The major active metabolite of primidone is phenobarbital. Clearance of both primidone and phenobarbital is prolonged in neonates, the elderly, and patients with hepatic and renal dysfunction. Phenobarbital is a potent hepatic enzyme inducer, and may affect the metabolism and levels of many other drugs metabolized by the same enzymes. Concurrent valproic acid use significantly decreases phenobarbital clearance.

Carbamazepine (Tegretol®)

The anticonvulsant carbamazepine is used not only for seizures but also for treatment of trigeminal neuralgia and bipolar disorder. Monitoring of carbamazepine levels is useful due to its slow and unpredictable absorption. Age and hepatic function affect drug clearance. Dose-related toxic effects include blurred vision, paresthesias, ataxia, nystagmus, and drowsiness. Carbamazepine is metabolized to the active metabolite, carbamazepine 10,11-epoxide. Children are known to accumulate the epoxide metabolite and, as a result, may present with toxicity overlapping efficacy with carbamazepine levels in the reference interval in some individuals. With chronic therapy, carbamazepine induces its own metabolism, and dosing adjustment becomes necessary.

Valproic Acid (Depakene®, Depakote®)

Valproic acid is used to treat all types of seizures. It is also used in the treatment of migraines and bipolar disorder. Valproic acid has a narrow therapeutic index. Dose-related adverse effects involve primarily central nervous system (CNS) depression. The average half-life of valproic acid is about 12 to 16 hours, but there is significant interindividual variability, and use of a sustained-release formulation is popular. The half-life of valproic acid is prolonged in neonates and in patients with liver dysfunction. Extensive protein binding accounts for the increased valproic acid toxicity observed in patients with uremia and cirrhosis.

Second-generation Antiepileptics

The second-generation antiepileptics encompass a range of drugs with different chemical structures and pharmacokinetics. Some are protein bound (lamotrigine is 55% bound to albumin) while others are not (levetiracetam is <10% protein bound). Common adverse effects include dizziness, ataxia, nausea, and vomiting. Decreased hematocrit and neutropenia can also be seen with lamotrigine. In general, the second-generation antiepileptics have a wider therapeutic index and fewer side effects than the first-generation drugs. HPLC and immunoassays are available. However, therapeutic and toxic ranges have not been established for all of these drugs. So, monitoring is generally conducted to define the individual level at which a patient is achieving therapeutic action with fewest side effects for future reference, for compliance, and for documentation of the level at which side effects are evident for that patient. The concept of individualized reference intervals is gaining popularity versus dosing to a target range based on the general population, since individualized ranges optimize dosage which best balances efficacy with toxicity for the patient's own pharmacokinetics.

Antidepressants

Tricyclic Antidepressants

Tricyclic antidepressants, for example, amitriptyline, nortriptyline (Pamelor®), imipramine (Tofranil®), and doxepin, are monitored for multiple reasons. There is significant interindividual variation in metabolism and elimination, such that standard dosing results in therapeutic levels in less than half of patients. Genetic variation accounts for some of this variability. The fraction of "poor metabolizers" is about 17% of Caucasians and 5% of other ethnic groups. Other indications for monitoring include a narrow therapeutic index, multiple drug interactions, and patient compliance.

Tricyclic antidepressants have a low margin of safety and cause anticholinergic toxicity, seizures, and arrhythmias in overdose. Although the correlation between toxicity and blood level is poor, there are general guidelines. Levels in excess of 500 µg/L may be associated with anticholinergic toxicity (flushing, tachycardia, fever, dilated pupils, dry mucous membranes, urinary retention, and absent bowel sounds). Cardiotoxicity is more likely to occur at levels greater than 1000 µg/L in acute overdose.

Lithium

Lithium is a univalent cation most commonly used to treat bipolar disorder. Lithium monitoring is useful due to its narrow therapeutic index and the wide interindividual variation in dose requirement.

Excretion of lithium is primarily renal. Children have increased clearance, while the elderly have decreased clearance. Lithium excretion parallels sodium excretion. Therefore, patients on stable doses of lithium may become toxic in states of sodium conservation such as fever, excessive sweating, lack of fluid intake, and diarrhea.

Toxicity is usually associated with levels in excess of 1.5 mmol/L. However, toxicity may occur at lower levels, especially in cases of chronic toxicity. Lithium overdose is characterized by lethargy, weakness, slurred speech, ataxia, tremor, and myoclonic jerks. Severe toxicity may result in seizure, hyperthermia, and coma. Management of patients who have ingested sustained-release lithium preparations is difficult, and serum measurements play a crucial role in the decision to instigate hemodialysis or whole bowel irrigation. Analytical methods involve the use of ion-specific electrodes, and spectrophotometry or colorimetric tests.

> Tricyclic antidepressants are monitored for multiple reasons. There is significant interindividual variation in metabolism and elimination, such that standard dosing results in therapeutic levels in less than half of patients. Genetic variation accounts for some of this variability.

Later-generation Antidepressants

Fluoxetine (Prozac®) was the first selective serotonin-reuptake inhibitor used to treat depression. Fluoxetine monitoring is useful when patient compliance is in question. Further monitoring is not likely to be beneficial since fluoxetine has a wide therapeutic index, and there is a poor correlation between blood levels and clinical response. Fluoxetine is metabolized by the liver to the active metabolite norfluoxetine.

Other serotonin-reuptake inhibitors/later-generation antidepressants—such as sertraline (Zoloft®), paroxetine (Paxil®), fluvoxamine (Luvox®), citalopram (Celexa®), escitalopram (Lexapro®), quetiapine (Seroquel®), trazodone (Deseryl®), and venlafaxine (Effexor®)—do not require routine monitoring due to their wide therapeutic indices.

Cardiac Drugs

Digoxin

Digoxin is a commonly used drug in the treatment of heart failure and arrhythmias, and it has a low therapeutic index. There is significant interindividual variation in digoxin absorption and distribution along with prolonged clearance in patients with impaired renal function. Digoxin overdose is characterized by gastrointestinal distress, confusion, visual changes, hyperkalemia, and life-threatening cardiac toxicity. Overdoses may be treated with an antidigoxin antibody antidote. Such treatment typically renders subsequent blood digoxin concentrations unreliable. Blood digoxin immunoassays are generally less reliable than immunoassays for other therapeutic agents. Interferences with digoxin immunoassays are frequently reported. These interferences are referred to as digoxin-like immunoreactive substances (DLIS).

Pain Management

Acetaminophen

> When it is used in the recommended doses, it is not necessary to measure acetaminophen levels. However, excess intake of acetaminophen can be associated with severe liver injury.

Acetaminophen is a therapeutic drug used as an analgesic and an antipyretic. When used in the recommended doses, it is not necessary to measure acetaminophen levels. However, excess intake of acetaminophen can be associated with severe liver injury. Thus, acetaminophen is representative of many compounds with a wide therapeutic window that does not require therapeutic monitoring when used in recommended doses. However, because toxicity can occur if the upper limit of the window is exceeded, monitoring acetaminophen levels in patients with excess intake is critical, particularly since an antidote, *N*-acetylcysteine, can be administered. **Table 6–5** presents an overview of the laboratory evaluation for acetaminophen toxicity. Immunoassays are available for the rapid determination of serum/plasma levels.

TABLE 6–5   Laboratory Evaluation for Acetaminophen Toxicity

Laboratory Tests	Results/Comments
Laboratory monitoring of acetaminophen concentration	The importance of laboratory monitoring is related to the use of *N*-acetylcysteine as a treatment for the acetaminophen overdose; it is important that the neutralizing effect of *N*-acetylcysteine be provided before acetaminophen metabolites produce liver injury. To determine whether the acetaminophen ingestion is likely to cause liver toxicity, a 4-h post ingestion serum concentration should be obtained; the serum concentration of the drug will be used to determine if the patient is likely to experience liver injury and, if so, treated with *N*-acetylcysteine. If the first acetaminophen level is obtained more than 4 h post ingestion, a nomogram can be used (available in many textbooks) to determine if the acetaminophen level at that time post ingestion is likely or not likely to be associated with liver injury.
Liver function tests	Hepatic necrosis becomes evident 24–48 h after the ingestion of the excess amount of acetaminophen if the patient is not treated; at that time, standard liver function tests such as AST (SGOT), ALT (SGPT), bilirubin, as well as the prothrombin time, can be used to assess the extent of liver injury.

Acetaminophen is rapidly absorbed from the gastrointestinal tract. The plasma concentration reaches its highest level 30 to 60 minutes after a dose. One of the compounds resulting from acetaminophen metabolism is an oxidation product that is hepatotoxic. Normally this metabolite, N-acetyl-p-benzoquinine imine (NAPQI), is detoxified by binding to glutathione in the liver. With excess intake of acetaminophen, the production of NAPQI exceeds the amount of hepatic glutathione, and this permits the NAPQI to produce liver injury. Renal damage also may occur as a result of injury by the same compound.

The recommended daily dose of acetaminophen is no more than 4 g per day. A single dose of 10 to 15 g may produce liver injury. Fatal disease is usually associated with ingestion of ≥25 g of acetaminophen. Acetaminophen at slightly more than the recommended 4 g per day can produce hepatotoxicity when the patient has also ingested ethanol. This response can be exacerbated if the patient had been fasting prior to ingestion of acetaminophen and ethanol, or takes another enzyme-inducing drug such as phenytoin. The ingestion of acetaminophen at greater than recommended doses produces corresponding elevations of acetaminophen in the blood, and the level of the drug in the blood correlates with the severity of hepatic injury.

> The recommended daily dose of acetaminophen is no more than 4 g per day. A single dose of 10 to 15 g may produce liver injury. Fatal disease is usually associated with ingestion of ≥25 g of acetaminophen.

Acute manifestation of excess acetaminophen intake typically occurs 2 to 3 hours after ingestion. Most often this includes nausea, vomiting, and abdominal pain. Cyanosis of the skin and fingernails may be observed as a result of methemoglobin generation from the overdose. The full extent of liver damage usually becomes apparent 2 to 4 days after drug ingestion. At that time, liver function test results, including the prothrombin time, become abnormal. A variety of associated abnormalities, including electrolyte disturbances, can occur if there is significant liver damage. Acute renal failure also may occur, even if liver failure is not observed.

Aspirin

Aspirin (acetylsalicylic acid) is a therapeutic drug that has been used for more than a century as an analgesic, antipyretic, anti-inflammatory, and antithrombotic agent. It is readily absorbed and rapidly metabolized by hydrolysis to salicylic acid. Peak concentrations occur within 1 to 2 hours of a therapeutic dose. Between 50% and 90% is bound to albumin in a dose-dependent manner. Further metabolism produces salicyluric and gentisic acids and glucuronide conjugates that are renally excreted. Aspirin is contained in many preparations, including those with other analgesics. When used in therapeutic doses, it is not necessary to measure levels. However, chronic salicylate poisoning (salicylism) carries a high morbidity (30%) and mortality (25%), and is difficult to diagnose without monitoring levels since the patient may be too confused to provide a reliable history. **Table 6–6** presents an overview of the laboratory evaluation for salicylate toxicity. Immunoassays are available for the rapid determination of serum/plasma levels. Approximately 500 mg/kg as an acute dose is potentially lethal in comparison to a normal dose of 15 mg/kg. When taken in therapeutic doses, the half-life is 2 to 5 hours, but metabolism becomes saturated once the dose exceeds about 30 mg/kg, causing a delay in drug elimination. An early feature of toxicity is respiratory alkalosis through direct stimulation of the respiratory drive center, followed by vomiting. The latter mechanism of toxicity results from uncoupling of oxidative phosphorylation, leading to ketosis, metabolic acidosis, and pyrexia, with further dehydration and electrolyte imbalance. Hematologic consequences arise that manifest as an increased prothrombin time, GI bleeding, and occasionally DIC (disseminated intravascular coagulation).

Other Pain Management Drugs

Buprenorphine and methadone are analgesics that are commonly utilized for opiate withdrawal, but have found recent medical application in the management of chronic pain. Fentanyl and oxycodone are other drugs utilized in pain management that may be monitored. Serum/plasma levels of these drugs correlate poorly with clinical effect because of tolerance. The safety of these drugs in doses utilized for pain management does not typically require monitoring and dosing can be adjusted based on pain relief. However, these drugs have high abuse potential, so patients are often required to sign a pain management agreement stating that they will only use the drug as prescribed, and not use illegal substances, in addition to other stipulations. Urine tests are sometimes used to monitor for compliance and ensure that the patient is not diverting the drug for sale or other purposes. Immunoassays are available for analysis of these drugs in urine samples.

TABLE 6–6   Laboratory Evaluation for Aspirin Toxicity

Laboratory Tests	Results/Comments
Detection of aspirin metabolites in urine by color test (Trinder reagent); monitoring of serum salicylate concentration by enzymatic assay or immunoassay	The importance of these tests is to establish the diagnosis of poisoning. Since a number of preparations are available containing sustained-release aspirin, it is recommended that serial blood samples be drawn at 3-h intervals to determine whether the drug concentration is still rising.
	The Done nomogram interprets the serum salicylate concentrations taken at 6 h after acute ingestion as follows: • <50 mg/dL: asymptomatic • 51–110 mg/dL: mild-to-moderate toxicity • >110 mg/dL: serious toxicity
	The use of the Done nomogram is unreliable when: • There has been a previous ingestion within 24 h • Poisoning is chronic (concentrations >30 mg/dL indicate serious toxicity) • Enteric-coated or sustained-release preparations have been ingested • Renal failure is present
	Treatment for aspirin overdose is symptomatic and supportive—administration of repeat doses of oral activated charcoal may be given in an attempt to prevent further absorption and increase fecal elimination. Bicarbonate is used to counteract the metabolic acidosis, and calcium and electrolytes are administered to prevent seizures and cardiac failure. Hemodialysis may be indicated at concentrations above 100 mg/dL (>40 mg/dL in chronic salicylism), and to support renal function and electrolyte balance.
	Regular monitoring of renal function, blood gas and lactate, and coagulation assessment are important for patient care.

DRUGS OF ABUSE

Overview

Drug of abuse testing (DAT) includes testing for the use of illicit drugs (e.g., cocaine and phencyclidine [PCP]) and potentially addictive or harmful therapeutic agents (e.g., benzodiazepines, opiates, and amphetamine). The goal of DAT is to detect past exposure or use of a drug. Quantitative levels of a drug or its metabolite in fluids are not required. Laboratory analysis determines if a drug is above (i.e., "present") or below (i.e., "absent") a defined cutoff concentration in the sample.

DAT assays are designed to detect either the parent drug, or metabolite with a longer half-life. Cocaine, for example, has a blood half-life of less than 60 minutes, but the principal metabolite, benzoylecgonine, has an 8-hour half-life. By detecting the metabolite, cocaine abuse can be detected for several days after use as opposed to the parent drug that is cleared in less than 5 hours. **Table 6–7** lists the typical detection window for analysis of common drugs of abuse.

Drugs and their metabolites are much more concentrated in urine than in serum. Urine is the specimen of choice for DAT testing because of its ready availability. Other specimens have also been utilized for DAT. Meconium (an infant's first bowel movement after birth) has been utilized to detect in utero exposure of a fetus to drugs. Since meconium is made during the last trimester of fetal development, drug exposure can be detected from as early as the sixth month of gestation. Hair and nails have also been analyzed in attempts to detect drug use over a longer time frame than urine, but the clinical utility of specimens other than urine remains controversial.

Analysis for multiple drugs in a patient's sample can be labor intensive and expensive. Laboratory analysis for drugs of abuse thus takes a two-tier approach for efficiency. A simple, rapid assay that can be readily automated is used to first screen a sample for the presence of a class of drugs. These screening tests are sensitive and designed to detect a broad range of similar drugs that share a common chemical structure. Unfortunately, screening tests are generally not very specific and subject to a variety of cross-reactivities that can lead to false-positive test results. Thus, a second

Drug of abuse testing (DAT) includes testing for the use of illicit drugs, and potentially addictive or harmful therapeutic agents.

The goal of drug of abuse testing is to detect past exposure or use of a drug. Quantitative levels of a drug or its metabolite in fluids are not required. Laboratory analysis determines if a drug is above (i.e., "present") or below (i.e., "absent") a defined cutoff concentration in the sample.

TABLE 6–7   Detection Window for Commonly Abused Substances

Urine DAT Name	Time (Days)	Comments
Amphetamines	2–4	
Barbiturates	1 to >5	Depends on barbiturate
Benzodiazepines	2 to >8	Depends on benzodiazepine
Cocaine metabolite	2 to >7	Heavy users may remain positive for 6–10 days using sensitive immunoassays with a 150 ng/mL cutoff
Methadone	1–4	
Opiates	2 to >5	Heavy users may remain positive for up to 7–8 days
Phencyclidine	7–14	
THC (marijuana)	20–30	

tier of more specific testing is conducted to "confirm" the presence of a particular drug in samples that screen positive. Common screening tests are immunoassays that can be readily performed on chemistry instrumentation in a clinical laboratory or on point-of-care devices for testing in a variety of settings outside of a formal laboratory. **Table 6–8** lists the cutoffs and other characteristics of immunoassay tests. Most immunoassays detect a number of drugs within a class of agents, but some immunoassays are specific to a given compound, like the metabolite of cocaine, PCP, oxycodone, and 6-monoacetylmorphine.

The second-tier or "confirmatory" testing employs a chromatographic separation prior to mass-spectrometric detection to exactly identify the drug or metabolite in samples that generated a positive immunoassay screen. (See Chapter 2.) Confirmatory testing is expensive and time-consuming, but is absolutely required for forensic, legal, preemployment, and other applications of the test result that mandate definitive analysis. Confirmatory testing can take several days and will not assist in the immediate care and management of a trauma or acute overdose patient.

The lack of confirmatory testing on clinical samples can lead to misinterpretation of test results unless the clinician maintains an active dialogue with the laboratory regarding the likely causes of false-positive screening tests. Many laboratories append a comment to warn that positive urine immunoassay results have not been confirmed. Common causes of false-positive test results may also be listed with the result.

Common drugs that cause cross-reactivity and false-positive DAT results are listed in **Table 6–8**. Cross-reactivity and the causes of false-positives are dependent on the antibody specificity employed in the immunoassay, so cross-reactivities will vary from one manufacturer to another and between laboratories based on the method utilized for analysis. Clinicians should be familiar with the characteristics and limitations of the drug tests employed to analyze patient specimens.

Drugs of abuse have no reference or therapeutic range, because the drug should not be detected in the patient's sample. However, sometimes a positive drug test is desired by the ordering physician. Urine oxycodone, for example, is utilized for pain management, as a positive result may indicate that patients are compliant with their drug regimen. On the other hand, a negative result indicates that a patient is not taking the oxycodone as prescribed and may be diverting the drug for other purposes, including selling for monetary profit.

Screening for drugs of abuse does not detect every possible drug that the patient may have ingested. Laboratory analysis is limited to the specificity of the tests at hand. Patients may have access to a wide variety of plants that contain toxins or medications for which the laboratory does not test. In general, drug analysis is designed for rapid identification that may permit effective treatment (e.g., acetaminophen and its antidote) to reduce the toxic effects of the compound. Concomitant ingestion of different drugs is very common and may play a role in laboratory analysis for drugs of abuse. For example, ethanol and cocaine are often ingested together, and coingestion of these drugs can form a toxic metabolite called cocaethylene.

Screening for drugs of abuse does not detect every possible drug that the patient may have ingested. Laboratory analysis is limited to the specificity of the tests at hand.

TABLE 6–8   Characteristics of Immunoassay Tests for Drugs of Abuse (DAT)

DAT Name	Specificity	Drug Class Targeted	Typical Cutoff (Range) Level (ng/mL)	Causes of False-positives	Common Drugs Typically Detected	Comments
Primary tests						
Amphetamines	Class	Amphetamines	500 (300–2000)	Isometheptene Heptaminol Selegiline Propylhexedrin	Amphetamine, methamphetamine MDMA ("ecstasy")	Pseudoephedrine no longer interferes with current immunoassays
Barbiturates	Class	Barbiturates	200 (100–500)	—	Butalbital, barbital, secobarbital, phenobarbital	
Benzodiazepines	Class	Benzodiazepines	200 (100–300)	Oxaprozin	Diazepam, chlordiazepoxide, alprazolam, oxazepam	Many assays are insensitive to clonazepam and lorazepam
Cocaine	Compound	Cocaine metabolites	150 (100–300)	—	Cocaine metabolites	Actual false-positives are quite rare, despite information on the Internet
Opiates	Class	Morphine and related compounds	300 (300–2000)	Quinoline antibiotics	Heroin, morphine, codeine, hydromorphone, hydrocodone	Oxycodone and oxymorphone are poorly detected; methadone use does not cause a positive test
Oxycodone	Compound	Oxycodone	100 (100–300)	—	Oxycodone, oxymorphone	Used to assess compliance/diversion and/or cause of a positive opiate test
6-Monoacetylmorphine	Compound	Heroin metabolite	10	—	Heroin use	Specific for heroin use, negating the "poppy-seed" defense; used to assess cause of a positive opiate test
Phencyclidine	Compound	Phencyclidine	25 (10–25)	Dextromethorphan, tramadol	Phencyclidine	
THC	Class	Cannabinoids	50 (20–100)	See comments	Marijuana and hashish use	Nexium use may cause false-positives with some immunoassays

Specimen Collection and Laboratory Analysis

The potential for sample adulteration is a concern for any DAT. False-negative results can be caused by purposely "adulterating" a urine sample to prevent the immunologic or indicator reaction from working, leading to a false-negative result despite drug in the sample. Common household chemicals such as bleach, vinegar, sodium bicarbonate, Drano®, soft drinks, or hydrogen peroxide may be added to a urine sample in an effort to cause false-negative results. Many of these additives work by changing the sample pH, to denature the antibody proteins used in the assay or to shift the pH away from optimum assay conditions. Such adulteration can be detected by checking the pH of urine samples submitted for drug testing. Other adulterants include glutaraldehyde or nitrites, and can be analyzed using specific tests for adulteration in the laboratory.

Patients can take diuretics to temporarily enhance elimination. Diuretics cause an increase in urine output, so drugs that may be present will be diluted below the assay cutoff concentration in the urine sample. Alternatively, patients may substitute water as their urine sample, so as to avoid detection of drug use. Collection facilities can deter sample dilution by monitoring the temperature of samples just after collection. Samples outside a physiologic temperature range should be suspected of dilution. Facilities can also cap hot water faucets and add bluing agents to the toilet water as additional deterrents. Laboratories can test for urine osmolality and look for specimen dilution by analysis of urine creatinine.

Patients may also try to avoid detection by substituting specimens. Submission of someone else's urine as a patient sample is perhaps the hardest for laboratories to detect. Sources of drug-free urine are readily available via the Internet, and these materials are used by patients trying to avoid detection of their drug use. In nearly all standard tests, these materials act like normal, unadulterated human urine. Without close monitoring of a patient during urine sample collection, sample substitution is nearly undetectable by laboratory methods.

When evaluating a patient for drug use, collecting an appropriate specimen is an important step to detecting the presence of a drug.

- Most drugs and metabolites are concentrated in urine after use. Urine is appropriate for qualitative analysis (presence/absence of drug) and for determining recent use of amphetamines, benzodiazepines, barbiturates, cannabinoids, cocaine metabolites, opiates, and their metabolites (including codeine and morphine), oxycodone, and PCP. Urine is easy to collect and noninvasive, but subject to adulteration, dilution, and sample substitution. Monitoring of urine collection is intrusive of patient privacy, so facilities collecting urine samples should take steps to deter adulteration (capping hot water faucets and using bluing agents in the toilets) and have patients remove coats and bulky clothing, and keep purses and backpacks out of the bathroom during collection.
- Serum/plasma and blood samples provide a single time point of drug in the patient's system. Since blood is in equilibrium with tissue and organ receptors at steady state, quantitative blood levels of drug can assess for intoxication and toxicity. Serum, plasma, and blood concentration are useful for analyzing alcohol intoxication, management of analgesic overdose (including acetaminophen and salicylates), and evaluation of TDM side effects and toxicity. Collection of blood requires a needlestick and phlebotomy, but is not subject to sample adulteration like urine samples.
- Other body fluids may prove useful: meconium for evaluation of in utero exposure to drugs, vitreous humor for postmortem examination, hair and nails for past exposure to certain drugs of abuse and toxins, and sweat or oral fluid that can be collected without invasion of privacy and are less prone to adulteration.

It is essential that specimens are collected at an appropriate time following ingestion and that the sample is properly preserved. Serial measurements over time may be necessary because of delayed gastric emptying or prolonged absorption from sustained-release preparations in overdose cases. Blood levels do not necessarily correlate with the severity of toxicity because many compounds distribute into specific body compartments or cells, and are therefore less detectable in blood. The detection of drugs in urine will depend on the patient's renal function and urine output, the time since last dose, chronic use of the drug, the patient's hydration state, and metabolism. Thus, urine collection within the first several hours after use has a better chance of detecting drug than urine collected several days after use. Not all drugs are equally stable in a body fluid. Alcohols should be collected anaerobically, as they are volatile compounds that will dissipate when exposed to air. Appropriate steps should be taken to preserve the drug in the specimen after collection prior to analysis.

Selected Drugs of Abuse

Amphetamines

Amphetamines are stimulants and common class of abused drugs. Methamphetamine (crank, speed), 3,4-methylenedioxymethamphetamine (a derivative of methamphetamine, also known as MDMA or ecstasy), and several other amphetamine derivatives are used orally and intravenously

> Sources of drug-free urine are readily available via the Internet, and these materials are used by patients trying to avoid detection of their drug use. In nearly all standard tests, these materials act like normal, unadulterated human urine.

as illicit drugs. A smokable form of methamphetamine is known as "ice." Amphetamine-like drugs also can be used as prescription medications for treatment of a variety of conditions and disorders. These include weight loss, narcolepsy, attention deficit disorders, and sinus congestion. Amphetamine-like drugs work primarily by activating the sympathetic nervous system via the CNS. Drugs in this class can produce toxicity at levels only slightly above the usual doses, but a high degree of tolerance can develop after repeated use. Patients who are intoxicated with amphetamine-like drugs present with CNS effects that can extend from euphoria to seizure and coma. More severe signs and symptoms are usually associated with greater amounts of drug ingestion. The acute peripheral manifestations extend from sweating and tremor to myocardial infarction, even if the coronary arteries are normal. Death in amphetamine users can be caused by ventricular arrhythmia. The ingestion of amphetamines and related drugs can be conclusively established by identification of these compounds in urine or in gastric samples. Quantitative serum levels often do not correlate with the severity of the signs and symptoms.

Barbiturates

Barbiturates are used clinically as hypnotic and sedative agents, for induction of anesthesia, and for treatment of epilepsy. Ultrashort-, short-, intermediate-, and long-acting barbiturates have different pharmacokinetic properties. All barbiturates cause a generalized depression of neuronal activity in the brain. The toxic dose of barbiturates depends on the specific barbiturate used, the route and rate of administration, and individual patient tolerance. Toxicity is likely to appear when the dose administered exceeds 5 to 10 times the hypnotic dose, but chronic use may result in marked tolerance. The patient with mild-to-moderate intoxication of barbiturates often presents with lethargy, slurred speech, nystagmus, and ataxia. With greater amounts of drug ingestion in overdose, hypotension, coma, and even respiratory arrest can occur. Barbiturates can be detected in both urine and serum to document their ingestion.

Benzodiazepines

Benzodiazepines are sedatives, and antiepileptic and antianxiety medications. The different benzodiazepines vary in potency, duration of effect, and conversion to active and inactive metabolites. Benzodiazepines produce a generalized depression of spinal reflexes and may cause coma. Death from benzodiazepine overdose is rare unless the drugs are used in combination with other compounds, such as alcohol. Oral overdoses of diazepam (Valium®) have been reported in excess of 15 to 20 times the therapeutic dose without serious depression of consciousness. However, if the same drug is given at a much lower concentration with rapid intravenous injection, respiratory arrest can occur. Although there is variability among benzodiazepines, the onset of CNS depression is typically observed 30 to 120 minutes after ingestion. Drug levels can be obtained from both serum and urine specimens. However, because levels are rarely of value in emergency management, only qualitative analysis is most often conducted. Of the benzodiazepines, clonazepam (Klonopin®), used in the treatment of absence seizures, is the most often monitored quantitatively, especially in children, although most patients are managed without monitoring. There is little evidence for a therapeutic window, probably because receptor effects do not mirror plasma concentrations, and tolerance can develop with continued use. HPLC is used for quantitative analysis in serum/plasma, but the presence of drug can be detected qualitatively in urine by immunoassay.

Cannabinoids

Cannabis derivatives include marijuana and hashish. Marijuana consists of the leaves and flowering parts of the plant *Cannabis sativa*. Marijuana is usually smoked in cigarettes or pipes, and can be ingested in food. Dried resin from the plant can be compressed into blocks to make hashish. The primary psychoactive cannabinoid in marijuana is delta-9-tetrahydrocannabinol (THC). THC is also available in capsule form as a treatment for nausea in patients being treated with chemotherapeutic agents and those undergoing treatment for glaucoma. The effects of THC are related to the dose and time after consumption. THC may be a stimulant, a sedative, or a hallucinogenic compound. A typical marijuana cigarette contains 1% to 3% THC, but some may contain up to 15% THC. Hashish contains 3% to 6% THC, and an oil extract can be prepared from hashish with 30% to 50% THC. Significant variability in toxicity exists between individuals, which is influenced by prior exposure to the drug and degree of tolerance. The clinical presentation of a patient after use of THC can vary from euphoria and a heightened sensory awareness to impaired short-term memory, depersonalization, visual hallucinations, and acute paranoid psychosis. THC use can be established by detection of the drug in urine. However, drug levels correlate poorly with the degree of intoxication. Since THC is hydrophobic and distributes into fat cells, a urine test for cannabinoids may be positive for 10 to 25 days after the last exposure in moderate to heavy users due to slow continued distribution from fat cells into the circulation prior to clearance by the kidneys. In fact, there are well-documented reports of true-positive test results in chronic users more than 80 days after last exposure to THC.

Cannabis for medical and recreational use has been legalized in many states. With legalization, there is an increasing need to determine intoxication when an individual is suspected of driving under the influence, in a manner similar to ethanol. Currently, there is no set level of cannabinoid concentration to indicate impairment, as the compounds detected by the current blood and oral fluid tests remain for days post ingestion. At present, police have to rely on field sobriety tests to assess intoxication, which are nonscientific, subjective measures. Identification of a marker of cannabis ingestion with a short half-life and tests that can be performed in the field are needed for law enforcement.

> A urine test for cannabinoids may be positive for 10 to 25 days after the last exposure in moderate to heavy users. In fact, there are well-documented reports of true-positive test results in chronic users more than 80 days after last exposure to THC. There is no reliable test for short-term cannabis induced intoxication for use by law enforcement for accident investigation or driving under the influence.

Cocaine

Cocaine is a stimulant drug. It may be sniffed into the nose, smoked, or injected intravenously. The "free base" form of cocaine is preferred for smoking because it volatilizes at a lower temperature and is not as easily destroyed by heat as the hydrochloride salt of the drug. Crack cocaine is a dried form of the drug that has been mixed in alkaline aqueous solution to generate the free base. Cocaine can also be combined with heroin and injected as a "speed ball." The primary effect of cocaine is generalized sympathetic stimulation, very similar to that produced by amphetamines. There is also a depression of cardiovascular function as a result of decreased cardiac contractility. The toxic dose depends significantly on the tolerance of the individual to the drug, the route of administration, and whether the cocaine is administered with other compounds. A dose that produces only euphoria when swallowed or snorted can produce convulsions and cardiac arrhythmias when rapidly injected intravenously or smoked. The initial euphoria from exposure to cocaine can be followed by anxiety, agitation, hyperactivity, and seizures. With high doses, respiratory arrest can occur. Death can result from fatal arrhythmia, status epilepticus, intracranial hemorrhage, or hyperthermia. Cocaine use can be detected through analysis of the primary metabolite, benzoylecgonine, in the urine, although parent drug and metabolites can also be analyzed in plasma/serum or in vitreous humor in death investigations.

Opiates and Opioids

Opiates are narcotic sedatives and analgesics used for pain management. They are naturally occurring compounds extracted from the poppy *Papaver somniferum*. Opioids include the naturally occurring opiates and their derivatives (morphine and codeine) and the synthetic opioids (dihydrocodeine, heroin, hydrocodone, hydromorphone, oxycodone, and oxymorphone). Many prescription medications contain opioids. Mixtures of aspirin or acetaminophen with an opioid compound, such as codeine, are in common use. Dextromethorphan is an opioid derivative that is used to suppress cough. Loperamide is another opioid, known under its brand name as Imodium, and is used to treat diarrhea. These compounds can be obtained without prescription as they have no analgesic or addictive properties.

Morphine is an opiate that is widely used in medicine to reduce pain. The best known drug of abuse in this category is heroin. In general, opiates and opioids cause sedation and respiratory depression. Toxicity is related to respiratory failure that can lead to death. The toxic dose varies widely with the opioid administered, its route and rate of administration, and the individual's tolerance to the drug. Diagnosis of opiate intoxication may be established clinically when the typical signs and symptoms are present—pinpoint pupils, and respiratory and CNS depression. These symptoms are reversed by administration of the opioid antagonist naloxone. Opioid use can be determined in urine using immunoassay. Specific immunoassays can detect the presence of methadone, fentanyl, and buprenorphine while chromatographic techniques can analyze meperidine and tramadol. Levels of these compounds in serum/plasma, however, are not usually analyzed, because opiate concentration correlates poorly with clinical effects.

Oxycodone is synthesized from thebaine, a natural constituent of opium. It is available in a number of compound analgesics, with acetaminophen and aspirin. Oxycodone abuse has grown over the last decade, and specific immunoassays are available for this drug, since most broad-spectrum opiate class screening immunoassays fail to detect oxycodone in the clinically relevant concentration range.

Phencyclidine

PCP is an anesthetic agent that became popular as an inexpensive street drug in the late 1960s. It is most often smoked, but it can be snorted, ingested orally, or injected. It is commonly used in combination with other illicit drugs. Ingestion of PCP produces a generalized loss of pain perception and can cause hallucinations, euphoria, and disinhibition. Ingestion of large amounts can produce death, often from self-destructive behavior or from complications of hyperthermia. PCP use can be detected in urine using immunoassays. PCP levels in the serum are not clinically valuable, because drug levels do not correlate with the degree of intoxication.

Alcohols: Ethanol, Methanol, Ethylene Glycol, and Isopropanol

Ethanol is the most common drug of abuse. Many patients presenting to hospitals with altered mental status suffer from excess ethanol ingestion. Ethanol is present not only in beverages but also in many medications. Ethanol intoxication is associated with many different types of accidental injury, particularly those involving motor vehicles. Chronic abuse of ethanol can lead to pancreatic disease and liver cirrhosis.

Ethanol is rapidly absorbed from the gastrointestinal tract. It distributes into the total body water and diffuses freely into the tissues. Peak blood ethanol levels occur 30 to 75 minutes after ethanol ingestion. Food ingestion can delay absorption. A useful rule of thumb is that 1 oz of 80 to 100 proof spirits, 4 oz of wine, or 12 oz of beer increases the blood alcohol concentration by 25 to 30 mg/dL when ingested over a period of several minutes. The blood ethanol level in a nonchronic alcoholic decreases at a rate of 15 to 25 mg/dL/h once ethanol ingestion is discontinued. The blood ethanol levels required to induce fetal alcohol syndrome have not been determined. Pregnant women who abuse ethanol have a high risk of delivering an infant with fetal alcohol syndrome. These infants have prenatal growth retardation, dysfunction of the CNS, and characteristic craniofacial abnormalities. Because an acceptable lower limit of alcohol intake in pregnancy has not been defined, pregnant women are generally advised to abstain from ethanol.

Metabolism of ethanol occurs by an oxidative pathway to acetaldehyde and acetic acid, and, also, by a nonoxidative pathway to fatty acid ethyl esters. When the acetaldehyde is subsequently converted to acetic acid, acidosis can occur. The major metabolizing enzyme for oxidation of ethanol to acetaldehyde is alcohol dehydrogenase, and a second group of enzymes is the cytochrome P450 system. The cytochrome P450 enzymes are liver microsomal enzymes involved in the metabolism of several drugs. Cytochrome P450 enzymes can be induced to higher levels of activity by ethanol. Ingestion of ethanol can thus alter the metabolism of a number of drugs, which are metabolized by this same system. Induction may increase or decrease the therapeutic and/or toxic effect of drugs. Ethanol can also compete with drugs for metabolism by the cytochrome P450 enzymes.

The measurement of blood ethanol concentration can be performed by breath analysis, or more accurately, by a specific enzymatic assay or by gas chromatography that can also measure ethanol, methanol, and isopropanol, individually (**Table 6–9**). Methanol and isopropanol are also toxic, primarily as a result of oxidative metabolism. Methanol metabolism can generate formic acid leading to blindness, while isopropanol is metabolized to acetone causing ketosis. Ethylene glycol, another volatile compound, is oxidized by similar metabolism to oxalic acid causing acute kidney failure. Gas chromatography under different laboratory conditions is required to detect ethylene glycol. The clinical presentation, sources for ingestion, and laboratory detection and quantitation of methanol, ethylene glycol, and isopropanol are shown in **Table 6–10**.

Ethanol is the most common drug of abuse. Many patients presenting to hospitals with altered mental status suffer from excess ethanol intake.

The measurement of blood ethanol concentration can be performed by breath analysis, or more accurately, by an enzymatic assay for ethanol specifically or a gas chromatographic test that can measure ethanol, methanol, and isopropanol, individually.

TABLE 6-9 **Laboratory Evaluation for Ethanol Intake**

Laboratory monitoring: acute intake	Blood ethanol level (see below)
Laboratory monitoring: chronic intake	Long-term markers of ethanol intake include elevated gamma-glutamyl transferase (GGT), carbohydrate-deficient transferrin, and fatty acid ethyl esters
Liver function tests	AST (SGOT), ALT (SGPT), and bilirubin assess ethanol-induced liver injury (see Chapter 16 for a discussion of cirrhosis)
Pancreatic function tests	Amylase and lipase can be used to assess ethanol-induced pancreatic injury (see Chapter 17 for a discussion of pancreatitis)
Blood Ethanol Concentration (mg/dL) (Ranges Overlap Because of Person-to-person Variability)	**Influence of Blood Alcohol Concentration in Individuals Who Are Not Chronic Ethanol Abusers**
10–50	Sobriety
40–120	Euphoria
90–250	Excitement
180–300	Confusion
270–400	Stupor
350–500	Coma
>450	Death can be produced by ingestion of 300–400 mL of pure ethanol or 600–800 mL of 100 proof whiskey in <1 h

Data from Dubowski KM. Alcohol determination in the clinical laboratory. *Am J Clin Pathol.* 1980;74:747–750.

TABLE 6-10 **Methanol, Ethylene Glycol, and Isopropanol Toxicity and Laboratory Monitoring**

	Methanol	Ethylene Glycol	Isopropanol
Sources for ingestion	Methanol, methanol-contaminated alcohols, and antifreeze	Antifreeze	Rubbing alcohol
Time until onset of symptoms	12–48 h	0.5–12 h	Minutes
Fatal dose of the pure compound	60–250 mL in most cases	Approximately 100 g	Approximately 250 mL
Clinical features	Impaired vision up to blindness, vomiting, seizures, coma	Anuria, vomiting, seizures, coma	Vomiting, abdominal pain, hematemesis, melena, coma
Antidote administration	4MP; ethanol	4MP; ethanol	None (hemodialysis >400 mg/dL)
Laboratory monitoring			
Presence in blood	Yes	Yes	Yes
Osmolality (mOsm = [mg/dL alcohol]/[10 × molecular weight])	Elevated	Elevated	Elevated
Hypoglycemia	Yes	Yes	No
Acidosis (blood pH)	Severe	Severe	Mild
Oxalate crystals (urine)	No	Yes (because ethylene glycol is metabolized to oxalate)	No
Anion gap	Large	Large	Normal

4MP, 4-methylpyrazole.

ENVIRONMENTAL TOXINS

Overview

Monitoring of environmental toxins is a significant challenge because so many substances that can produce illness and even death are encountered in daily life. Occupational exposure to heavy metals, gases, and caustic compounds can occur in the workplace, and leaching of toxins from an industry can contaminate soil and groundwater, leading to exposure of food sources, drinking water supplies, and livestock. Carbon monoxide, mercury, cyanide, and insecticides are some of the notable environmental toxins. Lead exposure can occur from occupational and nonoccupational sources (such as paint chips) and produce subclinical to life-threatening illness, depending on the amount ingested. Low-level exposure in children can produce serious disease and affect long-term mental development.

Laboratory analysis of an environmental toxin may not always measure the compound directly. In some cases, the toxin impairs flow through a metabolic pathway. Accumulated metabolites can be measured that reflect the toxic effects rather than a direct analysis of the toxin. Insecticide exposure, for instance, can be measured indirectly by cholinesterase enzyme activity rather than direct analysis of the insecticide levels in the body.

Carbon Monoxide

Description

Carbon monoxide poisoning is responsible for up to 4000 deaths per year in the United States and is the leading cause of accidental and deliberate poisonings. Approximately 10% of the cases involve children. The heart, CNS, and lungs are the organs most immediately affected by the toxic effects of carbon monoxide. Carbon monoxide can also impair vision, hearing, and peripheral nerve conduction. The poisoning may be sublethal and cause cardiac dysrhythmias, myocardial ischemia, headache, and a variety of other signs and symptoms. Survivors can suffer permanent, severe neurologic impairment.

The principal pathologic consequence of carbon monoxide poisoning is the binding of carbon monoxide to oxygen-binding sites in the hemoglobin molecule. The binding of carbon monoxide to hemoglobin results in the formation of carboxyhemoglobin. Carbon monoxide has a higher affinity for hemoglobin than oxygen and decreases hemoglobin's ability to deliver oxygen to the tissues producing ischemia.

The normal range of carboxyhemoglobin for nonsmoking adults is 0.1% to 0.9% of total hemoglobin. When hemolytic disease is present with increased breakdown of hemoglobin, the carboxyhemoglobin levels can increase to approximately 2%. Values at this level can have adverse clinical effects in patients with preexisting heart disease. There is a poor correlation between carboxyhemoglobin levels and clinical findings. **Table 6–11** shows the relative consequences of various amounts of carboxyhemoglobin, but individual patients demonstrate considerable variability

> Carbon monoxide poisoning is responsible for up to 4000 deaths per year in the United States and is the leading cause of accidental and deliberate poisonings. The principal pathologic consequence of carbon monoxide poisoning is the binding of carbon monoxide to oxygen-binding sites in the hemoglobin molecule.

TABLE 6–11   Clinical Presentation of Carbon Monoxide Toxicity

Carboxyhemoglobin Relative to Total Hemoglobin (%)	Clinical Findings in Adults[a]
0.1–0.9	Normal range for nonsmoking adults
1.5–10	Smoking adults
10–30	As concentration elevates, increasingly severe headache and greater dyspnea on exertion
40–50	Very severe headache and dyspnea with tachycardia; may be fatal
60–70	Coma, seizures, often fatal
80	Rapidly fatal

[a]Children are more sensitive and can present differently.

TABLE 6–12 **Laboratory Tests Used in the Evaluation of a Patient for Carbon Monoxide Poisoning**

Laboratory Test	Comments
Carboxyhemoglobin (% relative to total hemoglobin)	See **Table 6–11**
CBC/relevant microbiology studies	Anemias and infections can increase the concentration of carboxyhemoglobin and should be identified if present
Indicators of ischemic damage to skeletal and cardiac muscle	Creatinine kinase, troponin I, troponin T, lactate dehydrogenase, and/or aldolase may be elevated; myoglobin may be detectable in the urine if there is muscle damage

in clinical symptoms. Children are much more susceptible to acute carbon monoxide poisoning and have a different clinical picture that mimics gastroenteritis. Like adults, they can also have serious neurologic sequelae and myocardial ischemia. Patients are often unaware of their exposure to carbon monoxide because it is odorless and nonirritating. There is no pathognomonic feature of carbon monoxide intoxication. A rapid diagnosis of carbon monoxide poisoning is important in order to institute appropriate management and identify sources of carbon monoxide before other exposures can occur.

Diagnosis

Laboratory monitoring of carbon monoxide poisoning is performed by measurement of the carboxyhemoglobin levels (**Table 6–12**). A co-oximeter is a spectrophotometric device that measures the absorbance of light by blood at multiple wavelengths. The various forms of hemoglobin absorb light at characteristic wavelengths, allowing for the measurement of specific hemoglobins for example, carboxyhemoglobin. The patient also must be evaluated for possible underlying cause(s) of an increased carbon monoxide level (<10%), such as the presence of anemia, infection, and smoking that can increase carboxyhemoglobin levels. Because carbon monoxide can cause ischemic damage to skeletal and cardiac muscle, evaluation of ischemic muscle damage may also be appropriate.

> Laboratory monitoring of carbon monoxide poisoning is performed by measurement of the carboxyhemoglobin levels.

Lead

Description

Lead poisoning is primarily a disease of childhood. As research about lead toxicity has increased, the threshold for defining lead poisoning has decreased over the past 20 years. Prior to 1970, lead poisoning (plumbism) was defined by blood levels greater than 60 µg/dL. In 1971, the threshold was lowered to 40 µg/dL. By 1975, the acceptable level was 25 µg/dL and since 1985, blood levels of 10 to 15 µg/dL have been recognized to impair cognitive and behavioral development. Most recently, the Centers for Disease Control and Prevention have recommended lead levels in children of <5 µg/dL. As recently as 1992, 17.2% of children in the United States between the ages of 6 months and 5 years were estimated to have a blood lead level in excess of 15 µg/dL, although this pales in comparison to those observed in developing countries. These children were primarily from low-income families in large urban settings. The sources of lead for these children included not only lead paint but also lead-contaminated household dust, soil, and workplace clothing; the use of lead-containing cookware; exposure to lead in storage batteries, in fishing and curtain weights; and even lead-contaminated water from the use of lead-soldered pipes in older buildings. Some canned food has been reported to contain lead. Lead-containing costume jewelry, medicines, toys, and cosmetics (such as surma or kohl) imported to the United States from other countries have been demonstrated to contain lead. Obviously, the investigation of lead poisoning cases is important to identify the precise source of lead ingestion so that exposure can be eliminated.

> As understanding has increased about the toxicity of lead, the threshold for the definition of lead poisoning has decreased over the past 20 years.

There is a significant effort nationally to screen children, particularly those between the ages of 6 months and 5 years who live in, or are frequent visitors to, older housing built prior to 1960. Exposure to lead at high doses can produce persistent seizures, mental retardation, and chronic

TABLE 6–13   **Laboratory Monitoring of Children for Lead Poisoning (http://www.cdc.gov/nceh/lead/ casemanagement/caseManage_chap3.htm, Summary of Recommendations for Children with Confirmed [Venous] Elevated Blood Lead Levels)**

Blood Lead Level (μg/dL)*			
<5	5–44	45–69	≥70
Lead education • Dietary • Environmental	Lead education • Dietary • Environmental	Lead education • Dietary • Environmental	Hospitalize and commence chelation therapy (following confirmatory venous blood lead test) in conjunction with consultation from a medical toxicologist or a pediatric environmental health specialty unit
Lead risk assessment and environmental sampling if appropriate	Follow-up blood lead monitoring Complete history and physical exam Laboratory studies: • Iron status • Consider hemoglobin or hematocrit Environmental investigation Lead hazard reduction Neurodevelopmental monitoring Abdominal x-ray (if particulate lead ingestion is suspected) with bowel decontamination if indicated	Follow-up blood lead monitoring Laboratory studies: • Hemoglobin or hematocrit • Iron status • Free erythrocyte protoporphyrin Environmental investigation Lead hazard reduction Neurodevelopmental monitoring Abdominal x-ray (if particulate lead ingestion is suspected) with bowel decontamination if indicated Oral chelation therapy; consider hospitalization if lead-safe environment cannot be assured	Proceed according to actions for 45–69 μg/dL

*The following actions are **not** recommended at any blood lead level: searching for gingival lead lines; testing of neurophysiologic function; evaluation of renal function (except during chelation with EDTA); testing of hair, teeth, or fingernails for lead; radiographic imaging of long bones; x-ray fluorescence of long bones. For adults, it is recognized that accumulation of lead occurs, and blood lead concentrations <25 μg/dL do not require action.

behavioral dysfunction. Most of the absorbed lead is stored in the bones. However, lead can also be found in soft tissues and erythrocytes. Lead interferes with the enzymes involved in heme synthesis, so lead exposure can lead to anemia. Renal toxicity is also observed in some cases of chronic lead poisoning. Any child with developmental delay, behavioral disorders, seizures, learning disabilities, iron deficiency, hearing impairment, renal disorders, and recurrent vomiting and abdominal pain should be considered for lead toxicity.

Diagnosis

A whole blood lead level reflects the lead burden of the body. For small children, a finger-stick sample is usually sent for analysis. **Table 6–13** describes the laboratory monitoring for children suspected of lead poisoning relative to the presenting blood lead level. If the blood lead level is greater than 5 μg/dL, testing of a sample taken by venipuncture is recommended to rule out skin contamination. If this "clean" specimen contains more than 5 μg/dL lead, parental education on possible exposure sources is recommended. While initial testing is often performed by anodic stripping voltammetry, confirmation testing especially for concentrations above 40 μg/dL is generally performed by atomic absorption or mass spectrometry. Free erythrocyte protoporphyrin (zinc protoporphyrin) is formed from heme synthesis as a result of lead toxicity. The measurement of free erythrocyte protoporphyrin is, however, an insensitive screening test for lead exposure because it does not detect lead poisoning in children with lead levels less than

A whole blood lead level reflects the lead burden of the body. For small children, a finger-stick sample is usually sent for analysis. If the blood lead level is greater than 5 μg/dL, testing of a sample taken by venipuncture is recommended to rule out skin contamination.

25 µg/dL, and identifies less than 50% of children with blood levels greater than 25 µg/dL. The utility of free protoporphyrin measurement is primarily to detect ongoing lead exposure. Because the anemia from lead poisoning may resemble iron deficiency anemia, studies for iron deficiency (such as serum ferritin and the red cell distribution width in the complete blood count) should be obtained to differentiate anemia of lead poisoning from iron deficiency anemia.

A portion of this chapter on TDM is also found in a newsletter to the physicians at the Massachusetts General Hospital in Clinical Laboratory Reviews, 1999;8:1.

SELF-ASSESSMENT QUESTIONS

1. Which of the following drugs is rarely monitored to determine if a drug being taken by the patient is in a safe and/or therapeutic concentration?
   A. Tacrolimus
   B. Phenytoin
   C. Erythromycin
   D. Digoxin

2. Identify one of the choices from the following that is not an indication for therapeutic drug monitoring.
   A. Patient compliance with the prescribed drug regimen is uncertain.
   B. The prescribed drug has a low margin of safety, with toxic blood concentrations only slightly greater than therapeutic ones.
   C. The prescribed drug has minimal pharmacokinetic variability.
   D. The prescribed drug has frequent drug–drug interactions.

3. Which of the following organs is the primary site for drug metabolism?
   A. Kidneys
   B. Liver
   C. Lungs
   D. Gastrointestinal tract

4. Impaired function of which of the following organs requires dose adjustment because of reduced elimination for many therapeutic drugs?
   A. Kidneys
   B. Skin
   C. Gastrointestinal tract
   D. Lungs

5. Which of the following is a trough drug level?
   A. A sample drawn just prior to the next dose
   B. A sample drawn 4 hours after administration of a drug
   C. A sample collected 5 minutes after drug administration
   D. A sample drawn once per month to determine if a drug concentration is in the therapeutic range

6. Which of the following drug class–drug name pairs is incorrect, for these drugs that are monitored with laboratory testing?
   A. Antibiotics—Aminoglycosides
   B. Antiepileptics—Phenobarbital
   C. Immunosuppressants—Cyclosporine
   D. Antidepressants—Methotrexate

7. A patient is suspected of an overdose of acetaminophen (Tylenol). Which of the following laboratory tests should be selected to reveal toxicity if it is present?
   A. Alanine aminotransferase (ALT)
   B. Blood urea nitrogen (BUN)
   C. Amylase
   D. Troponin

8. Which of the following therapeutic drugs is less commonly abused than the others?
   A. Benzodiazepines
   B. Oxycodone
   C. Vancomycin
   D. Amphetamines

9. Which is the most appropriate sample to determine the presence or absence of a drug rather than quantification of the drug level?
   A. Sweat
   B. Urine
   C. Plasma
   D. Whole blood

10. Which of the following compounds is not an alcohol?
    A. Methanol
    B. Ethylene glycol
    C. Isopropanol
    D. Acetaldehyde

11. Which one of the following organs is least likely to be damaged by excess ethanol intake?
    A. Liver
    B. Pancreas
    C. Lungs
    D. Heart

12. A patient with the blood ethanol concentration of 400 mg/dL, who is not a chronic alcoholic, is most likely to experience which of the following?
    A. Euphoria
    B. Excitement
    C. Confusion
    D. Stupor or coma

13. A patient has the following laboratory values: severe acidosis, hypoglycemia, an elevated osmolality, and oxalate crystals in the urine. Which of the following four alcohols is the one most likely ingested by this patient?
    A. Ethanol
    B. Methanol
    C. Isopropanol
    D. Ethylene glycol

14. Which of the following environmental toxins is the leading cause of accidental and deliberate poisonings?
    A. Lead
    B. Mercury
    C. Cyanide
    D. Carbon monoxide

15. At which range of blood lead levels (µg/dL) is hospitalization absolutely required?
    A. Greater than 45
    B. Greater than 70
    C. Greater than 100
    D. Greater than 150

FURTHER READING

Advisory Committee on Childhood Lead Poisoning Prevention. *Low Level Lead Exposure Harms Children: A Renewed Call for Primary Prevention.* Atlanta, GA: US Department of Health and Human Services, CDC, Advisory Committee on Childhood Lead Poisoning Prevention; 2012. Available at http://www.cdc.gov/nceh/lead/acclpp/final_document_010412.pdf. Accessed March 2013.

Best CA, Laposata M. Fatty acid ethyl esters: toxic non-oxidative metabolites of ethanol and markers of ethanol intake. *Front Biosci.* 2003;8:e202–e217.

Dasgupta A. Therapeutic drug monitoring of digoxin: impact of endogenous and exogenous digoxin-like immunoreactive substances. *Toxicol Rev.* 2006;25:273–281.

Hammond S, et al. Laboratory assessment of oxygenation in methemoglobinemia. *Clin Chem.* 2005;51:434–444.

Johnson JA, et al. Clinical Pharmacogenetics Implementation Consortium (CPIC) guideline for pharmacogenetics-guided warfarin dosing: 2017 update. *Clin Pharmacol Ther.* 2017;102:397–404.

Leibovici L, Vidal L, Paul M. Aminoglycoside drugs in clinical practice: an evidenced based approach. *J Antimicrob Chemother.* 2009;63:246–251.

Moeller KE, et al. Urine drug screening: practical guide for clinicians. *Mayo Clin Proc.* 2008;63:66–76.

Morris RG. Cyclosporin therapeutic drug monitoring—an established service revisited. *Clin Biochem Rev.* 2003;24:33–46.

Newmeyer MN, et al. Free and glucuronide whole blood cannabinoids' pharmacokinetics after controlled smoked, vaporized, and oral cannabis administration in frequent and occasional cannabis users: identification of recent cannabis intake. *Clin Chem.* 2016;62:1579–1592.

Oellerich M, Armstrong VW. The role of therapeutic drug monitoring in individualizing immunosuppressive drug therapy: recent developments. *Ther Drug Monit.* 2006;28:720–725.

Olson KR, ed. *Poisoning & Drug Overdose.* 6th ed. New York, NY: McGraw-Hill Education; 2012.

O'Malley GF. Emergency department management of the salicylate-poisoned patient. *Emerg Med Clin North Am.* 2007;25:333–346.

Ostad Haji E, Hiemke C, Pfulmann B. Therapeutic drug monitoring for antidepressant drug treatment. *Curr Pharm Des.* 2012:18:5818–5827.

Patsalos PN, et al. Antiepileptic drugs—best practice guidelines for therapeutic drug monitoring: a position paper by the subcommission on therapeutic drug monitoring, ILAE Commission on Therapeutic Strategies. *Epilepsia.* 2008;49:1–38.

Roberts JA, Norris R, Paterson DL, Martin JH. Therapeutic drug monitoring of antimicrobials. *Br J Clin Pharmacol.* 2012;73:27–36.

Scheidweiler KB, Andersson M, Swortwood MJ, Sempio C, Huestis MA. Long-term stability of annabinoid in oral fluid after controlled cannabis administration. *Drug Test Anal.* 2017;9:143–147.

Schnur J, John RM. Childhood lead poisoning and the new Centers for Disease Control and Prevention guidelines for lead exposure. *J Am Assoc Nurse Pract.* 2014:26:238–247.

Schumacher GE, Barr JT. Therapeutic drug monitoring: do the improved outcomes justify the costs? *Clin Pharmacokinet.* 2001;40:405–409.

Sullivan LE, Fiellin DA. Narrative review: buprenorphine for opioid-dependent patients in office practice. Ann Intern Med. 2008;148:662–670.

Vale A. Alcohols and glycols. *Medicine.* 40:2012;89–93.

Wallemacq P et al. Opportunities to optimize tacrolimus therapy in solid organ transplantation: report to the European consensus conference. *Ther Drug Monit.* 2009;31:139–152.

Whyte IM, Francis B, Dawson AH. Safety and efficacy of intravenous *N*-acetylcysteine for acetaminophen overdose: analysis of the Hunter Area Toxicology Service (HATS) database. *Curr Med Res Opin.* 2007;23:2359–2368.

Willie S, Cooreman S, Neels H, Lambert L. Relevant issues in the monitoring and the toxicology of antidepressants. *Crit Rev Clin Lab Sci.* 2008;45:25–89.

Diseases of Infancy and Childhood

Paul Steele

CHAPTER OUTLINE

INTRODUCTION

It is difficult to precisely identify the diseases of infancy and childhood because many disorders that begin in childhood become clinically evident in adulthood if a long period of time is required to generate a pathologic lesion. The topics chosen for inclusion in this chapter are disorders presenting almost exclusively in childhood. However, they obviously represent only a small fraction of "childhood disorders." Many disorders in other sections of this book, such as hemophilia and numerous infections, occur or are diagnosed primarily in childhood. The chapter begins with an overview of prenatal and neonatal laboratory testing.

PRENATAL AND NEONATAL LABORATORY TESTING

Prenatal Testing and Screening

The disorders that can be diagnosed before birth number in the thousands. In families in which there is a history of a particular disorder, it is not uncommon to test prenatally for that particular disorder, often with DNA-based diagnostic tests. However, for the vast majority of families without a history of a specific illness, prenatal screening may also be undertaken. A screen differs from a test, in that it does not provide a definitive diagnosis but rather an assessment of the risk of a diagnosis. For most of these families, screening is preferred as an initial step because it is less invasive; for example, there are several maternal serum screening *assays* (see below) for fetal Down syndrome (also known as trisomy 21), but *testing* for fetal Down syndrome requires an invasive procedure such as chorionic villus sampling or collection of amniotic fluid. The decision to screen is a personal one for families and includes considerations such as parental age and desire to avoid having a diseased child.

Neonatal Screening

Neonatal screening was originally developed to detect diseases such as phenylketonuria (PKU) and congenital hypothyroidism, for which early detection and intervention could prevent catastrophic consequences such as intellectual disability (mental retardation). Improvements in assay methodology, such as decreases in cost and the availability of tandem mass spectrometry for single assay detection of many abnormalities, have expanded the neonatal screening menu to include assays for diseases that are not preventable but are often treatable. All 50 US states screen for over 30 disorders, including amino acidurias (such as PKU and maple syrup urine disease), organic acidemias (such as isovaleric acidemia), fatty acid disorders (such as medium-chain acyl-CoA dehydrogenase [MCAD] deficiency), hemoglobinopathies associated with hemoglobin S, congenital hypothyroidism, congenital adrenal hyperplasia, cystic fibrosis, and classical galactosemia, among others. As new methods and new assays are developed, some variation between states' neonatal screening menus will inevitably continue to exist; these variations are tracked on a website maintained by the National Newborn Screening & Global Resource Center.

> Neonatal screening was introduced as a means to detect disorders in which immediate treatment can result in the prevention of catastrophic consequences.

As with any screening program, positive results require follow-up confirmation testing; false-positives do occur. Suggested actions and algorithms for neonatal screen positives are published online by the American College of Medical Genetics and Genomics (ACMG). Urgent intervention is required for some of these disorders, to preserve life or prevent intellectual disability.

Neonatal Testing

The laboratory evaluation of an infant who appears clinically well in the first 24 hours of life but develops signs of illness on the second or third day may include:

- Blood gases to detect metabolic acidosis/alkalosis
- Urinalysis to detect ketonuria
- Complete blood count to detect abnormalities in blood cells
- A blood glucose test to detect hypoglycemia
- A blood ammonia test to detect elevated ammonia
- Liver function tests to detect hepatic dysfunction

TABLE 7-1   Routine Laboratory Screening for Inherited Metabolic Disease

Laboratory Test	Specimen
Lactate	Blood, CSF if indicated
Pyruvate	Blood
Amino acids	Urine, blood, CSF if indicated
Organic acids	Urine
Reducing sugars	Urine
Glucose	Blood, urine, CSF if indicated
Ketones and pH	Urine
Liver enzymes, electrolytes, uric acid, ammonia	Blood
Acylcarnitine profile	Blood
Mucopolysaccharide screen	Urine

CSF, cerebrospinal fluid.

- Prothrombin time and partial thromboplastin time to detect coagulopathies
- Blood lactate to detect lactic acidosis

Table 7-1 lists a number of screening laboratory tests that are typically ordered when there is suspicion that a neonate (or older child) is suffering from an inborn error of metabolism.

The results of these tests only suggest specific disorders, with additional testing required to identify a specific metabolic defect. Definitive tests to make a conclusive diagnosis of a metabolic disorder often involve the measurement of specific enzyme activities or various metabolites in a pathway. Because sepsis is often suspected, it must be ruled out in the sick infant if there are any signs or symptoms of infection.

A major cause of neonatal mortality and morbidity is preterm labor and delivery.

PREMATURITY

Description

A major cause of neonatal mortality and morbidity is prematurity, defined as birth prior to 37 weeks of gestation. When preterm labor or premature rupture of membranes causes prematurity, the underlying etiology is not often apparent, although it is believed to be commonly associated with infection or inflammation. Maternal correlates of prematurity include diabetes, obesity, intervention for infertility, genital or urinary infection, periodontal disease, low socioeconomic status, and other factors. Conflicting information exists about the value of intervention such as use of antibiotics for infection or infection risk.

Another cause of prematurity is iatrogenic, when the medical condition of the mother and/or fetus compels intervention to produce early delivery. The timing of such elective intervention for early delivery is influenced by the risk for fetal organ immaturity. Principal among these concerns is lung immaturity that is associated with the development of respiratory distress syndrome in the newborn.

Diagnosis

Risk of preterm delivery can be assessed by measurement of fetal fibronectin in cervical or vaginal fluid. This glycoprotein is produced by fetal membranes and appears in the cervix and vagina early in pregnancy as implantation develops, but normally disappears by week 20. Its reappearance in the third trimester often precedes labor and delivery. Its chief clinical value lies in its negative predictive value; that is, patients thought to be at risk for preterm labor who are negative for fetal fibronectin in their cervicovaginal fluid are very unlikely to deliver within 1 week of the laboratory result. The major barrier to the widespread use of the fetal fibronectin test, when positive, is that clinical interventions to end preterm labor are only partially successful.

In those instances when fetal or maternal health dictates early delivery, there are several tests available to assess fetal lung maturity. A simple and inexpensive test is to count lamellar bodies in amniotic fluid, using the platelet channel in a conventional hematology automated analyzer. These lamellar bodies are surfactant-containing products of Type II pneumocytes. The finding of greater than 50,000 lamellar bodies per microliter of amniotic fluid predicts lung maturity. If fewer bodies are present, further testing on the amniotic fluid sample is warranted. Other tests include identification of the presence of phosphatidylglycerol (PG), and determination of the ratio of lecithin to sphingomyelin (L/S ratio). The use of these lung maturity tests (and the amniocentesis required to perform them) for routine clinical care has declined markedly in recent years. If there is a medical need to deliver a preterm fetus, that delivery will proceed regardless of a lung maturity result. In late preterm pregnancy with uncertain gestational dates, advances in ultrasound technology have largely eliminated the routine need for lung maturity assays.

DOWN SYNDROME

Description

Down syndrome is the most commonly encountered, clinically significant autosomal chromosome aberration affecting individuals beyond infancy. This genetic defect, which can be detected by cytogenetic analysis, is trisomy 21. More than 90% of Down cases occur as a result of meiotic nondisjunction. Down syndrome is characterized by intellectual disability, cardiac malformations, malformations of the digestive tract, eyes, and ears, and the development of an Alzheimer-like disease process in later life.

The overall birth prevalence of Down syndrome is approximately 1 in 1000 births. However, a woman's individual risk to deliver an infant with Down syndrome depends substantially on her age. The risk increases significantly past age 35 years, with an incidence in the range of 1:270 to 1:100 by age 40 years.

Screening and Diagnosis

The neonatal diagnosis of Down syndrome is clinical, with metaphase chromosome analysis on peripheral blood serving merely to confirm the diagnosis.

Noninvasive fetal screening for Down syndrome involves many more tests (**Table 7–2**) that are used in combination to develop a risk assessment of Down syndrome during pregnancy.

> Down syndrome is the most commonly encountered, clinically significant autosomal chromosome aberration affecting individuals beyond infancy. This genetic defect, which can be detected by cytogenetic analysis, is trisomy 21. The neonatal diagnosis of Down syndrome is clinical, with metaphase chromosome analysis on peripheral blood serving merely to confirm the diagnosis.

TABLE 7–2   Laboratory Evaluation for Down Syndrome

Laboratory Test	Result/Comment
First-trimester screen	
Pregnancy-associated plasma protein A (PAPP-A)	Low in pregnancy with Down syndrome fetus
Free beta hCG	Elevated in pregnancy with Down syndrome fetus
Nuchal translucency	Ultrasound exam; permits evaluation of each fetus in multiple gestation pregnancy
Quadruple screen	**Second-trimester screen**
Alpha-fetoprotein (AFP)	Low in pregnancy with Down syndrome fetus; elevated with fetal neural tube defect
hCG	Elevated in pregnancy with Down syndrome fetus
Unconjugated estriol (UE3)	Low in pregnancy with Down syndrome fetus
Inhibin A	Elevated in pregnancy with Down syndrome fetus
DNA sequence of circulating cell-free fetal DNA	Can detect trisomy 21 as well as other defects including trisomy 18 and trisomy 13
Metaphase chromosome analysis	Diagnostic test; can be performed on chorionic villus sample, cells from amniotic fluid, and newborn blood

Definitive diagnosis of fetal Down syndrome during pregnancy is established by an invasive test, namely, metaphase analysis of cells from either chorionic villus sampling (typically limited to first trimester) or amniotic fluid collection. The decision to engage in fetal screening for Down syndrome or to move from screening tests to invasive diagnostic testing once a risk assessment is completed depends on patient preference. The invasive tests to assess for Down syndrome during pregnancy do carry a risk of miscarriage.

First-trimester screening typically consists of measurement of two analytes in maternal serum: pregnancy-associated plasma protein A (PAPP-A) and the free beta subunit of human chorionic gonadotropin (fβhCG); the former is low and the latter high in mothers carrying a Down syndrome fetus. A third part of first-trimester screening is ultrasound assessment for nuchal translucency, which is increased as a result of fluid accumulation in the neck of a Down syndrome fetus. This first-trimester screening is associated with a sensitivity of approximately 85%, with a 5% false-positive rate. Nuchal translucency alone is not recommended in singleton pregnancy because its sensitivity is only about 70%. However, in multiple gestation pregnancies, the interpretation of maternal serum markers can be problematic, while the nuchal translucency test permits evaluation of each fetus. Determination of nuchal translucency is highly operator-dependent and requires specific training.

Second-trimester screening typically consists of the so-called quadruple screen of maternal serum, consisting of measurement of the following analytes: alpha-fetoprotein, unconjugated estriol (both decreased in mothers carrying a Down syndrome fetus), and total hCG and inhibin A (both increased in such mothers). The quadruple screen has a detection rate of approximately 81% with a 5% false-positive rate. Maternal serum results are typically described in the form of "multiples of the median" (or MoM); the normal range is highly dependent on several factors including gestational age, number of gestations, maternal weight, and race.

Combining first- and second-trimester screens can provide an even higher level of detection. One approach is to sequentially conduct the tests; that is, inform the patient of the results of the first-trimester screen as soon as they are available (this permits her to choose a more definitive diagnostic method if indicated), and later perform the quadruple screen in the second trimester if appropriate. A noninvasive test that rivals the sensitivity and specificity of invasive testing is DNA sequencing of circulating cell-free fetal DNA (ccffDNA) in maternal serum. This test could also identify other chromosome aneuploidy syndromes such as trisomy 18, trisomy 13, and sex chromosome aneuploidy. Current recommendations for follow-up of positive ccffDNA sequencing results are to confirm the abnormality by invasive testing (metaphase chromosome analysis on chorionic villus or amniotic fluid samples), but a negative ccffDNA sequencing test in a patient whose first- or second-trimester screen is positive for Down syndrome may provide an option to forgo invasive testing.

A final point about maternal serum screening is that the alpha-fetoprotein assay in the quadruple screen, if elevated, provides a measure of increased risk for neural tube defects such as spina bifida. These cases can be further studied by amniotic fluid collection, with assessment of acetylcholinesterase as well as alpha-fetoprotein (both elevated with neural tube defects) and high-resolution ultrasound examination.

INFECTIOUS DISEASES IN THE PERINATAL PERIOD

Description

A number of maternal infections affect the fetus and newborn. Bacterial vaginosis, sexually transmitted diseases, and others increase the risk of preterm labor. Rubella and syphilis are associated with congenital anomalies. Neonatal death has been linked to a number of infections, including cytomegalovirus (CMV), group B streptococcus, herpes simplex, *Listeria*, parvovirus, among others. Postnatal disease in the offspring occurs with many infections, such as hepatitis B and C, human immunodeficiency disease (HIV), CMV, rubella, toxoplasmosis, and syphilis.

Screening and Diagnosis

Routine prenatal care is designed to screen for several of these infections, for the purpose of identifying pregnant women who need intervention or identifying susceptibility for a poor outcome

A number of maternal infections affect the fetus and newborn. Neonatal death has been linked to a number of infections, including cytomegalovirus (CMV), group B streptococcus, herpes simplex, *Listeria*, parvovirus, and others.

in the mother. The results of maternal screening tests may have implications for the fetus, especially when they indicate maternal infection during pregnancy. An example of the latter is rubella serology screening of maternal serum. Routine testing includes serologic testing for syphilis, hepatitis B and C, and HIV. Routine rectovaginal culture for group B streptococcus is performed late in the third trimester. Detection through nucleic acid testing and/or culture is carried out for *Chlamydia* and for gonorrhea in high-risk mothers, and for herpes simplex in mothers with genital lesions.

HEMOLYTIC DISEASE OF THE NEWBORN

Description

Hemolytic disease of the newborn (HDN), also known as erythroblastosis fetalis, is a syndrome in which the newborn becomes anemic from the destruction of his/her RBCs in utero. This RBC destruction is a result of maternal IgG antibodies formed against a red cell antigen, most commonly the Rh antigen (also known as D antigen), which are then delivered into the fetal circulation across the placenta. Antibody production by a mother who is Rh-negative results from exposure to Rh-positive fetal cells during pregnancy and, to a much greater extent, at delivery. Therefore, the women at greatest risk for delivering infants with HDN are Rh-negative mothers who conceive Rh-positive babies, and are in the second or subsequent pregnancies. It is general practice to identify risk of sensitization during pregnancy and treat the mother prophylactically by rapidly removing Rh-positive fetal cells through passive immunization with Rh immune globulin. Such immunizations are almost always effective in preventing the mother's immune system from developing these alloantibodies. Treatment is employed not only following delivery, when fetal to maternal bleeding is expected, but also during pregnancy itself.

> Hemolytic disease of the newborn (HDN), also known as erythroblastosis fetalis, is a syndrome in which the newborn becomes anemic from the destruction of his/her RBCs in utero.

Other red cell alloantibodies may be involved, although much less commonly. A form of HDN, usually mild, results from transplacental passage of IgG-class antibodies against A or B red cell antigens, to a Type A, B, or AB fetus. This disorder may occur with the first pregnancy, as it involves maternal antibodies that normally arise without the requirement of a previous pregnancy or incompatible blood transfusion.

Neonatal disease related to maternal antibody may occasionally involve targets other than RBC antigens; examples include neonatal alloimmune thrombocytopenic purpura (NAIT) with maternal antiplatelet antibodies.

Screening and Diagnosis

ABO/Rh typing is used in routine prenatal care to identify the mother's blood type. An antibody screen against a standard panel of red cells, employing the indirect antiglobulin method (see Chapter 2), is also routinely performed to determine if there are maternal alloantibodies (such as anti-Rh) that might be a threat to the fetus.

Testing for fetal blood type (which establishes presence or absence of fetal susceptibility in that pregnancy), as well as monitoring for fetal anemia and hyperbilirubinemia (the latter a consequence of the RBC destruction), typically requires invasive procedures such as amniocentesis (withdrawal of amniotic fluid) or cordocentesis (withdrawal of blood from the cord, in utero). Both of these carry some risk of pregnancy loss or fetal damage. A new, noninvasive approach is possible with genetic testing for the antigen genes. Genotyping of the father that reveals homozygosity of the antigen gene implies fetal antigen positivity. Heterozygosity in the father implies a 50% chance of fetal antigen negativity, in which case there would be absence of risk for HDN. Confirmation of fetal antigen negativity can be accomplished by genotyping of fetal DNA that is present in maternal plasma. Titering the quantity of maternal antibody as a disease predictor in the fetus has been used, but the amount of antibody does not always correlate with the severity of the disease. Testing of amniotic fluid for bilirubin by spectrophotometric analysis can be performed to help manage the disease; fetuses at high risk of severe anemia, based on the amniotic fluid bilirubin, would be delivered if tests of fetal lung maturity on the amniotic fluid sample (see above) reveal a low risk of respiratory distress syndrome. Otherwise, intrauterine blood transfusion and exchange could be performed. A noninvasive ultrasound test can detect fetal middle cerebral artery blood flow rates that correlate well with the presence of fetal anemia. This test has been shown to be more sensitive, specific, and accurate than the invasive amniotic fluid bilirubin measurement.

TABLE 7–3   Laboratory Evaluation of the Mother and Newborn for Hemolytic Disease of the Newborn (HDN)

	Result/Comment
To predict HDN during pregnancy	
Maternal ABO and Rh type	Provides screening for possible HDN risk
Maternal antibody screen	Detects many common anti-red cell antibodies
Maternal antibody titer	Significant elevation implies risk of HDN
Genotyping of father	Homozygosity for antigen gene implies fetal risk; heterozygosity for antigen gene requires further testing to assess fetal susceptibility
Genotyping of fetus	Presence of antigen gene can be assessed; specimen may be amniotic fluid or cord cells (both invasive) or maternal plasma
To assess for HDN during pregnancy	
ΔOD_{450}	Invasive; spectrophotometric assessment of bilirubin through assessment of change (delta) of optical density at 450 nm from expected to observed
Fetal hematocrit	Invasive; requires cordocentesis
Fetal middle cerebral artery flow	Noninvasive; peak velocity of systolic blood flow increases progressively with fetal anemia
To evaluate disease in the newborn	
Clinical findings	Infant may appear normal to very abnormal; jaundice is common; cardiorespiratory problems may occur; severely affected fetuses may die in utero or at delivery
Reticulocyte count	At 7 days of life, an elevated level is consistent with HDN
Nucleated red blood cells	A persistently high percentage of nucleated red blood cells is consistent with increased red blood cell production
Unconjugated bilirubin	Markedly elevated, but other entities, such as liver immaturity, can cause an increased unconjugated bilirubin in neonates
Haptoglobin	Low value indicates intravascular hemolysis
Direct antiglobulin test	Positive result indicates maternal antibodies to red blood cells in the newborn circulation

Laboratory evaluation of newborns for HDN includes complete blood count and direct antiglobulin test (DAT) on cord blood. The latter test detects the presence of immunoglobulin and/or complement deposited on the surface of red blood cells. See **Table 7–3** for a list of tests that are helpful in the laboratory evaluation of HDN.

CYSTIC FIBROSIS

Description

Cystic fibrosis is an autosomal recessive disease that results from a mutation in the cystic fibrosis transmembrane conductance regulator (CFTR) gene on the long arm of chromosome 7. The clinical presentation is dysfunction of exocrine glands, from abnormal chloride conduction across the apical membrane of epithelial cells, and subsequently chronic obstructive lung disease and exocrine pancreatic insufficiency. The most commonly found mutation in the CFTR gene is ΔF508 (loss of a phenylalanine codon at position 508), and it is present in approximately 70% of cases. However, approximately 2000 mutations in this gene have been described, most of which are rare; many are not yet unequivocally associated with disease.

Cystic fibrosis is an autosomal recessive disease that results from a mutation in the cystic fibrosis transmembrane conductance regulator (CFTR) gene on the long arm of chromosome 7.

The incidence of cystic fibrosis is approximately 1 in 2500 to 3400 Caucasian births, 1 in 17,000 births from individuals of African descent, and 1 in 90,000 Asian births. As many as 1 in 29 Caucasians may be a carrier for cystic fibrosis.

Screening and Diagnosis

Extending an offer to screen the carrier status of all couples planning for pregnancy is now recommended; access to a genetic counselor should be offered when one or both members of a couple have a family history of cystic fibrosis. The carrier screen is a molecular genetic test designed to

TABLE 7-4   Laboratory Evaluation for Cystic Fibrosis

Laboratory Test	Result/Comment
Quantitative pilocarpine iontophoresis sweat chloride test	Sweat chloride concentration >60 mEq/L confirms the diagnosis, in the presence of supporting clinical and laboratory information; differential diagnosis for a positive sweat test result includes untreated adrenal insufficiency, hereditary nephrogenic diabetes insipidus, hypothyroidism, pancreatitis, and malnutrition
Genetic testing	Used for carrier testing, disease testing, and newborn screen follow-up testing
72-h fecal fat level	Elevated
Fecal elastase	Decreased
Immunoreactive trypsinogen	Elevated in newborn screening test

detect the most common mutations; the number of mutations detected in typical carrier screening assays is growing (from 23 mutations originally, to well over a hundred for some assays) as the assay cost is progressively decreasing.

Screening newborns for the disease is increasingly common. The usual approach is to screen blood spots for immunoreactive trypsinogen (IRT) and then follow up elevated values with either a multiple-mutation DNA test or repeat IRT on a new sample.

Laboratory evaluation for screen-positive patients includes the same test used in the assessment of patients clinically suspected of having the disease: quantitative sweat chloride. This analysis involves testing to determine whether the patient exhibits elevated levels of chloride in sweat samples; these samples are typically elicited with the use of pilocarpine and iontophoresis.

Genetic testing for disease detection (as opposed to screening) involves a larger number of mutation investigations, typically more than 75. The initial genetic test for disease detection may be the same assay employed for carrier detection (see above): whereas the carrier assay is designed to detect a mutation in one gene i.e from one parent; the disease assay is designed to detect mutations in two genes. If no, or only one, mutation is detected in a suspected CF patient, nucleotide sequencing of the gene can be performed. Once a proband's genetic mutations have been documented, family members can be tested exclusively for these mutations, if family studies are desired.

Six classes of gene mutations, each specific for a different type of CFTR malfunction, have been described. The development of CFTR-modulating drugs, specific for a particular class of mutations, makes the genetic characterization of CF all the more important. **Table 7-4** presents the laboratory evaluation of cystic fibrosis.

AMINO ACIDURIAS

Description and Diagnosis

Amino acidurias are defects in the metabolism of amino acids that lead to their accumulation. The primary amino acidurias are a result of an inherited enzyme defect within a degradative pathway for a specific amino acid, or in a transporter in the renal tubules, that alters the reabsorption of the amino acid. Selected primary amino acidurias associated with impaired amino acid degradation are shown in **Table 7-5**. The defective enzymes and the amino acid or other compound in elevated concentration are listed for the individual disorders. In contrast to primary amino acidurias, secondary amino acidurias are accumulations of amino acids that arise when the organs responsible for their elimination or degradation, notably the liver and kidney, are functionally impaired. The diagnosis of a primary amino aciduria may be made by demonstrating a decrease in a specific enzyme activity required for the metabolism of the amino acid or by finding the associated abnormality in the gene coding for the enzyme. The presence of characteristic clinical signs and symptoms for the individual disorders is highly contributory toward establishing a diagnosis. The different amino acidurias vary from essentially benign, with no apparent disease, to lethal disorders. Furthermore, the clinical features can vary widely within a single disease, because some of the amino acidurias have multiple forms and because some enzyme deficiencies can result in an elevation of the same amino acid.

Amino acidurias are defects in the metabolism of amino acids that lead to their accumulation. The primary amino acidurias are a result of an inherited enzyme defect within a degradative pathway for a specific amino acid, or in a transporter in the renal tubules, that alters the reabsorption of the amino acid.

TABLE 7–5   Selected Amino Acidurias

Disorder	Defective Enzymes	Amino Acid or Other Compound in Elevated Concentration (Most Prominent Ones)
For enzymes outside the urea cycle		
Phenylketonuria (multiple forms of the disorder with different enzyme deficiencies)	Phenylalanine hydroxylase Dihydropteridine reductase Defect in biopterin synthesis	Phenylalanine
Tyrosinemia (multiple forms of the disorder with different enzyme deficiencies)	Fumarylacetoacetate hydrolase Tyrosine aminotransferase	Tyrosine
Alkaptonuria	Homogentisic acid oxidase	Homogentisic acid
Homocystinuria (multiple forms of the disorder with different enzyme deficiencies)	Cystathionine β-synthase Methylenetetrahydrofolate reductase (MTHFR) Methyltransferase	Homocysteine
Histidinemia	Histidase	Histidine
Maple syrup urine disease	Branched-chain ketoacid decarboxylase	Leucine, isoleucine, alloisoleucine, valine, and corresponding ketoacids (in acute attacks)
Nonketotic hyperglycemia	Block in glycine cleavage enzyme system	Glycine
Methylmalonic acidemia	Methylmalonyl-CoA mutase	Glycine and methylmalonic acid
Cystathioninuria	γ-Cystathionase	Cystathionine
Carnosinemia	Carnosinase	Carnosine
Hyperprolinemia (multiple forms of the disorder with different enzyme deficiencies)	Proline oxidase Δ^5-Pyrroline-5-carboxylic acid dehydrogenase	Proline
For enzymes within the urea cycle		
Citrullinemia	Argininosuccinate synthetase	Citrulline, ammonia, and alanine
Argininosuccinic aciduria	Argininosuccinate lyase	Argininosuccinic acid and citrulline; ammonia after meals
Argininemia	Arginase	Arginine; ammonia after meals
Hyperornithinemia	Ornithine decarboxylase	Ornithine, glutamine, and alanine; ammonia after meals
Ornithine transcarbamylase deficiency	Ornithine transcarbamylase	Ammonia and glutamine
Carbamoylphosphate synthetase deficiency	Carbamoylphosphate synthetase	Ammonia, glycine, and glutamine

LYSOSOMAL STORAGE DISEASES

Description and Diagnosis

Lysosomal storage diseases, like the amino acidurias, are inborn errors of metabolism. The lysosomal storage diseases result from the lysosomal accumulation of compounds that should otherwise be degraded by the enzymes in the lysosome. The diagnosis of a lysosomal storage disease is made by identifying the products stored in the tissues or excreted in the urine. Demonstration of an enzyme deficiency is usually sufficient for diagnosis of a specific lysosomal storage disease. DNA analysis for the mutation producing the enzyme deficiency for these and all other inborn errors also can be performed and may provide differentiation of severe from mild disease or even indicate lack of disease (so-called pseudodeficiency). As with the amino acidurias, a number of lysosomal storage disorders have subtypes, because different enzyme deficiencies may result in the accumulation of similar or identical compounds. **Table 7–6** provides a list of selected lysosomal storage disorders grouped into those associated with impaired degradation of sphingolipids

TABLE 7–6 **Selected Lysosomal Storage Disorders**

The Compound Stored in the Lysosome and Associated Disease	Enzyme Deficiency
Sphingolipidoses[a]	
Niemann–Pick disease	Sphingomyelinase
Gaucher disease	β-Glucosidase
Krabbe disease	Galactosylceramide β-galactosidase
Metachromatic leukodystrophy	Arylsulfatase A
Fabry disease	α-Galactosidase (X-linked)
Tay–Sachs disease	β-N-Acetylglucosaminidase A
Sandhoff disease	β-N-Acetylglucosaminidase A and B
Generalized gangliosidosis	β-Galactosidase
Mucopolysaccharidoses (MPS)[b]	
Hurler syndrome	α-L-Iduronidase
Scheie syndrome	α-L-Iduronidase
Hunter syndrome	Iduronate sulfatases (X-linked)
Sanfilippo syndrome (multiple forms of the disorder with different enzyme deficiencies)	Heparan N-sulfatase α-N-Acetylglucosaminidase α-Glucosaminide-N-acetyltransferase N-Acetylglucosamine-6-sulfate sulfatase
Morquio disease (multiple forms with different enzyme deficiencies)	Galactosamine-6-sulfate sulfatase β-Galactosidase
Maroteaux–Lamy disease	Arylsulfatase B
Glucuronidase deficiency	β-Glucuronidase
Glycogen storage disorders[c]	
Pompe disease	α-Glucosidase

[a]Accumulation of sphingolipids (which includes sphingomyelins, glucosylceramides, galactosylceramides, sulfatides, and gangliosides) due to deficiencies of enzymes required for their degradation.
[b]Accumulation of mucopolysaccharides (glycosaminoglycans) due to enzyme deficiencies required for their degradation.
[c]Accumulation of glycogen due to an enzyme deficiency required for its degradation.

The lysosomal storage diseases result from the lysosomal accumulation of compounds that should otherwise be degraded by the enzymes in the lysosome. The diagnosis of a lysosomal storage disease is made by identifying the products stored in the tissues or excreted in the urine.

(the sphingolipidoses), mucopolysaccharides (also known as glycosaminoglycans) (the mucopolysaccharidoses), and glycogen. As a class of disorders, the lysosomal storage disorders are rare. The one with the highest prevalence is Gaucher disease, which affects 1 in 600 in the Ashkenazi Jewish population. Each lysosomal storage disorder has its own characteristic clinical features, and most signs and symptoms of these diseases are expressed early in life. Many of these disorders can even be diagnosed in utero or in the period immediately after birth. There is often an urgency to establish the diagnosis so that appropriate treatment can be instituted as soon as possible.

NEUROBLASTOMA

Description

Neuroblastoma is a solid tumor that affects infants and toddlers. It is the most common malignancy under 1 year of age, and most patients are diagnosed by age 2 years. It presents either as a mass, often in the abdomen or neck, or with signs and symptoms of tumor spread, including bone pain or spinal cord dysfunction. Neuroblastoma is one of the "small round cell" tumors of childhood, and it must be distinguished from other tumors of that type, which include lymphoma, rhabdomyosarcoma, Ewing sarcoma, and primitive neuroectodermal tumor (PNET).

Diagnosis

Measurement of urinary catecholamines can be used to alert clinicians to the likelihood that an infant's tumor mass is a neuroblastoma, as the other "round cell tumors" listed above do not excrete catecholamines. Unlike pheochromocytoma (see Chapter 22), urinary metanephrines are usually not helpful, as most neuroblastomas do not produce an abundance of epinephrine. For the diagnosis and monitoring of neuroblastoma, vanillylmandelic acid (VMA) and homovanillic acid (HVA) are typically measured in urine by high-performance liquid chromatography (HPLC) methodology. For the subset of patients who are VMA/HVA negative, testing a panel of catecholamines and their metabolites may identify one or more other compounds that could then be used instead to follow urine levels longitudinally for treatment monitoring.

Detection of metastases in bone marrow samples of these patients is challenging with histologic methods as there are often very few tumor cells, but molecular studies are now being used to detect minimal residual disease. Examples of such assays being used for this purpose include reverse transcriptase-polymerase chain reaction (RT-PCR) for tyrosine hydroxylase (an enzyme involved in catecholamine synthesis) and for the proto-oncogene MYCN. The latter gene is of interest because its copy number in neuroblastoma tumor samples has prognostic significance. Amplification of MYCN is associated with a poorer prognosis in these patients. There is interest in developing other biomarkers for neuroblastoma; chromogranin A and neuron-specific enolase are two, among several, in use or in development.

> Neuroblastoma is a solid tumor that affects infants and toddlers. It is the most common malignancy under 1 year of age, and most patients are diagnosed by age 2 years.

SELF-ASSESSMENT QUESTIONS

1. Which of the following tests can be used to assess the risk of preterm delivery?
   A. Human chorionic gonadotropin (hCG) in serum
   B. Fetal fibronectin in the cervical or vaginal fluid
   C. Luteinizing hormone (LH) in urine
   D. Progesterone in serum

2. Which one of the following choices is not a component of the quadruple screen for Down syndrome, used as a second-trimester screen for the syndrome?
   A. Nuchal translucency
   B. α-Fetoprotein (AFP)
   C. Unconjugated estriol
   D. Inhibin A

3. Hemolytic disease of the newborn is a syndrome in which the newborn becomes anemic from the destruction of his/her red blood cells in utero. This red blood cell destruction is a result of maternal IgG antibodies formed against a red blood cell antigen. Which of the red blood cell antigens below is most commonly associated with hemolytic disease of the newborn?
   A. Kell antigen
   B. Duffy antigen
   C. Rh antigen
   D. Kidd antigen

4. Which of the following tests is less commonly used than the others to evaluate a patient for cystic fibrosis?
   A. Sweat chloride
   B. Immunoreactive trypsinogen
   C. Mutational analysis of the membrane chloride channel known as CFTR
   D. Amino acid profile

5. Which of the following pairs of (category of disease—disease name) is incorrect?
   A. Amino aciduria—Maple syrup urine disease
   B. Lysosomal storage disease—Phenylketonuria
   C. Glycogen storage disorder—Pompe disease
   D. Mucopolysaccharidosis storage disorder—Hurler syndrome

FURTHER READING

Brewington J, et al. Diagnostic testing in cystic fibrosis. *Clin Chest Med*. 2016;37:31–46.

Cappelletti M, et al. Inflammation and preterm birth. *J Leukoc Biol*. 2016;99:67–78.

Carter SC, et al. Pharmacogenetics of cystic fibrosis treatment. *Pharmacogenomics*. 2016;17:1453–1463.

DeFranco EA, et al. Improving the screening accuracy for preterm labor: is the combination of fetal fibronectin and cervical length in symptomatic patients a useful predictor of preterm birth? A systematic review. *Am J Obstet Gynecol*. 2013;208:233.e1–233.e6.

Skrzypek H, et al. Noninvasive prenatal testing for fetal aneuploidy and single gene disorders. *Best Pract Res Clin Obstet Gynaecol*. 2017;42:26–38.

Valle D, et al., eds. Part 8: Amino acids; lysosomal disorders. In: *The Online Metabolic & Molecular Bases of Inherited Disease*. New York, NY: McGraw-Hill; 2017.

Verly IRN, et al. Catecholamines profiles at diagnosis: increased diagnostic sensitivity and correlation with biological and clinical features in neuroblastoma patients. *Eur J Cancer*. 2017;72:235–243.

Yarbrough ML, et al. Fetal lung maturity testing; the end of an era. *Biomark Med*. 2014;8:509–515.

Blood Vessels

Michael Laposata

INTRODUCTION

Because blood vessels are present in all organs and tissues, vascular disease is not restricted to a limited group of signs and symptoms. All organs and tissues are potential targets of injury in vascular disease, and most patients present with signs and symptoms indicative of injury to a specific organ or tissue, usually as a result of diminished blood flow. For example, if there is decreased blood flow to the heart, the patient presents with signs and symptoms related to cardiac dysfunction. The decrease in blood flow could be the result of a lesion that originates in the blood vessel wall, and therefore a vascular disease, or an obstruction by a blood clot inside the blood vessel. The disorders originating within the blood vessel wall include atherosclerotic vascular disease, hypertensive vascular disease, vasculitis, tumors, and aneurysms. Blood vessel disorders that may result from an abnormality that is not within the blood vessel wall include deep vein thrombosis

(DVT), and what the DVT may generate if any of the clot moves to the lungs, pulmonary embolism (PE). DVT and PE are also discussed in this chapter. A first-time DVT or PE is nearly always the result of clot formation inside a normal vein. However, if an abnormality in vein anatomy exists, such as congenital atresia of the inferior vena cava, the defects within the blood vessels themselves can be highly contributory to the development of a DVT.

- Atherosclerotic vascular disease is one of the most predominant illnesses in the Western world. The goal of clinical laboratory testing is to identify the cause of atherosclerosis. This is usually related to excess dietary lipid or a disorder of lipid metabolism. This chapter provides information on dietary fat and disorders of lipid metabolism that lead to atherosclerosis.
- Hypertensive vascular disease is also common. The role of clinical laboratory testing is to determine if there is a correctable cause for hypertension. Because more than 90% of hypertension cases are "essential," there is currently no correctable cause. Treatment with antihypertensive medical therapy is important and beneficial, but it does not treat the underlying cause for hypertension in most cases. Some causes of hypertension, however, are identifiable and correctable, often surgically. An example of a surgically correctable form of hypertension is one in which a tumor secretes a hormone responsible for the elevation of blood pressure. Removal of the tumor often results in normalization of the blood pressure. The section "Hypertension" focuses on the correctable causes of hypertension and the laboratory tests useful in identifying them.
- Vasculitis represents a less commonly encountered group of disorders with inflammation in the blood vessel wall. Clinical laboratory testing has a limited role in establishing the diagnosis of a particular form of vasculitis. The diagnosis is made by the specific clinical features of the patient, the results of antineutrophil cytoplasmic antibody (ANCA) testing for some forms of vasculitis, and, on occasion, histopathologic review of a blood vessel biopsy specimen.
- DVT and PE are primarily diagnosed with imaging studies. However, an important test in the clinical laboratory, used primarily to rule out DVT and PE when the result is negative, is the D-dimer test.

ATHEROSCLEROSIS

Dietary Fat

Most of the lipid in the diet is in the form of triglycerides. Humans ingest grams of triglycerides daily. Nearly all (97%) of the mass of the triglyceride molecule is made up of the three fatty acids bound to the glycerol backbone. The triglyceride molecules are degraded in the gastrointestinal tract by lipases which liberate the fatty acids from the glycerol backbone of the triglyceride. Fatty acids are long chain carbon molecules with a carboxyl (COOH) end and a methyl (CH_3) end. Commonly encountered fatty acids in the diet are as long as 22 carbons. If there are no double bonds in the carbon chain, the fatty acid is saturated. If there is a single double bond, the fatty acid is monounsaturated. Two or more double bonds make the fatty acid polyunsaturated. For those fatty acids with a double bond, the number of carbons between the double bond and the methyl end identifies the family to which the fatty acid belongs. When the double bond nearest the methyl end of the fatty acid is three carbons inward, the fatty acid is known as an omega-3 or n-3 fatty acid. Similarly, if it is six carbons from the methyl end, it is known as an omega-6 or n-6 fatty acid. Other families of fatty acids include omega-9 and omega-7. Oils are composed of mostly omega-6 fatty acids (e.g., vegetable oil), omega-9 (e.g., olive oil), or omega-3 (e.g., fish oil). Humans are unable to synthesize omega-3 or omega-6 fatty acids, and for this reason they are known as essential fatty acids because they are essential in the diet. Saturated fatty acids and fatty acids in the omega-9 and omega-7 family are essential for life, but because these fatty acids can be made from smaller molecules in humans, they are known as nonessential fatty acids. There is strong evidence that saturated fatty acids are not healthy; polyunsaturated fatty acids can be healthy, but it depends to some extent upon the family. Notably, omega-3 fatty acids have beneficial effects for reducing cardiovascular risk and, as an adjunct therapy, for patients with depression. Omega-3 fatty acids are present in higher amounts in certain fish, especially those that swim in cold water. The two major omega-3 fatty acids, which are highly unsaturated, are EPA (eicosapentaenoic acid) which has 20 carbons and 5 double bonds and DHA (docosahexaenoic acid) which has 22 carbons and 6 double bonds. Omega-6 fatty acids, even though they are polyunsaturated, can lead to the generation of compounds which promote inflammation. Another classification is made for only those fatty acids with a double bond. If the hydrogen atoms are on the same side of the double bond in an unsaturated fatty acid, the fatty acid is known as a *cis* fatty acid. This is the natural form of the double bond. Alternatively, when the hydrogens are on the opposite sides of the double bond, the fatty acid is known as a *trans* fatty acid. Trans fatty acids are not healthy, and although small amounts are generated endogenously, much of the trans fatty acid in humans is from the diet, despite the growing restriction of trans fatty acids in commercially prepared food.

Unlike triglycerides which are eaten in grams daily, only milligrams of cholesterol are ingested. When cholesterol is bound to a fatty acid, it becomes a cholesterol ester. Cholesterol ester molecules are highly insoluble in water. Therefore, when cholesterol is delivered into the blood vessel wall, it is much more easily removed than a cholesterol ester molecule, which is created after the cholesterol is delivered into a growing plaque. Atherosclerotic plaques contain significant amounts of cholesterol esters.

Lipoproteins carry triglycerides and cholesterol esters because they are insoluble in the blood. The lipoprotein has a shell of phospholipid which has enough polarity to interact with water. Free cholesterol, that is cholesterol not bound to a fatty acid, is also polar and resides in the shell of the lipoprotein. Inside the shell, in the core of the lipoprotein, interacting with the nonpolar portion of the phospholipid molecule, are cholesterol ester and triglyceride. Lipoproteins also have certain apolipoproteins which affect their metabolism and distribution.

Description

Atherosclerotic vascular disease is a major cause of mortality and morbidity in the Western world. It is the consequence of an accumulation of lipid in large arteries including the aorta and, thereby, a narrowing of the lumen of the arteries, which results in decreased blood flow. When an atherosclerotic plaque ruptures, a thrombus can form over the ruptured plaque and totally occlude blood flow. Atherosclerotic disease is vascular in origin, in that lipid deposition and cell proliferation occur within the blood vessel wall. The end-organ damage depends on the anatomic location of the occluded artery. It is common to have generalized atherosclerosis with multiple vascular beds affected.

The causes of atherosclerotic vascular disease include:

- Ingestion of excess or atherogenic dietary fat, which is primarily saturated fatty acids and cholesterol. This is the most common cause of atherosclerotic vascular disease.
- Primary lipid disorders, also known as primary hyperlipidemias, which result in an increase in cholesterol, triglyceride, or both in the plasma. Many of these disorders are a result of genetic mutations that perturb the metabolism of cholesterol. They are not uncommon.
- Nonlipid disorders causing elevations in the concentration of plasma lipids, usually cholesterol and/or triglyceride. These are called secondary hyperlipidemias. Disorders or conditions that adversely affect lipid metabolism include hypothyroidism, nephrotic syndrome, liver disease, diabetes, obesity, and alcohol abuse. In addition, many medications can alter plasma lipid levels.
- Though not common, elevated levels of lipoprotein(a) (Lp(a) and pronounced "L-P-little a") with or without other lipid or lipoprotein abnormalities.
- Also not common, disorders that are associated with direct damage to the blood vessel wall, independent of lipid levels, such as high circulating concentrations of homocysteine.

Diagnosis

The initial approach to the patient for routine evaluation or for monitoring the status of atherosclerotic vascular disease is to determine if the patient has an elevation in serum or plasma cholesterol, and if so, to first determine if the cause is excess intake of dietary fat.

The initial approach to the patient for routine evaluation or for monitoring the status of atherosclerotic vascular disease is to determine if the patient has an elevation in serum or plasma total cholesterol and LDL cholesterol concentrations, and a low HDL cholesterol concentration, and if so, to first determine if the likely cause is excess intake of dietary fat.

TABLE 8–1   **The Major Plasma Lipoproteins**

Lipoprotein Class	Lipid Components of Core	Synonyms for Lipoprotein Classes	Predominant Apolipoproteins[a]
Chylomicrons	Triglycerides >> cholesterol esters	None	**B48** (also in chylomicron remnant), A-I, A-IV, C-I, C-II, C-III, E
Very-low-density lipoproteins (VLDL)	Triglycerides > cholesterol esters	Pre-beta lipoproteins	**B-100**, C-I (especially in hyperlipidemic patients), C-II (especially in hyperlipidemic patients), C-III, E (especially in hyperlipidemic patients)
Low-density lipoproteins (LDL)	Cholesterol esters > triglycerides	Beta lipoproteins	**B-100**
High-density lipoproteins (HDL)	Cholesterol esters > triglycerides	Alpha lipoproteins	**A-I**, A-II, A-IV, C-I (especially in normolipidemic patients), C-II (especially in normolipidemic patients), C-III, E (especially in normolipidemic patients)

[a]Major apolipoprotein in bold.

An elevated total cholesterol level (>200 mg/dL) prompts the need to determine the basis for the elevation. For plasma or serum concentrations of low-density lipoprotein (LDL) cholesterol, a high level is bad, and for high-density lipoprotein (HDL) cholesterol, a high level is good. **Table 8–1** describes the lipoproteins that transport lipids in the plasma.

Late in 2013, the American College of Cardiology and the American Heart Association, in conjunction with the National Heart, Lung, and Blood Institute, developed new guidelines. These contained substantial changes from the previous guidelines that were established more than a decade earlier by the Adult Treatment Panel III(ATP III). Previous targets for LDL cholesterol of 100 mg/dL, with the optional goal of less than 70 mg/dL, were removed as indicators of treatment success. Instead, four treatment groups for statin therapy have been identified. They are individuals with clinical atherosclerotic vascular disease; those with LDL cholesterol levels greater than 190 mg/dL; those with diabetes between 40 and 75 years old with LDL cholesterol levels between 70 and 189 mg/dL without evidence of atherosclerotic vascular disease; and individuals without evidence of cardiovascular disease or diabetes who have LDL cholesterol levels between 70 and 180 mg/dL and a 10-year risk of atherosclerotic vascular disease greater than 7.5%. The risk for stroke has been added to the coronary events traditionally covered by cardiovascular risk assessments. Specific recommendations on lifestyle for cardiovascular disease prevention include eating a diet rich in fruits, vegetables, whole grains, fish, low-fat dairy, lean poultry, nuts, legumes, nontropical vegetable oils with restriction of saturated fats, trans fats, sweets, sugar sweetened beverages, and sodium; and engaging in aerobic physical activity of moderate to vigorous intensity lasting 40 minutes per session three to four times per week. With regard to weight loss, the new recommendation is that patients with a BMI of 25, not 30 as in the past, who have even one comorbidity, such as an elevated waist circumference, should begin treatment for weight loss.

LDL Cholesterol

The most common method for determining LDL cholesterol is a calculation that requires the use of a fasting sample with a triglyceride level less than 400 mg/dL. The LDL is calculated according to the Friedewald formula, which is: calculated LDL cholesterol = total cholesterol − HDL cholesterol − (triglycerides/5). The very-low-density lipoprotein (VLDL) fraction is represented by (triglycerides/5) with the assumption that there is very little triglyceride in LDL and HDL. Because the plasma and serum triglyceride concentration increases with ingestion of dietary fat, a fasting sample is required for an accurate calculation of LDL cholesterol using the Friedewald formula. Although it is acceptable to drink water, the patient may not ingest any calories 8 to 12 hours before the blood sample is collected. If the patient does not fast, and the triglyceride is elevated above baseline, the calculated LDL cholesterol will be falsely low. Another challenge to an accurate determination of LDL cholesterol is that there is substantial biological variability, independent of any change in dietary habits, in the total cholesterol level. This would also have a significant impact on the calculated LDL value. For that reason, testing for total cholesterol and LDL cholesterol should be repeated on a second sample drawn 1 to 8 weeks later. The mean value from these two samples is used, as long as the differences between them are less than 30 mg/dL in total cholesterol. If the difference is greater than 30, a third sample should be obtained and the mean of the three samples calculated. The day-to-day variability in total cholesterol within a single individual is typically at least 10% and can be as high as 30%. This level of variability, in a patient whose LDL cholesterol is calculated using the Friedewald formula, could span a range of values from 125 to 165 mg/dL if the patient has a true value of 145 mg/dL. The Friedewald calculation fails if the triglyceride concentration in the fasting sample is higher than 400 mg/dL. At such high concentrations, the (triglyceride concentration/5) is no longer a reasonable estimate of the VLDL cholesterol concentration.

Assays that directly measure LDL are also available. These are not dependent on the Friedewald formula, and are therefore independent of the triglyceride concentration. For that reason, fasting is not required if a direct LDL assay is performed. The direct LDL cholesterol assay circumvents the issues associated with the calculated LDL cholesterol when it is greater than 400 mg/dL. However, even though these assays are routinely used, some studies have shown substantial imprecision with the assay, although this conclusion has been challenged by other studies. Direct LDL cholesterol measurement is not useful in patients with a dyslipidemia.

HDL Cholesterol

Low levels of HDL cholesterol (<40 mg/dL) represent a cardiac risk factor. However, an elevated HDL cholesterol concentration greater than or equal to 60 mg/dL reduces cardiovascular risk. The patient does not need to fast prior to sample collection for performance of the HDL cholesterol.

Total Cholesterol

The total cholesterol concentration is the sum of HDL cholesterol, LDL cholesterol, VLDL cholesterol, intermediate-density lipoprotein cholesterol (IDL cholesterol), and cholesterol associated with Lp(a). In the vast majority of patients, the cholesterol in IDL and in Lp(a) is very small relative to the other lipoproteins. The patient does not need to fast prior to sample collection for performance of the total cholesterol. Like HDL cholesterol, total cholesterol is not affected by recent dietary intake.

Non-high-density Lipoprotein Cholesterol

Non-HDL cholesterol is the difference between the total cholesterol concentration and the HDL cholesterol concentration. The remaining lipoprotein particles—LDL, VLDL, IDL, and Lp(a)— are all atherogenic. In some clinical trials, non-HDL cholesterol was shown to be superior over LDL cholesterol as a measurement of cardiovascular risk. Because neither the total cholesterol nor the HDL cholesterol is affected by the triglyceride level or ingestion of dietary fat, non-HDL cholesterol can be calculated on nonfasting specimens. Use of non-HDL cholesterol measurements instead of calculated LDL cholesterol measurements avoids the problem of calculating LDL cholesterol in patients who have triglyceride concentrations greater than 400 mg/dL.

High-sensitivity C-reactive Protein

The level of persistent inflammatory processes relates to the risk of cardiovascular events. Patients who have an existing inflammatory process typically have CRP levels greater than 3.0 mg/L. Transient elevations in CRP associated with benign processes occur frequently, and for that reason repeat testing within 2 weeks of an elevated value is recommended to determine if the CRP level exceeds 3.0 mg/L. The American Heart Association and the National Cholesterol Education Panel concur that CRP levels should be measured only after traditional lipid parameters have been assessed completely, with the CRP levels used to classify only those patients who are considered to have borderline cardiovascular risk. Values for CRP of less than 1.0 mg/L represent low risk; 1.0 to 3.0 mg/L is intermediate cardiovascular risk; in patients with greater than 3.0 mg/L CRP is considered to be at high cardiovascular risk. The CRP assay was not originally designed for a high-sensitivity analysis, and previously was only used to measure much higher values than the levels used in cardiovascular risk assessment.

Metabolic Syndrome

Metabolic syndrome is present when a series of risk factors for developing heart attack stroke and diabetes are present. In the United States, metabolic syndrome is extremely common, affecting more than 40% of people above the age of 60. Patients with the metabolic syndrome do not have physical symptoms. However, patients who have the metabolic syndrome, over time, commonly develop atherosclerotic vascular disease (myocardial infarction and stroke), kidney dysfunction, and type 2 diabetes with its associated risks and complications. Different expert groups have established the risk factors and their levels that are part of the metabolic syndrome from the American Heart Association and the National Cholesterol Educational Program.

> *Waistline*: For men, greater than 40 in; for women, greater than 35 in
> *Elevated triglycerides*: Equal to or greater than 150 mg/dL
> *Reduced HDL cholesterol*: For men, less than 40 mg/dL; for women, less than 50 mg/dL
> *Elevated blood pressure*: Equal to or greater than 130/85 mm Hg or use of a medication for hypertension
> *Elevated fasting glucose*: Equal to or greater than 100 mg/dL or use of a medication for hyperglycemia

Assessment of Cardiovascular Risk

Patients for whom testing for lipid status and inflammation is most useful include those with factors that increase cardiovascular risk, such as cigarette smoking, hypertension, diabetes mellitus, obesity, physical inactivity, or a family history of coronary heart disease, who are currently asymptomatic and have no history of coronary heart disease. As noted below in the scoring calculations for cardiovascular risk, decisions about patient management involve an assessment for both non-laboratory-test- and laboratory-test-associated risk factors. There are a number of risk calculations based on a combination of data from clinical history, signs and symptoms, and laboratory test results. The following are risk scores and their associated parameters. Collectively, they represent a risk for developing atherosclerotic plaques and to a much lesser extent, with inflammatory markers included, the risk of plaque rupture.

> *The Framingham score*: total cholesterol, HDL cholesterol, age, gender, smoking status, and blood pressure.
> *The Reynolds score*: high-sensitivity C-reactive protein (hs-CRP), total cholesterol, HDL cholesterol, age, gender, parental history, smoking status, and blood pressure. In women with diabetes, the hemoglobin A1C result is also included.
> *The PROCAM score*: LDL cholesterol, HDL cholesterol, triglycerides, family history of coronary artery disease, smoking status, age, and presence of diabetes. This score is validated only in men.
> *Systematic coronary risk evaluation (SCORE)*: total cholesterol, HDL cholesterol, age, gender, smoking status, and blood pressure.

Genetic Disorders Classified by Causation of an Excess or Deficiency of a Specific Class of Lipoprotein

Genetic abnormalities are much less common explanations for high blood lipid levels than excess intake of dietary fat. Described below are selected dyslipidemias and dyslipoproteinemias.

- *LDL-associated abnormalities:*

  High LDL-cholesterol
  Familial hypercholesterolemia: Defects in the LDL receptor gene cause an accumulation of LDL particles in the plasma. Patients have an elevated plasma LDL cholesterol and premature coronary artery disease. Gene with defect: LDLR (LDL receptor).
  Familial defective apolipoprotein B: The defective apolipoprotein B has a reduced affinity for the LDL receptor. Affected individuals usually have an elevated LDL cholesterol,

but there is wide variability in the LDL cholesterol levels. Gene with defect: APOB (apolipoprotein B).

Low LDL-cholesterol

Hypobetalipoproteinemia: Hypobetalipoproteinemia results from a mutation within the apolipoprotein B gene that results in truncation of the mature apolipoprotein B. This condition is not associated with an increased risk of cardiovascular disease. Gene with defect: APOB (apolipoprotein B).

Abetalipoproteinemia: This condition is caused by mutation in a gene coding for a protein required for assembly of apolipoprotein B-containing lipoproteins in the plasma. Affected patients suffer from mental and developmental retardation as children. Gene with defect: MTTP (microsomal triglyceride transfer protein).

- *Triglyceride-rich lipoprotein (VLDL and chylomicrons [CM]-associated) abnormalities:*

High triglyceride

Lipoprotein lipase deficiency: These patients have severe hypertriglyceridemia with associated complications such as pancreatitis, xerostomia, and xerophthalmia. The hypertriglyceridemia results from either a markedly reduced or absent level of lipoprotein lipase activity. Gene with defect: LPL (lipoprotein lipase).

Apolipoprotein C-II deficiency: These patients have familial chylomicronemia due to the absence of the activator of lipoprotein lipase, which is apolipoprotein C-II. Gene with defect: APOC-II (apolipoprotein C-II).

Dysbetalipoproteinemia: This disorder is characterized by an accumulation in the plasma of remnant lipoprotein particles, mostly from CM and VLDL. The excess plasma lipoprotein results in pathognomonic tuberous xanthomas and palmar striated xanthomas. Gene with defect: APOE (apolipoprotein E).

- *HDL-associated abnormalities:*

Low HDL-cholesterol

Apolipoprotein A-1 gene defects: Defects in genes for apolipoprotein A-I, C-III, and A-IV can all decrease the production of HDL particles. Some of these defects are associated with premature cardiovascular disease. However, other mutations appear to confer longevity despite very low HDL levels. Gene with defect: APOA1 (apolipoprotein A1).

Lecithin cholesterol acyltransferase (LCAT) deficiency: A deficiency of LCAT results in reduced conversion of cholesterol to cholesterol esters in the plasma. This results in low HDL cholesterol levels, corneal opacities, and hemolytic anemia. Gene with defect: LCAT (lecithin-cholesterol acyltransferase).

Tangier disease: Individuals with this disorder have reduced cellular cholesterol efflux. The mutation is in the gene that codes for the protein known as ATP-binding cassette A1 (ABCA1), which is a transporter protein. Many different mutations within this gene have been associated with Tangier disease, which is associated with an increased risk for coronary artery disease and extremely low HDL levels. Gene with defect: ABCA1 (ATP binding cassette subfamily A member 1).

High HDL-cholesterol

Cholesterol ester transfer protein (CETP) deficiency: Patients with this deficiency have extremely elevated HDL cholesterol levels, which are primarily cholesterol esters. A deficiency of this enzyme causes accumulation of cholesterol esters within the HDL particles, and, therefore, this deficiency is not associated with premature coronary artery disease. Gene with defect: CETP (cholesterol ester transfer protein).

HYPERTENSION

Description

Hypertension is a very common chronic disease, particularly in Western countries. In the United States, approximately one-half of adults suffer from hypertension. Most of these individuals have no identifiable cause for their hypertension. The 2017 guidelines from the American Heart Association and the American College of Cardiology are as follows. A normal blood pressure is <120 mm Hg systolic, **and** <80 mm Hg diastolic. Elevated blood pressure is between 120 and 129 systolic **and** <80 diastolic. Systolic blood pressures between 130 and 139 **or** diastolic blood pressures between 80 and 89 are considered stage 1 hypertension. Stage 2 is a systolic blood pressure >139 **or** a diastolic blood pressure >89. A hypertensive crisis with a systolic pressure above 180 **or** a diastolic pressure above 120 can damage blood vessels. Causes of a hypertensive crisis include not taking blood pressure medications, stroke, and acute myocardial infarction. The crisis can be life-threatening.

In evaluating a patient with hypertension, one question is whether there is an identifiable cause for the hypertension or whether it is idiopathic or "essential." Another important question is whether the hypertension has resulted in damage to the organs commonly injured in hypertensive individuals, namely, the brain, the heart, and the kidneys.

Hypertension with a potentially correctable cause is suggested by certain symptoms, such as flushing and sweating (which are associated with pheochromocytoma), findings on physical examination such as a renal bruit (which is associated with renal artery stenosis), and laboratory abnormalities such as hypokalemia, which can be found in patients with hyperaldosteronism. Among children, up to 85% with hypertension have a secondary cause and, therefore, require a careful evaluation of the patient for correctable cause. In children up to the age of 18 years, coarctation of the aorta and renal parenchymal disease are common etiologies for hypertension. Among adults, 5% to 10% for patients with hypertension have a secondary cause. Young adults with secondary hypertension are often explained by abnormalities in thyroid function and fibromuscular dysplasia. In middle-age adults, the most common secondary cause of hypertension is hyperaldosteronism. In older adults, atherosclerotic renal artery stenosis, renal failure, and hypothyroidism predominate as secondary causes. Obesity is a contributing factor to increased blood pressure at all ages. The increased blood volume increases arterial pressure. Other lifestyle factors which can increase blood pressure include using tobacco, too much salt in the diet, too little potassium in the diet, and excess ethanol intake (>2 drinks/day for men and 1 drink/day for women). There are many drugs causative for an elevation in blood pressure in some patients. Notable ones include oral contraceptives, selected nonsteroidal anti-inflammatory drugs such as ibuprofen, a variety of drugs used to treat psychiatric disorders such as tricyclic antidepressants, steroids such as methylprednisolone, and many herbal medicines and illicit drugs.

To understand the causes of hypertension, it is necessary to understand the mechanism by which blood pressure is regulated (see Chapter 22 for a related discussion on adrenal gland hormones). In response to decreased arterial pressure from a variety of causes, there is decreased blood flow to the kidney, causing the kidney to secrete renin. Renin released within the renal circulation converts angiotensinogen to angiotensin I, which is subsequently converted to angiotensin II. This molecule acts on the adrenal cortex to release aldosterone. Aldosterone increases sodium retention by the kidney, and thereby expands the extracellular fluid volume and returns the blood pressure to normal. Any alteration in this pathway, such as an increase in aldosterone or a decrease in blood flow to the kidney, will activate the renin–angiotensin system, lead to inappropriate fluid accumulation, and increase the blood pressure. This is why many of the diseases producing hypertension listed in **Table 8–2** are associated with kidney dysfunction. The renal disorders that are associated with hypertension can be renovascular, in which case the blood flow to the kidney is decreased, or they can be parenchymal. Parenchymal diseases include chronic kidney infections, glomerulonephritis, and polycystic kidney disease, among many others. Most of these conditions are treatable, and treatment of the underlying disorder may reduce the hypertension. Abnormalities in the adrenal gland, such as a pheochromocytoma or an aldosterone-secreting tumor (discussed in Chapter 22), also can lead to hypertension, and may be surgically correctable.

Diagnosis

The hypertensive patient undergoing evaluation is first studied using a number of routine tests including:

- Complete blood count to determine if the patient is anemic or polycythemic.
- Electrolyte measurements to measure the potassium and bicarbonate levels.
- Creatinine concentration in plasma or serum and creatinine clearance to assess renal function.

- Glucose (usually a fasting level) to diagnose diabetes, because diabetic patients have an approximately twofold higher incidence of hypertension than nondiabetic patients.
- Urinalysis to detect the presence of diabetes by glucose in the urine; urinalysis also may indicate the presence of significant parenchymal disease in the kidney if proteinuria, hematuria, or pyuria is present.

The tests to further investigate the cause of hypertension beyond the screening tests are more invasive, costly, or esoteric. These are noted in **Table 8–2**.

VASCULITIS

Description

The systemic vasculitides are disorders in which there is inflammation of the blood vessels and tissue necrosis. The different forms of vasculitis are classified by the size of the vessels affected. The classification of the different forms of vasculitis remains controversial and suboptimal, largely because of the low prevalence of these diseases, which are anatomically, epidemiologically, and clinically distinct. Vasculitis is known as primary vasculitis when there is no identifiable underlying etiology. Secondary vasculitis represents vasculitides in which there is an underlying

TABLE 8–2 **Evaluation of the Patient for Hypertension to Determine if Hypertension Is Essential or Correctable**

Disorder	Test Results Supporting the Diagnosis Results
Drug-induced hypertension	Positive history for ingestion of sympathomimetics, corticosteroids, mineralocorticoids, vasopressin, or cocaine, among other drugs, which have a hypertensive effect
Renal and vascular causes of hypertension	
Renal artery stenosis	Angiography and imaging studies consistent with stenosis; increase in serum creatinine after starting angiotensin-converting enzyme inhibitor or angiotensin receptor blocker; renal bruit
Chronic renal disease of multiple etiologies	Elevated BUN and creatinine
Polycystic kidney disease	Radiologic studies that confirm cystic disease of the kidney
Renin-secreting tumors (renal or extrarenal)	Elevated plasma renin activity, normal renal angiogram, low serum potassium, and elevated urinary aldosterone secretion
Coarctation of the aorta (decreased blood flow to kidney resulting from a defect in the aorta)	Imaging studies; arm to leg blood pressure difference >20 mm Hg
Adrenal causes of hypertension	
Primary hyperaldosteronism	Low or borderline serum potassium and elevated urinary aldosterone secretion
17-Alpha hydroxylase deficiency	Reduction in activity of 17-alpha hydroxylase (see Chapter 22); similar to primary hyperaldosteronism but with virilization and precocious puberty in males
11-Beta hydroxylase deficiency	Reduction in activity of 11-beta hydroxylase (see Chapter 22); similar to primary hyperaldosteronism but with virilization and precocious puberty in males
Cushing syndrome	Test results consistent with one of the different forms of Cushing syndrome (see Chapter 22 for diagnostic tests)
Pheochromocytoma	Test results that demonstrate an excess of catecholamines (see Chapter 22 for diagnostic tests)
Thyroid disorders	Abnormal thyroid-stimulating hormone (TSH) test as a screening assay for thyroid function

BUN, blood urea nitrogen.

condition. The underlying condition may be an infection such as HIV, or hepatitis B or hepatitis C, or an underlying connective tissue disease such as lupus or rheumatoid arthritis. The basis for identifying a specific form of vasculitis is histopathologic examination of the blood vessel, but this is often not feasible because of the blood vessels involved and the danger of obtaining tissue from them. It is for this reason that the classification must rely on criteria other than histopathology.

The large number of different vasculitides, which are sometimes overlapping in their clinical or anatomic characteristics, often makes the diagnosis of a specific form of vasculitis challenging. In general, a diagnosis is made by (1) the presence of characteristic clinical findings for the particular form of vasculitis and (2) inflammation within a specific size of blood vessels, as shown in **Table 8–3**. There are vasculitides that are infectious in origin that are not included in **Table 8–3**. Rocky Mountain spotted fever, syphilis, aspergillosis, herpes, and neisserial infections can all be associated with vasculitis. (See Chapter 5 for information on organisms and infections that can cause vasculitis.)

> Inflammation in the blood vessel wall is known as vasculitis. The large number of different vasculitides, which are sometimes overlapping in their clinical or anatomic characteristics, often makes the diagnosis of a specific form of vasculitis challenging.

Diagnosis

The laboratory testing is different for each of the vasculitides listed in **Table 8–3**. ANCA are autoantibodies, typically IgG, directed against antigens in neutrophils (most commonly) and monocytes. Because they are detected in patients with some forms of systemic vasculitis, known as the ANCA-associated vasculitides, they have been used diagnostically to identify patients with these particular forms of systemic vasculitis. These include granulomatous polyangiitis, formerly Wegener's granulomatosis, microscopic polyangiitis, and eosinophilic granulomatous

TABLE 8–3   Laboratory Evaluation for Selected Noninfectious Causes of Vasculitis

Vasculitic Disorder	Vessels with Inflammation	Clinical Laboratory Testing
Large vessel vasculitis: Giant cell arteritis	Aorta and large- to medium-sized arteries	Elevated erythrocyte sedimentation rate (ESR) or C-reactive protein (CRP) in most patients
Large vessel vasculitis: Takayasu arteritis	Aorta and large- to medium-sized arteries	Elevated ESR or CRP in most patients; BUN, creatinine, and urinalysis to assess and monitor renal disease
Medium vessel vasculitis: Polyarteritis nodosa	Medium-sized arteries; small arteries without pulmonary or glomerular involvement	Small aneurysms strung like beads of a rosary making the "rosary sign"; no specific lab tests
Medium vessel vasculitis: Kawasaki disease	Large- to medium-sized arteries; small arteries	Laboratory testing is not informative with self-limited form of the disease; if cardiac complications occur, tests for damage to cardiac muscle may be useful (see Chapter 9)
Small vessel vasculitis, ANCA-associated: Granulomatous polyangiitis, formerly Wegener's granulomatosis	Small arteries, arterioles, capillaries, venules, veins	Antiproteinase 3 (anti-PR3) ANCA (c-ANCA) detectable in the large majority of patients with active disease; a much smaller percentage have antimyeloperoxidase (anti-MPO) ANCA (p-ANCA)
Small vessel vasculitis, ANCA-associated: Eosinophilic granulomatous polyangiitis, formerly Churg–Strauss syndrome	Small arteries, arterioles, capillaries, venules, veins	Antimyeloperoxidase p-ANCA detectable in most patients; eosinophilia
Small vessel vasculitis, ANCA-associated: Microscopic polyangiitis	Small arteries, arterioles, capillaries, venules	Antimyeloperoxidase p-ANCA (more common) or antiproteinase 3 c-ANCA (less common) detectable in most cases; BUN, creatinine, and urinalysis to assess and monitor renal abnormalities
Small vessel vasculitis, immune complex associated: IgA vasculitis, also known as Henoch–Schönlein purpura	Arterioles, capillaries, venules; immune complex-mediated vasculitis, involving IgA	BUN, creatinine, and urinalysis to assess and monitor renal abnormalities; palpable purpura from small hemorrhages
Small vessel vasculitis, immune complex associated: Cryoglobulinemic vasculitis	Arterioles, capillaries, venules; immune complex-mediated vasculitis caused by cryoglobulins	Serum cryoglobulin with identification of type and quantitation, if present (see discussion on cryoglobulinemia in Chapter 3)
Single organ vasculitis: Cutaneous leukocytoclastic angiitis	Capillaries, venules, arterioles	May have underlying autoimmune, neoplastic, or infectious process or an accompanying vasculitis of a different type; laboratory testing is directed at detection of underlying diseases

ANCA, antineutrophil cytoplasmic antibody; BUN, blood urea nitrogen.

polyangiitis, formerly Churg–Strauss syndrome, as shown in **Table 8–3**. Immunofluorescence on ethanol-fixed neutrophils helps to differentiate the different ANCA patterns. Although there are subtypes, the principal forms of staining are p-ANCA (which is perinuclear staining), c-ANCA (which is cytoplasmic staining), and atypical ANCA. The most common target of p-ANCA antibodies is myeloperoxidase, a neutrophil granule protein involved in the generation of oxygen radicals. Less commonly these antibodies will recognize lactoferrin, elastase, and cathepsin G. The c-ANCA antigen is specifically proteinase 3 (PR3). There is a strong association between systemic vasculitides and HLA-DQB1 and HLA-DQA2.

Some of the vasculitides will affect the kidney, and for those, monitoring of renal function is important. The diagnosis of a particular form of vasculitis can be supported by a variety of other test results.

DEEP VEIN THROMBOSIS AND PULMONARY EMBOLISM

Description

DVT and PE are common disorders. The major concern for patients with DVT is the risk of embolism to the lungs (PE). The presence of a thrombosis in a deep vein in the leg is a risk factor for PE, but a thrombosis in a superficial vein in the leg is not. Clots in the superficial veins cannot embolize to the lungs. A DVT in the leg that is above the knee presents a significantly greater risk for PE than does a thrombosis in a deep vein that is below the knee. If the DVT has extended above the knee, patients are more likely to experience soft tissue swelling and discomfort, distention of the vein (a palpable "cord" on physical examination), Homans sign (pain on dorsiflexion of foot), erythema, and warmth. Upper extremity (usually arm) DVTs are much less common than lower extremity (leg) DVTs. A lower extremity DVT, especially if it is small, is often asymptomatic. Thrombosis in the pulmonary circulation can occur independently of DVT, but thrombosis in the pulmonary vasculature commonly results from thrombi originally developed in the deep veins of the leg.

> The major concern for patients with DVT is the risk of embolism to the lungs. A lower extremity DVT, especially if it is small, is often asymptomatic.

Both DVT and PE are commonly associated with one or more congenital or acquired risk factors for thrombosis. The acquired factors include trauma, immobilization, the postoperative state, antiphospholipid antibodies, malignancy, myeloproliferative disorder, pregnancy, and the postpartum state, among many others. The most commonly encountered congenital risk factors, described in detail in the section "Hypercoagulable States" in Chapter 11, include the factor V Leiden mutation that produces activated protein C resistance, the prothrombin G20210A mutation, and deficiencies of protein C, protein S, and antithrombin.

Diagnosis

As a thrombus is degraded, degradation products of cross-linked fibrin are generated. One of these degradation products is the D-dimer. The D-dimer levels are typically elevated in patients with DVT and PE. However, the D-dimer level can be elevated in many other clinical conditions associated with fibrin formation and degradation. These include malignancy, trauma, disseminated intravascular coagulation, and the postoperative states. Because of this, the diagnostic strength of the D-dimer test is its effectiveness in ruling out DVT and PE, when the result is negative. The assays for D-dimer measurement involve the use of monoclonal antibodies that specifically recognize the D-dimer. There are many different clinical assays with different sensitivities and specificities, but despite the variability in available assays for D-dimer, there are now many that can be used effectively in ruling out thrombosis in patients who do not have a high clinical probability of DVT and PE.

Clinical decision rules have been useful in standardizing the evaluation of patients with suspected DVT or PE, before the determination of the D-dimer. One commonly used clinical decision rule is the Wells score for DVT. Information from the medical history and physical examination are obtained, and points are assigned based on the presence of these individual parameters. For PE, two extensively validated clinical decision scores are the Wells score and the revised Geneva score. These two decision scores vary in the items that are included in the evaluation and the number of points assigned when the individual parameters are present.

TABLE 8–4   Tests for the Diagnosis of Deep Vein Thrombosis (DVT) and Pulmonary Embolism (PE)

Tests for DVT or PE	Description	Advantages	Disadvantages	Comments
Compression ultrasonography (for DVT)	Vein is visualized by ultrasound; then external compression is applied to the skin surface above the vein; normal veins collapse and thrombosed veins are not compressible	Useful for symptomatic proximal lower extremity DVT; noninvasive; highly specific	Less sensitive for asymptomatic DVT and distal lower extremity DVT	Most commonly used imaging procedure for initial evaluation of the patient suspected of having a DVT
Computed tomography (CT) scan for PE	X-rays are used to generate 3-dimensional images of the body	Convenient for diagnosing pulmonary embolism	Intravenous contrast material required	
Computed tomography (CT) scan for DVT	Filling defect is shown on delayed contrast-enhanced scan	Correlates well with ultrasonography and good diagnostic accuracy	Radiation dose, cost, and scanning time	For patient with leg swelling and negative or uncertain ultrasound results
D-dimer measurement (for ruling out DVT and PE)	D-dimer is a specific degradation product of cross-linked fibrin that is produced by physiologic fibrinolysis of thrombi	Simple blood test in a patient with a low risk for DVT or PE; using a sensitive method, a negative D-dimer test has a high negative predictive value in excluding DVT and PE	A positive result has to be confirmed by a more specific imaging test	Insensitive methods including manual latex agglutination must not be used to rule out DVT or PE

Imaging studies provide definitive diagnostic information in the evaluation of patients for DVT and for PE. In patients suspected of acute DVT, with a clinical decision rule score that makes DVT unlikely, the D-dimer test is performed first. If the test is negative in a patient with low likelihood for DVT, DVT is ruled out, but if the test is positive, a compression ultrasonography study is performed. A positive compression ultrasonography test confirms the DVT, and a negative test rules out DVT. In patients who have an evaluation with clinical decision rules that makes a DVT likely, the compression ultrasound is performed before the D-dimer. A positive compression ultrasound confirms the DVT, but a negative compression ultrasound prompts the performance of the D-dimer. A negative D-dimer test rules out the DVT, but a positive D-dimer test prompts a repeat compression ultrasound in 1 week. Computed tomography (CT) scanning for DVT can be used to evaluate the patient with leg swelling and equivocal compression ultrasonography.

Patients suspected of acute PE but with an unlikely diagnosis by clinical decision rules are evaluated first with a D-dimer test, just like for DVT. A negative D-dimer rules out the PE, but a positive result leads to the performance of a CT pulmonary scan. This imaging study involves injection of intravenous contrast material. The presence of intraluminal filling defects in the pulmonary arteries confirms a diagnosis of PE. In patients suspected of acute PE whose clinical decision rule analysis suggests PE, the imaging study is performed without the D-dimer test, and the result of the imaging study determines whether the PE is present or absent.

There are a variety of other imaging studies that can be performed to evaluate patients for DVT or PE, but these are much less commonly used. PE is also discussed in Chapter 14.

Table 8–4 presents the imaging studies and the D-dimer tests and their use in the diagnosis of DVT and PE.

STROKE

Description

A stroke occurs when the brain is deprived of oxygen, causing neurons to die. According to the National Stroke Association in 2016, 10% of people who suffer a stroke recover almost completely and 25% recover with minor impairments. However, 40% of those who experience a stroke experience moderate to severe impairments that would require special care. Depending upon the area of the brain that is affected by the stroke, specific functions are lost. For example, a stroke in one part of the brain might cause motor and sensory defects on the left side of the body, while another stroke in a different location of the brain results in facial droop and word finding difficulty. The failure to deliver oxygen and nutrients to neurons within the brain may be a result of an ischemic event (80%–85%) or a hemorrhagic event (15%–20%). In the former, there is a blockage of the blood vessel, and in the latter, the blood vessel ruptures and can no longer carry blood to tissues beyond the site of the rupture.

The principal cause of an ischemic stroke is atherosclerotic vascular disease. The most commonly affected vessels in patients with stroke are the large arteries in the neck and the large and small arteries within the brain. The accumulation of atherosclerotic plaques in these areas diminishes blood flow, and just as in the coronary arteries, when a plaque ruptures, the blood vessel is occluded by platelets intermixed with fibrin. Patients suffering an ischemic stroke who present for treatment within 4 to 6 hours after vessel occlusion can be treated with fibrinolytic agents such as intravenous tissue plasminogen activator to attempt to dissolve the clot and reestablish blood flow. In some cases, the major cause for thrombosis in these blood vessels is not related to an atherosclerotic plaque. One example is a prothrombotic condition known as the antiphospholipid syndrome. In this case, the blood is hypercoagulable, and patients can develop thrombi in blood vessels in the brain leading to stroke without a coexisting atherosclerotic plaque.

Ischemic strokes may be a result of a thrombosis formed at the site of the occlusion or occur as a result of an embolism. With an embolism, the occluding material is delivered to the site of the occlusion from another vascular location. A major cause for thrombosis in the blood vessels of the brain is caused by a thromboembolism from a venous site, such as the deep veins in the leg. Because 20% to 25% of individuals have a patent foramen ovale, and some percentage of these individuals can allow passage of small thrombi from the right side of the heart to the left side of the heart bypassing the lungs, venous thrombi can travel from a distant site where they are formed, and enter the brain to produce an occlusion that results in a stroke.

When there is a temporary disruption of the blood supply to the brain, from any of these causes, the result is called a transient ischemic attack or TIA. This is a warning of high risk for a stroke with permanent deficits. The causes for transient ischemic attack are the same as those for stroke. A history of multiple strokes can lead to vascular dementia. This form of dementia is similar to that found in Alzheimer's disease with defects in thinking, speaking, reasoning, and memory. Even mild cognitive impairment may be a result of occlusion of blood vessels in the brain.

Hypertension is another major cause for stroke. The increase in the pressure of blood flowing through the arteries produces damage and narrowing, and this contributes to the development of atherosclerosis in the arteries. In these patients, hypertension produces an ischemic stroke. When hypertension leads to rupture of a blood vessel supplying the brain with oxygen, the result is a hemorrhagic stroke. A hypertensive crisis is a severe increase in blood pressure, and it can also lead to stroke by causing leakage of blood out of the blood vessel. Patients are at very high risk when the systolic pressure is above 180 or the diastolic pressure is above 120.

Common causes of a hemorrhagic stroke include hypertension, ruptured brain aneurysm, and arteriovenous malformation. Approximately half of those who suffer a hemorrhagic stroke die within a matter of days. Early treatment is essential to reduce permanent damage to the brain if the patient does survive.

Diagnosis

The diagnosis of stroke is made when the patient appears with characteristic motor and/or sensory defects, along with cognitive difficulties. Unlike the troponin test useful as a diagnostic marker for acute myocardial infarction, there is no comparable test for stroke. Imaging studies to determine if the stroke is ischemic or hemorrhagic are highly important immediately upon presentation because the treatments of these two forms of stroke are essentially the opposite. For an ischemic presentation, the goal is to reduce the ability to form clots. For a hemorrhagic stroke, the goal is to promote the ability to form clots.

Laboratory tests for stroke have utility in determining the underlying cause that led to the stroke. For example, the patient who has a patent foramen ovale and an apparent embolus from a lower extremity as a cause for the stroke, merits testing for hypercoagulability in the veins. This would include tests for the factor V Leiden mutation, the prothrombin 20210 mutation, and the activities of protein C, protein S, and antithrombin, as well as antibodies to anticardiolipin and anti-beta-2 glycoprotein 1.

TABLE 8–5   The Role of the Clinical Laboratory for Patients with Stroke

To identify the underlying cause for stroke	Examples include tests that demonstrate high risk for atherosclerotic vascular disease and tests for hypercoagulability
To monitor effectiveness of antiplatelet therapy	Examples include tests to specifically assess the antiplatelet impact of clopidogrel and aspirin; and other platelet aggregation based tests to assess the effectiveness of any antiplatelet drug used for treatment of the stroke

Another important role for the clinical laboratory in the stroke patient is the monitoring of the antiplatelet drugs used to treat an ischemic stroke. Both clopidogrel and aspirin are used in the treatment of ischemic stroke, and these antiplatelet medications can be demonstrated as effective inhibitors of platelet function by laboratory tests. These monitoring tests for drugs used to treat ischemic stroke were developed because a segment of the population is unresponsive to clopidogrel, and patients receiving 81 mg of aspirin may not absorb enough of the aspirin to produce an antiplatelet effect. It is possible to create an antiplatelet effect with other drugs, such as prasugrel and ticagrelor, which can be used in place of clopidogrel, using several different tests for platelet function which are based upon platelet clumping in response to stimuli (**Table 8–5**).

SELF-ASSESSMENT QUESTIONS

1. One of the four major plasma lipoproteins has a lipid core in which the cholesterol esters are in higher concentrations than the triglycerides, and the shell contains only apolipoprotein B-100. Which one of the following lipoproteins has this composition?

    A. Chylomicrons
    B. Very-low-density-lipoprotein (VLDL)
    C. Low-density lipoprotein (LDL)
    D. High-density lipoprotein (HDL)

2. Which one of the following statements is true?

    A. A high concentration of HDL is desirable.
    B. A high concentration of LDL is desirable.
    C. A high concentration of C-reactive protein is desirable.
    D. A high concentration of total cholesterol is desirable.

3. All but one of the disorders or conditions below is associated with a correctable form of hypertension. Identify the choice that is not a correctable form of hypertension.

    A. Renal artery stenosis
    B. Pheochromocytoma
    C. Positive history for ingestion of corticosteroids
    D. Adenocarcinoma of the lung

4. All but one of the following tests is likely to be especially informative in the initial evaluation of the patient with hypertension. Which of the choices below represents the least informative test for evaluation of hypertension?

    A. Electrolyte measurements
    B. Creatinine concentration and plasma
    C. Urinalysis
    D. D-dimer

5. In the evaluation of the patient for a noninfectious causes of vasculitis, which of the following tests is least likely to be informative?

    A. Antibodies directed against antigens in neutrophils (ANCA)
    B. Determination of the specific size of blood vessel in which inflammation is present
    C. Prostate-specific antigen (PSA)
    D. C-reactive protein

6. Which of the following statements below regarding D-dimer testing to rule out pulmonary embolism is correct?

    A. A high sensitivity test is required so that the predictive value of a negative test approximates 100%.
    B. A high sensitivity test is required so that the predictive value of a positive test approximates 100%.
    C. A high specificity test is required so that the predictive value of a negative test approximates 100%.
    D. A high specificity test is required so that the predictive value of a positive test approximates 100%.

FURTHER READING

Al-Ansary LA, et al. A systematic review of recent clinical practice guidelines on the diagnosis, assessment, and management of hypertension. *PLoS One*. 2013;8:e53744.

Carey RM, et al. Prevention, detection, evaluation, and management of high blood pressure in adults: synopsis of the 2017 American College of Cardiology/American Heart Association hypertension guideline. *Ann Int Med*. 2018;168:351–358.

Dron JS, Hegele RA. Genetics of lipid and lipoprotein disorders. *Curr Genet Med Rep*. 2016;4:130–141.

Eckel RH, et al. 2013 ACC/AHA guideline on lifestyle management to reduce cardiovascular risk: a report of the American College of Cardiology/American Heart Association. *Circulation*. 2014;129(25 suppl 2):S76–S79.

Goff DC, et al. 2013 ACC/AHA guideline on the assessment of cardiovascular risk: a report of the American College of Cardiology/American Heart Association. *Circulation*. 2014;129(25 suppl 2):S49–S73.

Grau RG. Drug–induced vasculitis: new insights and a changing lineup of suspects. *Curr Rheum Rep*. 2015:17:71.

Grundy SM, et al; Coordinating Committee of the National Cholesterol Education Program. Implications of recent clinical trials for the National Cholesterol Education Program Adult Treatment Panel III guidelines. *Circulation*. 2004;110:227–239.

Grundy SM, et al., for the conference participants. Definition of metabolic syndrome: report of the National Heart, Lung, and Blood Institute/American Heart Association conference on scientific issues related to definition. *Circulation*. 2004;109:433–438.

Huisman MV, Klok FA. Diagnostic management of acute deep vein thrombosis and pulmonary embolism. *J Thromb Haemost*. 2013;11:412–422.

Jensen MD, et al. 2013 AHA/ACC/TOS guideline for the management of overweight and obesity in adults: a report of the American College of Cardiology/American Heart Association task force on practice guidelines and the Obesity Society. *Circulation*. 2014;129(25 suppl 2) S102–S138.

Laposata M. Fatty acids: biochemistry to clinical significance. *Am J Clin Path*. 1995;104:172–179.

Ortiz-Fernandez L, et al. Cross-phenotype analysis of immunochip data identifies KDM4C as a relevant locus for the development of systemic vasculitis. *Ann Rheum Dis*. 2018;77:589–595.

Reboussin DM, et al. Systematic review for the 2017 ACC/AHA/AAPA/ABC/ACPM/APhA/ASH/ASPC/NMA/PCNA guideline for the prevention, detection, evaluation, and management of high blood pressure in adults: a report of the American College of Cardiology/American Heart Association task force on clinical practice guidelines. *J Am Coll Cardiol*. Nov 7, 2017. pii: S0735-1097(17)41517-8.

Righini M, et al. D-dimer for venous thromboembolism diagnosis: 20 years later. *J Thromb Haemost*. 2008;6:1059–1071.

Rosafio F, et al. Platelet function testing in patients with acute ischemic stroke: an observational study. *J Stroke Cerebrovasc Dis*. 2017;26:1864–1873.

Stone NJ, et al. 2013 ACC/AHA guidelines on the treatment of blood cholesterol to reduce atherosclerotic cardiovascular risk in adults: a report of the American College of Cardiology/American Heart Association. *Circulation*. 2014;129(25 suppl 2):S1–S45.

Thomas SM, et al. Diagnostic value of CT for deep vein thrombosis: results of a systemic review and meta-analysis. *Clin Radiol*. 2008;63:299–304.

Whelton PK, et al. 2017 ACC/AHA/AAPA/ABC/ACPM/APhA/ASH/ASPC/NMA/PCNA guideline for the prevention, detection, evaluation, and management of high blood pressure in adults: executive summary: a report of the American College of Cardiology/American Heart Association task force on clinical practice guidelines. *J Am Coll Cardiol*. Nov 7, 2017. pii: S0735-1097(17)41519-1.

The Heart

Fred S. Apple

INTRODUCTION

There are many forms of cardiac disease. This chapter briefly covers the role of biomarkers in acute myocardial infarction (AMI) and congestive heart failure (CHF). The large numbers of other cardiac diseases are not discussed in this chapter because of the relatively minor role of diagnostic clinical laboratory tests in these disorders.

ACUTE MYOCARDIAL INFARCTION

Description

The term AMI is defined as an imbalance between myocardial oxygen supply (ischemia) and demand, resulting in injury to and the eventual death of myocytes. AMI should be used when there is evidence of myocardial necrosis in a clinical setting consistent with acute myocardial ischemia. Such necrosis is most often associated with a thrombotic occlusion superimposed on coronary atherosclerosis. It is now apparent that the process of plaque rupture and thrombosis is one of the ways in which coronary atherosclerosis progresses. Total loss of coronary blood flow results in a clinical syndrome associated with an ST-segment elevation MI (STEMI). Partial loss of coronary perfusion, if severe, can lead to necrosis as well, which is generally less severe and is known as non-ST-segment elevation MI (NSTEMI). Both STEMI and NSTEMI are considered type 1 MIs. In instances of myocardial injury with necrosis from a condition other than coronary artery disease (CAD), (e.g., coronary endothelial dysfunction, respiratory failure, hypotension, etc.), this MI is a type 2 MI that is secondary to ischemic imbalance. Other ischemic events of lesser severity without myocardial necrosis are designated as angina, which can range from stable to unstable.

Approximately 90 million (1 in 3) individuals in the United States have some form of heart disease. Seven million have had an MI and roughly 8.7 million have ischemic angina. Cardiovascular disease is responsible for more deaths and more hospitalizations in the United States than any other disease, over 5 million admissions yearly. Coronary heart disease (CHD) causes over one in seven deaths. Deaths that occur acutely result from ventricular arrhythmias or pump dysfunction and CHF with or without cardiogenic shock. The yearly financial burden of cardiovascular disease is in excess of $300 billion for CHD and stroke.

In many patients with AMI, no precipitating factor can be identified. The clinical history remains of substantial value in establishing a diagnosis. A prodromal history of angina can be elicited in 40% to 50% of patients with AMI. Of the patients with AMI presenting with prodromal symptoms, approximately one-third have had symptoms from 1 to 4 weeks before hospitalization; in the remaining two-thirds, symptoms predate admission by a week or less, with one-third having had symptoms for 24 hours or less. The pain of AMI is variable in intensity, and the discomfort is described as a squeezing, choking, vise-like, or heavy pain. It may also be characterized as a stabbing, knife-like, boring, or burning discomfort. Often the pain radiates down the left arm. In some instances, the pain of AMI may begin in the epigastrium and simulates a variety of abdominal disorders, which often causes AMI to be misdiagnosed as indigestion. In other patients, the discomfort of AMI radiates to the shoulders, upper extremities, neck, and jaw, again usually favoring the left side.

Diagnosis

The ideal biomarker of myocardial injury should (1) provide an early rule out of myocardial injury and AMI with an excellent clinical sensitivity and negative predictive value >99%, (2) provide early detection of myocardial injury and rule in for the diagnosis for an AMI, (3) serve as a risk stratification tool in patients presenting with ACS, (4) detect reocclusion and reinfarction, and (5) detect procedural-related perioperative MI during cardiac or noncardiac surgery. Ruling *out* AMI requires a test with high diagnostic sensitivity and negative predictive value (preferred by the ER physician in the urgent care, emergency setting as to not send anyone home with an AMI), whereas ruling *in* AMI requires a test with high diagnostic specificity and positive predictive value (preferred by the cardiologist following admission to avoid excessive and costly diagnostic evaluations in the non-AMI patient). It is the function of the laboratory to provide advice to physicians about cardiac biomarker/troponin characteristics.

Until 2000, the diagnosis of AMI established by the World Health Organization (WHO) required at least two of the following criteria: (1) a history of chest pain, (2) evolutionary changes on the ECG, and/or (3) elevations of serial cardiac biomarkers (total creatine kinase [CK] and CK-MB). The soon to be published 2018 Global Task Force for the Fourth Universal Definition of Myocardial Injury and Myocardial Infarction (September 2018) codifies the role of cTn testing (**Table 9–1**). The fourth universal definition of Myocardial Injury and Myocardial Infarction globally advocates that the diagnosis of AMI be made from evidence of myocardial injury based on cTnI or cTnT being increased above the 99th percentile upper reference limit (URL), indicating cardiac damage, in the appropriate clinical setting of ischemic symptoms. While the guideline does suggest that increases in troponin elicits a diagnosis of myocardial injury, it does not suggest that all increases of cTn should elicit a diagnosis of AMI, but only those associated with the appropriate clinical, ECG, and imaging findings. When cTn increases that are not caused by acute ischemia occur, the clinician is obligated to search for another etiology for the increase (**Table 9–2**). The initial ECG is diagnostic of AMI in only about 30% of AMI patients. The universal classification of different types of myocardial infarction is highlighted in **Table 9–3**.

Cardiovascular disease is responsible for more deaths and more hospitalizations in the United States than any other disease, over 5 million admissions yearly. Coronary heart disease (CHD) causes over one in seven deaths.

The fourth universal definition of Myocardial Injury and Myocardial Infarction globally advocates that the diagnosis of AMI be made from evidence of myocardial injury based on cTnI or cTnT being increased above the 99th percentile upper reference limit (URL), indicating cardiac damage, in the appropriate clinical setting of ischemic symptoms.

TABLE 9–1   Criteria for Diagnosis of Acute Myocardial Infarction

The term acute myocardial infarction (AMI) should be used when there is evidence of myocardial necrosis in a clinical setting consistent with acute myocardial ischemia. Under these conditions any one of the following criteria meets the diagnosis for MI:

- Detection of a rise and/or fall of cardiac biomarker values (preferably cardiac troponin [cTn]) with at least one value above the 99th percentile upper reference limit (URL) and with at least one of the following:
  - Symptoms of ischemia
  - New or presumed new significant ST-segment T-wave (ST-T) changes or new left bundle branch block (LBBB)
  - Development of pathological Q waves in the ECG
  - Imaging evidence of new loss of viable myocardium or new regional wall motion abnormality
  - Identification of an intracoronary thrombus by angiography or autopsy
- Cardiac death with symptoms suggestive of myocardial ischemia and presumed new ischemic ECG changes or new LBBB, but death occurred before cardiac biomarkers were obtained, or before cardiac biomarker values would be increased
- Percutaneous coronary intervention (PCI)-related MI is arbitrarily defined by elevation of cTn values (>5 × 99th percentile URL) in patients with normal baseline values (≤99th percentile URL) or a rise of cTn values >20% if the baseline values are elevated and are stable or falling. In addition, (i) symptoms suggestive of myocardial ischemia, (ii) new ischemic ECG changes, (iii) angiographic findings consistent with a procedural complication, or (iv) imaging demonstration of new loss of viable myocardium or new regional wall motion abnormality are required
- Stent thrombosis associated with MI when detected by coronary angiography or autopsy in the setting of myocardial ischemia and with a rise and/or fall of cardiac biomarker values with at least one value above the 99th percentile URL
- Coronary artery bypass grafting (CABG)-related MI is arbitrarily defined by elevation of cardiac biomarker values (>10 × 99th percentile URL) in patients with normal baseline cTn values (≤99th percentile URL). In addition, (i) new pathological Q waves or new LBBB, (ii) angiographically documented new graft or new native coronary artery occlusion, or (iii) imaging evidence of new low of viable myocardium or new regional wall motion abnormality are required

TABLE 9–2   Diagnoses with Increased Cardiac Troponin: Elevation of Cardiac Troponin Values Because of Myocardial Injury

Injury related to primary myocardial ischemia
- Plaque rupture
- Intraluminal coronary artery thrombus formation

Injury related to supply/demand imbalance of myocardial ischemia
- Tachyarrhythmias/bradyarrhythmias
- Aortic dissection or severe aortic valve disease
- Hypertrophic cardiomyopathy
- Cardiogenic, hypovolemic, or septic shock
- Severe respiratory failure
- Severe anemia
- Hypertension with or without Left Ventricular Hypertrophy (LVH)
- Coronary spasm
- Coronary embolism or vasculitis
- Coronary endothelial dysfunction without significant CAD

Injury not related to myocardial ischemia
- Cardiac contusion, surgery, ablation, pacing, or defibrillator shocks
- Rhabdomyolysis with cardiac involvement
- Myocarditis
- Cardiotoxic agents, for example, anthracyclines, Herceptin

Multifactorial or indeterminate myocardial injury
- Heart failure
- Stress (takotsubo) cardiomyopathy
- Severe pulmonary embolism or pulmonary hypertension
- Sepsis and critically ill patients
- Renal failure
- Severe acute neurological diseases, for example, stroke, subarachnoid hemorrhage
- Infiltrative diseases, for example, amyloidosis, sarcoidosis
- Strenuous exercise

TABLE 9-3   Universal Classification of Different Types of Myocardial Infarction

Type 1: spontaneous myocardial infarction
Spontaneous myocardial infarction related to atherosclerotic plaque rupture, ulceration, assuring erosion, or dissection with resulting intraluminal thrombus in one or more of the coronary arteries leading to decreased myocardial blood flow or distal platelet emboli with ensuing myocyte necrosis. The patient may have underlying severe CAD but on occasion nonobstructive or no CAD. These are either an ST-segment elevation MI (STEMI) or non-STEMI (NSTEMI)

Type 2: myocardial infarction secondary to an ischemic imbalance
In instances of myocardial injury with necrosis where a condition other than CAD contributes to an imbalance between myocardial oxygen supply and/or demand; for example, coronary endothelial dysfunction, coronary embolism, tachyarrhythmias/bradyarrhythmias, anemia, respiratory failure, hypotension, and hypertension with or without LVH

Type 3: myocardial infarction resulting in death when biomarker values are unavailable
Cardiac death with symptoms suggestive of myocardial ischemia and presumed new ischemic ECG changes or new LBBB, but death occurring before blood samples could be obtained, before cardiac biomarker could rise, or in rare cases when cardiac biomarkers were not collected

Type 4a: myocardial infarction related to percutaneous coronary intervention (PCI)
Myocardial infarction associated with PCI is arbitrarily defined by elevation of cTn values 5 × 99th percentile URL in patients with normal baseline values (<99th percentile URL) or a rise of cTn values >20% if the baseline values are elevated and are stable or falling. In addition, (i) symptoms suggestive of myocardial ischemia, (ii) new ischemic ECG changes or new LBBB, (iii) angiographic loss of patency of a major coronary artery or side branch or persistent slow- or no-flow or embolization, or (iv) imaging demonstration of new loss of viable myocardium or new regional wall motion abnormality are required

Type 4b: myocardial infarction related to stent thrombosis
Myocardial infarction associated with stent thrombosis is detected by coronary angiography or autopsy in the setting of myocardial ischemia and with a rise and/or fall of cardiac biomarkers values with at least one value above the 99th percentile URL

Type 5: myocardial infarction related to coronary artery bypass grafting (CABG)
Myocardial infarction associated with CABG is arbitrarily defined by elevation of cardiac biomarker values >10 × 99th percentile URL in patients with normal baseline cTn values (<99th percentile URL). In addition, (i) new pathological Q waves or new LBBB, or new LBBB, (ii) angiographically documented new graft or new native coronary artery occlusion, or (iii) imaging evidence of new loss of viable myocardium or new regional wall motion abnormality are required

cTn testing is most useful when patients are having nondiagnostic ECG tracings. Patients with AMI can be categorized into several groups based on time of presentation. First, there is the group of patients who present very early to the emergency department (ED), within 0 to 2 hours after the onset of ischemic symptoms that include chest pain, without diagnostic ECG evidence of AMI. For laboratory tests to be clinically useful, biomarkers (cTn is the gold standard) of MI must be released rapidly from the heart into the circulation to provide sensitive and tissue-specific diagnostic information. Further, the analytical assays using serum, plasma, or whole blood specimens must be rapid and sensitive enough to distinguish small changes within the reference interval. The high-sensitivity (hs) cTn assays have improved analytical sensitivity, and substantially improve early diagnostics. The second group of patients includes those presenting 2 to 6 hours after the onset of ischemic symptoms, without evidence of AMI on ECG. In this group of patients, the diagnosis of AMI requires serial monitoring of both cTn and ECG changes, with all cTn assays being useful to detect increased values at 6 hours. The third group of patients presents more than 6 to up to 48 hours after the onset of symptoms of ischemia with nonspecific ECG changes. cTn is also the ideal biomarker to detect myocardial injury in this group because it can persist in the circulation for 2 to 6 days, to provide a late diagnostic time window. The shortfall of cTn or any cardiac biomarker is its inability to distinguish recurrent injury from old injury based on a single result; thus, the importance of following serial results for a rising or falling pattern. The fourth group of patients includes those who present to the ED at any time after the onset of ischemic symptoms with clear ECG evidence of AMI, either a STEMI or Q-wave MI. In this group, detection with cTn is theoretically not necessary, but still cTn orders are obtained for completeness. **Figure 9-1** shows the kinetics of the rise and fall for a hs cTnI assay for type 1 MI, type 2 MI, chronic myocardial injury, and a non-myocardial injury patient, with the high-sensitivity (hs)-assay playing a substantial role in shortening the time for monitoring cTn to 3 hours, compared to 6 hours with contemporary assays.

Cardiac Troponin Biochemistry

Three troponin subunits, troponin T (the tropomyosinbinding component), troponin I (the inhibitory component), and troponin C (the calciumbinding component) form a complex that regulates the interaction of actin and myosin and thus regulates cardiac contraction. Troponins

Three troponin subunits, troponin T (the tropomyosin-binding component), troponin I (the inhibitory component), and troponin C (the calcium-binding component) form a complex that regulates the interaction of actin and myosin and thus regulates cardiac contraction.

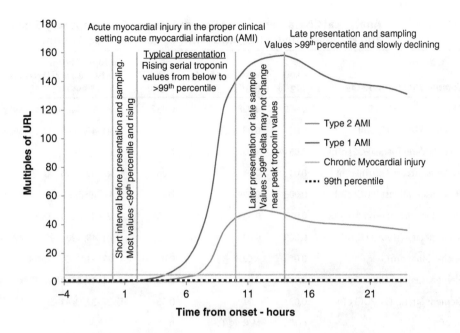

FIGURE 9-1 Representative profile of the rise and fall pattern of cardiac troponin for type 1 MI, type 2 MI, and chronic myocardial injury. (Reproduced with permission from the IFCC Task Force for Clinical Application of Cardiac Bio-Markers (TF-CB); prepared by Paul Collinson.)

are localized primarily in the myofibrils (94% to 97%) with a smaller cytoplasmic fraction (3% to 6%). cTnI and cTnT have different amino acid sequences encoded by different genes and differ from the Tns found in other muscle such as skeletal muscle. Human cTnI has an additional post-translational 31-amino acid residue on the amino terminal end compared with skeletal muscle TnI, giving it cardiac specificity. Only one isoform of cTnI has been identified and is not expressed in normal, regenerating, or diseased human or animal skeletal muscle. cTnT is also encoded by a different gene than the one that encodes skeletal muscle isoforms. An 11–amino acid amino terminal residue gives this biomarker cardiac specificity. However, during human fetal development, in some diseased human skeletal muscle (neuromuscular diseases), and in patients end-stage renal disease, small amounts of cTnT are expressed in skeletal muscle. There is evidence that injury to diseased skeletal muscle results in increases circulating cTnT immunoreactivity measured by the current hs cTnT (the FDA cleared 5th Generation of the cTnT) immunoassay used globally in clinical practice. The other troponin, troponin C, is not useful as a cardiac biomarker as the troponin C expressed in the heart is not specific for the heart. Following myocardial injury, multiple forms are elaborated both in tissue and in blood. The multiple forms of cTn include the T–I–C ternary complex, IC binary complex, and free I and T. Multiple chemical modifications of these forms can occur, involving oxidation, reduction, phosphorylation and dephosphorylation, and both C- and N-terminal degradation. The conclusions from these observations are that cTn immunoassays need to be developed in which the antibodies recognize epitopes in the stable region of cTnI and, ideally, demonstrate an equimolar response to the different cTn forms that circulate in the blood.

Analytical Methods for Measuring Cardiac Troponin

Numerous manufacturers have developed monoclonal antibodybased diagnostic immunoassays for the sensitive measurement of cTnI and cTnT. Most recently, improved analytics have led to the development of hs-cTnI and hs-cTnT assays. Assay times range from 5 to 30 minutes. **Table 9–4** shows analytical characteristics of representative assays (contemporary assays, hs-assays, and near bed-side point of care [POC] assays) approved for patient testing. In clinical practice, two obstacles limit the ease for switching from one cTnI assay to another or between cTnI and cTnT assays. First, there is currently no primary reference cTnI material available for manufacturers to

Numerous manufacturers have developed monoclonal antibody-based diagnostic immunoassays for the sensitive measurement of cTnI and cTnT.

TABLE 9–4   Analytical Characteristics of Representative Contemporary Sensitive, and High-sensitivity (hs), and Point-of-care Cardiac Troponin Assays

Company/Platform/Assay	LoD (µg/L)	99th Percentile (µg/L)	10% CV (µg/L)	Epitopes Recognized by Capture (C) and Detection (D) Antibodies
Abbott ARCHITECT cTnI	0.009	0.028	0.032	C: 87–91, 24–40; D: 41–49
Abbott i-STAT (POC) cTnI	0.02	0.08	0.10	C: 41–49, 88–91; D: 28–39, 62–78
Quidel (Alere) Triage (POC) cTnI	0.05	<0.05	NA	C: NA; D: 27–40
Beckman Access AccuTnI cTnI	0.01	0.04	0.06	C: 41–49; D: 24–40
Mitsubishi Pathfast (POC) cTnI	0.008	0.029	NA	C:41–49; D: 71–116, 163–209
Ortho-Clinical Diagnos Vitros cTnI	0.012	0.034	0.034	C: 24–40, 41–49; D: 87–91
Radiometer AQT90[a] (POC) cTnI	0.009	0.023	0.039	C: 41–49, 190–196; D: 137–149
Roche Cobas cTnT	0.01	<0.01	0.030	C: 125–131; D: 136–147
Siemens Centaur Ultra cTnI	0.006	0.04	0.03	C: 41–49, 87–91; D: 27–40
Siemens Stratus CS (POC) cTnI	0.03	0.07	0.06	C: 27–32; D: 41–56
hs-cTnI	ng/L	M/F, ng/L	ng/L	
Abbott ARCHITECT[a]	1.2	34/16	4.7	C: 24–40; D: 41–49
Beckman Access	2.3	12/20	<7.0	C: 41–49; D: 24–40
ET Healthcare Pylon	1.4	28/19	10	C: 27–40, D: 41–49
Ortho-Clinical Diagnostic Vitros	1.0	26/9	4.3	C: 87–91; D:24–40, 41–49
Singulex Clarity	0.09	9/8	0.88	C: 41–49; D: 27–41
Siemens ADVIA Centaur XPT	1.6	58/39	3.0	C: 30–35; D: 41–56, 171–190
hs-cTnT/Gen 5				
Roche cobas e601	3.0	22/14	11	C: 125–131; D: 136–147

LoD, limit of detection; POC, point of care; M, male; F, female. Note: µg/L in top portion of table and ng/L in bottom portion.

[a]Available outside the United States.

Data from Apple FS, Collinson PO; IFCC Task Force on Clinical Applications of Cardiac Bio-Markers. Analytical characteristics of high sensitivity cardiac troponin assays. *Clin Chem*. 2017:58:54–61.

The 2018 universal definition of Myocardial Infarction is predicated on cTn monitoring, with detection of a rising and/or falling cTn, and with at least one value above the 99th percentile URL.

use for standardizing assays. Second, concentrations fail to agree because of the different epitopes recognized by the multiple, different antibodies used in different assays. Therefore, standardization of cTnI assays remains elusive. For cTnT, there is only one manufacturer. While no standardization problems are expected, different instruments used to measure cTnT have shown variable results. Therefore, laboratories have to educate clinicians to better understand cTn assay-to-assay variability and understand that all assays are not created equal. In 2018, the IFCC Task Force on Clinical Applications of Cardiac Bio-Markers, along with the AACC Academy, readdressed quality specification aspects for cTn assays. These specifications were intended for use by the manufacturers of commercial assays and by clinical laboratories using cTn assays to establish uniform criteria so that all assays could be evaluated objectively for their analytical qualities and clinical performance. Factors addressed included antibody selection, calibration materials, imprecision characteristics at clinical decision values, effects of storage time and temperature, glass versus plastic tubes versus gel separator tubes, the influence of anticoagulants, and whole blood measurements (**Table 9–5**).

99th Percentile of the Upper Limit of the Reference Range (URL) as a Cutoff for Diagnosis of Acute Myocardial Infarction

The soon to be published 2018 Global Task Force for the Fourth Universal Definition of Myocardial Injury and Myocardial Infarction, which was preceded by The Global Task Force's 2012

TABLE 9–5   **Clinical Laboratory Practice Recommendations of the AACC Academy and IFCC Task Force Task on Clinical Applications of Cardiac Bio-Markers for the Use of Cardiac Troponin in Acute Coronary Syndromes**

1. For hs-cTn assays, laboratories should measure at least three different concentrations of QC materials at least once per day.
2. During initiation of hs-cTn testing, clinical laboratories should validate the limit of the blank (LoB), limit of detection (LoD), or limit of quantitation (LoQ) as applicable.
3. Report hs-cTn assays in whole numbers using ng/L without decimal points, reporting QC values to one decimal point.
4. Use a defined reference population to report 99th percentiles according to sex-specific cutoffs for hs-cTn assays.
5. For assays unable to detect cTn at concentrations at or above the LoD in at least 50% of healthy men and women, individually, they should be labeled as contemporary and not hs-cTn assays.
6. For hospitals using two or more cTn assays, differences in the sensitivity of the various cTn assays should be explained to the clinicians to better understand discrepancies when patients are transferred between facilities.
7. Cardiac troponin results should be reported within 60 minutes of a sample being received, with the first sample labeled 0 hour.
8. Determine the degree of serial changes for cTn values to assist in differentiating between patients who have acute cardiac injury, including AMI, from those that have chronic elevations, many of which may be related to structural heart disease.

From Apple FS et al, on behalf of the IFCC Task Force on Clinical Applications of Cardiac Bio-Markers. IFCC educational materials on selected analytical and clinical applications of high-sensitivity cardiac troponin assays. *Clin Biochem*. 2015;48:201–203 and Wu AHB et al. Clinical laboratory practice recommendations for the use of cardiac troponin in acute coronary syndromes: expert opinion from the Academy of the American Association for Clinical Chemistry and the Task Force on Clinical Applications of Cardiac Bio-Markers of the International Federation of Clinical Chemistry and Laboratory Medicine. *Clin Chem*. 2018;64:645–655.

"Third Universal Definition of Myocardial Infarction" guideline, is predicated on cTn monitoring, with detection of a rising and/or falling cTn, and with at least one value above the 99th percentile URL. The 99th percentile is the value below which 99% of the results are found (see **Figure 9–2**). As tests for troponin have improved, they have been able to detect much lower levels of troponin. The high-sensitivity test is able to measure much lower concentrations of troponin than the previous generations of troponin tests, and it has greater reproducibility on repeat measurement. Historically, if a heart attack was large, it was diagnosed by a troponin test result that was both detectable and increasing over 3 to 6 hours. On the other hand, those having smaller heart attacks had lower troponin values. Their diagnosis of acute MI was delayed because the older tests were relatively insensitive and 3 to 6 hours after the onset of ischemia was required for them to become high enough to measure and show serial increases with time. The one noteworthy downside to the improvement in detecting troponin is that the high sensitivity assays are now able to generate a measurable troponin value in healthy people. Many healthy people have very low levels of circulating troponin, sometimes below the limit of detection (LoD). With the new assays, minor troponin elevations can be observed which may reflect acute or chronic myocardial damage. For example, high blood pressure can cause damage to the heart and produce an elevated troponin level. For that patient, hospitalization is not necessary. The interpretation of the results is now much more complex than it has been in the past, so that not all patients with minor elevations in troponin are diagnosed with an acute MI.

Evidence indicates that the more analytically sensitive cTn assays (hs-cTnT assays) result in greater rates of cTn positivity, when compared with both contemporary and POC cTnT assays. This has been shown for hs-cTnT, but not for hs-cTnI assays. Milder and smaller MIs are now detected. Clinical cases prior to 2007 that were earlier classified as unstable angina can now be given a diagnosis of MI because of an increased and rising cTn. Further, procedure-related troponin increases (i.e., following angioplasty) are now given a diagnosis of MI (**Table 9–3**). The importance of small troponin increases has been confirmed by their association with a poor prognosis.

New clinical laboratory practice recommendations for the use of cTn assays in acute coronary syndromes (ACS) (**Table 9–5**) have been proposed in 2018 as an expert opinion from the AACC Academy and the IFCC Task Force-Cardiac Bio-Markers (TF-CB) focusing on (1) quality control (QC) utilization, (2) assay limits validating the lower reportable analytical limits, (3) units to be used in reporting measureable concentrations for patients and QC materials, (4) 99th percentile sex-specific upper reference limits to define normality, (5) criteria required to define

> Evidence indicates that the more analytically sensitive cTn assays (hs-cTnT assays) result in greater rates of cTn positivity, when compared with both contemporary and POC cTnT assays.

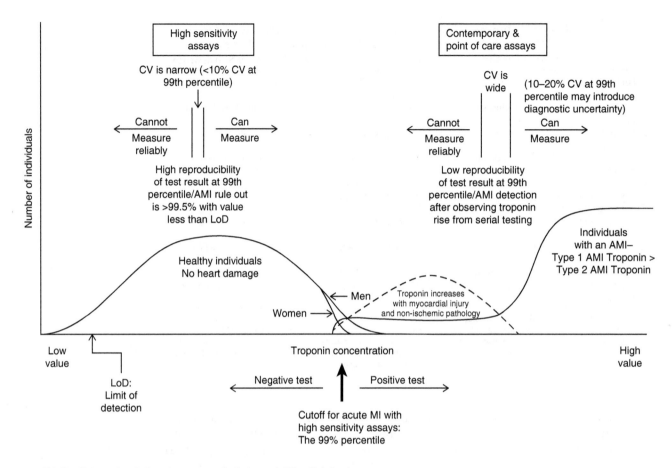

FIGURE 9–2 **Improvement in sensitivity of troponin assays over time and the clinical impact of the change.**

hs-cTn assays, (6) communication with clinicians and the role laboratories play in educating clinicians on the influence of preanalytical and analytical problems that confound assay results, (7) studies on hs-cTn assays and how authors need to document preanalytical and analytical variables, (8) harmonizing and standardizing assay results and the role of commutable materials, (9) time to reporting of results from sample receipt and sample collection, and (10) changes in hs-cTn concentrations over time and the role of both analytical and biological variabilities influencing results of serial blood collections.

Several biomarkers should no longer be used to evaluate cardiac disease. They include aspartate aminotransaminase (AST), total CK activity, CKMB isoforms, myoglobin, total lactate dehydrogenase (LD, same as LDH), and LD isoenzymes. These markers have poor specificity for the detection of cardiac injury because of their wide tissue distribution. Further, CKMB is no longer a recommended biomarker, and is suggested for clinical use only when cTn assays are not available. CKMB offers no additional diagnostic value to aid in the timing of the onset of myocardial injury, infarct sizing, or determination of reinfarction. There is no evidence to support dual testing for cTn and CKMB.

Several biomarkers should no longer be used to evaluate cardiac disease. They include aspartate aminotransaminase (AST), total CK activity, CKMB isoforms, myoglobin, total lactate dehydrogenase (LD, same as LDH), and LD isoenzymes.

Defining Healthy Reference Populations for Determining 99th Percentile URL

Representative 99th percentiles for contemporary, POC, and hs-assays are shown in **Table 9–4**. Defining what constitutes a healthy reference individual is challenging. Should individuals be apparently healthy, young individuals, or should they be age-matched patients hospitalized without known cardiovascular disease, similar to the demographics of patients who rule in for an AMI. How does one determine who is healthy? Should individuals be selected (a) via personal interview with questions addressing known cardiac medications, such as statins; (b) after obtaining information about known diseases associated with cardiovascular disease, such as renal disease or diabetes; or (c) via definitive physician evaluation of an individual after taking a history and physical examination, including an electrocardiogram, echocardiogram, or imaging? There are a number of conclusions about healthy reference individuals that are well accepted. Both younger and older apparently healthy reference groups should be recruited. Inclusion criteria should be based on data obtained from a history of medications (not on cardiac drugs, i.e., statins), known underlying diseases, and blood surrogate biomarker measurements: natriuretic peptide (NP) concentration for ruling out underlying myocardial dysfunction, an estimated glomerular filtration rate (eGFR) for defining underlying renal insufficiency, and HbA1C for undiagnosed diabetes. Men and women should be equally represented, with a diverse racial and ethnic mix. One study that has compared multiple assays ($n=19$) with the same reference group demonstrated substantial differences for both 99th percentiles and ability to measure concentrations above an LoD. Sex-specific 99th percentiles should be used for the hs-assays, as significantly higher concentrations have been shown for men versus women. Use of sex-specific 99th percentiles will have a substantial influence on detecting a great proportion of women at risk for myocardial injury.

Role of Cardiac Troponin in Early Rule Out of MI

In the appropriate low-risk clinical setting, hs-cTn assays now allow for a very early rule out of AMI. Numerous studies have documented that 20% to 50% of patients presenting to EDs can be safely discharged because of a baseline (single) hs-cTn concentration < LoD of an assay, with >99.5% negative predictive value and clinical sensitivity. The probability of acute MI or cardiac death in this group at 30 days is <0.5%.

Role of Cardiac Troponin for Risk Outcomes Assessment

Patients *with* Ischemia

In the environment of preventive and evidence-based medicine, the use of cTnI or cTnT measured in patients with ischemia allows clinicians to use biomarkers as both exclusionary and prognostic indicators. The results will assist in determining who is more at risk for AMI and death, and thereby determine who may benefit from early medical or surgical intervention. Such patients benefit from the use of anticoagulant therapy and the use of platelet antagonists, and an early invasive strategy. The goal of monitoring cTn in patients suggestive of ACS, with and without AMI, would be to effectively identify patients with unstable coronary disease and triage them to an appropriate therapeutic regimen. Optimal use of this strategy requires at least two blood samples for cTn measurement. General population screening of hospitalized patients with cTnI or cTnT is not recommended at present.

> The use of cTnI or cTnT measured in patients with ischemia allows clinicians to use biomarkers as both exclusionary and prognostic indicators

Patients *with* Nonischemic Presentations

Clinicians are often confronted with a clinical history of a patient without overt CAD and a low probability of myocardial ischemia. However, as a precautionary measure, serial cTns are ordered. A typical serial order set to rule in or rule out an AMI would include blood draws at 0 hour (presentation), 3 and 6 hours; with one additional 9- to 12-hour measurement if the earlier measurements are normal, when the clinical suspicion of AMI is high. When one or two of the serial cTn concentrations are found to be increased, the clinician would likely be confronted with the following concerns: (1) What does the increase mean in the clinical setting of a nonischemic patient? (2) Is the increase a false-positive finding resulting from an analytical error? (3) Why was the test ordered in the first place? As cTn assays with increasing low-end analytical sensitivity (hs-cTn assays) have been developed, the ability to detect minor degrees of myocardial injury in a variety of clinical conditions has widened and has led to a better understanding that cTn is not just a biomarker for AMI, but a sensitive biomarker for myocardial injury. The 20% of suspected ACS patients who clinically do not rule in for AMI, but display an increased cTn, represents patients with nonischemic pathologies (**Table 9–2**) in whom the mechanisms of injury are well defined (such as myocarditis, blunt chest trauma, and chemotherapeutic agents), as well as patients with increased cTn, in whom the mechanism of injury is not clear.

High-sensitivity Cardiac Troponin Assays

It is important to understand that the term "high sensitivity" (hs) reflects the assay's characteristics and does not refer to a difference in the form of cTn being measured. The term "high sensitivity," however, begs the question: how does one define an hs-assay? First, the total imprecision (CV) at the 99th percentile cTn value should be ≤10%. Second, measurable concentrations below the 99th percentile, for both men and women, should be attainable with a measureable concentration, that is greater than the assay's LoD for at least 50% of healthy individuals. None of the current US-marketed assays for both central laboratory contemporary or point-of-care assays meet this twofold hs criteria. Concentrations for hs-assays need to be expressed in nanograms per liter (ng/L), to distinguish them from the commonly published units of micrograms per liter of the contemporary/POC assays. The FDA is currently reviewing five different hs-assays for 510k clearance; so physicians will also soon use these hs-assays in clinical practice.

CONGESTIVE HEART FAILURE

Description

> CHF is a condition in which there is ineffective pumping of the heart leading to an accumulation of fluid in the lungs. Typically, it results from a loss of cardiac tissue and subsequent function.

CHF is a condition in which there is ineffective pumping of the heart leading to an accumulation of fluid in the lungs. Typically, it results from a loss of cardiac tissue and subsequent function. It is defined as the pathophysiological condition in which an abnormality of cardiac function is responsible for the failure of the heart to pump sufficient blood to satisfy the requirements of the metabolizing tissues. In the United States, CHF is the only cardiovascular disease with an increasing incidence. The National Heart, Lung, and Blood Institute estimates that the current prevalence is about 5 million Americans with CHF, with an incidence of approximately 400,000 new cases each year. CHF is the leading cause of hospitalization in individuals 65 years and older. Current prognosis is dependent on disease severity, but overall it is poor. The 5-year mortality is approximately 10% in mild CHF, 20% to 30% in moderate CHF, and up to 80% in end-stage disease.

Diagnosis

Natriuretic Peptides in Monitoring CHF

> Two biomarkers have been well studied to assist in these clinical settings: Brain natriuretic peptide (BNP) (the pharmacologically active hormone) and NT-proBNP (not pharmacologically active peptide).

Two biomarkers have been well studied to assist in these clinical settings: Brain natriuretic peptide (BNP) (the pharmacologically active hormone) and NT-proBNP (not pharmacologically active peptide). Both blood peptides are derived from cleavage of the myocardial proBNP peptide in response to myocardial stress and/or fluid overload. In general, the clinical evidence for utilization of either biomarker is very similar, but each has subtle analytical and physiological differences, depending on the pathophysiology of the individual patient. In the course of this chapter, both NPs are used interchangeably unless specifically noted.

The ACC/AHA practice guidelines for the evaluation and management of CHF indicate that the role of NP in the identification of CHF patients remains to be clarified. In contrast, the ESC has incorporated the monitoring of NPs into their practice algorithm at the time of patient presentation alongside the clinical history, physical examination, ECG, and chest x-ray. An abnormal NP finding would trigger an echocardiogram or an imaging modality. NP concentrations in patients diagnosed with CHF are substantially increased (>1000 ng/L for BNP or >1800 for NT-proBNP) when compared with patients who have minor increases (>300 ng/L) because of left ventricular (LV) dysfunction without acute CHF. CHF is more common in patients with advanced chronic renal disease. BNP and NT-proBNP are secreted in a pulsatile fashion from cardiac ventricles with an approximate half-life for BNP of 22 minutes in blood, and the NT-proBNP half-life on the order of 2 hours. While one mechanism of BNP clearance involves the renal parenchyma, the kidney is not thought to be the primary site for BNP clearance. The kidney more specifically affects NT-proBNP clearance. Thus, increases in BNP in hemodialysis patients are thought to represent both regulatory responses from the cardiac ventricle, resulting from increased wall tension, and a lack of renal clearance.

Importantly, NPs are not 100% specific for CHF. Increases have been described for other non-CHF etiologies involving filling pressure defects, including LV hypertrophy, inflammatory cardiac diseases, systemic arterial hypertension, pulmonary hypertension, acute and chronic renal failure, liver cirrhosis, and several endocrine disorders (e.g., hyperaldosteronism and Cushing syndrome). In CHF patients presenting to the ED, patients admitted tend to have higher BNP concentrations

(>500 ng/L) versus those who are discharged (mean >300 ng/L) at triage. Linear relationships with increasing BNP/NT-proBNP levels and the severity of CHF (NYHA classification I to IV) have been described. The largest prospective trial to date to evaluate the diagnostic value of BNP is "The *Breathing Not Properly* Multicenter Study," from which the level of BNP was found to be an independent predictor of CHF. Using a blood BNP cutoff concentration of 100 ng/L for CHF, there was a 90% clinical sensitivity and 75% clinical specificity, with an 81% accuracy. Without BNP monitoring, clinical judgment and traditional diagnostic methods demonstrated a diagnostic accuracy of only 74%. The knowledge of BNP reduced the proportion of patients in whom the clinician was uncertain of the diagnosis from 43% to 11%. Plasma BNP monitoring in the ED improved the treatment and evaluation of patients with early dyspnea, reducing the time to discharge and total cost of treatment. Similar data have been shown for the alternate biomarker NT-proBNP. After an AMI, NP increases in proportion to the size of the infarction, prompting investigators to explore the role of screening BNP for detection of LV dysfunction. In post-MI patients, BNP concentrations are inversely correlated with LV ejection fraction. However, there is inconclusive evidence for the role of BNP screening for asymptomatic LV dysfunction in the general population. In general, there does not appear to be a distinct advantage to use one biomarker (BNP or NT-proBNP) over the other in clinical practice. In the presence of a normal BNP or NT-proBNP, a diagnosis of CHF is highly unlikely.

In clinical practice, NP monitoring can best be used as a "rule-out" test for suspected cases of new CHF. It is not a stand-alone test and should not be a replacement for a full clinical assessment, including an echocardiogram when indicated. Monitoring NP may be useful in (1) guiding therapy, (2) monitoring the course of the disease, and (3) providing useful risk stratification information. NPs have been shown to be an independent predictor of cardiovascular mortality in patients with both CHF and ACS over a 1-year period. Further, BNP or NT-proBNP monitoring may assist in identifying patients with a lower risk of readmission within the next 30 days before discharge.

> In clinical practice, NP monitoring can best be used as a "rule-out" test for suspected cases of new CHF.

Analytical Methods for Measuring Natriuretic Peptides

Table 9–6 shows the current FDA-approved assays for BNP or NT-proBNP. For BNP and NT-proBNP, the commercial assays differ in standardization of measurements and antibodies used in the assay. The assays that use an antibody that recognizes the N-terminus labile region of BNP (e.g., Alere/Biosite, Beckman, and Abbott) demonstrate less analyte stability at room temperature (24 hours) than assays that use one of their antibodies recognizing the C-terminus (e.g., Siemens [Bayer]). The Roche NT-proBNP antibody configuration allows for 72 hours of sample stability at room temperature. **Figure 9–3** demonstrates the variable cross-reactivity that exists for BNP assays between the multiple forms of NPs that circulate after release from the heart. Just as for cTn assays, laboratorians and clinicians need to understand the lack of standardization between BNP assays, as well as between NT-proBNP assays from different manufacturers used in clinical practice, with the understanding that different assays should not be used in the same medical center for risk of misinterpretation of concentrations from one assay to the next.

> For BNP and NT-proBNP, the commercial assays differ in standardization of measurements and antibodies used in the assay.

Reference Intervals: Medical Decision Cutoff Values

A number of clinical factors affect the BNP and NT-proBNP concentrations, most importantly age, gender, obesity, and renal function. Significant differences are observed between men and women (higher), and there are increasing concentrations with age by decade. For BNP and

> A number of clinical factors affect the BNP and NT-proBNP concentrations, most importantly age, gender, obesity, and renal function.

TABLE 9–6   **Representative Commercial BNP and NT-proBNP Assays**

BNP
1. Abbott ARCHITEC
2. Alere/Biosite Triage
3. Beckman Coulter Access
4. Siemens Centaur

NT-proBNP
1. Roche Cobas
2. Siemens Centaur and Vista
3. Ortho-Clinical Diagnostics Vitros
4. Response Biomedical Ramp
5. Mitsubishi Pathfast

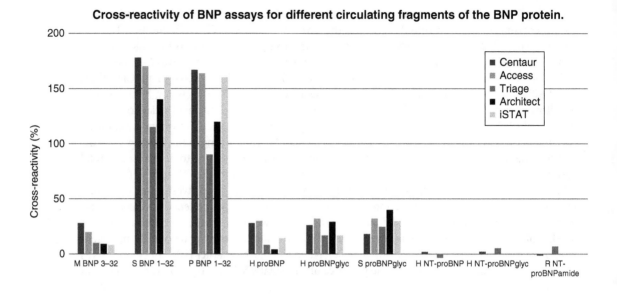

FIGURE 9–3 Representative cross-reactivity profile for BNP assays with BNP and NT-proBNP peptides. M, P, S, H, R are abbreviations for the source of the samples. The glycosylated- and amide-linked forms are noted with the terms glyc and amide. (With permission from Saenger AK, et al. Specificity of B-type natriuretic peptide assays: cross-reactivity with different BNP, NT-proBNP, and proBNP peptides. *Clin Chem.* 2017;63:351–358.)

NT-proBNP, the significance of the results for these assays in relation to the degree of left ventricle dysfunction remains a debate. For both analytes, there is an inverse relationship between values and body mass index. For NT-proBNP, establishing reference intervals has been challenging. Review of both the FDA-approved US package insert and the European assay package insert reveals substantial differences in what concentrations are considered normal by age and sex. For BNP, a cutoff of 100 ng/L has been endorsed as demonstrating optimal sensitivity and specificity. For NT-proBNP, the FDA-approved package insert describes a two-tier cutoff by age at ≤75 years: 125 ng/L and at >75 years: 450 ng/L. However, more evidence-based cutoffs have been derived from the PRIDE/ICON studies based on age and renal function, and are recommended as follows—age ≤50 years: 450 ng/L; age >50 years: 900 ng/L; all ages: best negative predictive value 300 ng/L; age >50 years and eGFR ≥60 mL/min: 450 pg/mL, and eGFR <60 mL/min: 1800 ng/L; age ≤50 years and eGFR ≥60 mL/min: 900 pg/mL, and eGFR <60 mL/min: 1800 ng/L.

Implications for Therapy Using Test Results for Natriuretic Peptides

The utility of serial measurements of NPs in guiding therapy for chronic heart failure has been the subject of numerous randomized controlled trials reported in the literature since 2000. The existing trial data suggest that adjustment of treatment in chronic heart failure according to NP measurements, used in conjunction with established clinical treatments, is likely to reduce cardiac mortality and hospital admissions with heart failure, at least in patients with systolic heart failure who are younger than 75 years and relatively free of comorbidities.

Biological Variability

As BNP and NT-proBNP become more widely used to monitor CHF patients following therapy, questions have addressed the usefulness of serial monitoring in assisting the success of drug therapy. In a study of 11 patients with CHF, the biological variation for BNP and NT-proBNP was evaluated using four different assays. The findings indicated that a change of 130% for BNP and 90% for NT-proBNP is necessary before results of serially collected data can be considered clinically and statistically significant. For example, these findings imply that a decrease from approximately 500 to 250 ng/L would be necessary for a clinician to conclude that therapy was successful in improving CHF features. Clinicians without this knowledge may inappropriately assume that a decrease from an admission BNP value of 500 ng/L to a 24-hour post-admission value of 400 ng/L may have been a result of successful patient management. It has been suggested that following the admission BNP value, a second BNP value be obtained within 24 hours of discharge to optimize the diagnostic utility of BNP in the overall assessment of patients with CHF.

> It has been suggested that following the admission BNP value, a second BNP value be obtained within 24 hours of discharge to optimize the diagnostic utility of BNP in the overall assessment of patients with CHF.

Novel Biomarkers for Heart Failure Risk Assessment

In addition to the advances in the understanding of established NP biomarkers in HF, there is an increased study of the elucidation of novel biomarkers potentially useful for the evaluation and management of patients with HF. Literature on candidate biomarkers from a number of studies will be growing over the next several years and include (a) myocyte stretch (with assays for ST2 [a member of the interleukin-1 receptor family]), GDF-15 (growth differentiation factor 15), and galectin-3 (a carbohydrate-binding lectin); (b) myocyte necrosis (with hs-cTn assays); (c) systemic inflammation (with assays for lipoprotein-associated phospholipase A2); (d) oxidative stress (with assays for myeloperoxidase); (e) extracellular matrix turnover (with assays for collagen propeptides); (f) neurohormones (with assays for chromogranin A); and (g) biomarkers of extracardiac processes, such as renal function (with assays for neutrophil gelatinase-associated lipocalin [NGAL]).

SELF-ASSESSMENT QUESTIONS

1. Among the choices below, there is one incorrect answer. Identify which answer is incorrect.
   An acute myocardial infarction is diagnosed when there is a rise or fall of a cardiac biomarker, preferably cardiac troponin, with at least one value above the 99th percentile upper reference limit and at least one of the following:
   A. Symptoms of cardiac ischemia
   B. Evidence of pulmonary embolism
   C. Development of pathological Q waves in the electrocardiogram
   D. Imaging evidence of new loss of viable myocardium

2. Which of the following biomarkers for myocardial infarction is preferred to establish the diagnosis?
   A. Creatine kinase-MB fraction (CK-MB)
   B. Lactate dehydrogenase (LDH)
   C. Cardiac troponin I or cardiac troponin T
   D. Aspartate aminotransferase (AST)

3. Which of the following biomarkers is most useful to identify congestive heart failure among other causes for shortness of breath?
   A. B-type natriuretic peptide (BNP)
   B. Troponin I
   C. D-dimer
   D. Troponin T

FURTHER READING

Apple FS, et al. Quality specifications for B-type natriuretic peptide assays. *Clin Chem*. 2005;51:486–493.

Apple FS, et al. Determination of 19 cardiac troponin I and T assay 99th percentile values from a common presumably healthy population. *Clin Chem*. 2012;58:1574–1581.

Apple FS, et al; for the IFCC Task Force on Clinical Applications of Cardiac Bio-Markers. Cardiac troponin assays: guide to understanding analytical characteristics and their impact on clinical care. *Clin Chem*. 2017;63:73–81.

Chapman AR, et al. Association of high-sensitivity cardiac troponin I concentration with cardiac outcomes in patients with suspected acute coronary syndrome. *JAMA*. 2017;318:1013–1924.

McFalls EO, et al. Long-term outcomes of hospitalized patients with a non-acute syndrome diagnosis and an elevated cardiac troponin level. *Am J Med*. 2011;124:630–635.

Peacock WF, et al; for the ADHERE Scientific Advisory Committee Study Group. Cardiac troponin and heart failure outcome in acute heart failure. *N Engl J Med*. 2008;358:2117–2126.

Saenger AK, et al. Specificity of B-type natriuretic peptide assays: cross-reactivity with different BNP, NT-proBNP, and proBNP peptides. *Clin Chem* 2017;63:351–358.

Sandoval Y, et al. Diagnosis of type 1 and type 2 myocardial infarction using a high-sensitivity cardiac troponin I assay with gender-specific 99th percentiles based on the Third Universal Definition of Myocardial Infarction classification system. *Clin Chem*. 2015;61:657–663.

Sandoval Y, et al. Present and future of high sensitivity cardiac troponin in clinical practice: a paradigm shift to high sensitivity assays. *Am J Med*. 2016;129:354–365.

Sandoval Y, et al. Rapid rule-out of acute myocardial injury using a single high-sensitivity cardiac troponin I measurement. *Clin Chem*. 2017;63:369–376.

Sandoval Y, et al. Single high-sensitivity cardiac troponin I to rule out myocardial infarction. *Am J MED*. 2017;130:1076–1083.

Tang WHW, et al. National Academy of Clinical Biochemistry practice guidelines: clinical utilization of cardiac biomarker testing in heart failure. *Circulation*. 2007;116:e99–e109.

Thygesen K, et al. Writing group on behalf of the Joint ESC/ACCF/AHA/WHF Task Force for the Universal Definition of Myocardial Infarction. Third Universal Definition of Myocardial Infarction. *J Am Coll Cardiol*. 2012;60:1581–1598.

Van Kimmenade RRJ, Januzzi JLJr. Emerging biomarkers in heart failure. *Clin Chem*. 2012;58:127–138.

Wu AHB, et al. Clinical laboratory practice recommendations for the use of cardiac troponin in acute coronary syndrome: expert opinion from the Academy of the American Association for Clinical Chemistry and the Task Force on Clinical Applications of Cardiac Bio-Markers of the International Federation of Clinical Chemistry and Laboratory Medicine. *Clin Chem*. 2018;64:645–655.

Diseases of Red Blood Cells

Daniel D. Mais

CHAPTER OUTLINE

ANEMIA

Definition

Anemia refers to a deficiency in red blood cells (RBCs) and implies a decline in oxygen-carrying capacity. The complete blood count (CBC) provides several measures of red cell quantity, including RBC count, hemoglobin (Hb) concentration, and hematocrit (Hct) (see description of RBC indices later in this chapter). Hb concentration is the parameter most widely used to diagnose anemia, based on 1967 World Health Organization (WHO) recommendations (**Table 10–1**). This definition is not universally accepted, and numerous alternatives have been proposed over the years, usually suggesting slightly higher values and race-specific values. It is important to remember also that the normal ranges for Hb and Hct are different for infants, children, adult men, adult women, pregnant women, and the elderly. Attention to age- and gender-appropriate normal ranges is important in the evaluation of anemia.

Anemia refers to a deficiency in red blood cells (RBCs) and implies a decline in oxygen-carrying capacity.

TABLE 10-1   WHO Definition of Anemia

Group	Hemoglobin (g/dL)
Infants and children, 6 months–6 years	<11.0
Pregnant females	<11.0
Children, 6–14 years	<12.0
Nonpregnant adult females	<12.0
Adult males	<13.0

TABLE 10-2   Classification of Anemia by Pathophysiology

Production Defect	Survival Defect
Proliferation defect • Anemia of chronic disease • Renal disease (low erythropoietin states) • Fanconi anemia • Blackfan–Diamond syndrome • Parvovirus infection • Drugs or toxins	*Hemolysis* • Hemoglobinopathies • Immune hemolytic anemias • Infectious causes of hemolysis • Membrane abnormalities • Metabolic abnormalities • Mechanical hemolysis • Drugs or toxins • Wilson disease
Maturation defect • Vitamin B$_{12}$ deficiency • Folate deficiency • Iron deficiency • Sideroblastic anemia • Lead poisoning	*Hemorrhage* *Hypersplenism*

Anemia may present with pallor, fatigue, dyspnea, or evidence of poor tissue oxygenation (chest pain due to poor cardiac oxygenation, altered mental status due to poor cerebral oxygenation). Often, particularly when anemia is mild or the patient is otherwise healthy, anemia presents simply as an abnormal CBC.

Anemia stimulates several compensatory mechanisms. The cardiopulmonary system compensates by attempting to make the most of the blood it has by exchanging more gases (tachypnea), and circulating more volume (tachycardia). The marrow responds with increased erythropoiesis, stimulated by an increase in renal production of erythropoietin (EPO) in response to hypoxia. If the means to create mature red cells are intact (i.e., if the underlying cause of the anemia is not a production or maturation defect), then this response can usually succeed. In addition to making more erythrocytes, the marrow begins to release immature erythrocytes into the circulation. Many of these still contain a network of ribosomes and rough endoplasmic reticulum involved in the making of Hb, which identifies them morphologically as reticulocytes (see description of reticulocyte counting later in this chapter). Over the next 3 to 4 days, this endoplasmic reticulum dissolves and a mature RBC results. In very brisk marrow responses, some red cells may be released that still contain a nucleus.

> Identifying the cause of anemia is usually fairly straightforward. Examination of the peripheral smear is especially important, since numerous clues can be found there.

Differential Diagnosis

Identifying the cause of anemia is usually fairly straightforward. There are several strategies for reaching the diagnosis (**Tables 10-2** and **10-3**), one of which is illustrated in the algorithms (**Figures 10-1** to **10-4**). Examination of the peripheral smear is especially important, since numerous clues can be found there (**Table 10-4**). **Figures 10-5** to **10-24** show many of the abnormal morphologies and intracellular inclusions of RBCs.

TABLE 10–3   Classification of Anemia by Mean Corpuscular Volume (MCV) and Red Blood Cell Distribution Width (RDW)

	Normal RDW	High RDW
Low MCV	Anemia of chronic disease Thalassemia Hemoglobin E	Iron deficiency anemia Sickle cell disease
Normal MCV	Acute blood loss Anemia of chronic disease Low erythropoietin states (renal failure)	Early nutritional (iron, B_{12}, folate) deficiency Sickle cell disease
High MCV	Aplastic anemia Liver disease Alcohol abuse	Folate and B_{12} deficiency Myelodysplasia Reticulocytosis (e.g., hemolysis)

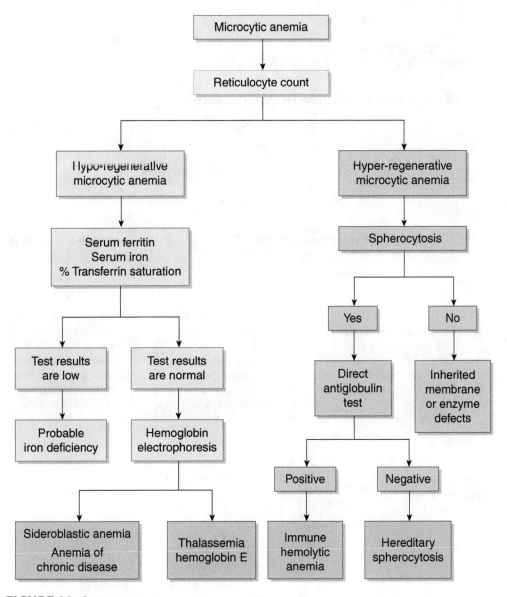

FIGURE 10–1 Diagnostic algorithm for microcytic anemia.

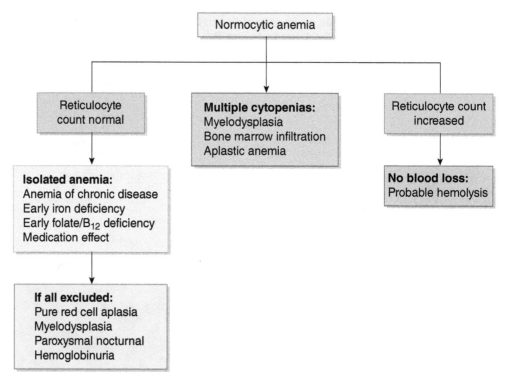

FIGURE 10–2 Diagnostic algorithm for normocytic anemia.

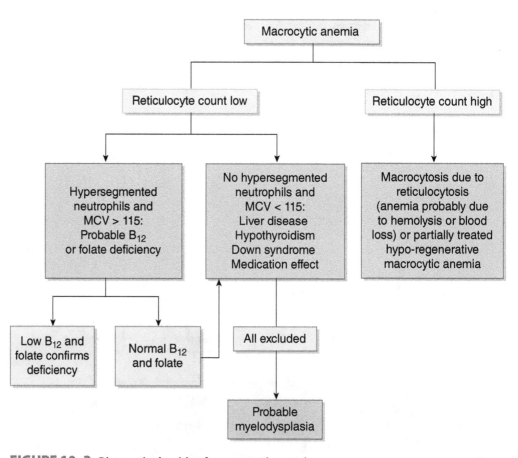

FIGURE 10–3 Diagnostic algorithm for macrocytic anemia.

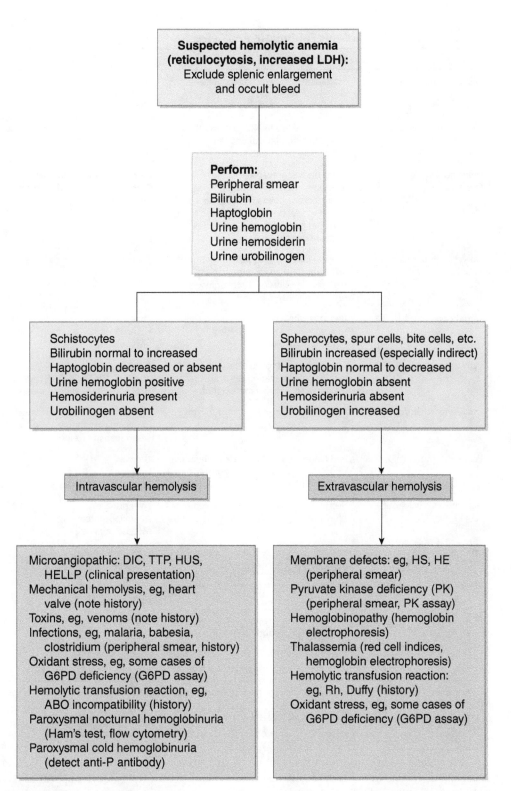

FIGURE 10–4 Diagnostic algorithm for suspected hemolytic anemia. DIC, disseminated intravascular coagulation; TTP, thrombotic thrombocytopenic purpura; HUS, hemolytic uremic syndrome; HELLP, hemolysis, elevated liver function tests, and low platelets; HS, hereditary spherocytosis; HE, hereditary elliptocytosis; G6PD, glucose-6-phosphate dehydrogenase.

TABLE 10–4   Morphologic Findings in Red Cells

Finding	Definition	Associated Conditions
Basophilic stippling	Small blue dots in red cells, due to clusters of ribosomes	Hemolytic anemias Lead poisoning Thalassemia
Pappenheimer bodies	Larger, more irregular, and grayer than basophilic stippling, due to iron-containing mitochondria	Asplenia Sideroblastic anemia
Heinz bodies Bite cells	Heinz bodies: gray–black round inclusions, seen only with supravital stains (crystal violet). Bite cells: sharp bite-like defects in red cells where a Heinz body has been removed in the spleen. Both are due to denatured hemoglobin	Oxidative injury as found in G6PD deficiency or with unstable hemoglobins
Howell–Jolly bodies Cabot rings	Howell–Jolly body: dot-like, dark purple inclusion. Cabot ring: ring-shaped dark purple inclusion. Both represent a residual nuclear fragment	Asplenia
Target cells	Red cells with a dark circle within the central area of pallor, reflecting redundant membrane	Thalassemia Hemoglobin C Liver disease
Schistocytes	Fragmented red blood cells, with forms such as helmet-shaped cells, due to mechanical red cell fragmentation	Microangiopathic hemolytic anemias (MHA): DIC, TTP, HUS, HELLP. Mechanical heart valves
Dacrocytes (teardrop cells)	Teardrop or pear-shaped erythrocytes	Can be seen in thalassemia and megaloblastic anemia Often seen in myelophthisis
Echinocytes (burr cells)	Red blood cells that have circumferential undulations or spiny projections with pointed tips	Uremia Gastric cancer Pyruvate kinase deficiency
Acanthocytes (spur cells)	Red blood cells that have circumferential blunt and spiny projections with bulbous tips	Liver disease Abetalipoproteinemia McLeod phenotype
Spherocytes	Red cells without central pallor due to decreased red cell membrane	Immune hemolytic anemia Hereditary spherocytosis
Elliptocytes	Red cells twice as long as they are wide	Iron deficiency Hereditary elliptocytosis
Stomatocytes	Red cells whose area of central pallor is elongated in a mouth-like shape	Alcohol abuse Dilantin exposure Rh null phenotype (absence of Rh antigens) Hereditary stomatocytosis

DIC, disseminated intravascular coagulation; TTP, thrombotic thrombocytopenic purpura; HUS, hemolytic uremic syndrome; HELLP, hemolysis, elevated liver function tests, and low platelets.

See **Figures 10–5** to **10–18** for peripheral smears with abnormal red blood cell morphology.

The reticulocyte count is an important piece of information. When markedly elevated, this is usually noticeable in a Wright-stained peripheral blood smear. Reticulocytes appear as large, polychromatophilic red cells, and when they are numerous, the smear is often described as having polychromasia. Anemia due to a production defect is associated with a normal to low reticulocyte count. Such hyporegenerative anemias include iron deficiency anemia, anemia of chronic disease (ACD), lead poisoning, folate deficiency, B_{12} deficiency, myelodysplastic syndrome, aplastic anemia, and pure red cell aplasia.

Regardless of the morphology or red cell size, anemia that is accompanied by reticulocytosis suggests either hemolysis or hemorrhage. Some exceptions should be noted. One is a partially treated production defect, such as in the early treatment of iron, folate, or B_{12} deficiency, in which one may find persistent anemia with reticulocytosis. Second, both hemolytic and blood-loss

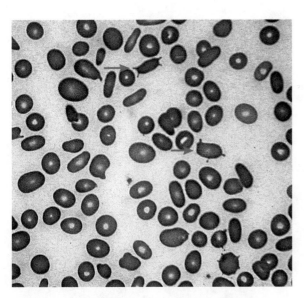

FIGURE 10–5 **Peripheral blood smear with acanthocytes.**

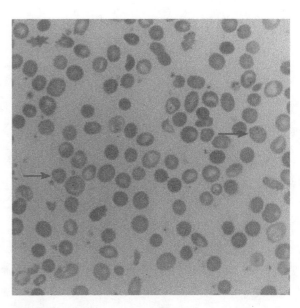

FIGURE 10–6 **Peripheral blood smear with the basophilic stippling.**

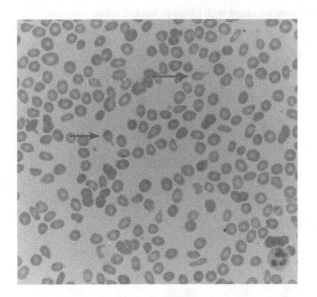

FIGURE 10–7 **Peripheral blood smear with dacrocytes.**

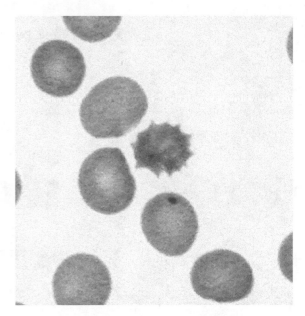

FIGURE 10–8 **Peripheral blood smear with echinocyte.**

anemia may eventually lead to depletion of iron, folate, or B_{12}, and they can present as a production defect. Lastly, paroxysmal nocturnal hemoglinuria (PNH) is a hemolytic anemia that may transform to aplastic anemia.

Hemolytic anemias are those in which red cell survival, normally 120 days, is shortened. The premature destruction of erythrocytes may occur within the bloodstream (intravascular hemolysis) or within the reticuloendothelial system (extravascular hemolysis). Intravascular hemolysis is caused by mechanical red cell trauma (e.g., microangiopathic hemolytic anemia [MHA] or mechanical heart valve), complement fixation on the red cell surface (e.g., ABO incompatibility), PNH, paroxysmal cold hemoglobinuria (PCH), snake envenomation, and infectious agents (e.g., malaria, babesiosis, *Clostridium*). Extravascular hemolysis is much more common and is typical

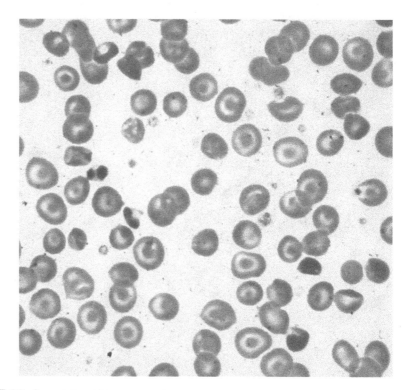

FIGURE 10–9   Peripheral blood smear from a patient with hemoglobin C disease.

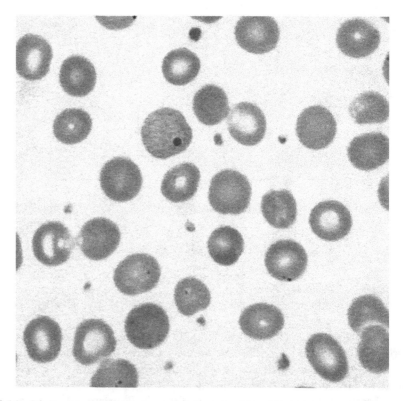

FIGURE 10–10   Peripheral blood smear showing a Howell–Jolly body.

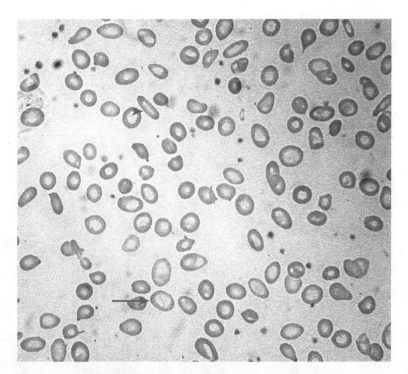

FIGURE 10–11 Peripheral blood smear from a patient with iron deficiency, showing hypochromic and microcytic red cells (arrow) and elliptocytes (arrowhead).

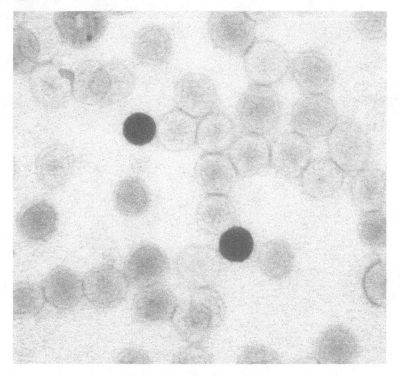

FIGURE 10–12 Slide showing the results of a Kleihauer–Betke test.

FIGURE 10–13 Peripheral blood smear from a patient with megaloblastic anemia and hypersegmented neutrophils.

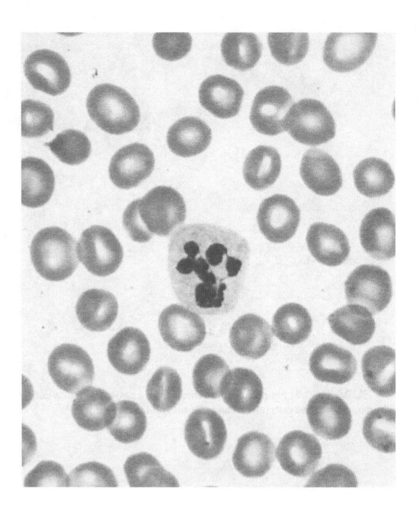

FIGURE 10–14 Peripheral blood smear from a patient with megaloblastic anemia and macroovalocytes.

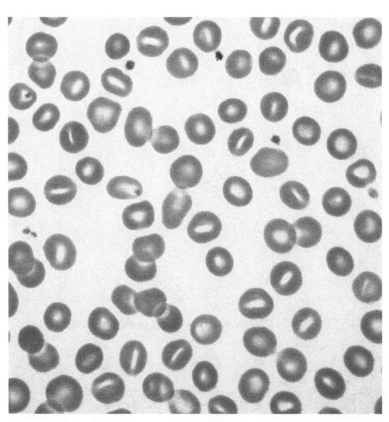

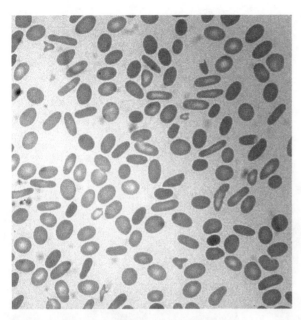

FIGURE 10–15 Peripheral blood smear from a patient with large numbers of elliptocytes.

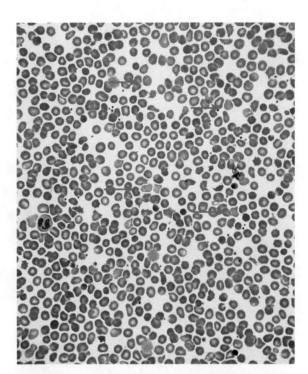

FIGURE 10–16 A peripheral blood smear stained with Wright stain showing reticulocytes.

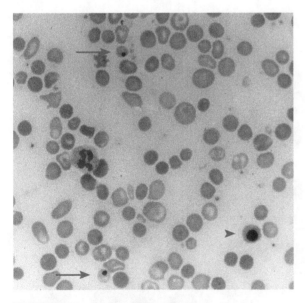

FIGURE 10–17 A peripheral blood smear showing circulating nucleated red blood cells (arrowheads), as well as Howell–Jolly bodies (arrows).

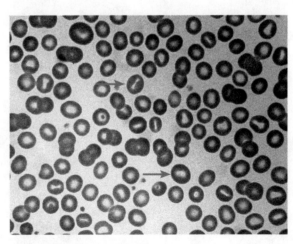

FIGURE 10–18 A peripheral blood smear from a patient with stomatocytes.

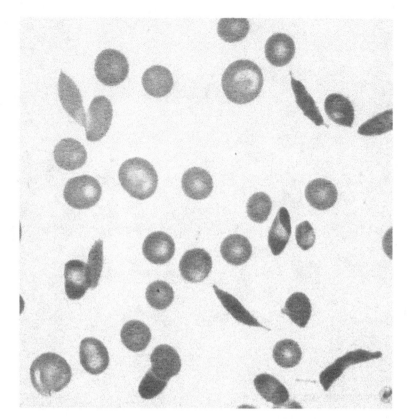

FIGURE 10–19 **Peripheral blood smear with sickle cells.**

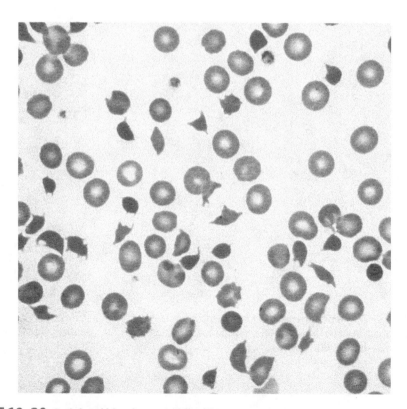

FIGURE 10–20 **Peripheral blood smear with schistocytes.**

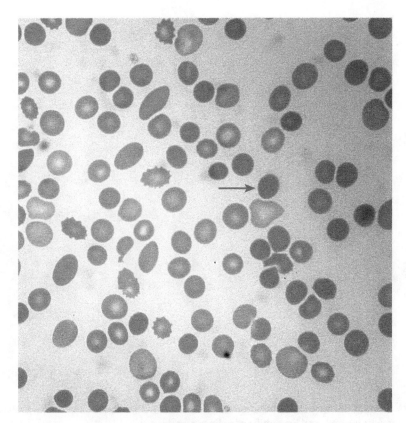

FIGURE 10–21 Peripheral blood smear with spherocytes.

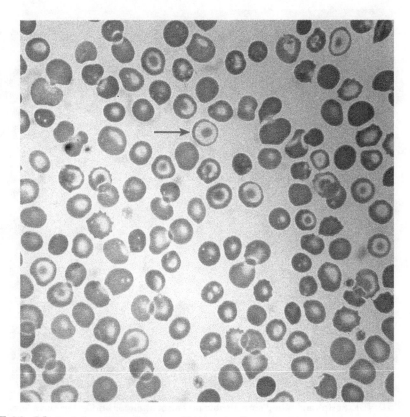

FIGURE 10–22 Peripheral blood smear with target cells.

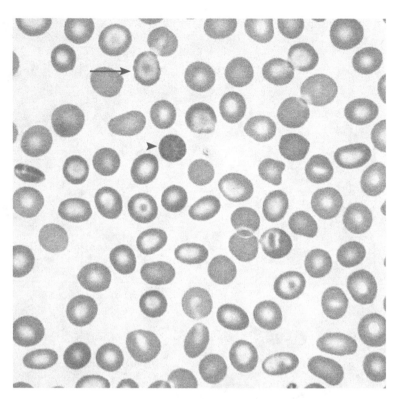

FIGURE 10–23 Peripheral blood smear from a patient with thalassemia, showing microcytic red cells, target cells (arrow), and basophilic stippling (arrowhead).

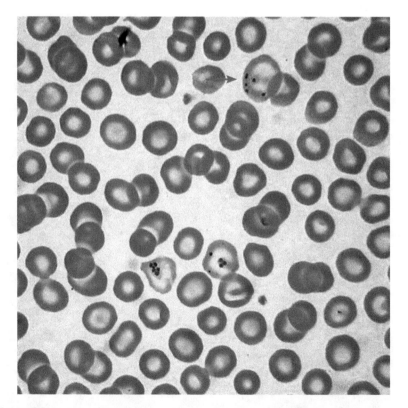

FIGURE 10–24 Peripheral blood smear showing Pappenheimer bodies (arrows). Sometimes mistaken for Howell–Jolly bodies (Figure 10—10).

TABLE 10–5 **Laboratory Distinction of Intravascular and Extravascular Hemolysis**

Intravascular Hemolysis	Extravascular Hemolysis
Schistocytes	Microspherocytes
↑ Lactate dehydrogenase (LD)	↑ LD
↓ Haptoglobin	Normal to ↓ haptoglobin
↑ Free hemoglobin, ↑ urine hemoglobin	↑ Indirect bilirubin
Hemosiderinuria	↑ Urine and fecal urobilinogen

for all remaining causes of hemolysis. The causes of hemolysis may be inherited or acquired. Inherited forms of hemolytic anemia usually, but not always, present in early childhood (**Table 10–5**).

Hemolytic anemia presents with jaundice, fatigue, tachycardia, and pallor. If chronic, enhanced excretion of Hb breakdown products often leads to the development of pigmented gallstones. Intravascular hemolysis may present with dark urine and back pain. Leg ulcers are common in sickle cell disease and hereditary spherocytosis (HS). Splenomegaly is a common finding in extravascular hemolysis. Laboratory findings in support of hemolysis include increased unconjugated bilirubin, increased lactate dehydrogenase (LD), and decreased haptoglobin. Reticulocytes, which are larger than mature red cells, are responsible for an unpredictability of the mean corpuscular volume (MCV). The blood smear may display helpful morphologic findings. Intravascular hemolysis is associated with hemoglobinuria and hemosiderinuria.

Acute Blood Loss

Description

Acute blood loss (hemorrhage) is seen most often as a result of surgery, trauma, or gastrointestinal pathology. Most often, hemorrhage is quite obviously present, but occasionally it is occult and internal (large retroperitoneal or pelvic hemorrhages). It can occur in the prehospital setting, and in that case its volume cannot be estimated.

The cardinal manifestations of acute blood loss—tachycardia, tachypnea, and hypotension—reflect not so much a decreased oxygen-carrying capacity as a decreased intravascular volume. A shift of water from the interstitial fluid compartment into the plasma leads to hemodilution and a lowered Hct. It is for this reason that the initial treatment is intravenous fluid resuscitation with normal saline; only if this is unsuccessful is blood transfusion considered.

Chronic slow blood loss is generally well tolerated and usually presents late in the disease process as iron deficiency anemia. Acute blood loss is not the only form of anemia that can present abruptly. Causes other than hemorrhage that may present as rapid-onset severe anemia include intravascular hemolysis and acute exacerbations of a chronic compensated hemolytic anemia, such as in sickle cell disease (**Table 10–6**).

> Acute blood loss (hemorrhage) is seen most often as a result of surgery, trauma, or gastrointestinal pathology.

TABLE 10–6 **Nonhemorrhagic Causes of Acute Severe Anemia**

Acute Intravascular Hemolysis	Acute Exacerbation of Chronic Hemolysis
Microangiopathic hemolytic anemia	Parvovirus B19 bone marrow infection (aplastic crisis)
Mechanical hemolysis (e.g., heart valve)	Splenic sequestration crisis
Toxins (e.g., venoms)	Hyperhemolytic crisis
Infections (e.g., malaria, *Clostridium*)	
Oxidant stress (especially in glucose-6-phosphate dehydrogenase deficiency)	
Hemolytic transfusion reaction (ABO incompatibility)	
Paroxysmal nocturnal hemoglobinuria	
Paroxysmal cold hemoglobinuria	

Diagnosis

The history and physical examination are the keys to arriving at the correct diagnosis. In perplexing situations, it may be necessary to exclude hemolysis. The main laboratory findings are a normocytic anemia with a marked reticulocytosis. The peripheral smear may be notable only for neutrophilia, a result of mobilization of granulocytes from marginal pools (demargination), which is a physiologic stress response. Somewhat later, there may be reactive thrombocytosis.

Iron Deficiency Anemia

Description

Within the cytoplasm of the marrow erythroblast, the predominant activity is the production of Hb molecules into which iron must be incorporated. Iron from the diet is absorbed principally in the duodenum. It is carried by transferrin to the marrow where it is internalized into erythroblasts and incorporated into protoporphyrin to yield heme. Iron not utilized in this way is stored bound to ferritin. When there is inadequate iron intake or excessive iron loss (**Table 10-7**), the ferritin–iron stores of the reticuloendothelial system become progressively depleted. Red cells are produced that contain an inadequate concentration of Hb, giving rise to the appearance of small, hypochromic red cells that are poorly equipped for the carriage of oxygen. Fewer mature red cells are subsequently produced, lowering the Hct (**Table 10-8**). The clinical manifestations include those directly attributable to anemia (fatigue, pallor), in addition to pica (a desire to ingest solids such as rock, dirt, or ice), atrophic glossitis, koilonychias, and esophageal webs. The coexistence of esophageal webs and iron deficiency has been called Plummer–Vinson syndrome. These latter manifestations are not commonly seen and follow prolonged, untreated iron deficiency.

Iron deficiency is the most common cause of anemia. Worldwide, the most common cause of iron deficiency is a dietary lack of iron. In the United States, iron intake is not usually problematic, although supply can lag demand in some populations, such as toddlers and pregnant women. The finding of iron deficiency produces an obligation to identify and treat the underlying cause. In American adults, this underlying cause is usually found within the gastrointestinal tract. Iron deficiency often is the first sign of an occult gastrointestinal malignancy.

> The finding of iron deficiency produces an obligation to identify and treat the underlying cause. In American adults, this underlying cause is usually found within the gastrointestinal tract. Iron deficiency often is the first sign of an occult gastrointestinal malignancy.

Diagnosis

In many cases, the CBC and peripheral blood findings are highly characteristic: low RBC count, low MCV, low mean corpuscular hemoglobin concentration (MCHC), and high red cell distribution width (RDW). The platelet count is often elevated. The peripheral blood shows hypochromic,

TABLE 10-7   **Causes of Iron Deficiency**

Mechanisms	Examples
Iron-poor diet	Strict vegetarians
Iron malabsorption	Celiac sprue Small bowel resection Achlorhydria Hookworm infection
Chronic blood (iron) loss	Menses Colorectal cancer Idiopathic pulmonary hemosiderosis

TABLE 10-8   **Stages of Iron Deficiency**

Stage	Laboratory Findings	Clinical Findings
Iron store depletion	↓ Serum ferritin, ↓ stainable marrow iron	None
Impaired erythropoiesis	All of the above plus ↑ TIBC, ↓ serum iron, and ↑ RDW	None
Iron deficiency anemia	All of the above plus microcytic, hypochromic anemia	Fatigue, pallor

TIBC, total iron-binding capacity; RDW, red blood cell distribution width.

microcytic red cells with scattered elliptocytes. This is in contrast to the most commonly entertained other diagnostic consideration, thalassemia, in which the RBC count is high, the RDW tends to be lower, elliptocytes are not seen, and target cells and basophilic stippling are more frequent.

To confirm the diagnosis of iron deficiency, the best single test is the serum ferritin. A ferritin above 15 µg/L essentially excludes iron deficiency, and the serum ferritin in iron deficiency is often below 10 µg/L. Lowered ferritin is the earliest finding in iron deficiency and persists throughout the course of the illness. The diagnostic difficulty with the use of ferritin is that it is an acute-phase reactant, an analyte that increases in response to inflammation. It may also be spuriously elevated in hepatic insufficiency, due to impaired clearance. Thus, other assays may occasionally be needed to make a diagnosis of iron deficiency anemia.

In established iron deficiency, the serum iron is typically low, the total iron-binding capacity (TIBC) is elevated, and the percent transferrin saturation is low. These findings are somewhat in contrast to those seen in ACD (see below). Serum soluble transferrin receptor is elevated whenever there are cells depleted of iron; thus, it is elevated in iron deficiency anemia and in erythroid hyperplasia (hemolytic anemia, polycythemia). Lastly, the zinc protoporphyrin (ZPP) and free erythrocyte protoporphyrin (FEP) are not only elevated in iron deficiency but also elevated in lead poisoning and ACD. As a last resort, marrow iron stores can be examined directly under the microscope if an adequate bone marrow aspirate is obtained.

Anemia of Chronic Disease

Definition

Sustained systemic inflammation alters iron utilization in the marrow, suppresses hematopoiesis, and blunts the response of EPO to anemia. This combination of factors leads to a mild, refractory, hyporegenerative anemia that is usually normocytic and normochromic, but is microcytic in up to one-third of cases. Although iron deficiency is the most common cause of anemia worldwide, ACD is the most common cause of anemia in both hospitalized and ambulatory hospital patients in the United States. The vast majority of cases are due to rheumatoid arthritis, collagen vascular disease such as lupus, chronic infection, and malignancy.

> ACD is the most common cause of anemia in both hospitalized and ambulatory hospital patients in the United States.

The means by which chronic inflammatory diseases cause anemia are still being elucidated. Marrow biopsies in patients with ACD display bountiful iron stores in the face of decreased iron uptake by erythroid precursors. Decreased transferrin receptors have been demonstrated on erythroblasts in ACD. In addition, patients with ACD have decreased production of EPO in response to anemia. Cytokines, including IFNγ, TNFα, IL-1, and hepcidin, have been shown to produce the conditions of ACD when injected into laboratory animals.

Diagnosis

The diagnosis of ACD is made difficult by the presence of numerous comorbid factors, in patients who, by definition, are ill. In such patients, ACD may be coincident with iron deficiency, folate deficiency, renal insufficiency, and/or frequent phlebotomy. Furthermore, in up to 30% of those with iron indices characteristic of ACD, no chronic illness can be identified.

The laboratory diagnosis of ACD depends on demonstrating a hypoproliferative (low reticulocyte count) normocytic or microcytic anemia in the presence of characteristic iron studies. The iron studies should document increased iron stores (normal to high serum ferritin or increased stainable iron in a bone marrow biopsy) and a low serum iron, low transferrin, and low TIBC.

A normal or elevated ferritin level is crucial for distinguishing ACD from iron deficiency. However, interpretation of the results for ferritin can be problematic because ferritin is an acute-phase reactant. Thus, while a low ferritin is essentially diagnostic of iron deficiency, a normal ferritin does not entirely exclude it. In confusing situations, the soluble serum transferrin receptor assay may be helpful. This analyte is increased in iron deficiency anemia and normal in ACD.

Thalassemia

Description

Mutations in the genes that encode globin chains may result in two broad categories of disease. Some mutations lead to the production of a structurally abnormal globin chain, resulting in a

Some mutations lead
to the production of a
structurally abnormal
globin chain, resulting in
a *hemoglobinopathy* such
as HbS (sickle cell disease
and sickle cell trait).
Other mutations lead
to reduced production
of a structurally normal
globin chain, resulting in
thalassemia.

hemoglobinopathy such as HbS (sickle cell disease and sickle cell trait). Other mutations lead to reduced production of a structurally normal globin chain, resulting in *thalassemia*.

An Hb molecule is composed of four polypeptide chains. The major adult Hb, hemoglobin A (HbA), is composed of two α chains and two β chains. The minor adult Hb (HbA2) is composed of two α chains and two δ chains. The major fetal hemoglobin (HbF) is composed of two α chains and two γ chains. The one constant feature of all Hbs is the α chain. The α chain genes are located on chromosome 16. Each chromosome 16 contains two separate α chain genes, for a total of four genes per normal cell, each transcriptionally active. Thus, to render an individual completely deficient of α chains, inheritance of four mutated genes is required. The β, γ, and δ chain genes are located on chromosome 11. Each chromosome 11 contains one β, one γ, and one δ gene. Should a mutation occur in the β chain, there can be a degree of compensation by increasing the production of γ, δ, or both. There is no such substitute for the α chain.

With decreased α chain production, α-thalassemia arises. Harm comes to the red cell, however, not from a deficiency of α chain, but from an excess of non-α chains (e.g., β). The excess chains form precipitates in the cell, leading to ineffective erythropoiesis, microcytosis, and enhanced splenic red cell destruction. Likewise, decreased β chain production (β-thalassemia) leads to precipitation of excess α chains and subsequent red cell destruction. Disease severity reflects the genotype (**Table 10–9**).

Diagnosis

Since α chains are present in utero, α-thalassemia can be diagnosed at birth. The diagnosis of β-thalassemia is somewhat delayed, since β chains are not produced to adult levels until 3 to 6 months of age. The CBC is notable for microcytosis, usually in the presence of a normal or high RBC count. The peripheral smear often displays target cells and may display basophilic stippling. When there is microcytosis, "thalassemic" indices, and normal iron studies, the diagnosis of thalassemia is essentially assured. In the case of β-thalassemia, an Hb electrophoresis displays

TABLE 10–9   Thalassemia Syndromes

Category	Syndrome	Genotype	Manifestations
Normal	Normal	αα/αα β/β	None
α-Thalassemia syndromes	α-Thalassemia (silent) carrier	αα/α∎ β/β	None
	α-Thalassemia minor	αα/∎∎ β/β	Mild
		α∎/α∎ β/β	
	Hemoglobin H	α∎/∎∎ β/β	Moderate to severe
	Hemoglobin Barts	∎∎/∎∎ β/β	Fatal
β-Thalassemia syndromes	β-Thalassemia minor	αααα β/β⁺	Asymptomatic
		αααα β/β°	
	β-Thalassemia intermediate	αααα β⁺/β⁺	Moderate to severe
		αααα β⁺/β°	
	β-Thalassemia major	αααα β°/β°	Severe; transfusion dependent

Notation: α, normal α gene; ∎, severely suppressed α gene; β, normal β gene; β⁺, moderately suppressed β gene; β°, severely suppressed β gene.

increased HbA2 and sometimes HbF (see description of Hb analysis later in this chapter and in Chapter 2). In α-thalassemia (recall that the α chain is needed for all Hb types), the proportion of hemoglobins appears normal. These findings are usually sufficient for the diagnosis. If further definition is required, molecular genetic testing is available.

Folate Deficiency

Description

Folate and vitamin B_{12} deficiency (described next) are the classical causes of megaloblastic anemia. The term *megaloblastic* refers to the appearance of hematopoietic precursor cells in the marrow. Their nuclei appear abnormally large and immature, resulting from nuclear maturation that lags behind cytoplasmic maturation. This megaloblastic change affects not only erythroblasts but other rapidly dividing cells as well, including maturing granulocytes, megakaryocytes, and enterocytes. It results from impairment of DNA synthesis and has more than just morphologic consequences.

> Folate and vitamin B_{12} deficiency are the classical causes of megaloblastic anemia.

Erythropoiesis becomes ineffective, resulting in a hypercellular marrow. Many erythroblasts are destroyed while still in the marrow. Thus, megaloblastic anemia is in part a hemolytic anemia; indeed, intramedullary destruction of maturing erythrocytes leads to increased LDH and bilirubin, as one would associate with hemolytic anemia. The red cells that do proceed to maturity are macrocytic, with the MCV in fully developed megaloblastic anemia exceeding 115 fL.

Folate deficiency does not cause the same neurologic defect that vitamin B_{12} deficiency causes. However, supplementation of folate in early pregnancy is known to reduce the incidence of neural tube defects. No clear mechanism for this effect has been established.

Dietary factors are a major cause of folate deficiency. Folate is found in leafy green vegetables, fruits, and legumes. Dietary folate is absorbed in the duodenum, and the body stores about a 4- to 5-month supply of it. Thus, within a relatively short time, poor diet, malabsorption, or excessive utilization can lead to folate deficiency (**Table 10–10**).

Diagnosis

The blood smear shows the classic features of megaloblastic anemia: marked oval macrocytosis, hypersegmented neutrophils, and large platelets. The diagnosis can be confirmed by measuring the serum or RBC folate. However, there are several confounding factors in the use of these tests. Several balanced meals can quickly normalize the serum folate, but the RBC folate reflects folate status better over time. Vitamin B_{12} deficiency can produce a falsely low RBC folate, but it does not affect the serum folate.

Vitamin B_{12} Deficiency

Description

Like folate deficiency, vitamin B_{12} deficiency leads to megaloblastic anemia. The main difference between the two conditions is that B_{12} deficiency may also produce a degenerative neurologic syndrome, the manifestations of which are attributable to demyelination of and loss of nerve fibers within the dorsal columns. The neurologic symptoms include paresthesia, weakness, and an unsteady gait. It is critical to make the diagnosis of B_{12} deficiency and treat it appropriately, because these neurologic changes are not reversible.

Malabsorption is the major cause of vitamin B_{12} deficiency (**Table 10–11**), most commonly from pernicious anemia. Pernicious anemia is a deficiency in gastric intrinsic factor (IF) due to

TABLE 10–10   **Causes of Folate Deficiency**

Inadequate intake	Malnutrition, chronic alcoholism
Malabsorption	Celiac sprue, small bowel resection
Increased demand	Pregnancy, chronic hemolysis
Renal loss	Dialysis

TABLE 10–11   Causes of Vitamin B$_{12}$ Deficiency

Inadequate intake	Strict vegetarians
Malabsorption	Pernicious anemia, achlorhydria, gastrectomy, ileal disease or resection, *Diphyllobothrium* infestation
Increased demand	Pregnancy, chronic hemolysis
Impaired transport	Trancobalamin deficiency

an autoimmune assault on the gastric mucosa. Unlike folate deficiency, B$_{12}$ deficiency is rarely due to a poor diet. This is because (1) B$_{12}$ is abundant in a wide range of dietary sources and (2) the body stores several years worth of vitamin B$_{12}$. Dietary deficiency thus requires multiple years of a highly restrictive vegetarian diet.

Diagnosis

The blood smear shows the classic features of megaloblastic anemia: marked oval macrocytosis, hypersegmented neutrophils, and large platelets. The diagnosis can be confirmed by measuring serum B$_{12}$ levels.

Identifying the cause of the deficiency is the next step in the evaluation. The Schilling test is designed for this purpose. The patient is given a parenteral dose of unlabeled B$_{12}$ followed by an oral dose of radiolabeled vitamin B$_{12}$. The purpose of the unlabeled dose is to fully saturate the body with B$_{12}$ so that the radiolabeled dose will be quickly excreted in the urine. A 24-hour urine sample is then collected. A low level of urinary radioactivity confirms B$_{12}$ malabsorption, but it does not identify the specific gastrointestinal defect. The second part of the Schilling test is then undertaken. The patient is given another oral dose of radiolabeled B$_{12}$ in addition to oral IF. Patients with pernicious anemia will demonstrate enhanced absorption (increased urinary radio-activity) in this second part of the test. The Schilling test has been largely supplanted by serologic tests for autoantibodies, including anti-IF and antiparietal antibodies.

Lead Poisoning (Plumbism)

Description

Lead toxicity affects RBCs, renal epithelium, and the nervous system. It generally presents insidiously, with nonspecific features such as abdominal pain and cognitive impairment. However, it may present abruptly with vomiting, seizures, and altered mental status. In addition, lead poisoning may present as a microcytic, hypochromic anemia. Exposure to lead occurs through environmental sources, such as lead-based household paint, contaminated soil, lead plumbing, and manufacturing facilities.

Lead exerts its hematologic effects in two ways: inhibition of heme synthesis in the maturing erythrocyte and decreased survival of mature erythrocytes. Lead has a strong affinity for certain amino acids, particularly the sulfhydryl group of cysteine, and certain organelles, particularly mitochondria. Since heme synthesis takes place within mitochondria, and two enzymes instrumental in this process, delta-aminolevulinic acid dehydratase (δ-ALA) and ferrochelatase, are rich in the sulfhydryl groups, this process is exquisitely sensitive to lead. Ferrochelatase catalyzes the insertion of iron into the protoporphyrin ring. Its inhibition leads to the accumulation of free (iron-free) erythrocyte protoporphyrin (FEP), much of which binds nonenzymatically to zinc to form ZPP. Separate from its effects on heme synthesis, lead inhibits ATPase-driven sodium channels, leading to increased osmotic fragility and hemolysis. Lastly, lead inhibits the enzyme 5′-nucleotidase, leading to basophilic stippling.

> Lead exerts its hematologic effects in two ways: inhibition of heme synthesis in the maturing erythrocyte and decreased survival of mature erythrocytes.

Despite all these vulnerabilities, anemia does not develop until blood lead levels are above 50 μg/dL. A blood lead level >10 μg/dL is considered elevated. Iron deficiency enhances the effects of lead toxicity in two ways. The absence of iron enhances the blockage of the ferrochelatase step in heme synthesis, and in an effort to absorb more iron, the gastrointestinal absorption of lead increases.

Diagnosis

Basophilic stippling is noted in the peripheral blood smear and in maturing erythroblasts in the marrow. The Centers for Disease Control and Prevention has defined lead poisoning as a blood lead level >10 μg/dL. Elevations in FEP and ZPP do not occur until blood lead levels exceed 35 μg/dL; thus, these assays are not sufficiently sensitive to screen for lead poisoning.

The advantage of FEP measurement, however, is that it can be performed reliably on small finger- or heel-prick samples. Furthermore, this assay can easily identify patients grossly intoxicated with lead. Elevated FEP and ZPP are not specific for lead poisoning and may also be seen in iron deficiency.

Sickle Cell Anemia and Other Hemoglobinopathies

Description

A hemoglobinopathy is a structural defect in Hb, usually resulting from a germline single-nucleotide point mutation in one of the Hb genes. There are examples of postsynthetic modifications in normally formed Hb, such as carboxyhemoglobin from carbon monoxide poisoning. The common hemoglobinopathies are listed in **Table 10–12**. In the United States, HbS is the most common abnormal Hb, followed by HbC, and HbE. Worldwide, HbS remains most common, but is followed closely by HbE (which is very common in Southeast Asia), followed by Hbs C, D, and G. In all, several hundred structurally abnormal Hbs have been described.

Homozygous sickle cell anemia (genotype SS, sickle cell disease) is associated with abnormal polymerization of Hb in red cells, leading to a cell with an altered shape that is rapidly cleared from the circulation. Polymerization of HbS is enhanced in hypoxic conditions. While normal red cells have a life span of about 120 days, the red cells in SS have an average life span less than 30 days. Hb electrophoresis shows that the red cells contain mostly HbS, with small quantities of HbF and HbA2. The clinical course in HbSS patients is one of chronic hemolysis punctuated by a wide range of complicating events (often called crises). Chronic hemolysis leads to a chronic anemia with growth retardation, delayed puberty, impaired exercise tolerance, jaundice, and cholelithiasis (due to the formation of pigmented gallstones). The patients are usually in need of intermittent transfusions. Episodic complications include vaso-occlusive events (e.g., stroke, avascular necrosis of bone, splenic autoinfarction), splenic sequestration crises, aplastic crises (due most often to marrow infection with parvovirus B19), bacterial sepsis, and hyperhemolytic crises. The risk of bacterial infection is related to an underlying functional asplenia that affects most sickle cell patients by late childhood. This confers a particular susceptibility to infection by encapsulated bacterial organisms such as *Haemophilus influenzae* and *Streptococcus pneumoniae*. The most common cause of death in sickle cell disease is infection, followed by stroke and other thromboembolic events.

Heterozygotes (genotype SA, sickle cell trait) are essentially asymptomatic and have normal red cell indices. The presence of sickle Hb can be detected by Hb electrophoresis, where it is found to represent about 35% to 45% of total Hb. When exposed to hypoxic conditions such as high

In the United States, HbS is the most common abnormal Hb, followed by HbC, and HbE. Worldwide, HbS remains most common, but is followed closely by HbE (which is very common in Southeast Asia), followed by Hbs C, D, and G.

TABLE 10–12 **Common Hemoglobinopathies**

Hemoglobin Gene Defects	Definition
Hemoglobin S	Change in sixth amino acid of the β chain from glutamate to valine (β_6 glu → val)
Hemoglobin E	Change in 26th amino acid of β chain from glutamate to lysine (β_{26} glu → lys)
Hemoglobin C	Change in 6th amino acid of β chain from glutamate to lysine (β_6 glu → lys)
Hemoglobin D	Change in 121st amino acid of β chain from glutamate to glutamine (β_{121} glu → gln)
Hemoglobin G	Change in 68th amino acid of α chain from asparagine to lysine (α_{68} asn → lys)

altitude, these patients are at risk for splenic infarcts. Interestingly, patients who are double heterozygotes for HbS and β-thalassemia are more severely affected than heterozygous SA, having red cells that contain >50% HbS. Conversely, double heterozygotes for S-α-thalassemia manifest less HbS (<35%) and less severe symptoms.

HbE is relatively benign clinically, in both heterozygous and homozygous forms. Patients with HbE have red cell indices, however, that closely resemble those of a thalassemic patient (microcytic with high RBC count). HbE is prevalent in Southeast Asia. Double heterozygotes for S and E (SE disease) manifest moderate-to-severe hemolysis.

HbC disease (genotype CC) is generally associated with mild hemolysis, and heterozygotes (CA) are clinically normal. In both, target cells tend to be numerous in the peripheral smear. Patients who are doubly heterozygous for S and C (SC disease) have manifestations intermediate between SS and SA. While manifestations are generally milder than SS, there is a greater incidence of avascular necrosis of bone and retinal damage in SC than in SS. The peripheral blood film shows both sickle cells and target cells.

Hbs D and G are benign Hb variants. They can lead to confusion in interpreting an abnormal Hb electrophoresis, since they appear in the same location as HbS. However, these patients are clinically well.

Diagnosis

The identification of variant Hbs is usually performed with Hb electrophoresis. However, many laboratories now use high-performance liquid chromatography (HPLC). One limitation of both of these techniques is that several different variants can give similar results, although this is significantly less problematic in HPLC. Findings must be correlated with knowledge of the patient's clinical status and red cell indices before a definitive diagnosis can be rendered.

There are a number of screening tests for sickle Hb. These are based on the tendency of HbS to polymerize. A positive sickle screen is not specific for sickle cell disease, however, and can be present in sickle cell trait, SC disease, and Hb C$_{harlem}$. Furthermore, a negative screening test does not entirely exclude HbS, particularly in infants who may still have significant quantities of HbF, which inhibits polymerization of HbS.

Hereditary Spherocytosis
Description

HS was once known as hereditary hemolytic jaundice. The cardinal features are chronic hemolysis, jaundice, and splenomegaly. It is a fairly common condition, particularly among people of Northern European descent, in whom it is the most common inherited red cell disorder. In the United States the incidence is about 1 in 5000. HS is usually transmitted as an autosomal dominant trait, but about 25% of affected families display autosomal recessive inheritance. This variation derives from the fact that HS can be caused by any one of several defects in RBC cytoskeletal proteins, including band 3, protein 4.2, spectrin, and ankyrin. A deficiency in any of these components leads to cytoskeletal instability. Subsequently, there is loss of the biconcave shape in favor of the stoichiometrically more attainable sphere.

The plurality of underlying molecular defects also contributes to clinical heterogeneity, with phenotypes ranging from mild to severe. HS may present early as neonatal jaundice, or it may present in late childhood with splenomegaly and mild anemia. While anemia in some cases is quite severe, in most cases the hemolytic anemia is mild and well compensated by the marrow. Some patients require splenectomy, which usually results in clinical remission. However, splenectomy carries with it an increased susceptibility to bacterial sepsis. As HS patients age, they are at risk for pigmented gallstones.

HS was once known as hereditary hemolytic jaundice. Its cardinal features are chronic hemolysis, jaundice, and splenomegaly. It is a fairly common condition, particularly among people of Northern European descent, in whom it is the most common inherited red cell disorder.

Diagnosis

The peripheral blood film shows numerous spherocytes. These appear as red cells that lack central pallor. Larger polychromatophilic cells are often numerous, reflective of an increased reticulocyte count. While spherocytes are typically smaller than normal red cells, the MCV may be low, normal, or high, owing to reticulocytosis. The MCHC is characteristically increased.

When numerous spherocytes are observed on a peripheral blood film, the two primary considerations are immune hemolysis and HS. Immune hemolysis can usually be excluded with a negative direct antiglobulin test (DAT, Coombs test).

The osmotic fragility test can be useful in supporting the diagnosis of HS. However, spherocytes from any cause will result in a positive test.

Hereditary Elliptocytosis (HE)

Description

This autosomal dominant disorder is due to defective tetramerization of cytoskeletal spectrin, resulting in elliptocytes, also called ovalocytes. There are several clinical variants. The common type of HE is seen primarily in African Americans and manifests as a mild lifelong hemolytic anemia. Hereditary pyropoikilocytosis is a variant of HE in which RBCs are exquisitely sensitive to damage from heat. The peripheral blood smear is notable for a profound degree of poikilocytosis with red cells of every size and shape. This condition is usually most pronounced in infancy and tends to abate with age, giving way to a phenotype of common HE. A stomatocytic type of HE exists that is also called Southeast Asian ovalocytosis. This phenotype confers some protection against infection by *P. vivax* malaria.

Diagnosis

There is no specific laboratory test for HE. The diagnosis depends on finding elliptocytes in the peripheral blood. By definition, these cells are twice as long as they are wide, and in HE they comprise more than 25% of all red cells. Elliptocytes are not unique to HE and may be seen in iron deficiency anemia and thalassemia. The proportion of elliptocytes is usually much less than 25% in these other conditions, and they are easily excluded on other grounds. Once these are ruled out, the diagnosis is made of HE.

Autoimmune Hemolytic Anemia

Description

When an antibody attaches to a red cell, the consequences depend largely on the nature of the antibody. Some antibodies are capable of activating complement and producing brisk intravascular hemolysis. Others behave as opsonins, promoting red cell destruction in the spleen. Some antibodies react only in a cold environment, some only in warmth. Some coat the red cell and do nothing more.

These disorders present with the typical manifestations of anemia, with variable rates of onset. Mild splenomegaly is common when hemolysis is extravascular. Dark urine, abdominal or back pain, and fever may accompany intravascular hemolysis. In severe IgM-induced cold autoimmune hemolytic anemia (CAIHA), the skin may have a livedo reticularis pattern, and there may be acrocyanosis on exposure to cold.

Warm autoimmune hemolytic anemia (WAIHA) is mediated by IgG autoantibodies that optimally bind RBCs at body temperature (37°C). The red cell antigens most commonly the target in WAIHA are the Rh antigens. IgG molecules must form cross-links to activate complement, and the target red cell antigens in WAIHA are usually insufficiently dense on the red cell surface to permit this. A higher-density antigen is involved in a condition known as PCH, described below. Thus, IgG antibodies opsonize the red cell in WAIHA, leading to membrane damage mediated by splenic macrophages with the formation of small, spherocytic cells (microspherocytes). In some cases, there is concomitant immune thrombocytopenia, and this association is known as Evans syndrome.

CAIHA, also called cold agglutinin disease, is mediated by IgM antibodies that bind RBCs at lower temperature ranges. The target antigens are usually the red cell antigens I or i. Those binding over a limited thermal amplitude (e.g., 0°C to 22°C) will obviously not produce clinical consequences. However, these antibodies may cause difficulty in the laboratory, where studies are routinely carried out at room temperature, which could be within this thermal amplitude. Antibodies with broader thermal amplitude may bind to red cells in the extremities, where temperature falls a bit below core body temperature, resulting in acrocyanosis. IgM antibodies are capable of activating complement. Most often, the clinical consequence is a result of opsonization by C3, leading to extravascular hemolysis similar to that seen in WAIHA. C3-mediated hemolysis

> Warm autoimmune hemolytic anemia (WAIHA) is mediated by IgG autoantibodies that optimally bind RBCs at body temperature (37°C). CAIHA, also called cold agglutinin disease, is mediated by IgM antibodies that bind RBCs at lower temperature ranges.

TABLE 10–13   Drug-induced Immune Hemolytic Anemia

Mechanism	Drug absorption (hapten)	Immune complex	AIHA
Type of hemolysis	Extravascular	Intravascular	Extravascular
Implicated drugs	Penicillin Ampicillin Methicillin Carbenicillin Cephalothin	Quinidine Phenacetin Thiazides Rifampin Sulfonamides	α-Methyldopa Mefenamic acid L-DOPA Isoniazid Procainamide Hydralazine Ibuprofen

is more of a hepatic process than a splenic one. Sometimes, however, the complete complement cascade is activated on the cell surface, resulting in intravascular hemolysis.

Both WAIHA and CAIHA are often idiopathic conditions. However, a significant number are secondary to another underlying condition, including lymphoid neoplasms (e.g., chronic lymphocytic leukemia), medication use, systemic autoimmune diseases (e.g., systemic lupus erythematosus), immunodeficiency (e.g., common variable immunodeficiency), and infection (infectious mononucleosis, HIV, and *Mycoplasma pneumoniae*).

PCH is caused by IgG antibodies that are directed at the red cell P antigen. The antibody responsible for PCH is called the Donath–Landsteiner antibody. This particular IgG antibody has peculiar tendencies, including the binding of red cells in colder temperatures (in the blood of the extremities) and the activation of complement, producing intravascular hemolysis. Originally described in association with syphilis, the antibody now is more often seen in children with viral infections. Mortality can be quite high, up to 30%.

Drug-induced immune hemolytic anemia arises through several pathophysiologic mechanisms (**Table 10–13**). An antibody may be raised against a drug that is capable of adhering nonspecifically to the red cell membrane (drug adsorption or hapten mechanism). Second, drug–antibody immune complexes may coat the red cell surface (immune complex mechanism). What distinguishes these first two mechanisms is that the antibody is directed against the drug, not a red cell antigen. Lastly, a drug may be responsible for eliciting a true autoimmune hemolytic anemia, with antibody against red cell antigens. This condition is clinicopathologically indistinguishable from AIHA, and it may or may not abate when the drug is discontinued.

Lastly, alloimmune hemolytic anemia is due to transfusion of red cells bearing an antigen foreign to the recipient. Most responsible antibodies arise as a result of prior sensitization, commonly prior transfusion or pregnancy, and most cause extravascular hemolysis of mild-to-moderate severity. In the case of ABO antigens, the antibodies are naturally occurring, and prior sensitization is not required for there to be a problem. Furthermore, ABO antibodies produce severe intravascular hemolysis, which can be fatal.

Diagnosis

The DAT, also known as the direct Coombs test, is pivotal for the diagnosis of immune hemolysis. This test is capable of demonstrating the presence of antibodies or complement on the surface of RBCs.

Additional laboratory findings include anemia, reticulocytosis, indirect hyperbilirubinemia, decreased haptoglobin, and an increased LDH. The peripheral blood smear often demonstrates spherocytes, polychromasia, and, in severe cases, nucleated red cells. In cold agglutinin disease, red cell clumping is seen.

An important consequence of red cell antibodies is their tendency to interfere with pre-transfusion testing.

Hemolytic Disease of the Fetus and Newborn (HDFN)
Description

If there is mingling of fetal and maternal blood (a fetomaternal hemorrhage), then the mother can become sensitized to antigens of the fetal blood cells. Some of these antigens are paternal in

> Drug-induced immune hemolytic anemia arises through several pathophysiologic mechanisms.

origin and may therefore be foreign to the mother, and a maternal antibody reaction may occur. If the antibody idiotype produced is one that can cross the placenta (most IgG subtypes can cross the placenta, IgM cannot), it can produce fetal hemolysis.

The severity of fetal hemolysis depends on several factors, including the identity of the immunizing antigen and the titer of maternal antibody. The pregnancy that creates sensitization is usually spared, as the initial reaction produces largely IgM that does not cross the placenta. In subsequent pregnancies, an IgG-mediated anamnestic response may be raised, producing HDN. Furthermore, pregnancy-induced maternal sensitization may complicate future transfusions.

When this syndrome was first recognized, it was most commonly associated with antibodies to the Rh antigen known as D. This D antigen is the basis for categorizing blood types as Rh+ or Rh−. However, prevention strategies have reduced the incidence of RhD HDFN to about 0.1% of all pregnancies. The incidence of maternal anti-Kell antibody now exceeds that of anti-D antibodies in many centers.

If a pregnant woman does have antibodies against a fetal antigen, the fetus is at risk for HDFN. Mild HDFN may only manifest as compensated hemolysis in which fetal erythropoiesis is capable of keeping up with the rate of red cell destruction. Severe HDFN manifests with fetal anemia, hyperbilirubinemia, and numerous circulating nucleated RBCs (erythroblastosis fetalis). Hypoproteinemia may ensue, leading to decreased serum osmotic pressure, and severe edema (hydrops fetalis). A pregnancy in which there is known sensitization (maternal antibodies to fetal red cell antigens have been detected) must be monitored to determine the severity of fetal hemolysis.

> If a pregnant woman does have antibodies against a fetal antigen, the fetus is at risk for HDFN.

RhD HDFN is prevented by the administration of Rh immune globulin (RhIg) to Rh-negative women during pregnancy. The RhIg binds to and effectively conceals D antigenic sites, precluding an immune response. RhIg is given routinely at 28 weeks, at term, and whenever a fetomaternal hemorrhage is suspected (amniocentesis, trauma, abortion, abruption, etc.).

Diagnosis

Several laboratory tests support the diagnosis and treatment of HDFN. First is blood typing to confirm the maternal, paternal, and neonatal Rh status.

Second, in Rh-negative women, a screening test for antibodies must be performed. This is a test in which maternal serum is incubated with a panel of red cells having known antigenic status. If an alloantibody is detected, its titer is determined by serially diluting the sample until reactivity is abolished. If a titer of >1:32 is present, the risk of HDN is considered sufficiently high to warrant fetal monitoring.

In Rh-negative women with alloantibodies, the fetus must be monitored to determine the severity of hemolysis. Amniocentesis is performed to determine the quantity of amniotic fluid bilirubin. When low, monitoring is continued. When high, consideration is given to therapeutic intervention, including intrauterine transfusion and, when possible, delivery.

In Rh-negative women without antibodies, laboratory tests are available to confirm and quantify a fetomaternal hemorrhage. These include the Kleihauer–Betke test, the erythrocyte rosette test, and others. If positive, a dose of RhIg may be given.

Microangiopathic Hemolytic Anemias

Description

This group of disorders shares the ability to create a microvascular environment capable of shredding red cells. They do this usually by inducing endothelial injury and thrombosis, generating a jagged lattice of fibrin against which red cells are thrust with the pressure of arterial blood. The result is intravascular hemolysis and the appearance of schistocytes in the peripheral blood film. Often the creation of thrombi is so brisk that thrombocytopenia results. The disorders associated with MHA include disseminated intravascular coagulation (DIC), thrombotic thrombocytopenic purpura (TTP), hemolytic uremic syndrome (HUS), and the pregnancy-associated syndrome of hemolysis, elevated liver enzymes, and low platelets (HELLP). A similar clinical picture can be created by malignant hypertension and macrovascular red cell trauma caused by mechanical heart valves.

Diagnosis

The peripheral blood smear shows schistocytes and, usually, thrombocytopenia. The associated conditions are clinicopathologic diagnoses for which there is no single diagnostic test.

Glucose-6-phosphate Dehydrogenase (G6PD) Deficiency

Description

This is the most common red cell enzyme defect. Since red cells lack a nucleus, they lack the capacity to make new enzymes. Even normal red cells have greater enzymatic capacity when young than when old. However, if the activity of a critical enzyme significantly degrades before the average red cell life span (120 days), then the cell dies prematurely. Red cells rely on G6PD to produce glutathione that absorbs oxidant stress to protect Hb from oxidation. Oxidized Hb forms precipitates within the red cell, known as Heinz bodies, whose excision by splenic macrophages results in bite cells.

There are numerous defective forms (disease-causing alleles) of G6PD. Most abnormal alleles result in a functionally normal enzyme but have a shortened life span within the red cell. Uncommon alleles result in decreased G6PD production, and even young cells have low activity in these cases. In most forms of the disease, young red cells, especially reticulocytes, have normal G6PD activity, whereas, in other forms, enzyme activity is universally decreased. Furthermore, the magnitude of this decrease varies. This heterogeneity results in three classes of G6PD deficiency: class 1, in which there is chronic low-level hemolysis; class 2, in which there is profound intravascular hemolysis following oxidant stress; and class 3, in which there is mild-to-moderate intravascular hemolysis following oxidant stress.

> Most G6PD-deficient persons are clinically well until exposed to excess oxidant (class 2 or 3). Such exposures arise in the form of ingestion (e.g., fava beans), medication use (e.g., nitrofurantoin, antimalarials, sulfa drugs), or infection.

Most G6PD-deficient persons are clinically well until exposed to excess oxidant (class 2 or 3). Such exposures arise in the form of ingestion (e.g., fava beans), medication use (e.g., nitrofurantoin, antimalarials, sulfa drugs), or infection. In most individuals, there is preferential destruction of older red cells.

Diagnosis

The peripheral smear shows a combination of bite cells and Heinz bodies. The latter require special (supravital) staining in order to be visualized. Laboratory assays are available for measuring G6PD activity. G6PD activity may appear normal during an acute episode, because only nonhemolyzed, younger cells are available to be assayed. If a normal result is obtained, consider repeating the assay in 3 months.

Pyruvate Kinase (PK) Deficiency

Description

A steady generation of ATP is needed to maintain the integrity of the red cell membrane. Red cells generate ATP principally via the glycolytic pathway, in which PK is an active enzyme. Deficient ATP production leads to progressive red cell dessication, causing predominantly extravascular hemolysis.

PK deficiency is usually a recessively inherited condition. The disease is worldwide in distribution but slightly more concentrated in particular populations, notably people of Northern Europe descent and the Pennsylvania Amish.

Diagnosis

Echinocytes are the classic peripheral smear finding, but these appear in large numbers only after splenectomy. An autohemolysis test is positive and corrects with the addition of ATP. A fluorescent spot test is performed in which red cells are incubated with NADH (which fluoresces) to check for conversion to NAD (which does not).

Paroxysmal Nocturnal Hemoglobinuria

Description

Complement activation occurs at a low level continuously in the blood, and formed C3b that does not bind to an available surface (bacterium, leukocyte, platelet, or RBC) is rapidly degraded.

Bound C3b can proceed to induce lysis of the cell to which it is attached. Thus, blood cells must have a mechanism for regularly shedding C3b to avoid lysis.

PNH is due to an acquired (somatic) mutation in the *PIG-A* gene of a hematopoietic stem cell, the major consequence of which is decreased production of the glycosylphosphatidylinositol (GPI) anchor. This is a molecule that functions as a transmembrane anchor for several surface proteins, many of which are involved in protecting the cell from complement lysis. Affected cells have decreased expression of, among others, CD16 (the F(c) receptor type III), CD55 (decay-accelerating factor [DAF]), and CD59 (membrane inhibitor of reactive lysis [MIRL]). Since this defect is found within an early stem cell, all cell lines (red cells, white cells, platelets) are affected.

PNH manifests as hemolysis, and its severity oscillates. Hemoglobinuria reflects the intravascular nature of the hemolysis. While hemolysis tends to be episodic (paroxysmal), some patients experience chronic hemolysis of uniform intensity. Furthermore, exacerbations are not usually nocturnal as implied in the original description. PNH is associated with a thrombotic tendency that can be the initial manifestation. Over time the disease may evolve to or present as aplastic anemia.

> PNH is due to an acquired (somatic) mutation in the *PIG-A* gene of a hematopoietic stem cell, the major consequence of which is decreased production of the glycosylphosphatidylinositol (GPI) anchor.

Diagnosis

A sucrose hemolysis test or acidified serum (Ham) test may be used to screen for PNH. In these assays, patient blood is exposed to an environment that promotes complement activation. Enhanced hemolysis in the patient sample as compared with a normal control is interpreted as a positive test. The preferred diagnostic modality is flow cytometry, a test that allows quantitation of the surface proteins known to be diminished in PNH.

Sideroblastic Anemia

Description

In the developing erythrocyte, it is within mitochondria that iron is incorporated into porphyrin to make heme. Ringed sideroblasts are the morphologic expression of the abnormal sequestration of iron within mitochondria. When increased ringed sideroblasts are found, the differential diagnosis includes myelodysplastic syndrome, alcohol abuse, copper deficiency (Wilson disease), lead toxicity, medication effect (isoniazid, pyrazinamide), pyridoxine (vitamin B_6) deficiency, and hereditary sideroblastic anemia.

Diagnosis

In the peripheral blood, one finds anemia with a dimorphic red cell population, that is, there are normocytic macrocytes and hypochromic microcytes. The diagnosis of sideroblastic anemia requires a bone marrow biopsy. Nonringed sideroblasts, defined as red cell precursors with one to four faint siderotic granules, are normal in the marrow. Ringed sideroblasts are defined as red cell precursors with at least 10 siderotic granules that surround at least one-third of the nucleus. Although they may be seen in small number in some normal individuals and in a wide range of disorders, when they are found in >15% of all red cell precursors, the diagnosis of sideroblastic anemia is made.

Pure Red Cell Aplasia

Description

Aplastic anemia is a term that refers to the complete absence of hematopoiesis, affecting granulocytic precursors, erythroid precursors, and megakaryocytes. A proliferative disorder may be isolated to a single cell line, however, as is the case in pure red cell aplasia. This condition may be acquired or congenital. Acquired pure red cell aplasia may be due to thymoma, EPO therapy, or infection with parvovirus B19.

Parvovirus B19 may cause a transient arrest of red cell production in healthy children and adults without serious consequences. Infection usually lasts about 2 weeks, and in those with a normal red cell life span of 120 days, this usually goes unnoticed. However, in those with chronic hemolytic anemia, a transient arrest of erythropoiesis may be catastrophic. The virus infects erythroid progenitor cells, causing a maturation arrest at the pronormoblast stage. Marrow examination finds numerous giant pronormoblasts, a reduction of the more mature forms, and viral nuclear inclusions.

Congenital pure red cell aplasia (Blackfan–Diamond syndrome) is a rare, constitutional red cell aplasia, which usually becomes evident by the age of 5 years. Erythroid precursors in the marrow are typically low or absent. HbF is increased.

Diagnosis

The diagnosis is made in a patient with isolated anemia, which is usually normocytic, with reticulocytopenia. The bone marrow biopsy shows an isolated decrement in erythropoiesis.

ERYTHROCYTOSIS

Definition

Erythrocytosis was traditionally defined as persistent elevation in the RBC mass. Since RBC mass is not easily measured, the current WHO definition relies on Hb, specifically Hb above 18.5 g/dL in men and 16.5 g/dL in women.

Differential Diagnosis

The primary considerations are myeloproliferative neoplasms (MPNs; polycythemia vera [PV]), reactive (secondary) erythrocytosis, and spurious erythrocytosis due to dehydration (Gaisbock syndrome) (**Table 10–14**). Secondary polycythemia is associated with low PaO_2 states (such as smoking and living at high altitudes), abnormal Hb variants, and certain neoplasms (renal cell carcinoma, cerebellar hemangioblastoma) that produce elevated EPO.

Polycythemia Vera

Definition

PV is an MPN that is due to a clonal neoplastic proliferation of erythroid precursors. It presents at a mean age of 60, most commonly with hypertension, thrombosis, pruritus, erythromelalgia, or headache. The erythrocytosis is usually normocytic. Neutrophilia and basophilia are common, and sometimes thrombocytosis is present. The cause of death is most commonly thrombosis. Some patients, however, progress to acute leukemia.

Diagnosis

The diagnosis of PV is made according to strict criteria (**Table 10–15**). The RBC mass is measured using isotope dilution, in which a sample of patient red cells is labeled with a radioactive isotope and reinfused. The red cell mass can then be calculated from the degree of dilution of the labeled red cells. This direct measurement of the red cell mass distinguishes reduced plasma volume from a true absolute erythrocytosis.

TABLE 10–14   Polycythemia Vera versus Secondary Erythrocytosis

Parameter	Polycythemia Vera	Secondary Erythrocytosis
RBC mass	↑	↑
PaO_2	Normal	Normal to ↓
Leukocytes and basophils	Normal to ↑	Normal
LAP score	↑	Normal
Serum vitamin B_{12}	↑	Normal
Serum EPO	↓	↑
Serum iron/stainable iron	↓	Normal

LAP, leukocyte alkaline phosphatase; EPO, erythropoietin.

TABLE 10–15   Criteria for Polycythemia Vera: A1 + A2 + Any Other A Criterion or A1 + A2 + Any Two B Criteria

A1	Increased RBC mass or Hb >18.5 g/dL (men), >16.5 g/dL (women)
A2	Erythrocytosis is primary—no familial erythrocytosis, hypoxemia (PaO$_2$ <92%), high-affinity hemoglobin variant, truncated erythropoietin (EPO) receptor, or tumor that is producing EPO
A3	Splenomegaly
A4	Clonal cytogenetic abnormality other than Philadelphia chromosome
A5	Endogenous erythroid colony formation in vitro
B1	Thrombocytosis >400 × 10^6/μL
B2	WBC >12 × 10^6/μL
B3	Panmyelosis on bone marrow biopsy
B4	Low serum EPO

Examination of the bone marrow shows a marked expansion of erythroid precursors. In PV, erythroid precursors are capable of spontaneous erythroid colony formation in vitro. In testing for endogenous erythroid colony formation, patient marrow is cultured. In PV, one can observe the spontaneous formation of erythroid colonies (without addition of EPO). In healthy patients or those with secondary erythrocytosis, erythroid colony formation requires exogenous EPO.

The janus kinase 2 (*JAK-2*) mutation has now been identified in >80% of PV cases. The *JAK-2* mutation is a valine to phenylalanine substitution at codon 617 (Val617Phe) that appears to confer cytokine-independent growth to cells bearing it.

The janus kinase 2 (*JAK-2*) mutation has now been identified in >80% of PV cases.

METHODS

Red Cell Indices

Measurement of total Hb is carried out most commonly through a chemical reaction. In the cyanohemoglobin (hemiglobin cyanide [HiCN]) method, Hb is converted to HiCN whose concentration is measured by spectrophotometry. The absorbance of the solution at 540 nm reflects the amount of Hb originally present.

The Hct can be measured directly (manual technique) by centrifuging a tube of whole blood. The ratio of the packed red cell column height to the total height is the Hct. Note that the Hct is a unitless value (a percentage), as the units cancel out in its calculation.

Erythrocytes (as well as leukocytes and platelets) can be counted manually, through the use of a hemocytometer. This is a labor-intensive method that is still used when, for various reasons, the automated analyzer gives erroneous results. RBC counts may be given in terms of cells per mm^3 (e.g., 5.5 × 10^6/mm^3), per μL (conventional units), or per L (SI units). When the Hct and RBC count are determined manually, the remaining red cell indices can be calculated. For example, MCV = Hct × 1000/RBC. The MCV is stated in femtoliters.

Automated techniques are widely used in clinical laboratories. On most instruments, the red cell count, MCV, and RDW are measured directly (as is the total Hb). The instrument then calculates the other indices, such as Hct. There are at least three different methods used by automated instruments to count cells: impedance (counts any particle of given size), optical methods (light scatter), or combination of impedance and light scatter.

In impedance counting, cells are suspended in a conductive diluent and passed one-by-one through an aperture across which a current is flowing. A cell within the aperture causes a momentary increase in electrical resistance (impedance). Voltage, a product of resistance and current ($V = I \times R$), increases when the resistance increases. The instrument interprets a momentary increase in voltage as a single cell. The amount of voltage change is proportional to the size of the cell. The instrument is programmed to count particles measuring between 36 and 360 fL as red cells. Of course, leukocytes, which are within this size range, will be counted as erythrocytes, but their relative number is so small (usually) that their effect is typically negligible. RBCs passing through the aperture come in a range of sizes (volumes), distributed in a roughly Gaussian curve. The mean of this distribution is taken as the MCV. The variance in the curve is the RDW. The rest of the red cell indices can be calculated as follows: Hct = MCV × RBC; MCHC = Hb/Hct × 100.

Reticulocyte Counting

Reticulocytes can be measured manually or by automation. In the manual method, a blood smear is stained with a supravital dye (e.g., new methylene blue) that highlights the endoplasmic reticulum that persists within reticulocytes. Red cells and reticulocytes are counted, and the result is given as a percentage (number of reticulocytes per 100 red cells).

Automated methods are more accurate, since many more cells can be counted. A blood sample is incubated with a supravital dye, and then passed through an automated counter in which they are exposed to a laser. Light scatter (which will be greatest in stained reticulocytes) is used to enumerate the reticulocytes.

Normally reticulocytes constitute less than 1.5% of all red cells. This proportion increases when red cells are lost or destroyed peripherally, reflecting a marrow response. A normal reticulocyte count in the face of anemia is indicative of an impaired marrow.

However, the reticulocyte percentage can be somewhat misleading in the presence of anemia. This is because anemia leads to increased EPO production, and EPO stimulates the proliferation of red cell precursors and stimulates the release of reticulocytes from the marrow. Even if the marrow capacity for proliferation is impaired, the latter effect can produce a transient appearance of reticulocytosis. Thus, to correct for this, one can calculate the reticulocyte index (RI): RI = reticulocyte percentage × (patient's Hct/normal Hct). A normal RI is <3%.

Hemoglobin Analysis

Electrophoresis is the separation of proteins through the application of voltage. Most proteins have a net charge, usually a net negative charge, and when placed into a semisolid medium (a gel) will move in response to a voltage. The distance that a protein moves depends on its size and the magnitude of its charge, so that different proteins can be separated from one another. The positively charged electrode attracts negatively charged proteins and is called the anode. Proteins that end up closest to the anode are called fast-migrating or anodal. Proteins that end up farthest from the anode are considered slow-migrating or cathodal.

If RBCs are lysed, the predominant protein within the lysate is Hb. In the normal adult, this Hb is largely HbA, with about 2% to 3% HbA2. When this lysate is applied to a gel across which a voltage is applied, the result is a prominent band (HbA) near the anode (fast-migrating) and a dim band (HbA2) near the cathode. Any deviation from this pattern is indicative of a hemoglobinopathy or thalassemia. Routine Hb electrophoresis is performed by placing a sample of lysed blood on a cellulose acetate gel at pH 8.6 (alkaline electrophoresis). The gel is subjected to electromotive force, fixed, and stained.

> If RBCs are lysed, the predominant protein within the lysate is Hb. In the normal adult, this Hb is largely HbA, with about 2% to 3% HbA2.

Thalassemia, being a quantitative defect in production of entirely normal Hbs, does not produce abnormal bands on the electrophoresis. Instead, β-thalassemia is diagnosed by the presence of "thalassemic indices" (low Hct, increased RBC count, low MCV) and a quantitatively increased HbA2. α-Thalassemia has "thalassemic indices" and normal HbA2.

True hemoglobinopathies are due to production of a structurally abnormal Hb molecule that usually produces a distinct band on electrophoresis. The identity of most, but not all, abnormal Hbs can be determined by routine electrophoresis, particularly when supplemented with some clinical information and CBC data. When there is uncertainty, electrophoresis on citrate agar at pH 6.2 (acid electrophoresis) produces a different set of electrophoretic positions that, in combination with the alkaline gel, can help identify an abnormal band.

Separation of hemoglobins by electrophoresis is still common practice, although the use of HPLC and capillary electrophoresis is increasing.

Screening Tests for Sickle Hemoglobin

Rapid detection of sickling Hb, without having to perform electrophoresis, is possible with one of two types of assay. In the first, the Hb solubility (dithionate) test, one can detect insoluble forms of Hb within a lysate of blood. Red cells are lysed in sodium dithionate buffer with saponin. After several minutes, marked turbidity indicates a positive screen. Note that this test detects free Hb with altered solubility and may be positive in a number of different genotypes: SS, SA, SC, SD, and some types of HbC. This test may be negative when the concentration of HbS is too small, for example, in neonates.

The second type of screening test, the sickling (metabisulfite) test, detects red cells with sickling Hbs. In this test, whole blood is subjected to metabisulfite, which encourages cells containing HbS to sickle. A smear is then examined microscopically for sickling. Like the solubility test, this test does not give genotypic information and may be positive in SS, SA, SC, S-other, and some types of HbC. The test requires at least 10% HbS to be positive. Thus, it may not be positive in neonates or those very aggressively transfused.

> Rapid detection of sickling Hb, without having to perform electrophoresis, is possible with one of two types of assay.

Osmotic Fragility Test

All red cells expand and eventually undergo lysis in a hypotonic environment, and spherocytic red cells do so at a faster rate than normal biconcave red cells. This is the basis of the osmotic fragility test. Red cells are incubated in progressively more hypotonic solutions, parallel with normal controls. Enhanced lysis, as compared with controls, is a positive test. A positive osmotic fragility test is not diagnostic of HS, however, since red cells that are spherocytic from any cause will give a positive result. The most common acquired cause of red cell spherocytosis is autoimmune hemolytic anemia.

Direct Antiglobulin Test (Coombs Test)

The reagent used in this test is an antibody, obtained from rabbit or goat, that reacts with (binds to) human globulins (antihuman globulin [AHG]). Specifically, these antibodies may have reactivity with IgG, complement protein C3, or both. Patient blood is mixed with AHG and then observed for agglutination (clumping). Depending on the reagent used, agglutination suggests that the patient's red cells are coated with IgG, C3, or both. Furthermore, since these were not added to the red cells in vitro, agglutination indicates that coating occurred in vivo.

In the usual case of WAIHA, the red cells agglutinate mainly with anti-IgG. There may or may not be reactivity with anti-C3. In cold agglutinin disease, red cells agglutinate only with anti-C3. While the titer of a warm autoantibody provides little useful clinical information, the titer of a cold agglutinin can be helpful. The cold agglutinin titer is the highest dilution of patient serum that causes agglutination of normal RBCs.

Kleihauer–Betke Test

The Kleihauer–Betke (acid elution) test is based on the observation that a weak acid is capable of eluting normal HbA out of red cells. In contrast, HbF is resistant to acid elution and remains within red cells. Thus, if blood is subjected to a weak acid, and then smeared and stained, the cells containing HbA will appear as pale "ghosts," whereas cells containing HbF appear bright red. In a pregnant woman, the presence of red cells with HbF is indicative of a fetomaternal hemorrhage.

SELF-ASSESSMENT QUESTIONS

1. Which one of the following parameters of the complete blood count does not provide a measurement of red blood cell quantity?

   A. Hemoglobin
   B. Red blood cell count
   C. Mean corpuscular volume (MCV)
   D. Hematocrit

2. All but one of the following is an anemia associated with a defect in the maturation of the red blood cell. Which of the following is not associated with a maturation defect?

   A. Folate deficiency
   B. Iron deficiency
   C. Lead poisoning
   D. Immune hemolytic anemia

3. Which of the following causes of anemia is not associated with a high value for MCV?
   A. Vitamin B_{12} deficiency
   B. Iron deficiency anemia
   C. Folate deficiency
   D. Alcohol abuse

4. Which one of the four choices below corresponds to the description of the following inclusion in red blood cells?
   In a Wright stain peripheral blood smear, the inclusions are blue dots within red cells that are larger than basophilic stippling and represent iron-containing mitochondria; they are commonly found in patients who are asplenic.
   A. Heinz bodies
   B. Pappenheimer bodies
   C. Howell–Jolly bodies
   D. Cabot rings

5. Which one of the four choices below corresponds to the description of the following abnormal red blood cell?
   In a Wright stain peripheral blood smear, the red blood cells have an area of central pallor that is elongated in a mouth-like shape.
   A. Spherocytes
   B. Target cells
   C. Stomatocytes
   D. Acanthocytes (spur cells)

6. Which of the following abnormal blood cells is most likely to be found in a patient with immune hemolytic anemia?
   A. Spherocytes
   B. Target cells
   C. Elliptocytes
   D. Dacrocytes (teardrop cells)

7. One of the following choices is unlikely to be present in the patient suffering from intravascular hemolysis. Identify the choice more likely to be associated with extravascular hemolysis than intravascular hemolysis.
   A. Schistocytes
   B. Markedly decreased haptoglobin
   C. Increased urinary urobilinogen
   D. Increased free hemoglobin

8. Which of the following choices below is unlikely to be a cause of iron deficiency?
   A. Small bowel resection
   B. Colorectal cancer with chronic blood loss
   C. Strict vegetarian diet
   D. Pulmonary embolism

9. Identify the one test below which is unlikely to be informative in a patient being evaluated for iron deficiency anemia.
   A. Serum ferritin
   B. Serum iron
   C. White blood cell count
   D. Peripheral blood smear

10. Which is the most common cause of anemia in both hospitalized and ambulatory patients in the United States?
    A. Anemia of chronic disease
    B. Iron deficiency anemia
    C. Immune hemolytic anemia
    D. Sickle cell anemia

11. Which of the following genotypes below represents the α-thalassemia syndrome known as hemoglobin H, characterized by moderate-to-severe impairment of red blood cell production?
    A. One normal α gene, and three severely suppressed α genes; two normal β genes
    B. Two normal α genes, and two severely suppressed α genes; two normal β genes
    C. Four severely suppressed α genes; two normal β genes
    D. Three normal α gene, and one severely suppressed α gene; two normal β genes

12. Which of the following is associated with pernicious anemia?

    A. Folate deficiency
    B. Vitamin B$_{12}$ deficiency
    C. Lead toxicity
    D. Iron deficiency

13. Which of the following hemoglobinopathies, shown as the two types of hemoglobin present in the red blood cells, is the most clinically severe disease?

    A. Hemoglobin S/Hemoglobin A
    B. Hemoglobin C/Hemoglobin C
    C. Hemoglobin S/Hemoglobin S
    D. Hemoglobin E/Hemoglobin E

14. Cold autoimmune hemolytic anemia (CAIHA), also called cold agglutinin disease, is mediated by antibodies that bind red blood cells at lower temperature ranges (well below 37°C). What is the antibody type that binds to the red blood cells to produce CAIHA?

    A. IgG
    B. IgM
    C. IgA
    D. IgE

15. Three of the drugs below have long been associated with drug-induced hemolytic anemia. Select the one which is not commonly associated with drug-induced hemolytic anemia.

    A. Erythromycin
    B. Penicillin
    C. α-Methyl dopa
    D. Quinidine

16. There are several laboratory tests that support the diagnosis of hemolytic disease of the newborn in Rh-negative women. Among the choices below, only one of the tests is not useful in this evaluation. Identify this test.

    A. A screening test for red blood cell antibodies in the mother's plasma or serum.
    B. The fetus must be monitored for severity of hemolysis, which may involve collection of amniotic fluid by amniocentesis.
    C. A Kleihauer–Betke test is useful to confirm and quantify the severity of fetomaternal hemorrhage.
    D. A screening test for antibodies to red blood cell antigens in the father's plasma or serum.

17. Which of the following statements about glucose-6-phosphate dehydrogenase (G6PD) deficiency-associated anemia is not true?

    A. Most G6PD-deficient patients are well until exposed to excess oxidant.
    B. The peripheral blood smear shows a combination of target cells and sickle cells.
    C. One ingested oxidant recognized to produce a hemolytic response in G6PD patients is fava beans.
    D. Red blood cells depend on G6PD to produce glutathione which neutralizes oxidant stress to prevent oxidation of hemoglobin.

18. Which of the following is true about sideroblastic anemia?

    A. Red blood cells known as sideroblasts contain mitochondria with abnormal sequestration of iron.
    B. The primary defect in sideroblastic anemia is the absence of the enzyme pyruvate kinase.
    C. Sideroblastic anemia shows episodic (paroxysmal) hemolysis.
    D. Sideroblastic anemia is associated with a complete absence of hematopoiesis.

19. Polycythemia vera is associated with which mutation below in more than 80% of cases?

    A. *btk* mutation
    B. Janus kinase 2 (*Jak-2*) mutation
    C. Prothrombin 20210 mutation
    D. α-Globin gene mutation

20. A person with no apparent disease provides a sample for hemoglobin electrophoresis. The most prominent band on the gel represents which of the following?

    A. α-Globin chain
    B. Hemoglobin A$_2$
    C. β-Globin chain
    D. Hemoglobin A

21. Which of the following is a test to assess red blood cell lysis in a hypotonic environment?

    A. The direct antiglobulin test
    B. The osmotic fragility test
    C. The Kleihauer–Betke test
    D. The sickle cell hemoglobin screening test

FURTHER READING

Annibale B, et al. Gastrointestinal causes of refractory iron deficiency anemia in patients without gastrointestinal symptoms. *Am J Med*. 2001;111:439–445.

Beutler E. The common anemias. *JAMA*. 1988;259:2433.

Beutler E, Waalen J. The definition of anemia: what is the lower limit of normal of the blood hemoglobin concentration? *Blood*. 2006;107:1747–1750.

Bianchi P, Fermo E, Vercellati C, et al. Diagnostic power of laboratory tests for hereditary spherocytosis: a comparison study on 150 patients grouped according to the molecular and clinical characteristics. *Haematologica*. 2012; 97:516–523.

Bilgrami S, Greenberg BR. Polycythemia rubra vera. *Semin Oncol*. 1995;22:307.

Bolton-Maggs PH, Langer JC, Iolascon A, et al. Guidelines for the diagnosis and management of hereditary spherocytosis—2011 update. *Br J Haematol*. 2012;156:37–49.

Bowie LJ, et al. Alpha thalassemia and its impact on other clinical conditions. *Clin Lab Med*. 1997;17:97.

Cash JM, Sears DA. The anemia of chronic disease: spectrum of associated diseases in a series of unselected hospitalized patients. *Am J Med*. 1989;87:638–644.

Fitzsimons EJ, et al. Erythroblast iron metabolism and serum soluble transferrin receptor values in the anemia of rheumatoid arthritis. *Arthritis Rheum*. 2002;47:166–171.

Gehrs BC, Friedberg RC. Autoimmune hemolytic anemia. *Am J Hematol*. 2002;69:258–271.

Geifman-Holtzman O, et al. Female alloimmunization with antibodies known to cause hemolytic disease. *Obstet Gynecol*. 1997;89:272–275.

Goddard AF, et al. Guidelines for the management of iron deficiency anaemia. British Society of Gastroenterology. *Gut*. 2000;46(suppl 3–4):IV1–IV5.

Harkness UF, Spinnato JA. Prevention and management of RhD isoimmunization. *Clin Perinatol*. 2004;722:721–742.

Kettaneh A, et al. Pica and food craving in patients with iron-deficiency anemia: a case-control study in France. *Am J Med*. 2005;118:185–188.

Lane PA. Sickle cell disease. *Pediatr Clin North Am*. 1996;43:639.

Manci EA, et al. Causes of death in sickle cell disease: an autopsy study. *Br J Haematol*. 2003;123:359–365.

Marchand A, et al. The predictive value of serum haptoglobin in hemolytic disease. *JAMA*. 1980;243:1909–1911.

Nilsson-Ehle H, et al. Blood haemoglobin values in the elderly: implications for reference intervals from age 70 to 88. *Eur J Haematol*. 2000;65:297–305.

Nissenson AR. Prevalence and outcomes of anemia in rheumatoid arthritis: a systematic review of the literature. *Am J Med*. 2004;116:50S–57S.

Perrotta PL, Snyder EL. Non-infectious complications of transfusion therapy. *Blood Rev*. 2001;15:69–83.

Rivera S, et al. Hepcidin excess induces the sequestration of iron and exacerbates tumor-associated anemia. *Blood*. 2005;105:1797–1802.

Rosse WF, Ware RE. The molecular basis of paroxysmal nocturnal hemoglobinuria. *Blood*. 1995;86:3277.

Wilson A, et al. Prevalence and outcomes of anemia in inflammatory bowel disease: a systematic review of the literature. *Am J Med*. 2004;116:44S–49S.

Wolf AW, et al. Effects of iron therapy on infant blood lead levels. *J Pediatr*. 2003;143:789–795.

Bleeding and Thrombotic Disorders

Elizabeth M. Van Cott and Michael Laposata

LEARNING OBJECTIVES

1. Learn the basic molecular events in clot formation and fibrinolysis.

2. Understand the basic classification of disorders in hemostasis.

3. Identify the appropriate laboratory tests for evaluation of the bleeding patient and the thrombotic patient.

4. Learn the prominent clinical and laboratory features of the individual disorders of hemostasis.

CHAPTER OUTLINE

The coagulopathies are grouped into disorders of bleeding and thrombosis. The hemorrhagic diseases are further subdivided into the two major categories of coagulation factor disorders and platelet disorders. To understand the diseases with abnormal coagulation that follow, a brief introduction to normal hemostasis precedes the discussions of the diseases.

INTRODUCTION TO HEMOSTASIS

Normal hemostasis is the controlled activation of coagulation factors and platelets leading to clot formation, with subsequent clot lysis, in a process that stops hemorrhage without excess clotting (thrombosis). Effective hemostasis is a rapid and localized response to an interruption in vascular integrity (vessel wall injury), such that clots are formed only when and where they are needed.

Clot Formation

Clot formation involves platelet activation and the subsequent generation of fibrin via the coagulation cascade. The two processes are discussed separately in the sections that follow.

Platelet Plug Formation

Platelet plug formation is initiated in vivo by exposure of platelets to vascular subendothelium when a vessel is injured. The platelets adhere to the subendothelium, spread out along the surface, and release substances that promote the aggregation of other platelets at that site. The platelets also accelerate fibrin clot formation by providing a reactive surface for several steps in the coagulation cascade.

Adhesion of platelets to the subendothelial surface is facilitated by a plasma protein, von Willebrand factor (vWF), especially in vessels with high shear forces (e.g., the fast blood flow in arteries has a higher shear force than slow blood flow in veins). vWF binds to a specific receptor on the platelet surface. Deficiency of vWF results in poor adherence of platelets to subendothelium. The severity of bleeding in von Willebrand disease (vWD) varies widely among patients. Another related platelet adhesion defect occurs in patients whose platelets lack the receptor for vWF. This bleeding disorder, known as Bernard–Soulier disease, results from an inability of platelets to bind vWF.

Platelet activation occurs from interaction of platelet agonists, most of which are soluble, with specific receptors on the platelet membrane. Physiologically important agonists include adenosine diphosphate (ADP), thrombin, epinephrine, collagen, and thromboxane A_2, which is derived from arachidonic acid. A sequence of membrane and cytoplasmic events is initiated by the agonist–receptor interaction, involving an increase in cytoplasmic calcium ion concentration and a platelet shape change from a disc to a spiny sphere. The change in cytoplasmic calcium concentration leads to contractile events in the platelet, causing alpha and delta granules (also known as dense bodies) to fuse with the platelet plasma membrane and release their granule contents into the extracellular space. Successful granule release requires the formation of thromboxane A_2 from endogenous arachidonate via the enzyme cyclooxygenase. This enzyme is inhibited irreversibly by aspirin and inhibited reversibly by a number of other anti-inflammatory agents. Treatment with aspirin can cause a platelet secretion defect (reduced release of granule contents) that is often clinically significant in patients with underlying coagulopathies. Alpha granules contain vWF, fibrinogen, Factor V, two platelet-specific proteins—platelet factor 4 (PF4) and beta-thromboglobulin—as well as a number of other proteins. Delta granules contain serotonin, adenosine triphosphate (ATP), ADP, pyrophosphate, polyphosphate, and calcium. The release of some of these substances, in particular ADP, activates unstimulated platelets nearby. Absence or deficiency of alpha or delta granules occurs as a feature of several congenital and acquired platelet function disorders, collectively known as storage pool disorders. Individuals whose platelets possess appropriate numbers of intact granules that cannot be released on appropriate stimulation have a platelet release defect, and on that basis also may have a bleeding tendency. Aspirin is a common cause of a platelet release defect, because it impairs thromboxane production.

Release of platelet granule contents is followed by platelet aggregation, that is, the binding of platelets to one another to form the platelet plug. Normal aggregation requires fibrinogen binding to platelets via the fibrinogen receptor, which is the glycoprotein IIb/IIIa complex (GP IIb/IIIa), on the platelet surface. Congenital absence of GP IIb/IIIa results in a bleeding diathesis known as Glanzmann thrombasthenia (GT).

The platelet surface serves as a site for certain coagulation pathway enzyme reactions (see below). For example, the platelet membrane can bind the Factor Xa/Factor Va complex that activates prothrombin to thrombin. Thus, platelet activation and fibrin formation via the coagulation cascade are interactive biological processes.

Clot formation involves platelet activation and the subsequent generation of fibrin via the coagulation cascade.

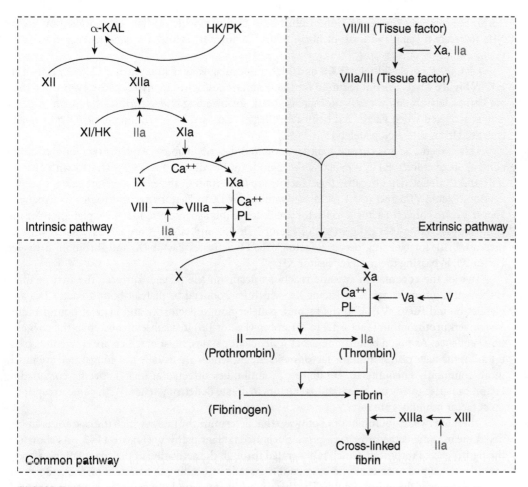

FIGURE 11–1   **The coagulation cascade. α-KAL, alpha-kallikrein; PK, prekallikrein; HK, high-molecular-weight kininogen; PL, phospholipid.**

Fibrin Clot Formation

The coagulation factor pathway is an enzymatic cascade with sequential conversion of proenzymes (zymogens) to fully activated enzymes, which then convert other zymogens to their activated forms (**Figure 11–1**). The final steps directly preceding fibrin formation can be activated through both the intrinsic and extrinsic pathways; hence, this part of the pathway is called the common pathway. Numerous positive and negative feedback mechanisms exist in the coagulation pathways so that the cascades do not proceed in an uncontrolled fashion. The pathways are now known to be extremely complex, with multiple interactions between factors in the intrinsic, extrinsic, and common pathways. The following description is a version of coagulation factor interactions that highlights the fundamental reactions.

The coagulation cascade is activated by the appearance of tissue factor (also historically known as Factor III), which is not normally exposed. Tissue factor is presented when a blood vessel is injured. It binds with Factor VII and small amounts of circulating active Factor VII (Factor VIIa), resulting in a complex of Factor VII or VIIa and tissue factor. The Factor VII in the complex can be autoconverted to Factor VIIa, resulting in a greater number of Factor VIIa–tissue factor complexes. This complex activates Factor IX to Factor IXa in the intrinsic pathway, with some activation of Factor X to Factor Xa in the common pathway. Factor IXa, with support from Factor VIII as a cofactor (or Factor VIIIa, which is a much more effective cofactor), activates Factor X to Factor Xa. Factor Xa with the assistance of Factor V or, more effectively Factor Va, converts prothrombin (Factor II) to thrombin (Factor IIa). At this point, the coagulation cascade is markedly amplified because thrombin activates Factor VIII to Factor VIIIa, a more effective cofactor, and activates Factor V to its more effective Factor Va form. In addition, thrombin activates Factor XI to Factor XIa, which, like Factor VIIa and tissue factor, activates Factor IX to Factor IXa.

Thrombin catalyzes the conversion of fibrinogen to fibrin, which is then cross-linked by Factor XIII to create a stabilized form of fibrin (clot). Factor XIII is also activated to Factor XIIIa by thrombin.

Factor XII, prekallikrein (PK), and high-molecular-weight kininogen (HMWK, shown as HK in **Figure 11–1**) are not required for the generation of fibrin in vivo because even when they are completely absent, there is no increased risk for bleeding. Nevertheless, the intrinsic pathway is activated when Factor XII contacts collagen (exposed by vessel injury) or polyphosphate (released from activated platelets).

This cascade, as it is currently understood and described above, explains two long-standing clinical observations. First, it explains the significant bleeding tendency associated with Factors VIII and IX deficiencies because these factors are important in the early stages of cascade amplification. Factor VIIa and tissue factor activate Factor IX to Factor IXa, and Factor IXa requires Factor VIII to convert Factor X to Factor Xa. Second, this scheme provides an explanation for the clinical observation that deficiencies of Factor XII, PK, and HMWK are not associated with an increased risk for bleeding because Factor VIIa/TF activates Factor IX, and thrombin activates Factor XI, bypassing the need for Factor XII.

Two of the coagulation cascade reactions occur on the platelet surface. The first of these is the activation of Factor X to Factor Xa, which is produced by platelet-bound Factor IXa and platelet-bound Factor VIIIa. In the second, platelet-bound Factor Xa and platelet-bound Factor Va convert prothrombin (Factor II) to thrombin (Factor IIa) in a subsequent step in the coagulation sequence. As noted below, single factor deficiency states, most of which are congenital, exist for all of the factors, but multiple factor deficiencies, which are usually not congenital, are much more commonly encountered. Inhibitors, as antibodies directed against a specific coagulation factor, can arise to any of the individual factors to create deficiency states. With some exceptions, most factor inhibitors are rare.

There are two major inhibitory pathways that determine the rate at which the cascade is amplified. One of these is the protein C–protein S anticoagulant pathway (**Figure 11–2**). As shown in the figure, excess thrombin, which is generated through the activation of the coagulation cascade, provides the signal to shut off the coagulation cascade by binding to a protein on the endothelial surface known as thrombomodulin. The thrombin/thrombomodulin complex converts protein C into its activated form. The activated protein C then binds free protein S as a cofactor. Protein S may be bound to C4b-binding protein and to a limited number of other proteins, in which case protein S becomes inactive. Once free (unbound) protein S binds to activated protein C, the activated protein C/protein S complex then proteolytically degrades Factors Va and VIIIa, reducing the flux through the coagulation cascade by removing these two activated cofactors. A mutation in the Factor V molecule, known as the Factor V Leiden mutation, makes Factor V resistant to proteolytic degradation by the activated protein C/protein S complex. This condition is known as activated protein C resistance. This permits the prothrombotic action of Factor Va to persist and contribute to a hypercoagulable state.

> There are two major inhibitory pathways that determine the rate at which the cascade is amplified. One of these is the protein C–protein S anticoagulant pathway. An additional mechanism for control of the coagulation cascade involves the inhibitory action of antithrombin.

An additional mechanism for control of the coagulation cascade involves the inhibitory action of antithrombin (formerly known as antithrombin III) (**Figure 11–3**). Antithrombin has a limited anticoagulant effect on its own, but in the presence of heparin or selected other negatively charged heparin-like molecules, antithrombin adopts a new conformation that increases its inhibitory activity 1000-fold, permitting it to inhibit most of the activated coagulation factors in complexes where both antithrombin and heparin bind to the activated coagulation factor. Inhibition of Factor Xa, however, does not require the direct binding of the activated coagulation factor by heparin. Factor Xa can be neutralized when it is bound only to antithrombin, after antithrombin has been activated by heparin or related molecule. The antithrombotic action of short chains of heparin (low-molecular-weight heparin) is directed primarily against Factor Xa because short heparin chains inhibit predominantly only Factor Xa (longer chains are required for Factor IIa inhibition). Fondaparinux, a synthetic heparin-related pentasaccharide, inhibits Factor Xa exclusively. Apixaban, betrixaban, edoxaban, and rivaroxaban are new anticoagulants that inhibit factor Xa directly, without antithrombin involvement.

It should be noted that all of the coagulation factors in the coagulation cascade are synthesized in the liver, and that the activity of Factors II, VII, IX, and X is vitamin K-dependent. Tissue factor is constitutively expressed on some cell types, and in other cell types, such as endothelial

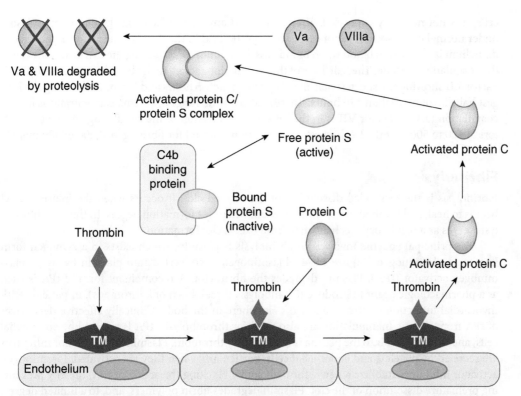

FIGURE 11–2 The protein C–protein S anticoagulant pathway. TM, thrombomodulin. (Redrawn with permission from Van Cott EM, Laposata M. Laboratory evaluation of hypercoagulable states. *Hematol Oncol Clin North Am.* 1998;12:1141–1166.)

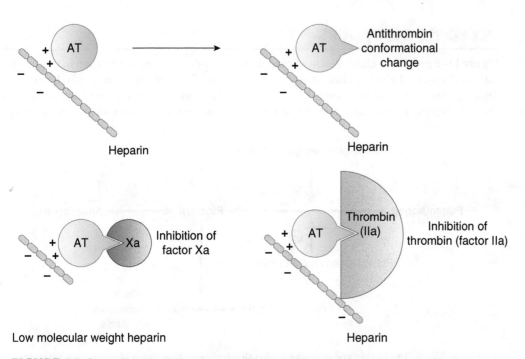

FIGURE 11–3 The anticoagulant action of antithrombin. AT, antithrombin. (Modified with permission from Kabakibi A, et al. The hypercoagulable state. *Turnaround Times* [a newsletter for physicians at the Massachusetts General Hospital, Boston]. 1994;3:1:1.)

Fibrinolysis is the controlled dissolution of the formed clot. It occurs when the injured vessel begins to heal, and is initiated to a limited extent when clot formation begins. In this way, fibrinolysis serves as a regulatory mechanism to limit excess clot formation.

cells, it is not normally expressed. There is little (if any) tissue factor in the circulating plasma under normal conditions. It is not exclusively synthesized in the liver. Tissue factor in the subendothelium is exposed to blood when blood vessels are injured, triggering the extrinsic pathway of the coagulation cascade. The half-lives of the coagulation factors in the blood vary markedly, with Factor VII showing the shortest half-life of approximately 5 hours and Factor XIII having the longest half-life of more than 120 hours. There is also a wide range of plasma concentrations for the coagulation factors. Factor VII is in the lowest concentration of the circulating coagulation factors at 100 to 500 ng/mL. The highest concentration is found for fibrinogen at 200 to 400 mg/dL.

Fibrinolysis

Fibrinolysis is the controlled dissolution of the formed clot. It occurs when the injured vessel begins to heal, and is initiated to a limited extent when clot formation begins. In this way, fibrinolysis serves as a regulatory mechanism to limit excess clot formation.

The principal enzyme involved in fibrinolysis is plasmin, which exists in a zymogen form known as plasminogen (**Figure 11–4**). Plasminogen is converted into plasmin by tissue plasminogen activator (tPA). Plasmin degrades the fibrin clot. A recombinant form of tPA is used as a pharmacologic agent to produce thrombolysis (breakdown of a thrombus), in patients with myocardial infarction or stroke, and clots elsewhere in the body. Clinically effective derivatives of tPA from genetic manipulation are also used for thrombolysis. tPA is released by endothelial cells, and its secretion into the plasma is increased by thrombin. Plasminogen activator inhibitors are secreted by platelets and endothelial cells, particularly when they are activated. Plasminogen activator inhibitors stabilize a newly formed clot by blocking the action of tPA, thereby preventing premature dissolution of the clot. Plasmin degrades fibrin polymers, and, to a limited degree, fibrinogen as well, by specific and sequential proteolytic cleavages, generating fibrin degradation products (FDP). These FDP (fragments X, Y, D, D-dimer, and E) may be detected in the plasma of patients experiencing fibrinolysis. Deficiency of plasminogen may predispose to thrombosis, and deficiency of plasminogen activator inhibitor may increase the risk for bleeding. Antiplasmin inhibits plasmin, but only when it is circulating and not when it is clot-bound. This prevents the circulation of a proteolytically active form of plasmin, while permitting clot lysis to proceed by plasmin within the clot. Deficiency of antiplasmin may result in a hemorrhagic tendency.

BLEEDING DISORDERS

Figure 11–5 provides a classification of coagulation disorders. The major division in the classification is between disorders associated with bleeding and disorders associated with thrombosis. There are two major subdivisions of bleeding disorders—those associated with coagulation factor and fibrinolytic pathway factor deficiencies, and those associated with an abnormal platelet

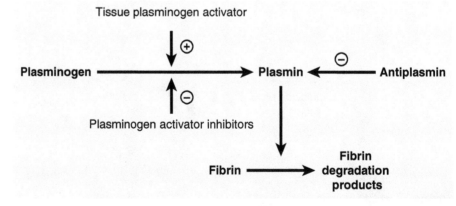

FIGURE 11–4 **The fibrinolytic pathway. A plus sign indicates that tissue plasminogen activator converts plasminogen into plasmin. A minus sign indicates inhibitory action. (Redrawn with permission from Kabakibi, A et al. The hypercoagulable state. *Turnaround Times* [a newsletter for physicians at the Massachusetts General Hospital, Boston]. 1994;3:1:1.)**

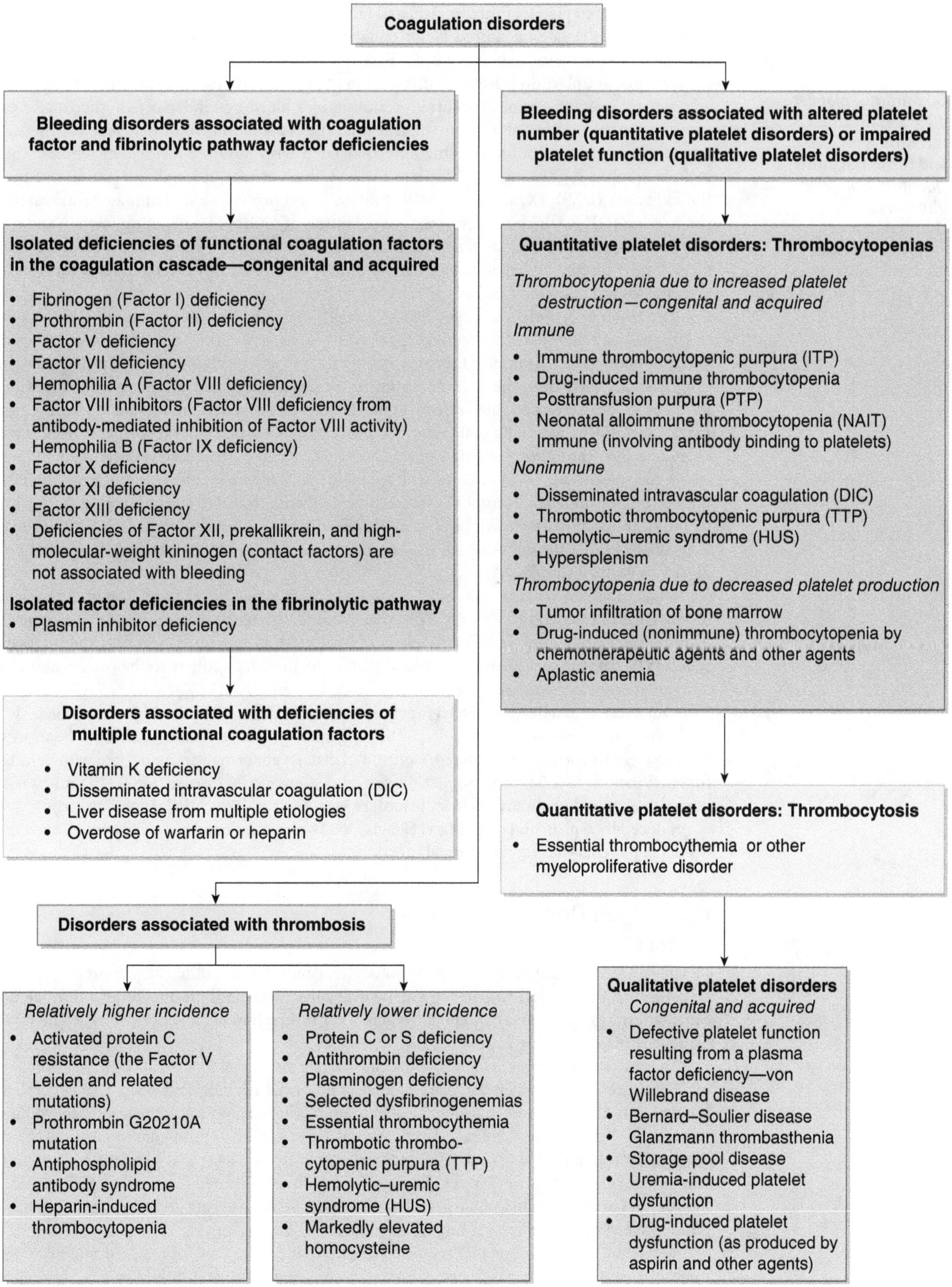

FIGURE 11–5 A classification of coagulation disorders.

Quantitative platelet disorders include thrombocytopenia and thrombocytosis. *Qualitative platelet disorders* are characterized by abnormal platelet function in the presence of a normal platelet count.

count or impaired platelet function. Isolated factor deficiencies are usually congenital, although occasionally an isolated acquired factor deficiency develops. An example of an acquired isolated coagulation factor deficiency is the Factor X deficiency associated with amyloidosis. The deficiency of antiplasmin is listed in this section because its absence permits increased plasmin activity and overactive clot dissolution, resulting in a bleeding tendency. Another major category of coagulation factor abnormalities is multiple coagulation factor deficiencies. There are several commonly encountered situations associated with multiple factor deficiencies. These include vitamin K deficiency or warfarin intake (which results in a reduced amount of functional Factors II, VII, IX, and X as well as protein C and protein S); disseminated intravascular coagulation (DIC), which results in the consumption of multiple coagulation factors; and liver disease that results in decreased synthesis of coagulation factors. Several activated coagulation factors are inhibited by heparin. Heparin administration results in inactivation of most of the activated coagulation factors.

The group of disorders associated with platelets is divided first into quantitative platelet disorders and qualitative platelet disorders. *Quantitative platelet disorders* include thrombocytopenia and thrombocytosis. Thrombocytopenia can be produced as a result of increased platelet destruction, from a variety of immune or nonimmune causes, or decreased platelet production. Common causes of decreased platelet production include tumor infiltration of bone marrow from metastases or a hematologic malignancy, and drug-induced thrombocytopenia as occurs with chemotherapy. Thrombocytopenia can also occur as a result of increased sequestration of platelets in the spleen, usually in patients with splenomegaly. Thrombocytosis is much less common than thrombocytopenia. Thrombocytosis can be divided into reactive thrombocytosis, in which there is a transiently increased number of platelets from a stimulus to increase platelet production, or neoplastic thrombocytosis, as seen in myeloproliferative disease and, less commonly, myelodysplastic disorders.

Qualitative platelet disorders are characterized by abnormal platelet function in the presence of a normal platelet count. vWD is a disorder in which there is defective platelet function, but from a defect originating outside the platelet, since vWF is generated primarily in endothelial cells. vWF coats the surface of the activated platelet to allow it to adhere to the cut vessel surface and initiate platelet plug formation.

Other causes of defective platelet function result from abnormalities within the platelet. These disorders may be congenital or acquired. The congenital ones are extremely rare, and the acquired ones are very frequently encountered. Congenital platelet abnormalities associated with defective function include GT, Bernard–Soulier disease, and storage pool disease (SPD). The much more common acquired qualitative platelet disorders include drug-induced platelet dysfunction, such as produced by aspirin and clopidogrel (Plavix), and uremia-induced platelet dysfunction, which occurs in patients with impaired renal function.

Fibrinogen Deficiencies

Description

Fibrinogen is produced in the liver by hepatocytes. Abnormalities of fibrinogen production may be congenital or acquired and, in general, involve either decreased production of a normal molecule (afibrinogenemia and hypofibrinogenemia) or production of an abnormal molecule (dysfibrinogenemia) (see **Table 11–1**).

In *congenital afibrinogenemia and hypofibrinogenemia*, there is a reduced (hypofibrinogenemia) or absent (afibrinogenemia) production of a normal fibrinogen molecule. In general, the homozygous deficiency results in afibrinogenemia, and the heterozygous state results in hypofibrinogenemia. Both disorders are rare. Homozygotes suffer a mild-to-moderate spontaneous bleeding tendency. Manifestations include umbilical stump hemorrhage and bleeding from mucous membranes, among many other possible signs and symptoms related to blood loss. Severe bleeding may occur with trauma or surgery. Hypofibrinogenemic patients are usually asymptomatic, but may bleed significantly with surgery or trauma.

Congenital dysfibrinogenemia is a result of inheritance of a gene for an abnormal fibrinogen molecule, which is produced in normal or near-normal quantities. All the fibrinogen produced by a homozygote for dysfibrinogenemia is abnormal, and approximately half of the fibrinogen

TABLE 11-1   Laboratory Evaluation for Fibrinogen Deficiencies

| Laboratory Test | Results/Comments | | | |
| | Quantitative Deficiencies | | Dysfibrinogenemia (Qualitative Deficiencies) | |
	Afibrinogenemia	Hypofibrinogenemia	Homozygous	Heterozygous
PT	Markedly prolonged	Normal to slightly prolonged	Markedly prolonged	Slightly prolonged to normal
PTT	Markedly prolonged	Normal to slightly prolonged	Markedly prolonged	Slightly prolonged to normal
Functional fibrinogen	Low	Slightly low to normal	Low	Slightly low to normal
Immunologic fibrinogen	Low	Slightly low to normal	Normal	Normal
Thrombin time	Prolonged	Normal to prolonged	Prolonged	Prolonged
Reptilase time	Prolonged	Normal to prolonged	Prolonged	Prolonged

PT, prothrombin time; PTT, partial thromboplastin time.

in a heterozygote is abnormal. Hundreds of abnormal fibrinogens have been described. The true incidence of dysfibrinogenemia is not known because many forms of the disorder are asymptomatic. Homozygotes may have a mild bleeding tendency, perhaps because the fibrinogen molecule is cleaved too slowly to form fibrin monomers or because abnormal fibrin monomers polymerize too slowly. The bleeding tendency is characterized by easy or spontaneous bruising, menorrhagia, and prolonged or severe bleeding with surgery or trauma. Heterozygotes are usually asymptomatic, but may show excessive bleeding with surgery or trauma. Several types of dysfibrinogenemia (approximately 10% to 15% of cases) are associated with an increased risk of thrombosis rather than bleeding. A few types of congenital dysfibrinogenemia are associated with both bleeding and thrombosis.

Acquired hypofibrinogenemia is observed predominantly in patients with advanced liver disease, in patients with a consumptive coagulation disorder such as DIC, and in those treated with thrombolytic therapy.

Acquired dysfibrinogenemia represents the acquired production of an abnormal fibrinogen molecule in normal or near-normal quantities, most often in patients with acute or chronic liver disease, especially those with primary or metastatic hepatic malignancies. The patient may or may not be symptomatic, depending on (1) whether there is simultaneous production of normal fibrinogen in amounts sufficient to allow normal hemostasis and (2) whether the abnormal fibrinogen can polymerize like a normal fibrinogen molecule (see the section "Hemostatic Abnormalities in Liver Disease").

> *Acquired hypofibrinogenemia* is observed predominantly in patients with advanced liver disease, in patients with a consumptive coagulation disorder such as DIC, and in those treated with thrombolytic therapy.

Diagnosis

See **Table 11-1** for the laboratory evaluation of the patient with a fibrinogen deficiency.

Prothrombin (Factor II) Deficiency

Description

Prothrombin (Factor II) is the precursor to thrombin (Factor IIa), which converts fibrinogen into fibrin in the common pathway of the coagulation cascade. Deficiency of prothrombin, either inherited or acquired, may result in a hemorrhagic diathesis. Inherited abnormalities of prothrombin are rare. As with fibrinogen, abnormalities occur in two major forms. The first is reduced or absent production of a normal prothrombin molecule. The second is production of normal amounts of an abnormal prothrombin molecule with decreased activity (dysfunctional form or dysprothrombinemia). Heterozygotes usually have approximately 50% of normal activity and may be asymptomatic or have a bleeding tendency. In one study, 83% of a small cohort of heterozygotes had bleeding, with Factor II levels ranging from 21% to 35%. Homozygotes usually have 1% to 25% of normal activity and have a mild-to-severe hemorrhagic tendency. Acquired hypoprothrombinemia occurs most often along with deficiencies of Factors VII, IX, and X in

Abnormalities occur in two major forms. The first is reduced or absent production of a normal prothrombin molecule. The second is production of normal amounts of an abnormal prothrombin molecule with decreased activity (dysfunctional form or dysprothrombinemia).

vitamin K deficiency and with warfarin (Coumadin) therapy; with deficiencies of multiple coagulation factors in liver disease or DIC; as an isolated coagulation factor deficiency in some patients with lupus anticoagulant (LA); and in patients exposed to topical bovine thrombin who develop antibodies to prothrombin (and not uncommonly to Factor V also). Bleeding manifestations depend on the level of prothrombin activity; usually no bleeding occurs with a prothrombin level >50% of normal.

Diagnosis

See **Table 11–2** for the laboratory evaluation of the patient with a prothrombin (Factor II) deficiency.

Factor V Deficiency

Description

Factor V is a high-molecular-weight protein (approximately 300,000 Da) that acts as an accelerating cofactor for the enzymatic conversion of prothrombin to thrombin by Factor Xa. When Factor V is cleaved to Factor Va by thrombin, its cofactor activity is significantly increased. Factors Va and VIIIa are degraded by activated protein C. An isolated deficiency of Factor V is a rare cause of bleeding.

Apparent heterozygous and homozygous deficient states have been observed. Heterozygotes usually have levels of approximately 50% of normal and can experience bleeding or may be asymptomatic. In a cohort of 19 heterozygous patients, 50% had bleeding, with Factor V levels

TABLE 11–2   Laboratory Evaluation for Coagulation Factor Deficiencies

Deficient Factor(s)	PT Prolonged if Deficient?	PTT Prolonged if Deficient?	Other Tests Useful in Diagnosis/Comments
Fibrinogen—see Table 11–1			
Prothrombin (Factor II)	Yes	Yes (usually less prominent than the PT prolongation)	Factor II assay; selected other factor assays to determine if Factor II is low along with other factors, especially VII, IX, and X—this often establishes the cause of a low Factor II level A lupus anticoagulant test to determine if a low Factor II level is associated with a lupus anticoagulant
Factor V	Yes	Yes (usually less prominent than the PT prolongation)	Factor V assay; selected other factor assays to determine if a low Factor V level is accompanied by other factor deficiencies
Factor VII	Yes	No	Factor VII assay; selected other factor assays to determine if Factor VII is low along with other factors, especially II, V, IX, and X
Factor VIII	No	Yes	Factors VIII and IX assays, as these two deficiency states are clinically indistinguishable von Willebrand factor antigen and ristocetin cofactor to determine if a low Factor VIII level represents hemophilia A or von Willebrand disease
Factor IX	No	Yes	Factors VIII and IX assays as these two deficiency states are clinically indistinguishable; selected other factor assays to determine if Factor IX is low along with other factors, especially II, VII, and X
Factor X	Yes	Yes (usually less prominent than the PT prolongation)	Factor X assay; selected other factor assays to determine if Factor X is low along with other factors, especially II, VII, and IX
Factor XI	No	Yes	Factor XI assay
Factor XII	No	Yes	Factor XII assay
Prekallikrein	No	Yes	Prekallikrein assay
High-molecular-weight kininogen	No	Yes	High-molecular-weight kininogen assay
Factor XIII	No	No	The screening test for Factor XIII deficiency assesses the solubility of the patient's clot in urea—clots from patients with Factor XIII levels <2% dissolve; a quantitative assay not involving clot solubility is also available and can detect mild deficiencies of Factor XIII

PT, prothrombin time; PTT, partial thromboplastin time.

ranging from 21% to 55%. Homozygotes have variable levels below 50%; they are most likely to be symptomatic if the level is 10% or less.

As with the other coagulation factors, two major forms of the inherited deficiency are described: reduced or absent production of a normal Factor V molecule (absence form) and production of an abnormal molecule with reduced activity in normal amounts (dysfunctional form). A rare combined deficiency of Factors V and VIII is due to a genetic defect in intracellular transport of Factors V and VIII. Acquired deficiencies of Factor V occur with liver dysfunction or DIC.

Diagnosis

See **Table 11–2** for the laboratory evaluation of the patient with a Factor V deficiency.

Factor VII Deficiency
Description

Factor VII is a vitamin K-dependent coagulation factor precursor that, when activated by thrombin, Factor Xa, or Factor IXa, is converted to Factor VIIa. This activated factor then converts phospholipid-bound Factor X into Factor Xa in the presence of calcium and tissue factor. It also converts Factor IX to Factor IXa. Factor VII deficiency may occur as an inherited or acquired disorder.

The inherited deficiency state, which is rare, may be present as reduced or absent production of a normal molecule (absence form) or production of an abnormal molecule with decreased activity in normal amounts (dysfunctional form). An inherited isolated deficiency of Factor VII in heterozygotes is usually associated with a Factor VII activity level of approximately 50%. In a cohort of 88 heterozygous patients, 36% had a bleeding tendency, with Factor VII levels ranging from 21% to 69%. In homozygotes, there are variable Factor VII activity levels below 50%. The bleeding risk is difficult to predict in these patients because the factor activity level correlates poorly with the patient's tendency to hemorrhage, but in general values <10% can be associated with major spontaneous bleeding. A large proportion of patients with less than 2% Factor VII do not bleed. Acquired Factor VII deficiency occurs in vitamin K deficiency and with warfarin therapy along with deficiencies of Factors II, IX, and X; and in DIC or liver disease along with multiple other coagulation factor deficiencies.

Intracranial hemorrhage has been reported in Factor VII-deficient patients, most often occurring in infants <1 year of age. Elevated Factor VII levels have been associated with an increased risk of cardiovascular disease.

> The bleeding risk is difficult to predict because the factor VII activity level correlates poorly with the patient's tendency to hemorrhage. A large proportion of patients with less than 2% Factor VII do not bleed.

Diagnosis

See **Table 11–2** for the laboratory evaluation of the patient with a Factor VII deficiency.

Hemophilia A (Factor VIII Deficiency)
Description

Hemophilia A is a bleeding disorder resulting from a deficiency of Factor VIII procoagulant activity. Factor VIII circulates in the plasma bound to vWF. Approximately 90% of patients with hemophilia A synthesize low amounts of normal Factor VIII molecules, and 10% of patients with hemophilia A synthesize normal amounts of an abnormal (nonfunctional) Factor VIII. Hemophilia A is inherited as an X-linked trait, and 65% to 75% of patients have a positive family history. Disease prevalence in the United States is 1 in 10,000 males; the carrier state in females is rarely symptomatic. Hemophilia A and hemophilia B (Factor IX deficiency, see below) are clinically indistinguishable. The likelihood of hemorrhage depends on the amount of Factor VIII present; the majority of patients (approximately 50% to 70% of hemophilia A patients) have severe disease. The severity of disease is categorized as follows:

- In mild disease: the VIII level is 6% to 20% of normal, with rare spontaneous bleeding.
- In moderate disease: the VIII level is 1% to 5% of normal, with occasional spontaneous bleeding.
- In severe disease: the VIII level is <1% of normal, with frequent spontaneous bleeding.

> Hemophilia A is a bleeding disorder resulting from a deficiency of Factor VIII procoagulant activity. Factor VIII inhibitors are antibodies, usually IgG, that bind to Factor VIII and inhibit its coagulant activity.

All hemophilia patients (A and B) may experience severe hemorrhage following trauma or surgery if there is no prior treatment to elevate the factor level. Bleeding that is characteristic of hemophilia (A and B) includes intra-articular (joint), intracranial, and intramuscular hemorrhage. The latter can produce a compartment compression syndrome. Easy bruising and prolonged bleeding after minor cuts and abrasions are also characteristic. The onset of hemorrhage is typically delayed following injury, and pathologic bleeding may occur hours after injury. Primary hemostasis (dependent on platelet plug formation) is intact, but secondary hemostasis (dependent on the fibrin clot generated by the coagulation cascade) is defective. Up to 15% of hemophilia A patients develop an inhibitor to Factor VIII at some time during the course of their disease (i.e., an antibody against Factor VIII). The inhibitor develops only in those transfused with Factor VIII-containing products, and most often in patients with <1% Factor VIII. Factor VIII inhibitors may also spontaneously occur rarely in nonhemophiliacs (see the section "Factor VIII Inhibitors").

Diagnosis

See **Table 11–2** for information regarding the laboratory evaluation for Factor VIII deficiency.

Factor VIII Inhibitors

Description

Factor VIII inhibitors are antibodies, usually IgG, that bind to Factor VIII and inhibit its coagulant activity.

Factor VIII inhibitors have been found in several clinical situations.

- Inhibitors are diagnosed most commonly in patients with hemophilia A. Inhibitors occur in 10% to 15% of these patients and make the treatment of hemorrhage much more difficult. The vast majority of cases of Factor VIII inhibitors in hemophilia A patients occur in those with severe hemophilia A (<1% Factor VIII activity). Inhibitor formation is related to transfusion of exogenous Factor VIII, and usually develops before 100 treatment days if it appears. Two immune response patterns have been observed in hemophilia A patients. The first is a high response pattern. Inhibitors rise to a high titer in response to exposure to Factor VIII. The titer may not decline for months to years, even without further exposure to Factor VIII. Rapid anamnestic responses are often seen within 3 to 7 days of reexposure in these patients. In the second pattern, there is a low response. In addition, inhibitors usually remain at a low titer despite reexposure. They may occasionally disappear and reappear spontaneously. Little, if any, anamnestic response is likely found in a low responder.
- Spontaneous inhibitors to Factor VIII can occur in the postpartum patient. Usually they are recognized 2 to 5 months after the birth of the first child and disappear spontaneously after 12 to 18 months. However, the course is variable, and there are reports of death from hemorrhage in some patients. Antigenic differences between mother and fetus do not sufficiently explain the development of a Factor VIII inhibitor, and its cause remains unknown.
- Inhibitors may occur in those with allergic and enhanced immunologic reactions, including patients with:
  (a) Rheumatoid arthritis
  (b) Systemic lupus erythematosus
  (c) Reactions to drugs, such as penicillin, chloramphenicol, sulfonamides, and phenytoin
  (d) Malignancy
  (e) Asthma
  (f) Crohn disease
  (g) Ulcerative colitis
  (h) Pemphigus
  (i) Multiple myeloma
- Inhibitors may appear in patients without any obvious underlying disorder. These are usually older individuals, and the inhibitor may remit in several months, persist for years, or disappear with immunosuppressive therapy.

TABLE 11–3   Laboratory Evaluation for Factor VIII Inhibitor

Laboratory Test	Results/Comments
PT	Normal
PTT	Prolonged; normalizes in a 1:1 PTT mixing study of patient plasma and normal plasma with a 0-min incubation (i.e., PTT performed immediately after mixing), but becomes prolonged with a longer incubation of the mixed plasma (60 or 120 min) at 37°C; the PTT of the mixed plasma at 60–120 min incubation with a clinically significant inhibitor is typically at least 8 s longer than the PTT of the mixed plasma at 0-min incubation
Factor VIII activity	Decreased
Factor VIII inhibitor assay	Used for quantitation of inhibitor; inhibitor levels are expressed in Bethesda units (BU); 1 BU/mL is the amount of inhibitor that produces a 50% reduction in Factor VIII activity

PT, prothrombin time; PTT, partial thromboplastin time.

In a hemophilia A patient, a poor response to treatment with Factor VIII concentrate may be the first indication that an inhibitor is present, or there may be an increased frequency of bleeding episodes. In nonhemophiliacs, development of a new hemorrhagic tendency is usually the presenting feature of a spontaneous Factor VIII inhibitor. The most favorable prognoses are for patients with low titer inhibitors, peripartum women, and patients without an underlying disorder.

Hemophilia B is an inherited hemorrhagic disorder resulting from a lack of procoagulant activity of Factor IX.

Diagnosis

See **Table 11–3** for information regarding the laboratory evaluation for a Factor VIII inhibitor.

Hemophilia B (Factor IX Deficiency)

Description

Hemophilia B is an inherited hemorrhagic disorder resulting from a lack of procoagulant activity of Factor IX. Factor IX is a vitamin K-dependent factor that, in its active form (Factor IXa), is a serine protease of the intrinsic pathway of the coagulation cascade. Approximately 70% to 90% of hemophilia B patients have a deficiency of a normal coagulant protein, and 10% to 30% produce an abnormal Factor IX that is nonfunctional. Inheritance is sex-linked, with affected males, and female carriers. Of hemophilia B patients, 60% to 70% have a positive family history for bleeding. The prevalence of hemophilia B is much less than that of hemophilia A. Approximately 1 in 50,000 males in the United States has hemophilia B versus 1 in 10,000 males with hemophilia A. The hemophilia B carrier state in the female is usually asymptomatic, as is the case with hemophilia A. Acquired Factor IX deficiency may occur along with deficiencies of Factors II, VII, and X in patients with vitamin K deficiency or those receiving warfarin therapy, and with deficiencies of other coagulation factors in patients with liver disease, DIC, or nephrotic syndrome.

As previously noted, hemophilia B is clinically indistinguishable from hemophilia A. The severity of hemorrhage depends on the amount of Factor IX activity present:

- In mild disease: 6% to 20% of normal IX activity is present, with rare spontaneous bleeding.
- In moderate disease: 1% to 5% of normal IX activity is present, with occasional spontaneous bleeding.
- In severe disease: <1% of normal activity is present, with frequent spontaneous bleeding.

Profuse bleeding may occur in any hemophilia B patient with trauma or surgery if there is no prior treatment to elevate the factor level. Bleeding in hemophilia B resembles that found in hemophilia A and includes deep tissue bleeding, intra-articular bleeding (hemarthrosis), intracranial bleeding (which may be lethal), and intramuscular bleeding with potential compartment compression syndrome. Severe mucosal membrane bleeding can occur in hemophilia, particularly after dental surgery.

Inhibitors develop to Factor IX in 1% to 5% of hemophilia B cases. These antibodies often occur in high titer and frequently present a major bleeding problem despite treatment.

Diagnosis

See **Table 11–2** for information regarding the laboratory evaluation for patients with hemophilia B.

Factor X Deficiency

Description

An inherited isolated deficiency of Factor X is a rare disorder. Homozygotes and heterozygotes have been identified. Homozygotes usually possess <2% of normal activity. Heterozygotes usually possess 40% to 70% of normal activity. In a cohort of 15 heterozygous patients, 33% had a bleeding tendency, with Factor X levels ranging from 23% to 47%. Patients with Factor X values <10% can have a high risk of spontaneous major bleeding, and those with >40% are usually asymptomatic. Inherited Factor X deficiency, like the other factor deficiency states, occurs in two major forms: reduced or absent synthesis of a normal molecule (absence form) and synthesis of an abnormal molecule in normal amounts (dysfunctional form).

Acquired Factor X deficiency may result from warfarin or vitamin K deficiency (in the presence of deficiencies of Factors II, VII, and IX), from liver disease (with deficiencies of other factors synthesized in the liver), with DIC, or as an isolated deficiency in cases of amyloidosis. In amyloidosis, Factor X becomes irreversibly bound to amyloid fibrils in the extracellular space, and is thereby removed from the circulation.

Diagnosis

See **Table 11–2** for information regarding the laboratory evaluation of patients with Factor X deficiency.

Factor XI Deficiency

Description

Factor XI deficiency is a commonly encountered disorder. Homozygotes typically have less than 20% of normal Factor XI activity. Heterozygotes have 20% to 70% of normal Factor XI activity. The deficiency in almost all cases appears to be a reduced or absent production of a normal molecule, rather than production of an abnormal or dysfunctional molecule.

The vast majority of the cases of Factor XI deficiency are in people of Jewish descent, particularly those of Ashkenazi origin. The frequency of the homozygous deficient state is 0.2% to 0.3% in the Ashkenazi population, and the frequency of the heterozygous state is extremely high, at approximately 5.5% to 11.0%.

The hemorrhagic tendency is variable for both heterozygotes and homozygotes. Patients with Factor XI levels <15% to 20% uncommonly have spontaneous bleeding but frequently have postoperative bleeding, and patients with levels between 20% and 65% tend to be asymptomatic or have low rates of postoperative bleeding. Bleeding does not correlate well with the level of Factor XI activity. Some homozygotes have an abnormal partial thromboplastin time (PTT), a very low Factor XI level of less than 10%, and no bleeding, even with surgery. The bleeding tendency of a particular individual is more closely related to the bleeding tendency of the patient's kindred than to the measured Factor XI level. The explanation, which is true for all mutations affecting coagulation factors, is that certain mutations produce a low level of Factor XI and a prolonged PTT but are not clinically significant in vivo. This is because they only affect the activity of the factor in the in vitro clotting factor assays, which are not exact replicas of clot formation in vivo. Acquired decreases in Factor XI can occur with pregnancy, proteinuria, liver dysfunction, and DIC.

Diagnosis

See **Table 11–2** for information regarding the laboratory evaluation of patients with Factor XI deficiency.

Deficiencies of the Contact Factors

Description

The contact coagulation factors (so named because they were originally thought to activate the coagulation cascade by contacting the cut surface of the vessel wall) include Factor XII, PK, and HMWK. A deficiency of any of the contact factors prolongs the PTT because the PTT assay is constructed to involve these factors, even though the coagulation cascade in vivo does not depend on these factors. Bleeding diatheses have not been reported in patients with deficiencies at any level of Factor XII, PK, or HMWK. Factor XII deficiency is fairly common, with many thousands affected, especially individuals of Asian descent and children with tonsillitis. HMWK deficiency and PK deficiency are rare.

The PTT was performed *without* activation several decades ago, and the clotting times were very long. For that reason, an activator was added to the reagents used in the assay. Since this change occurred more than 50 years ago, and unactivated PTT tests have not been performed clinically over that time, the term PTT and partial thromboplastin time are used in this book, instead of aPTT or activated partial thromboplastin time.

> A deficiency of any of the contact factors prolongs the PTT because the PTT assay is constructed to involve these factors, even though the coagulation cascade in vivo does not depend on these factors. Bleeding diatheses have not been reported in patients with deficiencies at any level of Factor XII, PK, or HMWK.

Diagnosis

See **Table 11–2** for information regarding the laboratory evaluation for contact factor abnormalities.

Factor XIII Deficiency

Description

Factor XIII circulates in plasma as a zymogen and is converted to its active form (Factor XIIIa) by thrombin. Factor XIIIa catalyzes the formation of covalent bonds between chains of adjacent fibrin monomers. This stabilizes the fibrin clot, making it rigid and more resistant to the action of plasmin. Congenital deficiency of Factor XIII is rare. The bleeding tendency in homozygotes is characterized by umbilical stump bleeding in newborns (>90% of patients with clinically significant Factor XIII deficiency have this finding), intracranial hemorrhage, miscarriages, and post-traumatic hematomas, with bleeding often delayed hours to days after the trauma. Patients with mild or moderate deficiencies might have mucocutaneous bleeding or be asymptomatic. Patients with Factor XIII levels above 30% are usually always asymptomatic.

Diagnosis

See **Table 11–2** for information regarding the laboratory evaluation for Factor XIII deficiency.

Antiplasmin Deficiency

Description

Antiplasmin or plasmin inhibitor (formerly known as alpha-2 antiplasmin) is a glycoprotein (GP) that serves as a regulator of fibrinolysis in several ways (see **Figure 11–4**). It blocks the enzymatic activity of plasmin (the major fibrinolytic enzyme) and other serine proteases, some of which are coagulation factors, and it inhibits the binding of plasminogen to fibrin. A bleeding diathesis is associated with the congenital deficiency of plasmin inhibitor. It is an extremely rare disorder and only homozygotes with <10% of normal plasmin inhibitor activity appear to be clinically affected. Those who do bleed may experience mucosal membrane bleeding (particularly in the genitourinary tract), subcutaneous hematomas, spontaneous bruising, and severe bleeding with trauma. Most heterozygotes are asymptomatic, but those few who are symptomatic have only a mild bleeding tendency. Acquired deficiency of plasmin inhibitor can occur in liver disease, nephrotic syndrome, amyloidosis, DIC, and, most notably, following thrombolytic therapy. In thrombolytic therapy, plasminogen is purposefully converted to plasmin, which results in the formation of plasmin–antiplasmin complexes, thereby reducing the amount of available antiplasmin.

Diagnosis

See **Table 11–4** for information on the laboratory evaluation of plasmin inhibitor deficiency.

TABLE 11–4   Laboratory Evaluation for Antiplasmin Deficiency

Laboratory Test	Results/Comments
PT	Normal
PTT	Normal
Antiplasmin	Decreased

PT, prothrombin time; PTT, partial thromboplastin time.

TABLE 11–5   Laboratory Evaluation for Vitamin K Deficiency

Laboratory Test	Results/Comments
PT	Always prolonged
PTT	May be prolonged, depending on severity
Factors II, VII, IX, and X, protein C, and protein S	The combined deficiencies of Factors II, VII, IX, and X, protein C, and protein S are diagnostic of vitamin K deficiency or ingestion of a vitamin K antagonist, such as warfarin, especially if a non-vitamin K-dependent coagulation factor (e.g., Factor V) level is normal; Factor VII and protein C decrease before the others because they have the shortest half-lives in the plasma

PT, prothrombin time; PTT, partial thromboplastin time.

Vitamin K Deficiency

Description

In adults, vitamin K deficiency most often occurs secondary to disease or drug therapy; it rarely occurs as a dietary deficiency. Causes of vitamin K deficiency include:

- Warfarin therapy (reduces the amount of active vitamin K)
- Antibiotic therapy (capable of suppressing bowel flora that synthesize vitamin K)
- Malabsorption syndromes: cystic fibrosis, sprue, ulcerative colitis, Crohn disease, parasitic infections, short bowel syndrome, and ileojejunostomy (for morbid obesity)
- Dietary restriction with incidental decrease in vitamin K intake
- Long-term total parenteral nutrition
- Biliary obstruction

Vitamin K depletion can occur in as little as 2 weeks if both intake (enteral and parenteral) and endogenous production of vitamin K are eliminated. In early deficiency, Factor VII only, or Factors VII and IX only, may be decreased due to their shorter half-lives. Vitamin K deficiency may present as an asymptomatic prolongation of the PT in mild cases or as a major spontaneous hemorrhage in severe deficiencies. The degree of prolongation of the PT does not accurately predict the risk of hemorrhage.

Most antibiotics destroy bacterial flora and must be considered as a possible cause of vitamin K deficiency in the bleeding patient. However, certain cephalosporins produce vitamin K deficiency much more rapidly than other antibiotics. Cephalosporins with an *N*-methylthiotetrazole (MTT) group in position 3 directly inhibit the vitamin K-dependent carboxylase that is responsible for converting Factors II, VII, IX, and X to their active form. Cephalosporins in the MTT group include cefamandole, cefoperazone, cefotetan, moxalactam, cefmetazole, and cefmenoxime. Weekly prophylaxis with vitamin K has been recommended when MTT-cephalosporins are given to patients at high risk for vitamin K deficiency.

Diagnosis

See **Table 11–5** for information on the laboratory evaluation for vitamin K deficiency.

In adults, vitamin K deficiency most often occurs secondary to disease or drug therapy; it rarely occurs as a dietary deficiency.

TABLE 11-6 **Commonly Used Assays in the Laboratory Evaluation for Disseminated Intravascular Coagulation (DIC)**

Laboratory Test	Results/Comments
FDP or D-dimer	Elevated in essentially all cases, both acute and chronic; elevated due to fibrinolysis of fibrin deposits in the microvasculature
PT	Prolonged in most cases of clinically significant DIC, due to a decrease in fibrinogen, prothrombin (Factor II), and multiple other coagulation factors
PTT	Prolonged less often than the PT in DIC, but increases along with severity of DIC due to a decrease in fibrinogen, Factor VIII, and multiple other coagulation factors
Platelet count	Decreased in most cases of acute DIC due to consumption of platelets
Fibrinogen	Low or decreasing with serial samples in <50% of acute DIC cases, due to the conversion of fibrinogen into fibrin; the fibrinogen level can be normal or even elevated in DIC by a variety of mechanisms, one of which is increased fibrinogen synthesis in the liver as part of the acute-phase response to infection or other stimulus
Schistocytes	Present in the peripheral blood smear in approximately 50% of acute DIC cases; results from microangiopathic hemolysis of RBCs as they traverse through vessels that are partially occluded by fibrin strands

FDP, fibrin degradation products; PT, prothrombin time; PTT, partial thromboplastin time.

Disseminated Intravascular Coagulation

Description

DIC is a common acquired coagulation disorder that occurs secondary to a variety of underlying disorders. The most common cause is infection; 10% to 20% of patients with gram-negative sepsis develop DIC. Other causes of DIC include obstetrical complications (retained dead fetus, placental abruption, amniotic fluid embolism, hypertonic saline-induced abortion, and septic abortion), extensive tissue injury (including trauma, ischemia, infarction, and burns), liver disease, transfusion of ABO-incompatible blood, and adult respiratory distress syndrome. The clinical presentation varies from an asymptomatic condition, detectable only by laboratory abnormalities, to a severe coagulopathy with a mortality of up to 80%.

The major events in acute DIC, independent of the cause, are microvascular thrombosis with consumption of platelets and coagulation factors, and then hemorrhage as a result of low levels of platelets and coagulation factors and overactivation of the fibrinolytic system to remove the thrombi. Hemorrhagic symptoms can include any of the following—petechiae, ecchymoses, mucosal oozing, hematuria, gastrointestinal tract bleeding, bleeding into surgical wounds, and prolonged bleeding at venous access sites. Severe bleeding may contribute to hypotensive shock.

DIC may present as a more chronic, low-grade condition in patients with malignancy. These patients are at risk for macrovascular (large vessel) thrombosis as well, most likely as a deep vein thrombosis.

The prolongations of the PT and the PTT reflect a decrease in fibrinogen and other coagulation factors that are consumed by clotting. In addition, fibrinogen is degraded by excess plasmin activation in the fibrinolytic system. Platelets are also consumed, and, therefore, the platelet count is typically low. The presence of FDP, one of which is the D-dimer, indicates that fibrin clots have been formed and subsequently degraded. There is no single laboratory test that can diagnose or exclude DIC, and the diagnosis is made when the characteristic laboratory abnormalities are present along with a known stimulus for DIC. A practical approach to diagnosis of DIC is to perform the PT, the PTT, and a D-dimer assay, with serial measurements of fibrinogen and platelets. In severe acute DIC, most of the laboratory test results will be abnormal, although fibrinogen may be normal or even elevated. In chronic DIC, the laboratory abnormalities may be less pronounced or even absent because the liver and bone marrow can increase production of coagulation factors and platelets, respectively, to offset the losses from consumption.

> The major events in acute DIC, independent of the cause, are microvascular thrombosis with consumption of platelets and coagulation factors, and then hemorrhage as a result of low levels of platelets and coagulation factors and overactivation of the fibrinolytic system to remove the thrombi.

Diagnosis

See **Table 11-6** for information on the laboratory evaluation for DIC.

Hemostatic Abnormalities in Liver Disease
Description

Patients with acute and chronic liver disease often have laboratory evidence of a hemostatic abnormality. These patients may be asymptomatic or have only mild bleeding problems, but those with advanced liver disease may experience a severe hemorrhage.

Hemorrhage in patients with liver disease may be due to one or more of the following:

- Coagulation factor abnormalities: These are caused by decreased hepatic synthesis of vitamin K-dependent factors (II, VII, IX, and X) and non-vitamin K-dependent factors. Decreased fibrinogen is usually found only in patients with severe hepatic failure; in fact, patients with acute hepatitis without hepatic failure usually have an increased fibrinogen level.
- Thrombocytopenia: This frequently occurs as a consequence of sequestration in the spleen, impaired platelet production, or increased platelet destruction. It is not usually a severe decrease in platelet number.
- Platelet dysfunction: The dysfunction is usually mild and its clinical significance is uncertain; platelet dysfunction may be clinically important only in liver disease patients with severe thrombocytopenia or severe renal failure, which can result in uremia-induced platelet dysfunction.
- DIC or a DIC-like syndrome: There is no general agreement as to whether the coagulation abnormalities that occur in patients with liver disease are due to DIC, liver disease alone, or a combination of these and other mechanisms. A DIC-like syndrome occurs frequently in patients with acute hepatic failure. Laboratory abnormalities in these cases include hypofibrinogenemia, thrombocytopenia, increased FDP such as D-dimer, and decreased levels of Factors V and VIII.
- Acquired dysfibrinogenemia (in patients with selected liver diseases [see the section "Fibrinogen Deficiencies"]): Impaired fibrin polymerization may result and thereby predispose the patient to bleeding.
- Increased fibrinolysis: Hemostatic abnormalities in patients with cirrhosis may be due to increased fibrinolysis. This may occur as a result of decreased hepatic clearance of plasminogen activators and decreased synthesis of inhibitors of fibrinolysis (see **Figure 11–4**).

Diagnosis

The laboratory evaluation for hemostatic defects from liver disease is shown in **Table 11–7**.

Immune Thrombocytopenic Purpura (ITP)
Description

ITP (where the *I* formerly stood for idiopathic) exists in both an acute and a chronic form. The disorder is one in which accelerated platelet destruction occurs in the absence of other causes such as DIC, thrombotic thrombocytopenic purpura (TTP), drug-induced thrombocytopenia, and neonatal thrombocytopenia. Platelet production is also often reduced.

TABLE 11–7   Laboratory Evaluation for Hemostatic Defects in Liver Disease

Laboratory Test	Results/Comments
PT and PTT	Both will be prolonged, but the PT prolongation is usually greater than the PTT prolongation
D-dimer or FDP	Elevated due to decreased clearance by the liver
Fibrinogen	Most often slightly low or normal; can be elevated if underlying illness causes acute-phase reaction
Platelet count	Most often slightly low or normal
Coagulation factor assays	Used to investigate the extent of coagulation factor deficiencies; in the absence of a concomitant DIC

DIC, disseminated intravascular coagulation; FDP, fibrin degradation products; PT, prothrombin time; PTT, partial thromboplastin time.

The destruction of platelets in ITP is antibody-mediated. The amount of platelet-associated IgG is increased in the majority of patients with acute and chronic ITP. Many patients with chronic ITP have increased levels of antiplatelet antibodies in the serum, as well as on the platelet surface. It should be noted that there are a host of disorders unrelated to immune thrombocytopenias, which are associated with increased IgG on the platelet surface. *Helicobacter pylori* infection has been associated with ITP.

In acute ITP, the platelet may be an innocent target of an antipathogen antibody that cross-reacts with an epitope on the platelet membrane. Chronic ITP appears to be more of a classic autoimmune illness in which the target antigens for platelet autoantibodies are platelet GPs. Sequestration and destruction of antibody-coated platelets occur predominantly in the spleen.

Acute ITP usually presents as a childhood illness with peak incidence between 2 and 9 years. It is heralded by a prodromal illness, such as a viral respiratory infection, in 60% to 80% of cases. The infection occurs 2 to 21 days prior to onset of thrombocytopenia. The risk of hemorrhage is greatest during the first 1 to 2 weeks after the onset of acute ITP. Intracranial hemorrhage is the most feared complication of ITP. The majority of patients experience a spontaneous resolution of acute ITP 3 weeks to 3 months after onset. A small percentage of patients do not recover fully after 12 months, and advance to a diagnosis of chronic ITP.

Chronic ITP occurs most commonly between the ages of 20 and 50 years, and in females more often than in males (ratio of 2:1 to 3:1). It is characterized by the absence of a prodromal illness and the presence of mild bleeding that may continue for months before medical attention is sought. Manifestations include scattered petechiae or purpura, mostly on distal extremities, mild mucosal bleeding, easy bruising, epistaxis, and menorrhagia. ITP is often discovered in an asymptomatic patient found to have a low platelet count as part of a complete blood count (CBC). The diagnosis of ITP is made only after ruling out other causes for an isolated thrombocytopenia by history, physical examination, and laboratory studies.

> Acute ITP usually presents as a childhood illness with peak incidence between 2 and 9 years. Chronic ITP occurs most commonly between the ages of 20 and 50 years, and in females more often than males.

Diagnosis

See **Table 11–8** for information on the laboratory evaluation for ITP.

TABLE 11–8 **Laboratory Evaluation for Immune Thrombocytopenic Purpura (ITP)**

Laboratory Test	Results/Comments
Platelet count	In acute ITP, most cases have <20,000 platelets/µL; in chronic ITP, counts range from 5000 to 75,000/µL commonly, and, on average, are higher than platelet counts in patients with acute ITP
Platelet morphology	Large (young) platelets are often seen on peripheral smear
PT and PTT	Normal
Hemoglobin and hematocrit	May be low if an accompanying blood loss is severe or long-standing; if there is no evidence of blood loss but there is an anemia, the possibility of a concomitant autoimmune hemolytic anemia and thrombocytopenia (Evans syndrome) should be considered
Antiplatelet antibodies	A test for antiplatelet antibodies is not recommended for diagnosis of ITP; it is generally neither sensitive nor specific for ITP; most patients with acute or chronic ITP will have increased immunoglobulin on the platelet surface; however, many disorders have increased levels of platelet-associated antibodies, including sepsis, drug-induced thrombocytopenia, lymphoproliferative disorders, disseminated intravascular coagulation, and autoimmune diseases; the test for antiplatelet antibodies, using various methodologies, detects small quantities of antibody on the platelet surface (much less antibody than is found on RBCs in patients with a positive direct antiglobulin test result)
Bone marrow aspirate	Not required unless indicated on the basis of other signs/symptoms; the bone marrow shows normal RBC and WBC precursors, and a normal or increased number of megakaryocytes; bone marrow platelet production may be increased greatly in an attempt to compensate for rapid platelet destruction
H. pylori, HIV, and HCV testing	These infections can cause an ITP-like thrombocytopenia that resolves when the infection is treated

PT, prothrombin time; PTT, partial thromboplastin time; *H. pylori, Helicobacter pylori*; HIV, human immunodeficiency virus; HCV, hepatitis C virus.

Drug-induced Immunologic Thrombocytopenia

Description

Many drugs have been implicated in drug-induced immune thrombocytopenia. However, most cases can be attributed to relatively few drugs, notably heparin, quinidine/quinine, gold salts, and sulfonamides. Exposure to most of these compounds is readily ascertained. However, when obtaining the patient's history, one should include inquiries regarding consumption of over-the-counter medications and topical medications, as well as soft drinks, mixers, and aperitifs to rule out exposure to quinine. The pathogenesis of thrombocytopenia for most drugs involves both the drug and IgG (as the predominant class of antibody involved). A plasma protein bound to the drug serves as the antigen; the antigen combines with a specific antibody, and this complex binds to the platelet membrane. This is known as an "innocent bystander" effect. The antibody-coated platelet is then sequestered and destroyed. Certain other drugs (e.g., protamine, bleomycin, and ristocetin) can cause destruction of platelets by a direct toxic effect that is nonimmune. In heparin-induced thrombocytopenia (HIT), a complex of heparin and a circulating protein derived from the platelet, known as platelet factor 4 (PF4), acts as the antigen. The complex, along with bound antibody, binds to the platelet surface, causing platelet activation, and unlike other drug-induced thrombocytopenias, an increased risk for thrombosis.

The true incidence of drug-induced immunologic thrombocytopenia is not known. The incidence varies with the drug in question and the clinical condition or treatment of the patient. It may be as high as 1% to 3% of people exposed to the drug, as is the case with unfractionated (standard) heparin. Of quinidine users, approximately 1 in 1000 develop symptomatic thrombocytopenia. Drug-induced immunologic thrombocytopenia occurs most commonly in patients more than 50 years old, but it also has been reported in infants less than 1 year old. It is not possible to predict that patients will develop thrombocytopenia from drug treatment.

Ingestion of a drug that induces thrombocytopenia may produce flushing, fever, headache, and chills prior to onset of thrombocytopenia. The onset of thrombocytopenia may be abrupt following drug exposure or, if it requires antibody generation to lower the platelet count, it may be delayed for 4 to 15 days. Anamnestic responses may occur and if they arise, the delay is shorter. Bleeding may occur as early as 6 to 12 hours after exposure to the drug in highly responsive patients. Bleeding manifestations may include one or more of the following: petechiae, purpura (usually the first symptom), mucosal hemorrhagic bullae, gastrointestinal or genitourinary hemorrhage, intrapulmonary hemorrhage, and, lastly, intracranial hemorrhage, which is rare, but often lethal. HIT is unique in that bleeding is uncommon, and, as noted above, HIT patients are at risk for thrombosis rather than bleeding.

Diagnosis

See **Table 11–9** for information on the laboratory evaluation for drug-induced immunologic thrombocytopenia. Laboratory tests for drug-induced thrombocytopenia are not routinely available, with the exception of testing for HIT. If HIT is considered, a platelet count should be

TABLE 11–9   Laboratory Evaluation for Drug-induced Immunologic Thrombocytopenia

Laboratory Test	Results/Comments
Platelet count	Extremely low (<10,000/μL) to slightly low
Tests for drug-dependent antibodies bound to the platelet and for drug-dependent antiplatelet antibodies in the serum unbound to platelets	Not routinely available (except for HIT antibody testing); both test results are usually positive; however, they may be negative if the reaction is dependent on an in vivo drug metabolite, rather than the parent drug if only the parent drug is used in the laboratory test; an assay for platelet activation by the drug should be positive if the mechanism of thrombocytopenia, in the presence of the drug, includes activation of platelets by antigen–antibody complexes; an in vivo challenge with the suspected drug to confirm toxicity can be extremely dangerous and is rarely, if ever, indicated; there are a variety of methodologies for tests assessing drug-induced platelet activation, including flow cytometry and the measurement of serotonin released from activated platelets; an ELISA assay for HIT detects antibodies to heparin–platelet factor 4 complexes

HIT, heparin-induced thrombocytopenia.

Many drugs have been implicated in drug-induced immune thrombocytopenia. However, most cases can be attributed to relatively few drugs, notably heparin, quinidine/quinine, gold salts, and sulfonamides.

Heparin-induced thrombocytopenia is unique in that bleeding is uncommon, and HIT patients are at risk for thrombosis rather than bleeding.

performed first. If the platelet count decreases to 50% or less of its apparent baseline value, a test for antibodies to the heparin–PF4 complex or a functional test that shows platelet activation in the presence of heparin and the patient's plasma should be performed.

Posttransfusion Purpura (PTP)

Description

PTP is a rare syndrome characterized by the sudden onset of thrombocytopenia 7 to 10 days following transfusion of blood or blood products containing platelets or platelet material. The thrombocytopenia appears to be due to antibody-mediated destruction of autologous as well as transfused platelets. In over 90% of cases, the antibody that develops in the affected individuals is directed against the antigen HPA-1a, formerly known as P1^{A1}, on platelet membrane GP IIIa. In these cases, the recipient's own platelets are HPA-1a negative. It is not known why there is destruction of the patient's own HPA-1a-negative platelets following platelet transfusion with HPA-1a-positive platelets. Only 2% to 3% of the population in the United States lacks this antigen. Antibodies against other platelet-specific antigens have been reported in PTP, but they are much less commonly encountered. In almost all cases, the development of anti-HPA-1a antibody is thought to be an anamnestic response, with prior sensitization occurring through previous transfusion or pregnancy.

PTP occurs predominantly in females, perhaps due to the likelihood of sensitization through pregnancy. The interval between the first exposure to the HPA-1a antigen and the transfusion that incites the thrombocytopenia is greater than 3 years in most cases in which the information has been reported. The onset of thrombocytopenia is fulminant in most cases, with the platelet count decreasing to <10,000/μL. Hemorrhage usually begins with purpura and mucocutaneous bleeding, and may progress to gastrointestinal and genitourinary bleeding, epistaxis, oozing from intravenous access sites, and intracranial hemorrhage. In severely affected patients sustained with supportive therapy of red blood cells and/or platelets, the thrombocytopenia usually begins to resolve in 14 days (mean value with a range 1 to 35 days). Cases with less severe thrombocytopenia apparently require a longer recovery period (24 days average, range 6 to 70 days). The outcome is fatal in approximately 10% of cases, usually due to hemorrhage. The risk of fatal hemorrhage appears to be greatest at the onset of the disease. Recurrent PTP has been documented, with the recurrence appearing no sooner than 3 years after the first episode, even though antibody may persist in the patient's blood during the intervening time and there may be repeated challenges with exogenous platelets.

Diagnosis

See **Table 11–10** for information on the laboratory evaluation for PTP.

Neonatal Alloimmune Thrombocytopenia (NAIT)

Description

NAIT is a disorder in which there is destruction of platelets in the fetus and newborn. The destruction occurs following transplacental passage of maternal IgG antibodies directed against

TABLE 11–10   Laboratory Evaluation for Posttransfusion Purpura

Laboratory Test	Results/Comments
PT and PTT	Normal
Platelet count	Usually decreased to <10,000/μL
Tests for antiplatelet antibodies in the serum	Positive (see below)
Test for HPA-1a antigen on platelets in cases involving the HPA-1a antigen	The HPA-1a antigen is absent from the patient's platelets; anti-HPA-1a antibody is present in the patient's serum in the majority of cases and an attempt should be made to demonstrate the specificity of this antibody to HPA-1a

PT, prothrombin time; PTT, partial thromboplastin time.

TABLE 11-11 **Laboratory Evaluation for Neonatal Alloimmune Thrombocytopenia (NAIT)**

Laboratory Test	Results/Comments
PT and PTT	Normal
Platelet count (in infants)	Normal to slightly decreased at birth, continues to decrease after birth with gradual decline beginning several hours after birth; many cases show only mild thrombocytopenia, but most symptomatic cases have <30,000 platelets/μL; approximately 50% have <20,000 platelets/μL; returns to normal within 2–3 weeks
Hemoglobin/Hematocrit	May be decreased with hemorrhage
Anti-HPA-1a antibodies (in HPA-1a-related cases)	A mother with HPA-1a-negative platelets is positive for the anti-HPA-1 antibody in serum

PT, prothrombin time; PTT, partial thromboplastin time.

Neonatal alloimmune thrombocytopenic purpura is a disorder in which there is destruction of platelets in the fetus and newborn. The destruction occurs following transplacental passage of maternal IgG antibodies directed against a platelet-specific antigen present on fetal platelets and absent from the mother's platelets.

a platelet-specific antigen present on fetal platelets and absent from the mother's platelets. The antibody-coated platelets are removed from the circulation by the neonate's reticuloendothelial system around the time of birth. The estimated incidence ranges from 1 in 5000 to 1 in 2000 births, with an increasingly higher incidence in recent years attributed to improved surveillance and serologic testing for the disorder. The platelet-specific antigen implicated in 80% to 90% of all cases (and 95% of symptomatic cases) of NAIT is HPA-1a. As previously noted, this antigen is present on the platelets of 97% to 98% of the general population. In approximately 50% of cases, NAIT occurs during the first pregnancy; when it does occur, there is a 97% chance that the next pregnancy will be affected.

Affected newborns are usually the product of an otherwise uncomplicated pregnancy and delivery. Within hours after birth, petechiae and ecchymoses appear in a generalized distribution. Other clinical signs include neurologic abnormalities if intracranial hemorrhage occurs, and pallor from anemia, if the bleeding is severe. Intracranial hemorrhage is the leading cause of death in NAIT, with a 50% mortality. Overall mortality from NAIT is approximately 5% to 10%. Thrombocytopenia usually persists for approximately 2 weeks in untreated cases (range of 1 week to 2 months), and 1 week in treated cases.

Diagnosis

See **Table 11–11** for information on the laboratory evaluation for NAIT.

Discussions of TTP and hemolytic–uremic syndrome (HUS), which are thrombocytopenias associated with thrombosis, are presented among the thrombotic disorders.

Essential Thrombocythemia

Description

Essential thrombocythemia is a chronic myeloproliferative neoplasm, characterized by thrombocytosis arising from the clonal proliferation of a neoplastic multipotent stem cell. Life expectancy can be essentially normal with a median survival of 10 to 15 years, but the disease course is frequently complicated by both hemorrhage and thrombosis. A small percentage (<5%) of patients progress to acute leukemia, predominantly those patients previously treated with radioactive phosphorus or alkylating agents to reduce their platelet counts. At the time of diagnosis using older criteria, mild splenomegaly occurs in 30% to 50% of patients, and hepatomegaly in 15% to 20%. Using 2008 WHO diagnostic criteria, splenomegaly is present in only a minority of patients at diagnosis. The incidence of the disorder is higher in older age groups.

The principal diagnostic feature of essential thrombocythemia is a persistently elevated platelet count with bone marrow megakaryocyte hyperplasia. Patients with this disorder can progress to a "spent" phase, characterized by myelofibrosis and a low platelet count. The purpose of the laboratory testing is to eliminate other possible etiologies for the thrombocytosis. Other entities in the differential diagnosis of an elevated platelet count include reactive thrombocytosis and other myeloproliferative disorders—myelofibrosis, polycythemia vera, and chronic myelogenous leukemia.

TABLE 11–12 **Laboratory Evaluation for Essential Thrombocythemia (ET)**

Laboratory Test	Results/Comments
Platelet count	Sustained platelet count >450,000/µL[a]
Hemoglobin	Lack of elevation in hemoglobin helps exclude polycythemia vera[a]
DNA testing	*JAK2* V617F or other clonal marker[a]
	Absence of *BCR-ABL* (to exclude chronic myelogenous leukemia)[a]
Bone marrow biopsy	Proliferation mainly of the megakaryocytic lineage with increased numbers of enlarged, mature megakaryocytes. No significant increase or left shift of neutrophil or red cell lineages. Absence of fibrosis helps exclude myelofibrosis[a]
Platelet aggregation	Does not contribute to diagnosis, but platelets may be hypoaggregable or hyperaggregable
Acute-phase reactants	Elevated acute-phase reactants, such as C-reactive protein or fibrinogen, raise the possibility that the thrombocytosis is reactive rather than ET. Causes of reactive thrombocytosis include iron deficiency, splenectomy, surgery, infection, inflammation, connective tissue disease, malignancy, and other causes (if *JAK2* V617F is absent, the diagnosis requires absence of evidence for reactive thrombocytosis; however, the presence of reactive thrombocytosis does not exclude ET if all of the other requirements are present[a])

[a]Required for diagnosis according to 2008 WHO guidelines.

Diagnosis

See **Table 11–12** for information on the laboratory evaluation for essential thrombocythemia.

von Willebrand Disease

Description

vWD is caused by a quantitative deficiency of normal vWF in the majority of cases and a qualitatively abnormal vWF in the remainder of cases. vWF normally polymerizes to form multimers, which are aggregates of a single vWF polypeptide; in normal plasma, the multimers have a range of sizes. vWF has two major roles:

- Platelet adhesion: Large multimers of vWF (i.e., those with many units of the single polypeptide) effectively promote platelet adhesion to the subendothelium in injured vessels; if only small multimers are present, platelet plugs form poorly.
- Binding of Factor VIII: vWF circulates in the plasma with Factor VIII, the coagulant protein that is lacking in hemophilia A. vWF prolongs the half-life of Factor VIII by protecting it from rapid degradation. If vWF is reduced, Factor VIII coagulant activity is often reduced as well.

vWD prevalence estimates vary, with reported values as high as 1% of the general population. Unlike hemophilia A and B, vWD affects both men and women. It is likely to be the most common inherited bleeding disorder. There are three major types of vWD. The types were reorganized and renumbered with Arabic numerals in the 1990s (see **Table 11–13**). The most common type (type 1) is usually a mild bleeding disorder; it accounts for the majority of all cases of vWD. Type 2 vWD includes patients with qualitative vWF defects. Type 3 is rare and inherited as an autosomal recessive trait. It is associated with severe bleeding and very low to absent vWF levels. The types are distinguished from each other by laboratory testing.

It should also be noted that the mean vWF levels vary with blood type as shown in the second portion of **Table 11–14**.

More than 65% of patients with vWD have type O, presumably because patients with this blood type start from a lower baseline value for vWF.

The severity of bleeding is highly variable among patients, even within the same subtype of vWD, and even within an individual patient over time. Typically, bleeding manifestations such as easy bruising or epistaxis begin in early childhood. Other manifestations include menorrhagia and mucous membrane bleeding (from the gingiva, oropharynx, and gastrointestinal and genitourinary tracts). Profuse hemorrhage may occur with a significant hemostatic challenge such as trauma or surgery.

von Willebrand disease is caused by a quantitative deficiency of normal von Willebrand factor in the majority of cases and a qualitatively abnormal von Willebrand factor in the remainder of cases.

vWD prevalence estimates vary, with reported values as high as 1% of the general population. Unlike hemophilia A and B, vWD affects both men and women.

TABLE 11–13   Classification of von Willebrand Disease (vWD)

Type and Description of Defect

1: Partial quantitative deficiency of vWF

2: Qualitative defects in vWF

2A: Absence of high-molecular-weight multimers in plasma due to a defect in vWF

2B: Absence of high-molecular-weight multimers due to increased affinity of abnormal vWF for platelet glycoprotein Ib

2M: Decreased vWF function without the loss of high-molecular-weight multimers

2N: Decreased affinity for Factor VIII (can be misdiagnosed as hemophilia)

3: Severe quantitative deficiency of vWF

Platelet-type vWD: Absence of high-molecular-weight multimers in plasma due to increased affinity of abnormal platelet vWF receptor for normal vWF

Acquired vWD: Reduction in plasma vWF associated with the presence of an underlying disease that leads to removal of vWF from the circulation

vWF, von Willebrand factor.

TABLE 11–14   Laboratory Evaluation for von Willebrand Disease (vWD)

Laboratory Test	Results/Comments
Ristocetin cofactor activity (vWF:RCo)	A functional assay for vWF; assesses the ability of normal platelets to aggregate in the presence of ristocetin; normal aggregability to ristocetin requires large multimers of vWF
von Willebrand factor antigen (vWF:Ag)	An immunologic assay for vWF; assesses the quantity (not the function) of vWF
Factor VIII activity (Factor VIII)	Factor VIII becomes decreased secondary to the low vWF; if it is low enough, decreased Factor VIII activity is associated with a prolonged PTT
vWF multimer analysis	vWF multimer analysis assesses the size distribution of vWF multimers; loss of high-molecular-weight multimers occurs in type 2A and type 2B vWD
Low dose ristocetin–induced platelet aggregation	Platelets with high-molecular-weight von Willebrand multimers on their surface, as in type 2B vWD, aggregate at doses of ristocetin lower than doses typically used to stimulate platelet aggregation
Blood Group	**Mean vWF (%)**
O	75
A	106
B	117
AB	123

PTT, partial thromboplastin time; vWF, von Willebrand factor.

Diagnosis

> If the patient history strongly suggests vWD, and the test results are normal, the tests should be repeated at a later time because plasma levels for vWF are increased during pregnancy, stress, while receiving oral contraceptives, and during an acute illness or injury.

Laboratory test results vary with the type and subtype of vWD. Like the severity of bleeding, the laboratory values can also vary widely over time for an individual patient, and may sometimes be normal. Normal results from a single determination do not rule out the diagnosis. If the patient history strongly suggests vWD, and the test results are normal, the tests should be repeated at a later time because plasma levels for vWF are increased during pregnancy, stress, while receiving oral contraceptives, and during an acute illness or injury. Therefore, values obtained at these times may be unreliable for diagnosis. It is also not yet clear if the absolute level of vWF or the level relative to the mean vWF for the blood type of the patient is more important in establishing the diagnosis. Current guidelines note that the absolute level of vWF seems to be more important than the level relative to blood type.

See **Table 11–14** for information on the laboratory evaluation for vWD.

von Willebrand Disease Types, Subtypes, and Their Expected Test Results

- Type 1: vWF multimers of all sizes are decreased due to a defect in synthesis or release of vWF from the endothelium, the site of most vWF synthesis. Functional (ristocetin cofactor or vWF:RCo) and antigenic (vWF antigen or vWF:Ag) levels of vWF are usually proportionately decreased. Factor VIII activity might also be low. The vWF multimer pattern shows a normal distribution of multimers.

- Type 2A: Absence of large and intermediate-size vWF multimers from the plasma and platelet surface, due to a defect in the synthesis or polymerization of multimers, or from increased proteolysis of multimers. Functional activity (vWF:RCo) is decreased compared with antigenic levels (vWF:Ag). Therefore, vWF:RCo < vWF:Ag < Factor VIII is the most commonly observed pattern in type 2A. The vWF multimer pattern shows an abnormal distribution of multimers, with the absence of large and intermediate-size multimers.
- Type 2B: Marked deficiency of large vWF multimers from plasma. Intermediate-size and small multimers are present. Large multimers are present on the patient's platelets, due to increased affinity of the abnormal vWF molecule for the platelet surface. Functional and antigenic levels in plasma samples are similar to those in type 2A (vWF:RCo < vWF:Ag < Factor VIII). The vWF multimer pattern shows the absence of large multimers from plasma. The patient's platelets show increased aggregation at low concentrations of ristocetin that do not cause normal platelets to aggregate. The patient's platelets aggregate at low concentrations of ristocetin because they are coated with large vWF multimers.
- Types 2M and 2N are uncommon and are briefly described in **Table 11–13**.
- Type 3: Severe deficiency of all vWF multimers, due to a marked defect in synthesis. Factor VIII activity is less severely affected than vWF activity. Both functional and antigenic vWF levels are markedly reduced. The vWF multimer pattern shows a virtual absence of all-size multimers.
- Platelet-type Willebrand disease: vWF is qualitatively normal, but abnormal platelets have an increased affinity for large multimers of vWF due to a defect in platelet GP Ib. The laboratory test values are similar to those in type 2B.
- Acquired vWD: This disorder has been found in patients with systemic lupus erythematosus, multiple myeloma, Waldenström macroglobulinemia, lymphoproliferative disorders, and other diseases. Patients have no congenital or familial history of bleeding. Causes of the decrease in circulating vWF include adsorption of large multimers onto cells (e.g., lymphocytes or tumor cells) or the presence of antibodies to vWF. Acquired vWD resolves when the underlying disorder is effectively treated.

Bernard–Soulier Disease and Glanzmann Thrombasthenia

Description

Bernard–Soulier syndrome (BS) and GT are rare congenital hemorrhagic disorders that result from absent or defective specific platelet membrane GPs, impairing platelet function. BS is characterized by a decrease of functional GP Ib/IX/V, the platelet receptor for vWF. GT is characterized by a decrease of functional GP IIb/IIIa, the complex that mediates platelet aggregation by binding fibrinogen to the platelet surface when platelets are activated.

GT often decreases in severity with age. Manifestations include easy bruising, epistaxis, mucous membrane bleeding—particularly in the gastrointestinal tract—and menorrhagia. The amount of hemorrhage is highly variable among affected patients.

> Bernard–Soulier syndrome and Glanzmann thrombasthenia are rare congenital hemorrhagic disorders that result from absent or defective specific platelet membrane glycoproteins, impairing platelet function.

Diagnosis

See **Table 11–15** for information on the laboratory evaluation for BS and GT.

Platelet Storage Pool Disease

Description

Platelet SPD represents a group of disorders in which there is a deficiency of platelet granules. Decreased secretion of platelet granular contents at the time of platelet activation makes the platelets less hemostatically effective. The congenital forms of SPD include:

- Delta SPD: platelets have a decreased number of delta (dense) granules; these secretory granules contain ADP, polyphosphate, serotonin, and calcium.

TABLE 11–15   Laboratory Evaluation for Bernard–Soulier Disease and Glanzmann Thrombasthenia

Laboratory Test	Results/Comments
Platelet count	Slightly to moderately decreased in BS, occasionally normal; in GT, the platelet count is usually normal, but may be slightly decreased
Platelet morphology on peripheral smear	In BS, the platelets are very large (>80% of platelets are >2.5 mm in diameter) accounting for the synonym for this disorder as the "giant platelet syndrome"; in GT, platelets usually appear normal
PT and PTT	Normal
Platelet aggregation studies	In BS, there is decreased aggregation with ristocetin, but a normal response with epinephrine, ADP, arachidonic acid, and collagen; in GT, aggregation is absent (with nearly flat line tracings) with epinephrine, ADP, collagen, and arachidonic acid, but there is normal aggregation with ristocetin
Quantitative tests for platelet glycoproteins	BS patients have low amounts of glycoprotein Ib/IX; GT patients have low amounts of glycoprotein IIb/IIIa

ADP, adenosine diphosphate; BS, Bernard–Soulier disease; GT, Glanzmann thrombasthenia; PT, prothrombin time; PTT, partial thromboplastin time.

- Alpha-delta or alpha-partial delta SPD: decreased number of delta granules with either a complete or partial deficiency of alpha granules; alpha granules contain many proteins including fibrinogen, PF4, platelet-derived growth factor, and beta-thromboglobulin.
- Alpha SPD ("gray platelet syndrome"): decreased number of alpha granules, and a normal number of delta granules; platelets appear gray, large, and vacuolated on a peripheral blood smear.

> **Most patients with storage pool disease have mild bleeding symptoms. Bleeding manifestations of SPD include mild mucous membrane bleeding, easy bruising, menorrhagia, and excessive bleeding following dental or general surgery.**

SPD also may occur as an acquired abnormality, acutely in patients who have been supported on a cardiopulmonary bypass device and chronically in some cases of acute leukemia and myeloproliferative disorders. The molecular basis of most types of congenital SPD is unknown. It may result from abnormal granule morphogenesis or abnormal granule maturation in megakaryocytes. SPD may be a manifestation of a global defect in granule formation as in the Hermansky–Pudlak syndrome (see below). Hereditary SPD is the most common congenital qualitative platelet disorder, but it is still quite rare.

Most patients with SPD have mild bleeding symptoms. Bleeding manifestations of SPD include mild mucous membrane bleeding, easy bruising, menorrhagia, and excessive bleeding following dental or general surgery. SPD may also occur as a component of the following syndromes:

- Hermansky–Pudlak syndrome: Features include delta SPD, oculocutaneous albinism, pulmonary fibrosis, and the accumulation of ceroid-like material in cells of the reticuloendothelial system. One subtype is due to a defective gene (called HSP1) on chromosome 10.
- Chediak–Higashi syndrome: Features include delta SPD with giant platelet granules, photophobia, nystagmus, pseudoalbinism, lymphadenopathy, splenomegaly, and increased susceptibility to infection. It is attributed to defects in a gene called CHS1 on chromosome 1, affecting protein trafficking.
- Thrombocytopenia with absent radius: Features include alpha SPD and absence of the radius bone.
- Wiskott–Aldrich syndrome: Features of this X-linked recessive disorder include delta SPD with other metabolic platelet defects, recurrent infections, eczema, lymphocytopenia, multiple cellular and humoral immunologic defects, and thrombocytopenia with microplatelets (small platelets); the thrombocytopenia may resolve following splenectomy. It is attributed to a genetic defect in a gene called WASP on the X chromosome, affecting signal transduction and other functions.

Diagnosis

See **Table 11–16** for information on the laboratory evaluation for storage pool deficiency.

TABLE 11–16   Laboratory Evaluation for Storage Pool Deficiency

Laboratory Test	Results/Comments
PT and PTT	Normal
Platelet count	Variable
Peripheral blood smear	Shows thrombocytopenia with large, gray, vacuolated platelets in alpha SPD; giant granules in platelets, neutrophils, eosinophils, lymphocytes, and monocytes in Chediak–Higashi syndrome; microplatelets and thrombocytopenia in Wiskott–Aldrich syndrome
Platelet aggregation studies	Absent or extreme diminution of the secondary wave of aggregation with ADP and epinephrine
Platelet ATP/ADP ratio	Increase in delta granule deficiency due to low ADP in these platelets (this testing is not routinely available)
Electron microscopy of circulating platelets	May reveal a decrease in alpha granules, delta granules, or both
Alpha granule quantitation	Alpha granule contents may be assayed by measuring the amount of platelet beta-thromboglobulin or platelet factor 4, both of which are normally present in alpha granules (this testing is not routinely available)

ADP, adenosine diphosphate; ATP, adenosine triphosphate; PT, prothrombin time; PTT, partial thromboplastin time; SPD, storage pool deficiency.

TABLE 11–17   Laboratory Evaluation for Hemostatic Defects in Uremia

Laboratory Test	Results/Comments
PT and PTT	Normal
Platelet count	May be decreased, but it is rarely <80,000/µL; hemodialysis can exacerbate the thrombocytopenia, but the function of the platelets may improve
Platelet aggregation studies	No typical pattern of responses to platelet agonists; decreased response to ADP, collagen, and epinephrine often observed

ADP, adenosine diphosphate; PT, prothrombin time; PTT, partial thromboplastin time.

Hemostatic Defects in Uremia

Description

The bleeding tendency in uremia-induced hemorrhage is attributed to platelet dysfunction and endothelial cell dysfunction.

Bleeding manifestations may be mild or severe and can include petechiae, ecchymoses, epistaxis, and purpura. Paradoxically, chronic renal failure is also associated with an increased incidence of arterial and venous thrombosis, and, therefore, can influence hemostasis toward bleeding or clotting.

Diagnosis

See **Table 11–17** for information on the laboratory evaluation for hemostatic defects in uremia.

Drug-induced Qualitative Platelet Dysfunction

Description

Platelet dysfunction may occur on ingestion of a wide variety of drugs, particularly aspirin and clopidogrel (Plavix). Due to the ubiquity of aspirin in over-the-counter medications, many medications are implicated in platelet dysfunction. Some patients consume multiple drugs, such as aspirin and clopidogrel, with different and additive antiplatelet effects and thereby inhibit platelet function by more than one mechanism. Drug-induced platelet dysfunction can present a high bleeding risk in patients with existing hemostatic defects, but typically does not result in clinically significant bleeding in normal individuals. When hemorrhage does occur, there is usually

> The bleeding tendency in uremia-induced hemorrhage is attributed to platelet dysfunction and endothelial cell dysfunction. Bleeding manifestations may be mild or severe and can include petechiae, ecchymoses, epistaxis, and purpura.

TABLE 11–18   Drug-induced Qualitative Platelet Dysfunction

Laboratory Test	Results/Comments
Platelet count	The platelet count is necessary to identify an underlying thrombocytopenia, if one exists, which is aggravated by a drug effect
PT and PTT, von Willebrand factor antigen, and ristocetin cofactor	Abnormal only if there is an underlying coagulation factor abnormality
Platelet aggregation studies	Abnormal platelet aggregation may be observed in patients exposed to certain drugs in vivo, especially to weak platelet agonists such as epinephrine; however, the presence of abnormal aggregation does not correlate well with the risk of bleeding

PT, prothrombin time; PTT, partial thromboplastin time.

an underlying hemostatic disorder affecting either the platelets or coagulation factors, or an anatomic lesion, such as an ulcer, that predisposes the patient to bleeding.

Commonly encountered coagulopathies that place patients at risk for bleeding when there is a superimposed drug-induced platelet defect include vWD, thrombocytopenia of any cause, and anticoagulation therapy. Hemorrhagic manifestations can include petechiae and purpura, ecchymoses, mucosal membrane bleeding, hematuria, epistaxis, and oozing from intravenous access sites and surgical incisions.

Diagnosis

Laboratory tests are of little value in predicting the clinical significance of drug-induced platelet defects. They can confirm the presence of abnormal platelet function, but cannot assess the risk of bleeding. Furthermore, laboratory abnormalities in platelet function are not specific for a particular drug. See **Table 11–18** for information on the laboratory evaluation for drug-induced platelet defects.

THROMBOTIC DISORDERS

The disorders associated with thrombosis are grouped into those with a relatively higher prevalence and those with a relatively lower prevalence. Among those with a higher prevalence are activated protein C resistance, which is produced by the Factor V Leiden mutation, the prothrombin G20210A mutation, and the antiphospholipid antibody syndrome (an acquired disorder).

In this chapter, the disorders associated with thrombosis (**Figure 11–5**) are grouped into those with a relatively higher prevalence and those with a relatively lower prevalence. Among those with a higher prevalence is activated protein C resistance, which is produced by the Factor V Leiden mutation. This mutation is present in 3% to 5% of Caucasian populations. Other thrombotic disorders with a high prevalence are the prothrombin G20210A mutation, and the antiphospholipid antibody syndrome (an acquired disorder). The thrombotic disorders with a lower prevalence include protein C deficiency, protein S deficiency, and antithrombin deficiency. Elevated plasma homocysteine levels may also increase the risk for thrombosis. Plasminogen deficiency is also rare, and its association with thrombosis is controversial. Two other rare conditions, dysfibrinogenemia of certain types and essential thrombocythemia, can produce either thrombosis or bleeding. Also rare are TTP and HUS.

Hypercoagulable States
Description

Hypercoagulable states are associated with an increased risk for thrombosis (**Table 11–19**). There are both hereditary and acquired hypercoagulable states. Hereditary forms may arise from a quantitative or qualitative deficiency of a regulatory anticoagulant protein, such as protein C, protein S, or antithrombin (see **Figures 11–2** and **11–3**). Activated protein C resistance is caused by a mutation in the Factor V molecule (nearly always the Factor V Leiden mutation), which prevents activated protein C-mediated inactivation of Factor Va. The prothrombin G20210A mutation is prevalent in Caucasian populations, similar to Factor V Leiden. Prothrombin G20210A is a mutation in the promoter of the prothrombin gene, causing increased synthesis of prothrombin (Factor II). Hyperhomocysteinemia, a disorder in which there is an abnormally high level of

TABLE 11–19   Laboratory Evaluation for Hypercoagulable States

Hypercoagulable State	Incidence in General Population	Site of Thrombosis	Relevant Laboratory Test Results	Comments
Inherited				
Activated protein C resistance (nearly always associated with the presence of the Factor V Leiden mutation)	3%–5% in Caucasians	Predominantly venous	Positive activated protein C resistance test; DNA test positive for Factor V Leiden	Uncommon in those of African and Asian descent
Prothrombin G20210A mutation	1.5%–3% in Caucasians	Predominantly venous	DNA test positive for prothrombin G20210A	Uncommon in those of African and Asian descent
Hyperhomocysteinemia (especially congenital forms with extremely high values); can also be acquired	Markedly high values are extremely rare; mild elevations are common	Venous and arterial; often with atherosclerosis	At least moderately elevated homocysteine	It has been shown that vitamins do not decrease thrombotic risk
Protein C deficiency (congenital deficiency only)	0.2%–0.4%	Predominantly venous	Low functional and (if type I deficiency) antigenic protein C	Risk of warfarin-induced skin necrosis if anticoagulation is initiated with warfarin in the absence of heparin
Protein S deficiency[a] (congenital deficiency only)	0.2%–0.4%	Predominantly venous	Low functional and (if type I deficiency) antigenic protein S	Estrogen, pregnancy, and oral contraceptives cause acquired decreases, as do acute-phase reactions
Antithrombin deficiency[a] (congenital deficiency only)	0.01%–0.02%	Predominantly venous	Low functional and (if type I deficiency) antigenic antithrombin	Heparin use can cause an acquired deficiency
Acquired				
Antiphospholipid antibody (APA) (the presence of a lupus anticoagulant, an anticardiolipin antibody, and/or anti-beta-2 glycoprotein I antibody)	1%–5% in the general population; much higher incidence in groups with certain underlying conditions, especially systemic lupus erythematosus; higher incidence with age	Venous and arterial	Positive test results for lupus anticoagulant and/or anticardiolipin antibody, and/or anti-beta-2 glycoprotein I antibody	To make a diagnosis of antiphospholipid syndrome, test results for the lupus anticoagulant, anticardiolipin antibody, and/or anti-beta-2 glycoprotein I antibody must be positive on two separate occasions 12 weeks apart, in the setting of thrombosis, or specific pregnancy complications, occurring within 5 years of a positive test

Selected other acquired predisposing conditions for thrombosis

For venous thromboembolism: postoperative state, immobility, trauma, obesity, congestive heart failure, pregnancy and postpartum state, estrogen and progesterone use, nephrotic syndrome, L-asparaginase therapy, infection, prolonged travel, dehydration, smoking, and malignancy

For arterial thromboembolism: atherosclerosis, damaged endothelium, bypass grafts, cardiac emboli (from atrial fibrillation, mitral stenosis, or mural thrombus following myocardial infarction), and arteritis

For both venous and arterial thromboembolism: disseminated intravascular coagulation, malignancy, myeloproliferative disorders, systemic lupus erythematosus, paroxysmal nocturnal hemoglobinuria, and heparin-induced thrombocytopenia

[a]If both protein C and protein S are decreased, vitamin K deficiency or warfarin intake should be considered, especially if the prothrombin time is prolonged; if protein C, protein S, and antithrombin are all decreased, decreased synthesis of these proteins from liver disease, or recent/active clotting with consumption of the factors, may be the explanation.

plasma homocysteine, can be hereditary or acquired. Hyperhomocysteinemic individuals are at increased risk for coronary artery disease and deep venous thrombosis. However, studies have not yet shown that reducing slightly or moderately elevated homocysteine with vitamin therapy reduces the thrombotic risk. A block in the pathway at any one of the several steps results in the accumulation of homocysteine. When the homocysteine level is manyfold higher than the upper limit of normal, this very high value may contribute to the damaging effects on the blood vessel wall. Acquired hypercoagulable states arise from a diverse array of clinical conditions. They include malignancy, immobilization, surgery, trauma, obesity, smoking, infection, prolonged travel, and the use of oral contraceptives, estrogen replacement therapy, and progesterone, among many others. An acquired hypercoagulable state for which specific coagulation testing is available is the antiphospholipid antibody syndrome.

The presence of one hypercoagulable condition alone is not usually sufficient to initiate thrombosis. The presence of a second (or more), superimposed hypercoagulable condition (often called a "second hit") appears to be required to provoke a thrombotic event. For example, a person with activated protein C resistance may not experience a thrombotic event until suffering major trauma as a "second hit."

Diagnosis

Laboratory testing for hypercoagulable states is most often performed for patients presenting with a personal or family history of thrombosis. The laboratory evaluation for hereditary hypercoagulable states is best performed as a panel of test results. The most common disorders are activated protein C resistance (caused nearly always by Factor V Leiden) and prothrombin G20210A, and the less common are deficiencies of protein C, protein S, and antithrombin. Frequently, antiphospholipid antibody testing is performed in conjunction with the tests for hereditary hypercoagulable disorders. If all of these tests are negative and the clinical suspicion for a congenital hypercoagulable state remains high, additional testing for the more rare hypercoagulable disorders can be performed. There are many acquired conditions or treatments that reduce the level of protein C, protein S, and antithrombin in the test panel for hypercoagulability, but despite this, the risk for thrombosis is not significantly increased on that basis. For example, warfarin reduces the levels of protein C and protein S but reduces thrombotic risk. Antithrombin is lowered by heparin therapy. Pregnancy, oral contraceptives, and estrogen therapy can all decrease the activity of protein S, although they can induce a hypercoagulable state by other mechanisms. Active clot formation, liver dysfunction, or DIC can lower protein C, protein S, and antithrombin. In situations where such a confounding variable exists that alters the level of protein C, protein S, or antithrombin, the tests should be repeated (if possible) when the variable is no longer present to obtain the patient's true baseline values. This should allow determination of whether a heritable deficiency of any of these three proteins truly exists:

Laboratory testing for hypercoagulable states is most often performed for patients presenting with a personal or family history of thrombosis. The laboratory evaluation for hereditary hypercoagulable states is best performed as a panel of test results.

- Activated protein C resistance: Usually, the first assay performed is a functional assay for activated protein C resistance. If the result is abnormal, genetic analysis is performed to confirm whether Factor V Leiden is present in the heterozygous state, present in the homozygous state, or absent.
- Prothrombin G20210A: This mutation is identified by genetic analysis that can specifically identify heterozygous and homozygous states.
- Hyperhomocysteinemia: Plasma homocysteine levels are measured by a variety of automated methods. Hemocysteine is not commonly associated with thrombotic risk; only, possibly, with very high levels.
- Protein C, protein S, and antithrombin deficiencies: Individual functional assays to measure the activity of these endogenous anticoagulant proteins detect both qualitative (normal number of abnormally functioning molecules) and quantitative (low number of normally functioning molecules) deficiencies. In contrast, an antigenic (immunologic) assay, which measures only the quantity of protein present, can detect quantitative but not qualitative deficiencies. Therefore, the first assay performed should be a functional assay. If the result is abnormal, an antigenic assay can be performed to determine if the cause of the decreased activity is a quantitative or qualitative deficiency of the protein.

- LA (an antiphospholipid antibody): A variety of tests can be used to detect an LA. This antibody interferes with the cofactor action of phospholipid in the coagulation cascade in laboratory assays only (see the section "Antiphospholipid Antibodies: The Lupus Anticoagulant, Anticardiolipin Antibodies, and Beta-2 Glycoprotein I Antibodies" [Beta-2 GP I antibodies]). Various phospholipid-dependent coagulation test times, especially PTT-based or dilute Russell viper venom time (DRVVT) assays, can be used. The DRVVT is the clotting time obtained using Russell viper venom, which contains a Factor X activator.
- Anticardiolipin antibody or beta-2 GP I antibody (both are antiphospholipid antibodies): These antiphospholipid antibodies may or may not be associated with the presence of an LA (see the next section), and they are detected by enzyme-linked immunoassays.

See **Table 11–19** for characteristics of the hypercoagulable states.

Antiphospholipid Antibodies: The Lupus Anticoagulant, Anticardiolipin Antibodies, and Beta-2 Glycoprotein I Antibodies

Description

Antiphospholipid antibodies recognize specific phospholipid–protein complexes rather than phospholipid alone. They can be immunoglobulin type IgG or IgM, or, less commonly, IgA. The LA is an immunoglobulin that can interfere with phospholipid-dependent coagulation reactions in laboratory assays without inhibiting the activity of any specific coagulation factor. It targets phospholipids bound to prothrombin, beta-2 GP I, protein C, protein S, or other proteins bound to phospholipids. Anticardiolipin antibodies are another type of antiphospholipid antibody, which target beta-2 GP I bound to a particular phospholipid, cardiolipin; these can be detected by anticardiolipin antibody immunoassays. Anti-beta-2 GP I antibodies also target beta-2 GP I.

An antiphospholipid antibody may occur in apparently healthy individuals with no detectable illness. It also occurs in patients with a variety of clinical conditions or disorders including:

- Systemic lupus erythematosus and other autoimmune disorders
- Malignancy
- Following ingestion of selected drugs (procainamide, quinidine, phenytoin, chlorpromazine, valproic acid, amoxicillin, augmentin, hydralazine, streptomycin, and propranolol have all been reported to induce an LA)
- Infectious diseases—bacterial (including spirochetal and mycobacterial), viral, fungal, and protozoal infections
- Following vaccination

A lupus anticoagulant is the most common cause of a prolonged PTT that remains prolonged in a PTT mixing study (a PTT performed on a sample of mixed patient and normal plasma).

Estimates of prevalence have been highly variable because results are completely dependent on the test(s) used for detection of antiphospholipid antibodies, and some methods are more sensitive than others. Approximately 2% of patients with a prolonged PTT will have an LA as the cause of the prolongation. LA is the most common cause of a prolonged PTT that remains prolonged in a PTT mixing study (a PTT performed on a sample of mixed patient and normal plasma). It is estimated that 1% to 5% of the general population has an antiphospholipid antibody. The frequency of antiphospholipid antibody in systemic lupus erythematosus patients is in the 30% to 40% range. Antiphospholipid antibodies due to infections are typically transient and asymptomatic.

Although the LA acts as an anticoagulant in vitro, it does not appear to be associated with hemorrhage, even with surgical challenge. Rare cases of bleeding in patients with the LA can almost always be attributed to specific abnormalities in hemostasis that happen to be present along with the LA. Decreased prothrombin (Factor II) is occasionally found with the LA. The LA can bind directly to prothrombin, but typically the LA does not neutralize the procoagulant activity of prothrombin even when it does bind to it. In an occasional patient, however, antibody binding does reduce the prothrombin concentration by accelerated clearance of prothrombin/antiprothrombin complexes, and these patients can have hemorrhagic complications. Concomitant thrombocytopenia is not infrequently found in patients with the LA, and this also may be a cause for hemorrhage.

Antiphospholipid antibodies are associated with an increased risk for venous and arterial thrombosis. The role of the antiphospholipid antibody in thrombosis is not clear, although several mechanisms for thrombosis have been proposed. The incidence of clinically apparent thromboembolism in patients with the LA, with or without systemic lupus erythematosus, is difficult to determine because of the variety of tests used to detect the LA. However, data suggest that the percentage of patients with the LA who will develop thrombosis is 1% per year if there is no history of thrombosis and 5.5% per year if there has been at least one prior thrombotic event. High titers of anticardiolipin or anti-beta-2 GP I antibodies present a higher risk for complications than low titers, and IgG is thought to be higher risk than IgM or IgA. There is a greater risk for thrombosis if more than one of the three antiphospholipid antibody tests (LA, anticardiolipin antibodies, and anti-beta-2 GP I antibodies) are abnormal.

Recurrent spontaneous abortion has been reported to be increased in patients with antiphospholipid antibodies. There is evidence suggesting that thrombosis and infarction in the placenta mediate antiphospholipid antibody-associated spontaneous abortion in a significant number of women experiencing recurrent fetal loss or premature birth.

Diagnosis

There are no "gold standard" tests that unequivocally establish the presence of antiphospholipid antibodies:

- *For the LA*: A prolonged PTT and a PTT mixing study that does not correct into the normal range are clues to the presence of the LA, although some PTT reagents are not sensitive to the LA. Therefore, it should be noted that the routine PTT is not an appropriate screening test for the LA. A PTT- or DRVVT-based test with a reduced amount of phospholipid can be used as a screening test for the LA. If it is prolonged, a 1:1 mixing study and a confirmatory assay should be performed. In the presence of an LA, the PTT or DRVVT usually remains prolonged when equal portions of patient plasma and normal plasma are mixed. Confirmatory assays demonstrate that the clotting time shortens toward normal when excess phospholipid is added, overcoming the LA effect. The PT is not typically increased by the LA, unless the patient has an associated hypoprothrombinemia or the thromboplastin used in the PT is one that is particularly sensitive to inhibition by the LA.
- *For anticardiolipin or anti-beta-2 GP I antibodies*: An enzyme-linked immunosorbent assay (ELISA) is used that quantitates IgG and IgM antibody levels in arbitrary units. IgA is also measured in some kits.

Patients with antiphospholipid antibodies may have a false-positive serologic test result for syphilis (such as Venereal Disease Research Laboratories [VDRL] and rapid plasma reagin [RPR]). See **Table 11–19** for information on the laboratory diagnosis of antiphospholipid antibodies.

Thrombotic Thrombocytopenic Purpura
Description

TTP is a clinical syndrome that is characterized by a triad (1 to 3 below, more commonly) or pentad (1 to 5 below, less commonly) of signs and symptoms:

> Thrombotic thrombocytopenic purpura is a clinical syndrome that is characterized by a triad (more commonly) or pentad (less commonly) of signs and symptoms.

1. Thrombocytopenia with generalized purpura, and mucous membrane bleeding
2. Hemolytic anemia (microangiopathic) sufficient to cause jaundice or pallor
3. Neurologic abnormalities, which may include fluctuating weakness, dysphagia, headache, dementia/behavioral changes, obtundation, seizures, diplopia, paresthesias, and coma
4. Fever
5. Renal dysfunction, which may include hematuria, proteinuria, or renal insufficiency

The characteristic, but not pathognomonic, pathology includes platelet and fibrin "hyaline" thrombi in the small arteries, arterioles, and capillaries in a widespread organ distribution. Organ ischemia and infarction that arise from these thrombi are thought to give rise to the observed fever and organ dysfunction. The etiology for TTP has been shown to be a deficiency of vWF-cleaving protease. Nonfamilial cases of TTP are a result of an inhibitor to the vWF-cleaving protease; the familial form of TTP is apparently caused by a constitutional deficiency of the protease.

TABLE 11–20   Laboratory Evaluation for Thrombotic Thrombocytopenic Purpura

Laboratory Test	Results/Comments
Activity of von Willebrand factor-cleaving protease activity	A low value for this enzyme activity is the diagnostic hallmark for the disease, but the assay may not be available for rapid diagnosis of TTP. If the value is low, tests to detect an inhibitor to the protease can be performed
PT, PTT, and fibrinogen levels	Usually normal
Fibrin degradation products or D-dimer	Normal or slightly elevated
Hemoglobin/hematocrit	Mild-to-moderate decrease in most cases; hemorrhage and hemolysis can result in severe anemia in some patients
Haptoglobin	Low as a reflection of intravascular hemolysis
Platelet count	Decreased, often in the range of 10,000–50,000/μL
Peripheral blood smear	Shows schistocytes, nucleated RBCs, and decreased platelet number
Direct and indirect antiglobulin tests	Negative, ruling out an immune hemolytic anemia
Indirect bilirubin	Mild-to-moderate elevation
Serum lactate dehydrogenase (LDH)	Elevated, correlating with the severity of hemolysis and possibly tissue damage from ischemia
WBC count and differential	Shows a mild leukocytosis with a left shift
Urinalysis	Characterized by mild-to-moderate proteinuria and hematuria (without casts)
BUN and creatinine	May or may not be elevated, depending on the presence of renal impairment

BUN, blood urea nitrogen; PT, prothrombin time; PTT, partial thromboplastin time.

The unusually large forms of vWF in the plasma of patients with TTP promote the aggregation of platelets in vivo, which accounts for most of the clinical findings.

TTP can occur at any age but is most common between the ages of 20 and 50 years. Peak incidence is in the third decade. There is a female to male ratio of 3:2. TTP usually occurs as an acute, fulminant disease, but may also occur in a chronic form or in an acute relapsing form. The acute and acute relapsing types are often preceded by a viral prodrome. Nonspecific signs such as malaise, weakness, fatigue, and anorexia may predominate at first, until the above triad or pentad develops in days to weeks. The chronic type usually pursues an indolent, low-grade course, with ongoing disease activity for months.

Nonspecific manifestations in other organ systems resulting from ischemia may include:

- Cardiac: conduction defects, sudden death, and heart failure
- Pulmonary: lung infiltrates and acute respiratory failure
- Gastrointestinal: abdominal pain due to visceral ischemia, pancreatitis, and gastrointestinal mucosal hemorrhage

Diagnosis

See **Table 11–20** for information on the laboratory evaluation for TTP.

Hemolytic–Uremic Syndrome

Description

HUS is a clinical syndrome with presentation and manifestations similar to TTP. Despite the clinical similarity, evidence has shown that the low levels of vWF-cleaving protease found in TTP are not found in HUS. Thus, the pathogenesis of these two disorders is apparently completely different. HUS is characterized by fever, microangiopathic hemolytic anemia, thrombocytopenia, and renal dysfunction. It differs clinically from TTP in the following ways: neurologic symptoms are

TABLE 11–21 **Laboratory Evaluation for Hemolytic–Uremic Syndrome**

Laboratory Test	Results/Comments
PT, PTT, and fibrinogen	Normal
Fibrin degradation products or D-dimer	Absent or minimally increased
Hemoglobin/hematocrit	Decreased with microangiopathic changes on the peripheral blood smear (nucleated RBCs, schistocytes)
Platelet count	Mild-to-moderate decrease
Urinalysis	Hematuria, proteinuria, and red cell casts
Creatinine	Elevated
Lactate dehydrogenase (LDH)	Elevated
Indirect bilirubin	Elevated
Haptoglobin	Low
Direct antiglobulin test (DAT)	Negative
E. coli O157:H7	Commonly positive

PT, prothrombin time; PTT, partial thromboplastin time.

Hemolytic–uremic syndrome is a clinical syndrome with presentation and manifestations similar to TTP. Despite the clinical similarity, evidence has shown that the low levels of vWF-cleaving protease found in TTP are not found in HUS.

less pronounced or absent in HUS; renal function is usually more impaired in HUS than in TTP; HUS occurs in a younger population than TTP with a peak incidence between 6 months and 4 years, with males and females equally affected; HUS is a more common entity than TTP; as with TTP, hyaline thrombi may be found, but in most cases they tend to be confined to the glomerular capillaries and afferent arterioles.

HUS occasionally occurs in adults, and is often distinguished from childhood HUS because of its strong association in adults with obstetrical complications such as eclampsia. The prognosis is worse in adults than in affected children, with an adult mortality as high as 60%.

Acute HUS occurs in nonfamilial and familial forms, which may have different causes. Non-familial forms are most often associated with a diarrheal illness caused by a Shiga-toxin-producing *E. coli* (in particular, *E. coli* O157:H7). Familial forms have been linked to abnormalities in complement factor H and factor I. The majority of childhood cases resolve without sequelae, if children with acute renal failure receive dialysis when necessary. The prognosis depends on the duration of renal failure and the severity of the neurologic disturbance. Renal function returns to normal in approximately 90% of childhood cases.

Diagnosis

See **Table 11–21** for information on the laboratory evaluation for HUS.

Anticoagulant Therapies

Thrombosis can be treated and/or prevented with anticoagulant therapies, which are therapies that inhibit the coagulation cascade, thereby inhibiting fibrin clot formation. Since too little anticoagulation might allow new thrombosis to occur while too much anticoagulant can cause bleeding, laboratory tests can be used to determine how much anticoagulation is present in the patient, so that the dose can be adjusted if needed. For decades, heparin and warfarin were the only anticoagulants available for use. Heparin is given intravenously or subcutaneously, and warfarin is taken orally. As described previously, heparin inhibits multiple coagulation factors, and the effect of this inhibition is that heparin prolongs the PTT. Most PT reagents contain a heparin neutralizer that largely prevents significant PT prolongations for patients on heparin. Warfarin decreases the synthesis of active forms of Factors II, VII, IX, and X, which prolongs the PT. Different PT methods can demonstrate different degrees of prolongation with warfarin. Therefore, a formula is used to convert the PT into a more standardized number that takes into account the relative sensitivity of the PT

TABLE 11–22   Laboratory Monitoring of Anticoagulant Therapies

Anticoagulant	Mechanism	Tests to Monitor Anticoagulation
Warfarin	Decreases active forms of Factors II, VII, IX, X	INR
Heparin	Inhibits Factors IIa, Xa, IXa, XIa, Xa, XIIa	PTT[a]
LMWH	Inhibits Factor Xa	Anti-Factor Xa
Fondaparinux	Inhibits Factor Xa	Anti-Factor Xa
Rivaroxaban	Inhibits Factor Xa	Anti-Factor Xa
Apixaban	Inhibits Factor Xa	Anti-Factor Xa
Argatroban	Inhibits Factor IIa	PTT
Dabigatran	Inhibits Factor IIa	Dilute thrombin time
Bivalirudin	Inhibits Factor IIa	ACT for cardiac catheterization

INR, international normalized ratio; PTT, partial thromboplastin time; ACT, activated clotting time.
[a]For high doses during cardiac catheterization, the ACT is used.

reagent. This calculation is called the international normalized ratio (INR), and it is meant to provide similar results no matter what method is in use by the laboratory. To be sure the correct amount of anticoagulation is present, heparin is closely monitored with the PTT, and warfarin is closely monitored with INR measurements.

Newer anticoagulants have emerged that do not routinely need monitoring with laboratory tests. Nevertheless, laboratory monitoring may still be occasionally indicated. Low-molecular-weight heparin, fondaparinux, rivaroxaban, edoxaban, betrixaban, and apixaban inhibit Factor Xa. Therefore, these anticoagulants can be monitored with anti-Factor Xa assays. These are assays that can measure the concentration of the anticoagulant based on how much inhibition of Factor Xa is detected. Direct thrombin inhibitors (argatroban, bivalirudin, and dabigatran) inhibit thrombin, which prolongs the PTT and to a lesser extent the PT. A dilute thrombin time assay has been shown to have a linear relationship to therapeutic doses of dabigatran. The PTT can be useful to monitor argatroban. Bivalirudin is specifically approved for use during percutaneous coronary intervention (PCI), a cardiac catheterization procedure that requires anticoagulation that is monitored with a rapid, bedside whole blood clotting time test called the activated clotting time (ACT). If a patient has PCI with bivalirudin, the ACT is used.

Only warfarin, rivaroxaban, dabigatran, edoxaban, betrixaban, and apixaban are administered orally. The other anticoagulants are administered parenterally.

See **Table 11–22** for a summary of the mechanisms of action and the laboratory tests to measure the anticoagulation effect of these various anticoagulant therapies.

Antiplatelet Therapies

Patients with arterial thrombosis, in particular myocardial infarction or ischemic stroke, are usually treated with antiplatelet therapy, to inhibit platelet activation. Unlike many anticoagulant therapies, laboratory testing is not yet routinely used to monitor antiplatelet therapy. Studies are ongoing to determine if laboratory monitoring of platelet therapy is beneficial. A variety of platelet-inhibiting medications are available. Aspirin irreversibly inhibits cyclooxygenase in platelets, which prevents the generation of thromboxane A2 from arachidonic acid. This inhibits platelet aggregation because thromboxane A2 triggers the release of platelet granules and activates other platelets. Several GP IIb/IIIa inhibitors are available (abciximab, eptifibatide, or tirofiban). These agents inhibit platelet aggregation because GP IIb/IIIa on the platelet surface mediates platelet aggregation. Clopidogrel, prasugrel, and ticagrelor all inhibit an ADP receptor on the platelet surface, which ultimately inhibits activation of platelet GP IIb/IIIa. Dipyridamole inhibits platelets through multiple mechanisms.

A portion of this chapter, primarily the material in the section "Introduction to Hemostasis," was adapted with permission with modifications from Laposata M, Connor AM, Hicks, DG, Phillips DK. The Clinical Hemostasis Handbook. Chicago, IL: Year Book Medical Publishers; 1989.

SELF-ASSESSMENT QUESTIONS

1. Which of the following disorders of coagulation or conditions is associated with thrombosis rather than bleeding?
   A. von Willebrand disease
   B. Factor V deficiency
   C. Factor V Leiden mutation
   D. Immune thrombocytopenic purpura

2. Which of the following conditions or disorders is not associated with deficiencies of multiple coagulation factors?
   A. Hemophilia A
   B. Vitamin K deficiency
   C. Liver disease
   D. Disseminated intravascular coagulation (DIC)

3. All of the following are quantitative platelet disorders. One of them is immune mediated, that is, involves an antibody that binds to platelets. Identify the immune-mediated thrombocytopenia.
   A. Disseminated intravascular coagulation (DIC)
   B. Hemolytic uremic syndrome (HUS)
   C. Posttransfusion purpura
   D. Thrombotic thrombocytopenic purpura

4. Of the choices below, three represent quantitative platelet disorders and one represents a qualitative platelet disorder. Identify the qualitative platelet disorder characterized by defective binding of platelets to Fibrinogen.
   A. Glanzmann thrombasthenia
   B. Immune thrombocytopenic purpura
   C. Hypersplenism
   D. Essential thrombocythemia

5. A patient is known to have a congenital deficiency of a coagulation factor. The patient presents with a normal prothrombin time (PT) and a markedly elevated partial thromboplastin time (PTT). Which of the following factors is most likely to show a deficiency?
   A. Factor VII
   B. Factor XI
   C. Factor XIII
   D. Fibrinogen

6. Which of the following factors, even when markedly deficient and associated with a markedly prolonged PTT, does not predispose the patient to bleeding?
   A. Factor VIII
   B. Factor IX
   C. Factor XII
   D. Factor V

7. Vitamin K deficiency most often occurs secondary to disease or drug therapy rather than reduced dietary intake. Which of the following conditions does not predispose to vitamin K deficiency?
   A. Warfarin therapy
   B. Malabsorption associated with cystic fibrosis
   C. Antibiotic therapy
   D. Hepatitis A

8. Which of the following conditions is not a well-established cause of disseminated intravascular coagulation?
   A. Malignancy
   B. Pulmonary fibrosis
   C. Obstetrical complications such as fetal death in utero
   D. Severe infection

9. With regard to acute disseminated intravascular coagulation (DIC), which of the following statements is true?
   A. DIC commonly presents clinically as a bleeding disorder.
   B. DIC commonly presents as a thrombotic disorder.
   C. Approximately half of patients with DIC present with bleeding, and approximately half present with thrombosis.
   D. Even patients with very severe DIC rarely experience bleeding or thrombosis.

10. Which of the following coagulation abnormalities is not likely to be present in a patient suffering from severe liver disease associated with cirrhosis?

    A. Decreased production of coagulation factors
    B. Hyperactive platelet function
    C. Thrombocytopenia
    D. Increased D-dimer levels in the circulation

11. Which of the following statements about immune thrombocytopenia (ITP) is not true?

    A. The destruction of platelets in ITP is antibody mediated.
    B. Acute ITP usually presents as a childhood illness.
    C. Chronic ITP occurs most commonly in patients between ages 20 and 50.
    D. Chronic ITP is much more prevalent in males than in females.

12. Which of the following drugs is least often associated with drug-induced thrombocytopenia?

    A. Quinidine
    B. Heparin
    C. Sulfonamides
    D. Aspirin

13. Which of the following coagulation disorders has the highest incidence in the population?

    A. von Willebrand disease
    B. Factor V deficiency
    C. Essential thrombocythemia
    D. Platelet storage pool deficiency

14. Which of the following tests is least likely to be informative in the evaluation of the patient for von Willebrand disease?

    A. Factor VIII
    B. Ristocetin cofactor (an assessment for von Willebrand factor activity)
    C. von Willebrand factor antigen
    D. White blood cell count

15. A patient with von Willebrand disease is being evaluated to determine the subtype of the disorder. It has been shown that the patient's platelets have been coated with von Willebrand factor derived from the pool of circulating von Willebrand factor. It was also found that the patient's platelets aggregated to an extremely low dose of ristocetin added as an agonist in standard platelet-rich plasma aggregometry. What is the most likely subtype of von Willebrand disease in this patient?

    A. Type 1
    B. Type 2A
    C. Type 2B
    D. Type 3

16. Individuals with which of the following blood type have a lower baseline level of von Willebrand factor?

    A. Type O
    B. Type A
    C. Type B
    D. Type AB

17. A patient with a decreased functional platelet glycoprotein Ib/IX/V complex is most likely to have which diagnosis below?

    A. Glanzmann thrombasthenia
    B. Bernard–Soulier disease
    C. Platelet storage pool disease
    D. Cyclooxygenase deficiency

18. Which of the following heritable thrombotic disorders is the most commonly encountered among Caucasians?

    A. Protein C deficiency
    B. Antithrombin deficiency
    C. Factor V Leiden mutation
    D. Protein S deficiency

19. Which of the following tests for hypercoagulability does not yield reliable results for the baseline level in the presence of warfarin?

    A. Antithrombin
    B. Factor V Leiden mutation
    C. Protein C
    D. Prothrombin 20210 mutation

20. What protein is the target of "antiphospholipid" antibodies?
    A. β2 Glycoprotein 1
    B. Cardiolipin
    C. Phosphatidylserine
    D. Phosphatidylinositol

21. Which of the following is not an antiphospholipid antibody?
    A. Lupus anticoagulant
    B. Anticardiolipin antibody
    C. Anti-β2 glycoprotein 1 antibody
    D. Antinuclear antibody

22. Which of the following anticoagulants below selectively inhibits coagulation factor X?
    A. Warfarin
    B. Heparin
    C. Dabigatran
    D. Rivaroxaban

23. Which of the following anticoagulants is monitored with the international normalized ratio (INR)?
    A. Low-molecular-weight heparin
    B. Apixaban
    C. Unfractionated heparin
    D. Warfarin

24. The effect of which of the following drugs markedly affects the results of a platelet aggregation test?
    A. Dabigatran
    B. Apixaban
    C. Rivaroxaban
    D. Aspirin

25. Which of the following pairs listing a platelet inhibitor with its mechanism of inhibitory action is incorrect?
    A. Clopidogrel/Block of platelet ADP receptor
    B. Aspirin/Block of platelet thromboxane receptor
    C. Eptifibatide/Block of platelet fibrinogen receptor
    D. Ibuprofen/Block of platelet cyclooxygenase

FURTHER READING

Acharya SS, et al. Rare bleeding disorder registry: deficiencies of factors II, V, VII, X, XIII, fibrinogen and dysfibrinogenemias. *J Thromb Haemost.* 2004;2:248.

Adcock DM, Gosselin R. Direct Oral Anticoagulants (DOACs) in the laboratory: 2015 review. *Thromb Res.* 2015;136:7–12.

Arber DA, Orazi A, Hasserjian R, et al. The 2016 revision to the World Health Organization classification of myeloid neoplasms and acute leukemia. *Blood.* 2016;127:2391–405.

Avecilla ST, et al. Plasma-diluted thrombin time to measure dabigatran concentrations during dabigatran etexilate therapy. *Am J Clin Pathol.* 2012;137:572–574.

Boyce T, et al. *Escherichia coli* O157:H7 and the hemolytic–uremic syndrome. *N Engl J Med.* 1995;333:364.

Bussell JB, et al. Fetal alloimmune thrombocytopenia. *N Engl J Med.* 1997;337:22–26.

Castellone DD, Van Cott EM. Laboratory monitoring of new anticoagulants. *Am J Hematol.* 2010;85: 185–187.

Feinstein DI. Immune coagulation disorders. In: Colman W, et al, eds. *Hemostasis and Thrombosis: Basic Principles of Clinical Practice.* 4th ed. Philadelphia, PA: Lippincott Williams & Wilkins; 2001:1003.

Feinstein DI, Marder VJ, Colman RW. Consumptive thrombohemorrhagic disorders. In: Colman W, et al, eds. *Hemostasis and Thrombosis: Basic Principles of Clinical Practice.* 4th ed. Philadelphia, PA: Lippincott Williams & Wilkins; 2001:1197.

Finazzi T, et al. Natural history and risk factors for thrombosis in 360 patients with antiphospholipid antibodies: a four-year prospective study from the Italian registry. *Am J Med.* 1996;100:530.

Furlan M, et al. von Willebrand factor-cleaving protease in thrombotic thrombocytopenic purpura and the hemolytic–uremic syndrome. *N Engl J Med.* 1998;339:1578.

George JN, et al. Chronic idiopathic thrombocytopenic purpura. *N Engl J Med.* 1994;331:1207.

George JN, et al. Idiopathic thrombocytopenic purpura: a practice guideline developed by explicit methods for the American Society of Hematology. *Blood.* 1996;88:3.

Gill JC, et al. The effect of ABO blood group on the diagnosis of von Willebrand's disease. *Blood*. 1987;69:1691–1695.

Gillis S. The thrombocytopenic purpuras: recognition and management. *Drugs*. 1996;51:942.

Hoyer L. Hemophilia A. *N Engl J Med*. 1994:330:38.

Joist JH, George JN. Hemostatic abnormalities in liver and renal disease. In: Colman W, et al, eds. *Hemostasis and Thrombosis: Basic Principles of Clinical Practice*. 4th ed. Philadelphia, PA: Lippincott Williams & Wilkins; 2001:839.

Kempton CL, White GC Jr. How we treat a hemophilia A patient with a factor VIII inhibitor. *Blood*. 2009;113:11–17.

Khor B, Van Cott EM. Laboratory evaluation of hypercoagulability. *Clin Lab Med*. 2009;29:339–366.

Kottke-Marchant K. Platelet disorders. In: Kottke-Marchant K, ed. *An Algorithmic Approach to Hemostasis Testing*. Northfield, IL: College of American Pathologists Press; 2008:185–216.

Kurtzberg J, Stockman JA. Idiopathic autoimmune thrombocytopenic purpura. *Adv Pediatr*. 1994;41:111.

Laposata M, et al. *The Clinical Hemostasis Handbook*. St. Louis, MO: The CV Mosby Company; 1989.

Mackman N, Gruber A. Platelet polyphosphate: an endogenous activator of coagulation factor XII. *J Thromb Haemost*. 2010;8:865–867.

Miyakis S, et al. International consensus statement on an update of the classification criteria for definite antiphospholipid syndrome (APS). *J Thromb Haemost*. 2006;4:295–306.

Neunert C, et al. The American Society of Hematology 2011 evidence-based practice guideline for immune thrombocytopenia. Blood. 2011;117:4190–4207.

Nichols WL, et al. Diagnosis, evaluation, and management of von Willebrand disease. NIH publication number 08-5832. National Heart, Lung, Blood Institute (NHLBI); 2007.

Peyvandi F, et al. Classification of rare bleeding disorders (RBDs) based on the association between coagulant factor activity and clinical bleeding severity. *J Thromb Haemost*. 2012;10:1938–1943.

Provan D, et al. International consensus report on the investigation and management of primary immune thrombocytopenia. *Blood*. 2010;115:168–186.

Roberts HR, White GC Jr. Inherited disorders of prothrombin conversion. In: Colman W, et al, eds. *Hemostasis and Thrombosis: Basic Principles of Clinical Practice*. 4th ed. Philadelphia, PA: Lippincott Williams & Wilkins; 2001:839.

Rodeghiero F, et al. Standardization of terminology, definitions and outcome criteria in immune thrombocytopenic purpura of adults and children: report from an international working group. *Blood*. 2009;113(11):2386–2393.

Rothenberger SS, McCarthy LJ. Neonatal alloimmune thrombocytopenia: from prediction to prevention. *Lab Med*. 1997;28:592.

Saha M, McDaniel JK, Zheng XL. Thrombotic thrombocytopenic purpura: pathogenesis, diagnosis and potential novel therapeutics. *J Thromb Haemost*. 2017; 15:1889–1900.

Seitz R, et al. ETRO Working Party on Factor XIII questionnaire on congenital Factor XIII deficiency in Europe: status and perspectives. *Semin Thromb Hemostasis*. 1996;22:415.

Seligsohn U, et al. Inherited deficiencies of coagulation factors II, V, VII, X, XI and XIII and combined deficiencies of factors V and VIII and of the vitamin K-dependent factors. In: Lichtman MA, et al, eds. *Hematology*. 7th ed. New York, NY: McGraw-Hill; 2006:1887.

Shahani T, et al. Human liver sinusoidal endothelial cells but not hepatocytes contain factor VIII. *J Thromb Haemost*. 2014;12:34–35.

Siegler RL. The hemolytic uremic syndrome. *Pediatr Clin North Am*. 1995;42:1505.

Souid A, Sadowitz PD. Acute childhood immune thrombocytopenic purpura: diagnosis and treatment. *Clin Pediatr*. 1995;34:487.

Taaning E, Svejgaard A. Post-transfusion purpura: a survey of 12 Danish cases with special reference to immunoglobulin G subclasses of the platelet antibodies. *Transfus Med*. 1994;4:1.

Tarr PI, Gordon CA, Chandler WA. Shiga-toxin-producing *Escherichia coli* and haemolytic uraemic syndrome. *Lancet*. 2005;365:1073–1086.

Tsai H-M, Lian EC-Y. Antibodies to von Willebrand factor-cleaving protease in acute thrombotic thrombocytopenic purpura. *N Engl J Med*. 1998;339:1585.

Van Cott EM, Drouin A. von Willebrand disease. In: Kottke-Marchant K, ed. *An Algorithmic Approach to Hemostasis Testing*. 2nd ed. Northfield, IL: College of American Pathologists Press; 2016;241–252.

Van Cott EM, Eby C. Antiphospholipid antibodies. In: Kottke-Marchant K, ed. *An Algorithmic Approach to Hemostasis Testing*. 2nd ed. Northfield, IL: College of American Pathologists Press; 2016:327–336.

Van Cott EM, Laposata M. Laboratory evaluation of hypercoagulable states. *Hematol Oncol Clin North Am*. 1998;12:1141.

Verhovsik M, et al. Laboratory testing for fibrinogen abnormalities. *Am J Hematol*. 2008;83:928–931.

Waters AH. Autoimmune thrombocytopenia: clinical aspects. *Semin Hematol*. 1992;29:18.

Zhang B, et al. Genotype–phenotype correlation in combined deficiency of factor V and factor VIII. *Blood*. 2008;111:5592–5600.

Transfusion Medicine

Christopher P. Stowell

LEARNING OBJECTIVES

1. Understand the process of blood collection and the preparation of blood components and plasma derivatives.

2. Learn which tests must be performed to assure safe transfusion.

3. Learn the specific indications for transfusion of individual blood components and alternatives to allogeneic transfusion.

4. Understand the clinical complications that may arise after transfusion of blood components.

5. Learn about the collection and use of hematopoietic progenitor cells.

6. Learn the process of apheresis and its clinical indications.

CHAPTER OUTLINE

Transfusion medicine is the field of medicine that encompasses blood banking (the collection, preparation, testing, and storage of blood components and plasma derivatives) as well as the therapeutic uses of blood components, plasma derivatives, and apheresis technology. It also includes the collection, storage, and use of hematopoietic and other blood-derived cells. An overview of the steps from collection of the blood to transfusion of its components is

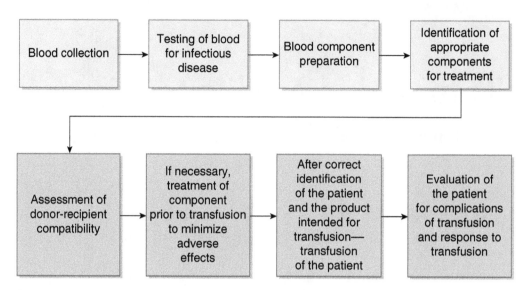

FIGURE 12–1   **An overview of blood collection, processing, and transfusion.**

shown in **Figure 12–1**. Briefly (with more complete descriptions to follow), blood is collected as whole blood or by apheresis from screened, volunteer donors, and samples of the blood are tested for infectious diseases and to determine the blood type. Whole blood may be fractionated into packed red blood cells (RBCs), platelets, and a plasma product. Alternatively, all three components can be collected by apheresis. Plasma can be further processed to provide albumin, clotting factor concentrates, and immunoglobulin preparations. The transfusion of blood components requires testing to be done to establish compatibility between the product and the intended recipient. Blood components may also be treated to reduce complications of transfusion (e.g., remove leukocytes to prevent febrile reactions). As complex, biologically derived therapeutic agents, blood components and derivatives are responsible for a variety of potential untoward effects that must be evaluated and managed. The entire process, from blood collection to transfusion and posttransfusion evaluation, is described in this chapter (see **Figure 12–1**).

> Whole blood may be fractionated into packed red blood cells (RBCs), platelets, and a plasma product.

COLLECTION OF BLOOD AND PREPARATION OF BLOOD COMPONENTS

Blood Collection

The cornerstone of a safe blood supply is the volunteer blood donor who is motivated by altruism. In the past, the use of paid donors was associated with increased levels of transfusion-transmitted hepatitis. Concerns remain about the impact of significant financial incentives on the frank disclosure of health problems or high-risk behaviors that might disqualify a potential blood donor. In the United States, virtually all of the blood is collected from volunteer donors. Regional blood centers collect and distribute more than 90% of the US blood supply while hospital blood banks collect the remainder. The Food and Drug Administration (FDA) Center for Biologics Evaluation and Research regulates all aspects of blood collection and processing, but most blood banks and donor centers are also accredited, on a voluntary basis, by the AABB, formerly known as the American Association of Blood Banks. Blood donors are screened for behaviors or medical conditions that might make blood donation unsafe for them (e.g., anemia, coronary artery insufficiency) or the donated blood hazardous for the transfusion recipient (e.g., exposure to viral hepatitis, use of a teratogenic medication). The AABB has developed, and the FDA has sanctioned, a Uniform Donor Health Questionnaire that is in wide use in the United States and reflects the consistency of donor criteria throughout the country. To qualify for blood donation, the prospective donor must also pass a basic physical screening that includes temperature, blood pressure, pulse, and examination of the arms for signs of intravenous drug use, and have a hemoglobin level determined on a finger-stick or venous blood sample which is at least 13.0 g/dL for males and

12.5 g/dL for females. The collecting agency must check its records to be sure that the donor has not previously been disqualified from donating.

In the process of blood collection, the venipuncture site is disinfected and a needle, which is connected to a collecting set, is inserted into a vein in the arm. The collecting set includes a primary collection bag and several integrally connected satellite bags that are used to make components. The primary collection bag contains a solution that includes an anticoagulant (citrate) and a variety of substances, such as phosphate, adenine, and dextrose, which improve the recovery of the RBCs when transfused and permit their storage in the refrigerator for 35 to 42 days. The typical donation is approximately 450 to 500 mL of whole blood, but may not exceed 10.5 mL/kg of the donor's weight, and must be collected in no more than 15 minutes if a unit of platelets is to be made. This volume of blood represents approximately 10% of the total blood volume of a donor weighing 70 kg, and its loss is well tolerated by healthy individuals. Samples of blood for serologic and infectious disease testing are also obtained at the time of donation, often by collecting the first 15 to 25 mL of blood drawn into a separate container (usually another satellite bag) which has the advantage of diverting the blood most likely to be contaminated with skin bacteria away from the collection bag. Once the collection has been completed, the needle is withdrawn from the donor's arm, and the tubing connecting the needle to the primary collection bag is heat-sealed off.

> The typical donation is approximately 450 to 500 mL of whole blood. This volume of blood represents approximately 10% of the total blood volume of a donor weighing 70 kg, and its loss is well tolerated by healthy individuals.

Component Preparation

Almost all of the whole blood collected is separated into its components—RBCs, platelets, and plasma—in order to be able to store each under optimal conditions. This separation process entails two centrifugation steps and relies on the system of integrally connected satellite bags to carry out all of the preparation steps in a closed, aseptic environment (see **Table 12–1** for a description of blood components, and Chapter 2 for a diagram of blood component preparation). In the procedure used in the United States, RBCs are separated from platelet-rich plasma by the first, relatively low *g* force, centrifugation step. The platelet-rich plasma is expressed from the primary collection bag into one of the satellite bags that is heat-sealed off from the packed RBCs in the primary collection bag. The packed RBCs remaining in the primary collection bag may be stored for up to 35 days at 1°C to 6°C (CPDA-1 RBCs). In some collection systems, additional additive–preservative solution from another satellite bag may be added to the packed RBC, creating a product with a lower hematocrit (but identical RBC mass) and an additional week of storage (42 days).

The platelet-rich plasma, which was expressed off the packed RBC after the first spin, is then separated into platelets and plasma by a second, higher *g* force, centrifugation step. The platelet-poor plasma is expressed into another satellite bag after this second centrifugation step and is usually frozen within 8 hours of collection (as fresh frozen plasma [FFP]) or within 24 hours of collection (24-hour plasma). The platelet pellet that remains is suspended in 40 to 60 mL of plasma and is called a platelet concentrate or whole blood-derived platelets. The term "random donor platelets," although commonly used, is inaccurate. Platelets are stored at 20°C to 24°C for up to 5 days, whereas the various plasma-derived components are stored frozen (≤−18°C for 1 year; ≤−65°C for 7 years). Since one transfusion dose for an adult patient consists of 4 to 10 units of platelet concentrates, it is common to use commercially available closed systems to pool and leukoreduce them.

FFP can be used to prepare another useful component, called cryoprecipitated antihemophilic factor (or "cryoprecipitate"). When FFP is thawed at 1°C to 6°C, a precipitate forms. Most of the plasma can be expressed into a satellite bag, leaving behind this cryoprecipitate that is suspended in 10 to 20 mL of plasma, refrozen, and then stored (≤−18°C for 1 year). Cryoprecipitate contains about half of the Factor VIII, von Willebrand factor, Factor XIII, and fibrinogen that was present in the original unit of plasma, but in a much smaller volume. The plasma remaining after the cryoprecipitate has been removed may also be refrozen. "Plasma–cryoprecipitate reduced" (or cryo-poor plasma) may be used as the starting material (source plasma) for the preparation of plasma derivatives such as albumin and immunoglobulins, and occasionally for replacement during plasmapheresis for patients with thrombotic thrombocytopenic purpura (see **Table 12–2**). Thus, each unit of whole blood can be separated into a unit of packed RBCs, a platelet concentrate, and either FFP or cryoprecipitate plus some other plasma product. The different plasma products (absent cryoprecipitate) may all be used as source plasma for the preparation of derivatives, such as albumin or immunoglobulin.

TABLE 12–1   Blood Component Descriptions and Indications

Category	Description of Product	Major Indications	Actions	Precautions
Packed RBCs	Packed RBCs are the product of a centrifugal separation of red cells from plasma; this component has a hematocrit of 55–80%	Packed RBCs are used for treatment of a symptomatic anemia; this component may also be used for exchange transfusion when treating sickle cell crisis or hemolytic disease of the newborn	Packed RBCs provide RBC mass and increase oxygen-carrying capacity in the blood	RBCs must be ABO- and Rh-compatible, and crossmatched
RBCs, leukoreduced	Packed RBCs may be modified by removal of leukocytes by filtration or washing; washing RBCs is less effective at removing leukocytes than filtration	The indications for this product are the same as for packed RBCs; leukoreduced RBCs are used for individuals who have experienced febrile reactions due to passenger WBCs in a blood component; they are also used to prevent alloimmunization in a patient who may require multiple platelet transfusions, or to prevent cytomegalovirus infection in a susceptible patient	Packed RBCs provide RBC mass and increase oxygen-carrying capacity in the blood	RBCs must be ABO- and Rh-compatible, and crossmatched
Fresh frozen plasma (FFP)	Plasma that is separated from the cellular components and frozen within 8 h of collection of whole blood is known as FFP; it may also be prepared from plasma collected by apheresis	Because FFP contains significant levels of all the plasma coagulation factors, including Factors V and VIII that are labile, it is useful to control bleeding in patients who have multiple coagulation factor deficiencies; FFP should not be used to correct a deficit of blood volume; other volume expanders that are less potentially infectious should be used	FFP restores plasma proteins, particularly coagulation factors, and this may result in control of a bleeding episode	This component should be ABO-compatible with the recipient's RBCs, but crossmatching is not performed prior to transfusion; Rh type is not a consideration
Cryoprecipitate	Cryoprecipitate is generated by thawing FFP at 1–6°C; the precipitate is collected and refrozen; a typical unit of cryoprecipitate contains at least 80 units of Factor VIII and at least 150 mg of fibrinogen in a volume of less than 25 mL	This component is used for patients with a deficiency of fibrinogen (often from disseminated intravascular coagulation), or deficiency of Factor XIII	Transfusion of cryoprecipitate to raise fibrinogen levels to 100 mg/dL may be useful to provide hemostasis for fibrinogen deficiency	Crossmatch testing is unnecessary; although ABO-compatible cryoprecipitate is preferred, it is not necessary; the Rh type is not a consideration
Platelets collected by apheresis	Platelets obtained by apheresis contain at least 3×10^{11} platelets/unit; the product has a volume between 200 and 400 mL	Platelet transfusions are indicated for patients who are thrombocytopenic due to decreased platelet production or blood loss and for those patients who do not have an adequate number of functioning platelets; platelet transfusions are not usually effective in conditions associated with rapid platelet destruction; platelets may be useful in preventing a bleeding episode if given as a prophylactic measure to patients with very low platelet counts	The elevation of the platelet count in a thrombocytopenic patient or the transfusion of functionally active platelets into a patient with dysfunctional platelets, can result in the cessation or prevention of bleeding	Although crossmatching is not necessary, platelet products that are ABO-compatible with the recipient are preferred to minimize the infusion of incompatible plasma

(Continued)

TABLE 12–1 **(Continued)**

Category	Description of Product	Major Indications	Actions	Precautions
Platelet concentrates (whole blood-derived platelets)	Platelet concentrates are obtained from a single unit of whole blood, and contain at least 5.5×10^{10} platelets; suspended in 40–60 mL of plasma, which is stored at 20–24°C; they are usually pooled (typically 4–6 units) to provide a dose equivalent to 1 unit of apheresis platelets	Same as for apheresis platelet	Same as for apheresis platelets	Same as for apheresis platelets
Granulocytes collected by apheresis	Granulocytes are collected from a single donor by apheresis; the product, which contains other blood cells as well, is in a volume of 200–300 mL	Granulocytes may be indicated for the patient who has both neutropenia and a documented infection that is not responsive to therapy; this product should not be used for prophylaxis against infection; in general, it has been more effective in infants than in adults	The granulocytes may contribute to the eradication of infection in a neutropenic recipient	Crossmatching must be performed before transfusion because of the large number of RBCs in the product; in addition, the granulocytes are very labile, so this product should be transfused as soon as possible after collection

TABLE 12–2 **Derivatives of Blood Components and Indications for Their Use**

Derivative	Description and Indication
Factor VIII	Prepared for treatment of hemophilia A; Factor VIII can be purified from pooled human plasma and treated to remove and inactivate infectious agents; recombinant Factor VIII products are available; some plasma-derived preparations contain significant amounts of von Willebrand factor and are suitable for treatment of this disease as well
Factor IX	Prepared using methods similar to those for Factor VIII; it is used for the treatment of patients with hemophilia B; recombinant factor IX is also available; concentrates that contain Factors II, VII, and X along with Factor IX are also available, and are known as prothrombin complex concentrates; some of these concentrates are potentially thrombogenic and are therefore not the preferred product for treatment of hemophilia B
Albumin	Prepared from pooled donor plasma as a 5% or a 25% solution in a manner that removes infectious agents; albumin is used as replacement fluid for plasmapheresis, for hypoalbuminemic patients with acute lung injury, in conjunction with large-volume paracentesis, for diuresis in patients with ascites unresponsive to diuretics, in selected patients with subarachnoid hemorrhage to prevent vasospasm, and in selected burn patients; it should not be used routinely for volume expansion when crystalloid or synthetic colloid volume expanders such as dextran and hydroxyethyl starch are available
Intravenous immunoglobulin (IV Ig)	The IgG fraction prepared from pooled donor plasma is processed to minimize IgG dimerization and remove or inactivate infectious agents; used as antibody replacement therapy in humoral immunodeficiency states (see Chapter 3) and in the treatment of selected autoimmune disorders such as idiopathic or immune thrombocytopenic purpura (ITP)
Rh immune globulin	The IgG fraction prepared from pooled plasma from donors with high-titer anti-D treated to remove or inactivate infectious agents; administered by intramuscular injection to Rh-negative women to prevent their alloimmunization during pregnancy and childbirth; Rh-negative women should receive this product at 28 weeks of gestation and again within 72 h of the birth of an Rh-positive baby, or at the time of abortion, miscarriage, vaginal hemorrhage, ectopic pregnancy, abdominal trauma, or invasive procedure such as amniocentesis or chorionic villus sampling; an intravenous formulation of this product is used for treatment of ITP
Antithrombin III concentrate	Prepared for treatment of patients with low amounts of circulating antithrombin III who are susceptible to thrombosis; antithrombin is purified from pooled human plasma and treated to remove or inactivate infectious agents
Recombinant, activated Factor VII	A recombinant version of activated Factor VII prepared for treatment of patients with acquired Factor VIII and Factor IX inhibitors and for patients with congenital Factor VII deficiency; the widespread off-label use in bleeding patients with complex coagulopathies is being tempered by the poor outcomes in randomized trials for this indication; should be used with caution in patients with prothrombotic tendencies

Blood components also may be donated by a procedure known as apheresis, in which whole blood is removed from the donor, the component of interest (plasma or platelets most commonly, but RBCs as well) is removed, and the remaining blood elements are returned to the donor (see Chapter 2 for a diagram of apheresis). This procedure may be done manually, but is now usually carried out using an automated device. Using an apheresis instrument, whole blood is drawn from the donor's vein as an anticoagulant solution (usually citrate) is added, and pumped into a centrifuge where it is separated into its components. The component of interest is drawn into a collection bag, and the rest of the blood is returned to the donor via the same or a different vein. This process may be discontinuous (filling the instrument, separating the components, returning the residual blood, and repeating the cycle) or continuous (using separate lines to draw blood into the instrument and return it to the donor). The entire extracorporeal circuit is sealed except at the points of contact with the donor's vein(s). Apheresis is commonly used to obtain plasma, usually for further processing into derivatives such as albumin, clotting factor concentrates, and immunoglobulins, as well as to obtain platelets. A unit of apheresis platelets (commonly called "single donor platelets") contains more platelets than a unit derived from a whole blood donation. Transfusion of a unit of apheresis platelets, which must contain at least 3×10^{11} platelets, usually elevates an adult patient's platelet count by 30,000 to 50,000 platelets/μL. Since 1 unit of whole blood-derived platelets must contain only 5.5×10^{10} platelets, the usual adult dose is 4 to 10 units or 1 unit/10 kg. Whole blood-derived platelets are less expensive to prepare than apheresis platelets because they do not require special equipment for their isolation. However, apheresis platelets can easily be prepared in such a way that they contain very few residual white blood cells ("process leukoreduced"), which is an advantage for some patient groups.

Granulocytes also can be harvested by apheresis for transfusion to patients who are neutropenic and suffering from severe infection. Instruments designed to collect RBCs by apheresis (typically 2 units at a time if the donor meets the somewhat more stringent size and hematocrit requirements) or various combinations of RBCs, platelets, and plasma are also in use. Finally, apheresis is used to collect peripherally circulating hematopoietic progenitor cells (HPCs) for autologous and allogeneic HPC transplantation.

Testing of Donated Blood

Donated blood is held in quarantine following collection while a variety of laboratory tests are performed using blood specimens obtained from the donor at the time of collection. The ABO and Rh types are determined on an RBC sample obtained at each donation, and the donor serum or plasma is screened for the presence of unexpected RBC alloantibodies. The concern is that such alloantibodies could cause destruction of a transfusion recipient's RBCs if they express the target antigen. Plasma or platelets from a donor with an alloantibody are not used for transfusion, although RBCs are generally safe, particularly if they have been saline washed. Records from any previous donations, including the results of ABO and Rh typing, are also checked, to reduce the opportunity for donor or unit misidentification.

Infectious Disease Testing

Transmission of viruses, bacteria, and parasites by transfusion of blood components has been well documented. To minimize infectious disease transmission, blood donors are screened for evidence of infection and for participation in activities that may have exposed them to infectious agents. In addition, each blood donation is subjected to several tests for infectious agents before it is made available for transfusion. The tests required for each donation are shown in **Table 12–3**. Platelets, which are stored at 20°C to 24°C, must also be screened for evidence of bacterial contamination, which is currently responsible for the majority of transfusion-transmitted infections. Several commercial systems have been licensed for the testing of leukoreduced apheresis and whole blood-derived platelets. Alternatively, apheresis platelets may undergo a process of pathogen inactivation which uses amotosalen, a psoralen, which is activated by ultraviolet light and crosslinks the RNA and DNA of contaminating microorganisms and leukocytes, thus inactivating them. Pathogen inactivated (PI) platelets do not need to be

TABLE 12–3   Infectious Disease Testing of Donated Blood

Required	Optional
Serologic test for syphilis	Antibody to cytomegalovirus
Antibody to HIV-1 and HIV-2 HIV-1 RNA	
Antibody to hepatitis C virus (HCV)	
HCV RNA	
Hepatitis B surface antigen	
Antibody to hepatitis B core antigen	
Antibody to HTLV-I and HTLV-II	
Zika virus RNA	
West Nile virus RNA[a]	
Antibody to *Trypanosoma cruzi*[b]	
Screen for bacteria (platelets only)	

HIV, human immunodeficiency virus; HTLV, human T-cell lymphotropic virus.

[a]Determined locally and may vary by season and/or for detection of WNV-infected mosquitoes by public health surveillance.

[b]Testing is done once on all donors and is only repeated if there is another exposure, that is, residence in an endemic area of South or Central America.

TABLE 12–4   RBC Compatibility

ABO Group of Patient	Isoagglutinins Present	Compatible Donor RBC Units	Incompatible Donor RBC Units
A	Anti-B	A, O	B, AB
B	Anti-A	B, O	A, AB
AB	Neither	A, B, AB, O	None
O	Anti-A, anti-B, anti-AB	O	A, B, AB
RBC D Antigen	**Acceptable Donor Units**	**Unacceptable Donor Units**	
Rh-positive	Rh(D)-positive, Rh(D)-negative	None	
Rh-negative	Rh(D)-negative	Rh(D)-positive	

further screened for bacterial contamination. All donors must be screened once for antibody to *Trypanosoma cruzi*, the organism that causes Chagas disease, and deferred indefinitely if they are positive. Thereafter, donors do not need to be retested unless they have a possible exposure, that is, residence in an endemic area of South or Central America. It is likely that screening for infection with *Babesia* spp. will become a requirement in 2018. Tests for the antibody to *Babesia* and for *Babesia* DNA are being evaluated but have not yet been approved for use. It is also not yet clear whether testing will be restricted to collection facilities in the states where *Babesia* infection is most prevalent, or be required throughout the country.

Transmission of viruses, bacteria, and parasites by transfusion of blood components has been well documented. To minimize infectious disease transmission, blood donors are screened for evidence of infection and for participation in activities that may have exposed them to infectious agents.

COMPATIBILITY TESTING

Pretransfusion Testing to Assess Donor/Recipient Compatibility for Blood Components Containing RBCs

Prior to transfusion, the compatibility of donor RBCs with the intended transfusion recipient must be established (see **Tables 12–4** and **12–5** for RBC compatibility issues). Part of this process involves various serologic tests. However, an equally important part of this process is the proper identification of the patient when the blood bank specimen is obtained, and again when

TABLE 12–5   Rh Haplotype Nomenclature (Fisher–Race)

CE Phenotype	D Phenotype	
	RhD Positive	RhD Negative "d"
C e	CDe = R_1	Cde = r'
c E	cDE = R_2	cdE = r"
c e	cDe = R_0	cde = r
C E	CDE = R_z	CdE = r^y

Misidentification of patients and mislabeling of specimens are the most common serious errors encountered in transfusion. ABO mistransfusion as a result of this kind of error is far more frequent than the transmission of HIV and all of the hepatitis viruses, combined.

the transfusion is initiated. Misidentification of patients and mislabeling of specimens are the most common serious errors encountered in transfusion. ABO mistransfusion as a result of this kind of error is far more frequent than the transmission of HIV and all of the hepatitis viruses, combined. Compatibility testing includes:

- The identification of patient and proper labeling of the specimen for compatibility testing. The blood bank specimen (tube of blood) must be labeled at the bedside using the patient's armband for identification. The label must include two patient identifiers (typically name and medical record number) and the date. There must also be some means of identifying the phlebotomist (commonly, but not necessarily, by signing or initialing the tube or requisition). The AABB recently established a new *Standard* for transfusion services regarding specimen collection and labeling. If the facility does not use an electronic method to verify the identity of the patient (i.e., a machine readable arm band), then two people must sign the sample: the person who drew the blood, and a second person who validated that the patient was identified correctly and that the sample was labeled correctly.
- The determination of the ABO and Rh type of the donor. The collecting facility determines the ABO group (by front- and back-typing as described below) and Rh type of the donated unit (and checks prior records). The hospital transfusion service must confirm the ABO group (front type only) and the Rh type of Rh(D)-negative units (only) that have been received from the collecting facility.
- The determination of the ABO and Rh type of the patient on a current specimen, and a comparison to previous records, if any. The ABO group (front and back types) and Rh type are determined on a current specimen. The specimen must be <3 days old for any patient who has been transfused or pregnant within the last 3 months; however, many transfusion services require new specimens every 3 days to keep things simple.
- A screen of the recipient's serum/plasma for unexpected RBC alloantibodies. If unexpected antibodies (i.e., not anti-A or anti-B) are found, as described below, the antigen specificity of these antibodies must be identified to establish the risk of a hemolytic transfusion reaction (HTR) and to help identify potentially compatible donor RBCs that lack the target antigen. A record check for previously identified alloantibodies must also be made.
- The performance of a crossmatch (see Chapter 2 for illustration of the crossmatch). Several techniques for performing the crossmatch are described below.
- The identification of the patient when the transfusion is initiated. The patient must once again be properly identified using the armband to be sure that the unit is intended for the patient. The armband is the only link between the patient, the specimen, and the blood component.

ABO Grouping

After the identification of the patient and the specimen for compatibility testing, the most important step in assuring the safety of an RBC transfusion is the determination of the ABO group of the donor unit and the intended recipient. The specificity of the A and B blood group antigens lies in the presence of carbohydrate structures that are borne by membrane-associated glycoproteins and glycolipids. The *A* gene encodes a glycosyltransferase that attaches an *N*-acetylgalactosamine residue to the core structure (called "H") while the *B* gene encodes an enzyme that transfers a

CHAPTER 12 Transfusion Medicine 329

galactose residue. These two different residues impart A or B serologic activity, respectively, to the glycoprotein or glycolipid core structure. The *O* gene, which is a phenotypic recessive, does not encode for an active enzyme, so the RBC of people who are group O are coated with an unmodified H structures. Since the *A* and *B* genes are codominant, people who inherit one copy of each will have both enzymes, and thus both A and B antigens will be expressed on their RBCs.

During the first year of life, individuals begin to make antibodies to whichever A and B antigens they lack. Thus, a person with A antigen on his or her RBCs (group A) has naturally occurring anti-B antibodies in the plasma (see **Table 12–4**). It is the presence of these antibodies (called isoagglutinins because of their ability to agglutinate RBCs in vitro) that makes ABO mistransfusion so hazardous. The isoagglutinins are largely IgM and fix complement readily. Hence, they can cause intravascular hemolysis.

Because determining the ABO group is so critical, it is required not only to test for A and B antigens on the RBCs but also to demonstrate the presence of the appropriate anti-A and anti-B isoagglutinins in the plasma or serum (see Chapter 2 for a diagram of ABO and Rh typing). The presence of A or B antigens on patient or donor RBCs is detected by combining them with reagent "anti-A" in one test tube and reagent "anti-B" in another test tube, and then assessing RBC agglutination. Agglutination with anti-A, for example, indicates the presence of A antigen on the RBCs. This test is called the "front" or "cell" typing. The plasma of a patient or donor is tested for the presence of anti-A or anti-B antibodies by combining the plasma with reagent RBCs known to be either group A or group B, and then assessing RBC agglutination. Agglutination of the reagent B cells indicates the presence of anti-B isoagglutinin in the plasma, which would be the expected finding in a person who is blood group A. This test is called the "back" or "serum" typing. The results of the front- and back-typing must be congruent.

Rh Typing

The second most important antigen system with respect to transfusion safety is the Rh system. Approximately 85% of Caucasians express the D (or Rh) antigen and are called D (or Rh)-positive (see **Table 12–4**). Rh-negative individuals, who lack the D antigen, are vulnerable to development of an alloantibody to the D antigen, the most immunogenic antigen on human RBCs, if they are exposed to D-positive RBCs by transfusion or, for a woman, by maternal–fetal hemorrhage. Anti-D is the most common cause of severe hemolytic disease of the newborn, although the frequency of this complication of pregnancy has been considerably decreased since the advent of Rh immune globulin. This product is an immunoglobulin fraction obtained by pooling the plasma of people with high-titer anti-D. When given by intramuscular injection to individuals who have been exposed to D-positive RBCs (e.g., women pregnant with a D-positive fetus), it reduces the chance of sensitization presumably by binding to D-positive fetal cells, leading to their rapid clearance from the maternal circulation before an immune response can be generated (see the section "Hemolytic Disease of the Newborn [HDN]" in Chapter 10).

The Rh type is determined by incubating the RBCs with a reagent antibody to the D antigen. Rh-positive cells expressing the D antigen are agglutinated by the reagent antibody. RBCs that do not agglutinate in the presence of the Rh antibody are incubated a second time, usually after the addition of an enhancer of agglutination. RBCs that do not agglutinate after this second step are considered to be Rh(D)-negative. A small number of people have RBCs that do not agglutinate in the first step but are agglutinated after the second, enhanced, incubation step. These individuals are considered to have the weak D (formerly D^u) phenotype. Donors, and usually patients as well, who are weak D are treated as if they are D-positive, since some weak D RBCs can elicit the formation of anti-D alloantibodies in D-negative individuals, or can be the target for anti-D alloantibodies.

The *RHD* gene is located on chromosome 1 immediately adjacent to the highly homologous *RHCE* gene, and the two are inherited as a haplotype exhibiting linkage disequilibrium. The *RHD* gene encodes for the D protein that expresses D ("Rh") antigenic activity. The most common mechanism for the Rh(D)-negative phenotype (especially among people of Caucasian background) is the complete absence of the *RHD* gene. This phenotype is often represented as "d," but in fact there is no "d" gene or "d" protein. These individuals lack the D gene and D protein altogether. The *RHCE* encodes for a protein that is structurally very similar to the D protein, but

After the identification of the patient and the specimen for compatibility testing, the most important step in assuring the safety of an RBC transfusion is the determination of the ABO group of the donor unit and the intended recipient.

carries two different antigens, each of which has two common, codominant alleles: C/c and E/e. Since these genes are inherited as a haplotype, a shorthand nomenclature (Fisher–Race) is in wide use and is shown in **Table 12–5**.

The Antibody Screen and the Indirect Antiglobulin Assay Used to Detect Antibodies

To determine if the patient has an alloantibody to a RBC antigen, an antibody screen is performed. In this test, the patient's serum or plasma is combined with two or three reagent RBCs that are specifically chosen because they bear a number of the antigens to which clinically significant RBC alloantibodies are made. These cells are group O so that they will not be agglutinated by the anti-A or anti-B isoagglutinins that may be present. If the patient serum does not produce agglutination of the reagent screening cells, then no unexpected RBC alloantibodies are present.

Although the anti-A and anti-B isoagglutinins are predominantly IgM and readily produce agglutination in vitro, most of the other clinically significant RBC alloantibodies are IgG and do not. To detect IgG alloantibodies, an assay called the indirect antiglobulin test (formerly the indirect Coombs test) is used for the antibody screen (see Chapter 2 for a diagram of the indirect antiglobulin test). In this technique, the patient's serum is combined with the reagent screening cells, often in the presence of an additive, such as low ionic strength saline or polyethylene glycol, which promotes binding of antibody to RBCs, and the mixture is incubated at 37°C. If an RBC alloantibody is present, it will bind to the screening cell with the target antigen. The cells are then washed with saline, and the "antiglobulin reagent" is added. Antiglobulin reagent consists of a mixture of antibodies to IgG and/or complement. These antibodies bind to any IgG or complement attached to the screening cell. By binding to IgG or complement on adjacent target cells, the anti-IgG "crosslinks" the RBCs and produces RBC agglutination in vitro. It is called the indirect antiglobulin test because it requires first an incubation with the alloantibody (the serum sample) followed by a second step when the antiglobulin reagent is added. The antiglobulin test is commonly performed in a test tube, but has also been adapted to assays based on solid phase or gel column techniques.

If one or more of the screening cells is agglutinated by the patient's serum, indicating the presence of an RBC alloantibody, steps must be taken to identify its specificity by determining its target antigen. This is accomplished again using the indirect antiglobulin test and adding the patient's serum to a panel of group O RBCs (typically around 10) that have been chosen to express the target antigens of the most commonly encountered clinically significant alloantibodies. The pattern of which panel cells are agglutinated in the indirect antiglobulin test can be used to determine the antigen to which the patient's alloantibody is directed. Based on the accumulated clinical experience with alloantibodies of a given specificity, it is usually possible to predict the likelihood that a particular alloantibody will cause an HTR or hemolytic disease of the newborn (see **Table 12–6**). If the alloantibody has the potential of causing hemolysis, donor RBCs that lack the target antigen must be chosen for transfusion. The typing of RBCs for specific antigens is accomplished in a manner similar to that used for the determination of the ABO and Rh type using commercial antisera directed at specific antigens. Patients who have multiple alloantibodies, or alloantibodies directed at high-frequency antigens, may pose the challenge that very few donors will lack the target antigen(s). Under these circumstances, the blood bank may have to screen the red cell inventory for antigen-negative units, request their blood supplier to do the same, or, in some instances, locate suitable units through a national rare blood registry.

The RBC Crossmatch

There are three crossmatch techniques in common use: the antiglobulin technique crossmatch, the immediate spin crossmatch, and the electronic crossmatch.

The antiglobulin crossmatch was the standard for years and still must be performed when a patient has an RBC alloantibody or even a history of having had one (see Chapter 2 for a diagram of the blood crossmatch). This crossmatch procedure is very similar to the antibody screen and is based on the indirect antiglobulin technique, except in this case the patient's serum is

There are three crossmatch techniques in common use: the antiglobulin technique crossmatch, the immediate spin crossmatch, and the electronic crossmatch.

TABLE 12-6   The Major RBC Antigens: Frequencies and Clinical Significance

System	Antigen	Population Frequencies			Implicated in	
		European	Sub-Saharan African	East Asian	Hemolytic Disease of the Newborn	Hemolytic Transfusion Reaction
Rh	D	0.85	0.92	0.99	Yes	Yes
	C	0.68	0.27	0.93	Yes	Yes
	c	0.80	0.98	0.47	Yes	Yes
	E	0.29	0.22	0.39	Yes	Yes
	e	0.98	0.98	0.96	Yes	Yes
Kell	K	0.09	0.02	Rare	Yes	Yes
	k	0.99	>0.99	>0.99	Yes	Yes
Duffy	Fy^a	0.66	0.10	0.99	Yes	Yes
	Fy^b	0.83	0.33	0.19	Yes	Yes
	Fy$^{(a-b-)}$	Rare	0.68	Rare	NA	NA
Kidd	Jk^a	0.77	0.92	0.72	Yes	Yes
	Jk^b	0.74	0.49	0.76	Yes	Yes
MNSs	M	0.78	0.74	0.50	Yes, few cases	Yes, few cases
	N	0.72	0.75	0.67	Yes, rarely	No
	S	0.55	0.31	0.09	Yes	Yes
	s	0.89	0.93	1.00	Yes	Yes
Lewis	Le^{a*}	0.22	0.23	0.19	No	Yes, few cases
	Le^{b*}	0.72	0.55	0.81	No	No
	Le$^{(a-b-)}$	0.06	0.22	0.12	NA	N

NA, not applicable.

*Not allelic pair.

combined with RBCs from the donor unit. If the patient has an alloantibody to the donor RBCs, the antibody will become bound to the donor RBCs during the incubation step, and the cells will be agglutinated by the antiglobulin reagent added in the final step. If agglutination occurs, the crossmatch is incompatible and the unit of RBCs should not be transfused to that patient. If the RBCs from this donor were mistakenly transfused, they would be destroyed prematurely, that is, an HTR would occur. If there is no agglutination, the patient does not have alloantibodies to the antigens present on this donor's RBCs, and the crossmatch is compatible.

The immediate spin crossmatch is done by combining the patient's serum with a sample of the donor RBCs intended for transfusion, centrifuging them without incubation or the use of the antiglobulin reagent, and observing them immediately for agglutination. This technique detects ABO incompatibilities, but is not sensitive to the presence of other RBC alloantibodies. It may only be used in patients who do not have unexpected alloantibodies (i.e., they have a negative antibody screen), in massive transfusion (transfusion of the equivalent of one entire blood volume), and in emergency circumstances when an abbreviated crossmatch procedure is imperative for providing blood rapidly.

In the electronic crossmatch, blood bank personnel rely on the computer to verify the ABO (and Rh) compatibility between donor RBCs and the patient. A number of requirements must be met by the information system and the bench procedures involved in the typing, and extensive validation must be performed. This technique is again only suitable for patients who do not have unexpected RBC alloantibodies, or in emergency situations.

Direct Antiglobulin Test (Formerly Direct Coombs Test)

This test detects the presence of IgG or complement that is bound, in vivo, to the patient's RBCs by using antiglobulin reagent specific for IgG or various complement components, including C3b, C3d, and/or C4d. In this technique, the patient's RBCs are washed with saline, and the antiglobulin reagent is then added directly (hence the name of the test) (see Chapter 2 for a diagram of the direct antiglobulin test). The cells are observed for agglutination after incubation. The presence of RBC coated with immunoglobulin and/or complement is evidence of immune-mediated hemolysis. Disorders associated with a positive direct antiglobulin test include hemolytic disease of the newborn, autoimmune hemolytic anemia, and drug-induced hemolytic anemia. A positive direct antiglobulin test result is also observed in patients experiencing an HTR where donor RBCs are circulating coated with the recipient's alloantibody. Note that most patients with positive direct antiglobulin tests do not have hemolysis. A positive direct antiglobulin test is found in many patients with lymphoproliferative and autoimmune disorders, or who are taking various medications such as procainamide, vancomycin, and drugs in the penicillin and cephalosporin families.

If a patient has an RBC autoantibody, especially if it is an IgG, it may interfere with routine serologic testing, especially any test that is based on the indirect antiglobulin technique such as the antibody screen and the crossmatch. Absorption techniques are used to remove the autoantibody from the patient's plasma, but leave any alloantibody behind. In the autologous absorption technique, the patient's RBCs (after treatment to remove any autoantibody) are incubated with the patient's own plasma. The autoantibodies bind to the patient's RBC, but any alloantibodies present do not, since the patient lacks those antigens, by definition. After absorbing out all of the autoantibody (which may take a few cycles with fresh batches of the patient's RBCs) the autoabsorbed plasma can be tested for alloantibodies using the conventional antibody screen described above. If the patient has been recently transfused, this absorption technique cannot be used, because the transfused cells might absorb some of the alloantibody as well as the autoantibody if they happen to bear the target antigen. In this case the RBCs used for the absorption may be phenotypically matched to the patient, or several cells may be chosen, each of which displays a different array of RBC antigens—hence the name, the heterologous absorption technique. The sample of patient plasma that was absorbed by the heterologous cells is then also tested for RBC alloantibodies using the conventional antibody screen described above.

Compatibility Testing for Other Blood Components That Do Not Contain RBCs

Compatibility testing for blood components without RBCs (i.e., platelets and plasma) is much less complex than it is for products with RBCs since no crossmatching is necessary. ABO grouping of donor units and the patient must be performed to avoid the transfusion of plasma that is ABO-incompatible with the recipient's RBCs. The amount of anti-A and/or anti-B isoagglutinin in a unit of apheresis platelets or FFP (200 to 300 mL) could lead to destruction of some of the recipient's RBCs if there were an ABO mismatch. Rh-negative recipients may receive plasma products or apheresis platelets from a donor of any Rh type, since these components do not contain RBCs. Whole blood-derived platelets from Rh-negative donors may be preferentially selected for Rh-negative patients, particularly if there is visible RBC contamination of the platelet product, to avoid the possibility of alloimmunization to the D antigen.

Molecular Techniques in Immunohematology

In the last 20 years, molecular techniques have greatly increased our understanding of blood group antigen structures and their genetics, and have explained many of the serologic conundrums that baffled blood bankers for decades. Although not in routine use in the hospital transfusion service at this point, a widening array of applications has been making its way into the clinical arena. Some of these applications include:

1. Genotyping blood donors—Microarray-based platforms and mass spectrometry techniques have been used to genotype large numbers of blood donors for a number of the most common clinically significant antigens. The availability of this information facilitates the identification of donor units for patients who require RBC with a specific phenotype.

2. Genotyping patients—Similar technology can be applied to individual patients in circumstances when it is difficult to obtain a reliable phenotype by serologic methods, for example, in patients who have already been transfused or who have autoantibodies.
3. Hemolytic disease of the newborn—Detection of the *RHD* gene in the fetus of an alloimmunized mother can be performed using amniotic fluid or maternal plasma, thereby establishing whether or not the fetus is at risk for hemolytic disease of the newborn. The absence of the *RHD* gene in the fetus also obviates the need for additional, more invasive testing of the fetus, such as per-umbilical blood sampling. It is also possible to determine whether or not the father is homozygous for the *RHD* gene.
4. Genotyping in the absence of serologic reagents—Typing sera for some clinically significant blood group systems, such as Scianna and Dombrock, are not routinely available, and others are periodically in short supply. Genotyping has been used as an alternative in these situations.

Other potential applications:

1. Extended electronic crossmatching—The use of the electronic crossmatch to insure ABO and RhD compatibility between donor RBC and recipient is well established. The extension of this technique for matching for other clinically significant antigens would be feasible if more extended genotype information was available for donors. This approach could be used in two circumstances:
   a. Alloimmunized patients—For example, the database could be searched for donor RBCs that were A, R_1r, and Kell (K1) negative for a patient who was group A with anti-E and anti-K. Only these units would require antigen confirmation (serologically according to current regulations) and crossmatching.
   b. Multiply transfused patients—Prospective genotype matching could be performed for transfusion-dependent patients, such as those with sickle cell disease, thalassemia, or aplastic anemia, to reduce the incidence of alloimmunization and delayed HTRs, especially the hyperhemolysis syndrome.
2. Autoimmune hemolytic anemia—The evaluation of patients with autoimmune hemolytic anemia is time-consuming and technically demanding, especially if they require autologous or heterologous absorptions. The goal of identifying units suitable for transfusion could be met, and perhaps more rapidly, by extended genotype matching.

INDICATIONS FOR TRANSFUSION

Table 12–7 is a list of indications for transfusion of RBCs, platelets, plasma, and cryoprecipitate.

Red Blood Cells

A National Institutes of Health (NIH) Consensus Conference established broad parameters for perioperative RBC transfusion. Although the conclusion of the conference was that "no single measure can replace good clinical judgment as the basis for decisions regarding perioperative transfusion," it was suggested that patients with hemoglobin levels exceeding 10 g/dL (100 g/L) rarely require transfusion, while those with hemoglobin levels less than 7 g/dL (70 g/L) frequently do. Several professional organizations have also established guidelines for RBC transfusion. There have been a number of randomized trials comparing the clinical outcomes of liberal and stringent RBC transfusion triggers in different patient groups that have consistently failed to demonstrate any benefit of transfusing patients for hematocrits of 30% (10 g/dL) compared with triggers as low as 21% (7 g/dL).

Platelets

Indications for platelet transfusion have also been addressed by an NIH Consensus Conference and various professional organizations. Of particular interest is the reassessment of the use of prophylactic platelet transfusions in thrombocytopenic patients with marrow failure. In general, the traditional trigger level of 20,000 platelets/μL for prophylactic transfusion has been replaced with

Hemoglobin levels exceeding 10 g/dL (100 g/L) rarely require transfusion, while those with hemoglobin levels less than 7 g/dL (70 g/L) frequently do.

TABLE 12-7 **Indications for Transfusion**

Packed RBCs

Hgb <7 g/dL or hematocrit <21% in a patient with uncompromised cardiovascular function

Hgb <10 g/dL or hematocrit <30% in a patient with cardiovascular disease, sepsis, or hemoglobinopathy

Platelets

Prophylactically for platelet count <10,000/μL (adults), or <50,000/μL (neonate)

<30,000 platelets/μL and bleeding or minor bedside procedure

<50,000 platelets/μL and intraoperative or postoperative bleeding

<100,000 platelets/μL and bleeding post cardiopulmonary bypass

Do not transfuse platelets in setting of thrombocytopenic thrombotic purpura, heparin-induced thrombocytopenia. Platelet transfusions are unlikely to be useful in idiopathic thrombocytopenic purpura or posttransfusion purpura.

Fresh frozen plasma

Bleeding in patients with INR ≥2

Bedside procedure and INR ≥2

Prophylaxis (nonbleeding) with INR ≥10

FFP is not indicated for patients with INR <1.5

Thrombotic thrombocytopenic purpura

Cryoprecipitate

Bleeding in the setting of:
- Dysfibrinogenemia
- Fibrinogen <100 mg/dL
- von Willebrand disease

Hgb, hemoglobin; INR, international normalized ratio.

In general, the traditional trigger level of 20,000 platelets/μL for prophylactic transfusion has been replaced with a level of 10,000 platelets/μL.

a level of 10,000 platelets/μL. There has even been a challenge to the utility of any prophylactic platelet transfusion, including before minor procedures such as line placement and lumbar puncture. This challenge suggests that platelets should only be administered in cases of actual bleeding. Appropriate uses of platelets in other settings are included in **Table 12-7**.

Fresh Frozen Plasma

Clinical situations in which FFP is likely to be useful also have been established by an NIH Consensus Conference and professional organizations. FFP has been used as replacement therapy for deficiencies of clotting factors and regulatory proteins, including protein C and protein S, for which specific concentrates or recombinant products are not available. The use of FFP to reverse mild coagulation abnormalities is not warranted. The risk of bleeding appears to be very low when the prothrombin time (PT) and the international normalized ratio (INR) derived from it are only mildly elevated (PT is <1.5 times the control or the INR is ≤1.5). The same can be said for mild elevations of the partial thromboplastin time (PTT) associated with coagulation factor deficiencies. It is also unlikely to provide any benefit to patients with mild elevations in the PT or PTT who are undergoing minor procedures (e.g., line placement). On the other hand, FFP is effective in the treatment of thrombotic thrombocytopenic purpura, reversing the effects of warfarin in an emergency situation, the treatment of the bleeding patient with disseminated intravascular coagulation, and massive transfusion cases.

Cryoprecipitate

The practice of using cryoprecipitate as a source of fibrinogen and Factor XIII is well accepted. In addition, cryoprecipitate can be mixed with thrombin to form topical fibrin "glue," which is used to initiate anatomic connections and control bleeding over large surfaces; however, products with standardized amounts of fibrinogen that have undergone viral inactivation procedures are now commercially available and are generally preferable. The role of cryoprecipitate in the treatment of bleeding in uremic patients is controversial. Cryoprecipitate is no longer recommended for treatment of hemophilia A or von Willebrand disease because of the availability of other products.

COMPLICATIONS OF BLOOD TRANSFUSION

An adverse effect of blood transfusion occurs in approximately 3% of transfusions in the United States. These complications of transfusion can be classified as immunologic, infectious, or due to the chemical or physical characteristics of blood components. Fatal complications of transfusion (and donation) must be reported to the Centers for Biologics Evaluation and Research branch of the Federal Food and Drug Administration. Recently, the Centers for Disease Control has developed a hemovigilance system whereby transfusion services report (electronically) complications of transfusion using standardized criteria which become part of a national database maintained by the National Healthcare Safety Network. Similar systems in Europe and Canada have been responsible for identifying emerging problems and assessing the effectiveness of specific interventions.

Immunologic Reactions

RBC Reactions

Hemolytic Transfusion Reactions

Although HTRs are much discussed, they are fortunately quite uncommon, reflecting the efficacy of the serologic and procedural techniques in place to prevent their occurrence. Although HTRs occur with less than 0.1% of the units transfused in the United States, they can be life-threatening. It bears noting that fatal, acute HTR due to ABO incompatibility is a more frequent adverse outcome of transfusion than infection with HIV or HCV, and it is more often the result of patient or sample misidentification than to serologic mishaps or exotic blood types.

HTRs are mediated by antibodies directed against alloantigens present on transfused RBCs. Most alloantibodies to RBC antigens, other than the AB isoagglutinins, develop in response to exposure to allogeneic RBCs by transfusion or maternal–fetal hemorrhage. There are hundreds of RBC antigens comprising more than 50 systems. Fortunately, only a small proportion of these are routinely clinically significant. In addition to the AB isoagglutinins, antibodies to antigens in the Rh, Kell, Duffy, Kidd, and MNSs systems are responsible for the preponderance of HTRs. Identification of these alloantibodies, by the techniques discussed above, is important because the degree and severity of hemolysis differs among them.

HTRs can be either acute, occurring within 24 hours of transfusion, or delayed, in a reaction that appears 5 to 7 days (range 3 to 21 days) after the transfusion. Acute reactions are usually more severe than their delayed counterparts, and occur in patients who already have antibodies to RBC alloantigens when they are transfused with RBCs bearing those target antigens. The most severe acute HTRs are due to ABO incompatibility because the AB isoagglutinins are present at a substantial titer and fix complement efficiently, being largely IgM. The A and/or B antigen sites are also abundant on RBCs (typically 1 to 2×10^6 antigen sites per cell). Antibodies to antigens in the Kell, Kidd, and Duffy systems also have been responsible for acute HTR.

Patients with an acute HTR typically present with temperature elevation, an important point, because they might initially be mistaken for a febrile-nonhemolytic transfusion reaction (FNHTR; discussed later). Nausea, vomiting, hypotension, low back pain, and substernal pressure may also signal the occurrence of acute hemolysis. Hemolysis is generally intravascular in this setting. The hemoglobin released into the plasma from the lysed RBCs is apparent as hemoglobinemia (red plasma rather than yellow) and hemoglobinuria (red urine that remains red after centrifugation). Disseminated intravascular coagulation and systemic hemodynamic instability may be triggered by the hemolysis. Together with the direct toxic effects of cell-free hemoglobin on the tubular cells of the kidney, these conditions are responsible for the impaired kidney function that often accompanies acute intravascular hemolysis. Therapy is largely supportive, but preservation of renal function is critical, and is often accomplished through the use of intravenous hydration and diuretics.

An adverse effect of blood transfusion occurs in an estimated 3.0% to 3.5% of transfusions in the United States. These complications of transfusion can be classified as immunologic, infectious, or due to the chemical or physical characteristics of blood components.

Delayed HTRs occur in two situations. In one, the patient is exposed to a foreign RBC allo-antigen by transfusion and mounts a primary immune response. As the amount of antibody in the plasma increases, hemolysis of the transfused RBCs with the inciting antigen may ensue. The second situation in which a delayed response may occur is when a patient is reexposed to an alloantigen to which he or she was sensitized in the past by previous transfusion or pregnancy (anamnestic response). Even if the alloantibody to this antigen is not detectable prior to the transfusion, exposure to the alloantigen can stimulate an anamnestic response. Antibodies to Kidd and Rh antigens are frequently responsible for such reactions. Hemolysis is typically extravascular in delayed HTR with the only clinical and laboratory signs being a decrease in the hemoglobin level, a rise in the bilirubin level, a low-grade temperature, and a feeling of malaise. When no hemolysis can be detected in a delayed HTR, the reaction is called a delayed serologic (rather than hemolytic) transfusion reaction.

Reactions to Plasma Components

Hypersensitivity Reactions—Allergic and Anaphylactic Transfusion Reactions

Allergic reactions occur in approximately 1% to 3% of patients receiving blood products containing plasma. In most cases, these hypersensitivity reactions are a host response to foreign plasma proteins in the donor blood components. The vast majority of these reactions consist of hives, pruritus, and erythema, and can be managed with antihistamines or steroids. More serious responses such as bronchospasm, laryngeal edema, gastrointestinal disturbance (nausea, vomiting, cramps, and diarrhea), and hypotension (anaphylactoid reaction) are much less frequent. IgA-deficient patients with anti-IgA antibodies in their plasma are at risk for serious reactions, including frank anaphylaxis if exposed to IgA in a transfused blood component. If transfusion is required, these patients should be provided with components from IgA-deficient donors, or, in an elective situation, store their own components for later use. Washing packed RBC can effectively remove IgA. Patients who are IgA deficient, but who do not have anti-IgA, do not require special preparations, but should be observed closely during transfusion.

White Blood Cell Reactions

Febrile-nonhemolytic Transfusion Reactions

These reactions are among the most common transfusion-related complications and accompany approximately 1% to 3% of transfusions of cellular components. They are more common in patients who are either multiparous or multiply transfused with nonleukoreduced, cellular components. An FNHTR usually presents with a temperature elevation of 1°C or more, during or shortly after a transfusion (usually within 1 to 2 hours), that is unlikely to be associated with the patient's underlying disease or therapy. The temperature elevation is often accompanied by chills, rigors, and generalized discomfort, and in some patients, nausea and vomiting as well. The majority of these reactions are mild and do not persist for more than 8 hours. Antipyretics may be administered, and occasionally meperidine may be required to treat severe rigors. These reactions have long been considered to be the product of antileukocyte antibodies present in the recipient's plasma, reacting with WBCs or WBC fragments in the transfused product. There may, however, be other etiologies for the FNHTRs, including the presence of cytokines released by lymphocytes in the donated unit during storage.

Transfusion-associated Graft Versus Host Disease (TA-GVHD)

Immunocompetent T lymphocytes present in cellular blood components may engraft in an immunoincompetent transfusion recipient, particularly if cellular immunity is compromised. The engrafted, allogeneic T cells mount an alloimmune response to cells in the skin and gastrointestinal tract, similar to what occurs in hematopoietic stem cell transplant-associated GVHD. However, in transfusion-associated GVHD, the donor T cells attack the host cells in the bone marrow as well, making this complication of transfusion lethal in most cases. Fortunately, T lymphocytes in cellular blood components can be inactivated by exposure to gamma irradiation, which effectively prevents this complication. Patients at risk for this rare complication include those undergoing HPC transplantation or who have hematologic malignancies. Low-birth-weight infants, infants with hemolytic disease of the newborn, and fetuses receiving intrauterine transfusions are also at risk. Patients with congenital T-cell immunodeficiencies (e.g., Wiskott–Aldrich and DiGeorge syndromes) have also developed this complication. Cellular components from blood

---

Febrile-nonhemolytic transfusion reactions are among the most common transfusion-related complications and accompany 1% to 3% of transfusions of cellular components.

relative donors are also routinely irradiated to prevent TA-GVHD that may occur in the circumstance when the donor is homozygous for an HLA haplotype shared with the transfusion recipient. In this situation, the transfused T cells remain immunologically invisible to the otherwise immunocompetent host and, rather than being cleared, they engraft and attack the host because they recognize the mismatched host haplotype antigens as foreign. Most of the reports of TA-GVHD in other patients, such as those with solid tumors or who were undergoing surgery, predate the awareness of this one-way haplotype match, which is the most likely explanation for the occurrence of this event in these immunocompetent patients.

Transfusion-related Acute Lung Injury (TRALI)

TRALI is characterized by the development of acute respiratory distress, hypoxia, and bilateral infiltrates on chest x-ray, often accompanied by fever and hypotension, during or within 6 hours of completion of a transfusion. To meet the current working definition of TRALI, there must be no preexisting form of acute lung injury or other risk factors such as sepsis, aspiration, or pneumonia. Most patients recover completely with supportive care, which may include mechanical ventilation. The pulmonary infiltrates usually resolve within 2 to 4 days without long-term sequelae; however, there is a 5% mortality rate. This complication is attributed to the presence of antileukocyte antibodies in the plasma of donor blood (often from females with a history of pregnancy) that react with the recipient's WBCs, should they bear the target HLA antigen. This results in the formation of immune complexes that are trapped in the pulmonary vasculature and lead to alveolar edema. At present, various steps are being taken to reduce the incidence of TRALI, including making FFP from predominately male donors or donors with no history of pregnancy or transfusion, or by testing donors for HLA antibodies.

Platelet Reactions

Posttransfusion Purpura (See the Section "Bleeding Disorders" in Chapter 11)

This rare complication occurs in patients who lack a common platelet antigen (often HPA-1A) and have developed an alloantibody by exposure through prior transfusion or pregnancy. When reexposed to HPA-1A by transfusion of a platelet product or an RBC product containing contaminating platelets, these patients appear to develop an anamnestic response and become severely thrombocytopenic 7 to 10 days later. Paradoxically, the patient's own platelets, which are HPA-1A negative, are also cleared. Several explanations have been offered, including the observation that there is an initial IgM response that reacts with GP IIb–IIIa (essentially a platelet autoantibody) but then "matures" with the production of an IgG with anti-HPA-1A specificity. The reaction is self-limiting, but may be complicated by severe hemorrhage. Steroids and intravenous immunoglobulin have been used successfully to manage this immunologic reaction.

> Transfusion-related acute lung injury is characterized by the development of acute respiratory distress, hypoxia, and bilateral infiltrates on chest x-ray, often accompanied by fever and hypotension, during or within 6 hours of completion of a transfusion.

Refractoriness to Platelet Transfusions

Patients may become sensitized to leukocyte and platelet antigens through transfusion or pregnancy. Transfused platelets will be cleared rapidly if given to a patient who has preformed antibodies directed at foreign platelet antigens or HLA Class I molecules, which are also expressed on the platelet membrane. As a result, it may be extremely difficult to raise the platelet count in such patients. A patient is considered to be refractory to platelet transfusion if the increment measured between 15 and 60 minutes after the platelet transfusion is lower than expected on two occasions. Note that counts done several hours afterward are not useful for determining which patients are immunologically refractory. The posttransfusion count may be corrected for the number of platelets administered and the patient's body surface area (the "corrected count increment") as follows:

$$\text{Corrected count increment} = \frac{\text{Platelets count increment} \times \text{Body surface area} \times 10^{11}}{\text{Number of platelets transfused}}$$

Here the default for number of platelets transfused is: 1 unit whole blood-derived platelets = 5.5×10^{10} platelets; 1 unit apheresis platelets = 3×10^{11} platelets.

A corrected count increment of <7500 is a strong evidence of immunologic refractoriness. Note that other causes of refractoriness should be ruled out, among them are: active bleeding, fever, sepsis, splenomegaly (splenic sequestration), disseminated intravascular coagulation, marrow transplantation, antibiotics (e.g., vancomycin), IV amphotericin B, thrombotic thrombocytopenic purpura, idiopathic or immune thrombocytopenic purpura, and heparin-induced thrombocytopenia.

Patients with immunologic refractoriness may respond well to platelets from donors who lack the HLA antigens corresponding to the patient's HLA alloantibodies (or to platelets that are HLA matched) or to platelets that have been chosen by platelet crossmatching.

Leukocytes in the transfused unit appear to be necessary for stimulating the immune response to both platelet and leukocyte antigens. Alloimmunization may be prevented by transfusion of cellular components from which leukocytes have been removed, usually by passage of the product through a filter that retains the leukocytes. Patients who are likely to need extensive platelet transfusion support, especially of platelets (e.g., for HPC transplants or hematologic malignancies) often receive leukoreduced cellular components to reduce the likelihood of alloimmunization.

Nonimmunologic Reactions

Complications Created by the Physical Characteristics of Blood

Hypothermia

Transfusion of small volumes of cold blood may be associated with minor discomfort. This complication can be averted by using blood warmers or blankets. In the setting of massive transfusion, however, the rapid transfusion of large amounts of blood that is at 1°C to 10°C contributes to hypothermia. Hemostasis is impaired when the circulating blood is below 37°C and in extreme situations, cardiac dysrhythmias and arrest may occur. In this setting, the use of high-throughput blood warmers is warranted.

Transfusion-associated Circulatory Overload (TACO)

Volume overload is a relatively common but often overlooked complication of transfusion. Patients with congestive heart failure or renal failure, the very young, and the very old are particularly at risk. It should be suspected in a patient who complains of dyspnea, orthopnea, cough, or chest pain, during or soon after transfusion, particularly if there are signs of hypoxia, rales, tachycardia, or hypertension. Supplemental oxygen and diuresis may be required. Future transfusions should be carried out slowly and perhaps with the aid of a diuretic.

Chemical Complications

Iron Overload

> Volume overload is a relatively common but often overlooked complication of transfusion. Patients with congestive heart failure or renal failure, the very young, and the very old are particularly at risk.

Each unit of packed RBC contains approximately 200 mg of iron. Chronic RBC transfusion can overwhelm the body's mechanisms for eliminating excess iron, resulting in iron accumulation in various tissues. An individual who has received 100 or more units of RBCs (20 g of iron) is at risk to develop various complications of iron overload, including cardiac dysrhythmias, pancreatic failure ("bronze diabetes"), and liver function abnormalities. Tissue iron can be mobilized and excreted using chelating agents such as deferoxamine or deferasirox. Chelation therapy is a slow process and is more effective if deployed well before tissue accumulation of iron is extensive.

Potassium Toxicity

Potassium leaks out of RBCs during storage as ATP levels decline and the ATPase-dependent Na^+/K^+ pump activity diminishes. Once the banked RBCs are transfused, they transport glucose, restore their ATP levels, and take up the K^+ that was lost during storage. In the short term, however, each unit of RBCs might contain as much as 7 mmol of extracellular K^+ at the time of expiration. There have been a handful of reports of neonates, or patients with renal failure, receiving large volumes of banked blood, who have developed life-threatening cardiac dysrhythmias. Neonates usually receive RBC units that have been stored for less than 1 week and have not yet accumulated much extracellular K^+. Washing RBC is also an effective means of removing extracellular K^+, although it is very rarely required.

Citrate Toxicity

Citrate is the anticoagulant used in the collection of all blood products and is therefore transfused with the blood product into the patient. Since the citrate is present in the plasma, most of it ends up in platelet and plasma components while there is relatively little in packed RBCs. Citrate is metabolized by every nucleated cell of the body, but in circumstances where large volumes of banked blood are being infused rapidly, as in massive transfusion, the rapid influx of citrate may overwhelm the body's metabolic capacity, leading to an accumulation in the patient's plasma. Most patients can receive up to 1 unit of FFP every 6 minutes without evidence of citrate toxicity. Patients with liver failure metabolize citrate more slowly, however, and are particularly susceptible. The accumulating citrate chelates calcium, causing the ionized calcium levels to drop and producing perioral tingling and extremity paresthesias. In extreme circumstances, it may produce severe hypo(ionized)calcemia that can lead to cardiac dysrhythmias.

Depletion of 2,3-Diphosphoglycerate (2,3-DPG)

With increasing storage time of RBCs, the intracellular level of 2,3-DPG decreases, producing a left shift of the oxyhemoglobin dissociation curve. Once banked RBCs are transfused, they restore the levels of 2,3-DPG over a period of 24 to 48 hours. It has been suggested that the high oxygen affinity of the hemoglobin in the 2,3-DPG-deficient banked RBCs might impair oxygen delivery, particularly to neonates. As a result, it has become a general practice to transfuse neonates with RBCs that have been banked less than 1 week. However, most of the literature demonstrating unfavorable outcomes for neonates receiving older units was based on studies with RBC storage systems in which maintenance of 2,3-DPG levels was not as effective as it is using the current systems.

Infectious Complications (See the Section "Infectious Disease Testing")

The Classic Pathogens

Transfusion transmission of the hepatitis viruses and the retroviruses has been substantially reduced through the interventions of donor education, screening on the basis of medical history and risk behaviors, and testing, including the use of highly sensitive techniques based on amplification of viral genetic nucleic acids. The residual risk of HIV or HCV infection through transfusion is in the range of one event per 1 to 2×10^6 units transfused. Viral transmission by pooled plasma products has also been largely eliminated by the use of robust viral inactivation techniques or replacement with recombinant proteins.

> Transfusion transmission of the hepatitis viruses and the retroviruses has been substantially reduced through the interventions of donor education, screening on the basis of medical history and risk behaviors, and testing.

The Current Significant Pathogens

At the present time, bacterial contamination of blood components is the most significant infectious complication of transfusion in developed countries, in terms of both the number of transmitted infections and the number of fatalities. It has been estimated that in the United States, approximately 1 in 500,000 units of RBCs, or 1 in 10,000 to 20,000 units of platelets, is associated with transfusion-transmitted sepsis. The organisms most frequently associated with septic RBC transfusions are psychrophilic gram-negative bacteria such as *Yersinia enterocolitica* and *Pseudomonas* spp., as well as *Enterobacter* spp. and *Serratia* spp. Platelet units have been reported to transmit gram-positive cocci (*Streptococcus aureus*, *S. epidermidis*, and *Staphylococcus* spp.) as well as gram-negative organisms (*Klebsiella* spp., *Serratia* spp., *Salmonella* spp., and *Enterobacter* spp.). The sources of these bacteria are thought to be skin commensals picked up and introduced into the blood donation with the venipuncture, or less commonly, cryptic bacteremia in clinically healthy donors. Even if the inoculum is quite small, blood is a superb culture medium, particularly when stored at room temperature, as is the case for platelets. Although donors are now questioned specifically about antibiotic use, the health history is neither a sensitive nor a specific screening tool. The implementation of tests to screen platelet products for evidence of bacterial contamination was discussed above and is now routine.

Cytomegalovirus (CMV) is a ubiquitous member of the herpes virus family to which approximately 30% to 60% of adults in developed countries have been exposed. CMV can be transmitted by transfusion of blood components that contain leukocytes, such as packed RBCs and platelets. Although primary infection rarely produces serious disease in immunologically intact hosts, it is associated with systemic infection in immunocompromised patients who are CMV-seronegative. The following groups of patients have been shown to be susceptible to transfusion-transmitted CMV primary infection and disease and should receive CMV reduced-risk cellular blood components:

1. Premature, low-birth-weight (<1200 g) neonates
2. CMV-seronegative pregnant women (including those undergoing intrauterine transfusions)

3. CMV-seronegative recipients of, or candidates for, hematopoietic or solid organ transplants
4. CMV-seronegative, HIV-infected patients

CMV reduced-risk blood components can be obtained by screening donors for CMV antibody (IgG) that indicates past exposure, or by removing the leukocytes that contain latent CMV by filtration with leukocyte reduction filters. These two approaches have been shown to be equally effective in preventing transfusion-transmitted CMV infection. Only cellular components need to be CMV reduced-risk, since intact mononuclear cells are required to transmit CMV.

Emerging Pathogens

The blood supply will always be vulnerable to the introduction of new pathogens into the donor population. In some instances, the pathogen may truly be a new organism, or one that has recently acquired the ability to infect humans, such as the SARS virus, various strains of avian flu, and the bovine prion responsible for variant Creutzfeldt–Jakob disease. Population shifts in response to natural or man-made catastrophes, or simply travel for business or pleasure, spread pathogens from one part of the world to another, such as the West Nile virus, *Plasmodium* spp., *Trypanosoma* spp. and, most recently, Zika virus. In some circumstances, questioning donors about exposure to a pathogen or a history of a characteristic illness, or the rapid development of a screening test has been an effective means of interdicting transfusion transmission of a new infectious agent. However, an effective response is more difficult in the circumstance where the organism has not been identified, its biology is unique, the routes of transmission are not well understood, or the clinical effects are not well defined. As a result, work continues to develop pathogen inactivation technology.

Transfusion Reaction Workup

If a reaction is suspected, the transfusion must be stopped immediately while maintaining venous access, and the patient must be assessed. Emergent airway and hemodynamic instability should be dealt with immediately and appropriate measures taken to alleviate the patient's major symptoms and concerns. If the assessment reveals that the patient's only symptoms are cutaneous manifestations of hypersensitivity (flushing, pruritus, and urticaria), then the transfusion may be resumed under careful observation. In all other situations, the transfusion of that unit should be stopped and a clerical check should be performed to verify that the correct unit (i.e., one labeled for that patient) has been administered. A transfusion reaction form should be filled out and a new blood bank specimen should be drawn from the patient. The transfusion reaction form, the unit involved, and the new specimen should be returned to the blood bank for evaluation. A posttransfusion urine specimen should also be obtained and sent for urinalysis.

> If a reaction is suspected, the transfusion must be stopped immediately while maintaining intravenous access, and the patient must be assessed.

The blood bank treats the transfusion reaction workup as a stat request. A clerical check is performed, and the posttransfusion specimen is compared to the pretransfusion specimen used for compatibility testing for the appearance of hemolysis or hyperbilirubinemia. The ABO and Rh type of the posttransfusion specimen is determined to confirm that the pretransfusion specimen was indeed from this patient and that the ABO and Rh type of the unit that was being transfused was appropriate. A direct antiglobulin test is also performed on the posttransfusion specimen looking for antibody-coated RBC (i.e., donor cells coated with recipient alloantibody) indicating an immune-based HTR. Any findings suggestive of an HTR trigger a more extensive investigation in the blood bank. If the workup rules out a hemolytic reaction, transfusion may resume.

ALTERNATIVES TO ALLOGENEIC TRANSFUSION

The 1980s saw extensive development of techniques to avoid allogeneic transfusion (transfusion with someone else's blood), particularly in elective surgery. The major driver was concern about the infectious complications of transfusion. Before the development of a screening test in 1985, HIV transmission rates may have been as high as 1 in 10,000 units transfused in some urban centers in the United States, while as many as 5% to 10% of transfusion recipients developed what was then called non-A, non-B hepatitis, and is now known to have been due primarily to HCV, which was only identified in 1989. Although demand for these blood-sparing techniques is not as great as it was 20 years ago, they are still in use and continue to be helpful for patients with unusual blood types or multiple alloantibodies for whom it is difficult to find compatible blood. In addition, the drive to avoid allogeneic blood exposure has reinforced common sense measures: treatment of medically correctable anemia, greater physician tolerance of asymptomatic anemia, meticulous surgical hemostasis, and the wider use of hemostatic medications. The licensing of recombinant erythropoietin also reduced the dependence of patients with renal failure, malignancies, and HIV infection on regular RBC transfusion.

Four techniques in particular were developed to reduce the dependence of surgical patients on banked RBC: preoperative autologous blood donation (PABD), acute normovolemic hemodilution (ANH), intraoperative blood recovery and reinfusion, and postoperative blood recovery and reinfusion.

PABD is suitable for patients undergoing elective surgical procedures for which RBC transfusion is commonly required, and in this setting can reduce allogeneic blood use. Since the blood may only be used by the donor/recipient, donor qualifications are simple and no testing (other than ABO/Rh typing) is required. Note that mistransfusion, bacterial contamination, and volume overload are just as likely to occur with an autologous unit as with an allogeneic unit. Since the hazards averted (especially infection) are very small, donors who might be put at even a small risk by donation (e.g., mild anemia and coronary artery insufficiency) should be discouraged from PABD.

ANH is a technique whereby several units of blood are removed from a patient in the operating room immediately before a procedure. The volume is replaced with crystalloid. The blood is returned if bleeding occurs, or at the end of the procedure. It has the advantage that little advance planning is necessary, but it is not very efficacious at reducing allogeneic RBC transfusions for patients with moderate anemia from whom only a few units can be withdrawn at the beginning of the procedure.

Blood recovered from the operative field can be collected, processed in some manner, and reinfused. Shed blood is collected by suction into a reservoir, usually with heparin or citrate, and then usually washed in a centrifugal device specially designed for this purpose. The washed RBCs are suspended in normal saline and pumped into a bag suitable for reinfusion to the patient. The washing procedure removes materials that might cause reactions such as cell debris, activated clotting factors, and complement. A similar process can be carried out manually. This technique is particularly helpful in procedures where large volumes of blood are lost. Although somewhat expensive, the recovery of 3 to 4 units of RBCs is usually adequate to recover the costs. This technique is suitable for elective as well as emergency procedures during which blood loss is extensive.

Devices are also available for collecting blood shed in the postoperative period. Many of them rely on filtration of the shed blood. The filtration technique is not adequate to remove materials that can provoke a reaction and is generally not worth risking for the small amounts of blood that can be recovered. A small, centrifugal device that washes the blood collected postoperatively is also available. Although it provides a much cleaner product, the small volumes of blood recovered in this manner do not make it cost-effective.

CELLULAR THERAPIES

Cellular therapies encompass the collection, processing, storage, and therapeutic use of hematopoietic cells, most commonly HPCs. In addition, mononuclear cell fractions from HPC donors have been used to enhance the graft versus tumor effect of allogeneic transplantation, and dendritic cells sensitized to tumor antigens have been used to treat solid tumors. Allogeneic HPCs have the advantage that they are free of malignancy and may have a significant graft versus tumor effect; they are preferred for most forms of leukemia, Hodgkin disease, and the myelodysplastic syndromes. Allogeneic transplantation has also occasionally been used to treat certain genetic disorders of the hematopoietic system, such as sickle cell disease and thalassemia. Autologous HPC transplants are not complicated by rejection and have a lower incidence of GVHD. They are performed in patients with some forms of non-Hodgkin lymphoma and multiple myeloma, and as rescue therapy after intensive chemotherapy for some solid tumors (e.g., testicular, breast, and ovarian cancer).

Cellular therapies encompass the collection, processing, storage, and therapeutic use of hematopoietic cells.

Potential allogeneic donors must in general meet the criteria for blood donation, including infectious disease testing, although some of these criteria may be waived if an alternate suitable donor cannot be found. Potential donors must be typed for HLA Class I and II antigens using molecular techniques. Class I mismatches pose an increased risk for rejection and failure to engraft, whereas Class II mismatches are associated with increased incidence of GVHD. A single Class I or II mismatch usually has little impact on survival. Two Class I mismatches, or a Class I and a Class II mismatch, are usually associated with poorer outcomes. Haploidentical sibling donors have been used successfully. If a suitable family member donor cannot be found (and only one in four siblings is likely to be a two haplotype match), a donor may be sought through the National Marrow Donor Program, a registry of people who have been HLA typed and have expressed a willingness to donate HPCs. The search may take a few months and is less likely to be successful for patients with unusual phenotypes. There has been considerable effort in the last few years to register donors from previously underrepresented minority populations. ABO or Rh matching is not necessary since the transplant recipient will convert to the donor type if engraftment is successful, although RBC engraftment may be delayed if donor RBCs are incompatible with the recipient's anti-A or anti-B isoagglutinins. Donor isoagglutinins may also cause hemolysis of residual recipient RBCs, or at least a positive direct antiglobulin test. The conversion from recipient to donor blood type does pose problems for the transfusion service that must provide blood that is compatible with both donor and recipient until the recipient's original RBCs and isoagglutinins are undetectable.

HPCs may be collected from peripheral blood by apheresis, from bone marrow by aspiration, or from cord blood. Apheresis collection now accounts for 90% of autologous transplants, and 50% of allogeneic transplants. Bone marrow aspiration is performed with multiple punctures and aspirations of the posterior iliac crest and must be performed in the operating room with the donor under general anesthesia. The aspirates are anticoagulated (heparin or citrate), filtered, and pooled into a bag that is then usually stored frozen until the time of the transplant.

Collection by apheresis is less invasive and less likely to recover residual malignant cells. In addition, it has been shown to be associated with quicker engraftment, although chronic GVHD is somewhat more likely to occur than with marrow transplantation. The number of HPCs in the peripheral blood is ordinarily very low, so autologous donors are prepared by the administration of granulocyte colony-stimulating factor or granulocyte–macrophage colony-stimulating factor at the point when their marrow is rebounding from a cycle of chemotherapy. Under these circumstances, the levels of HPCs (which can be determined by measuring the number of CD34-positive cells in the peripheral blood by flow cytometry) may be elevated 200- to 1000-fold. The pheresis instrument is configured to collect the mononuclear cell fraction. Large volume collections (with three blood volumes processed) are typically performed, which reduces the number of procedures needed to collect the targeted number of CD34-positive cells (typically 2 to 4×10^6 per kg patient weight). Large volume collection may also have the effect of recruiting HPCs from the marrow during the collection.

The HPC product undergoes extensive quality control testing, including ABO and Rh type, RBC and WBC counts (and differential), CD34 cell count, an assay to enumerate colony-forming units in vitro, cell viability, and testing for bacteria, fungi, and mycoplasma. Autologous HPC products are frozen (usually at a controlled rate) in the presence of 10% dimethylsulfoxide and 10% protein (plasma or albumin) as cryoprotectants, and stored in mechanical freezers or liquid nitrogen tanks. At the time of transplant, the units are thawed at 37°C, usually at the patient's bedside, and then administered intravenously, much like a conventional transfusion. Allogeneic HPC are usually maintained at 4°C and infused into the recipient within 24 hours.

Umbilical cord blood contains high levels of circulating HPCs, and this observation has led to the development of cord blood banking. If a mother meets the criteria for allogeneic blood donation (except for hemoglobin level and recent pregnancy because she has just delivered) including the usual infectious disease testing, and there is no history of genetic diseases in the family of either parent, she may give consent for the blood to be drained from the placenta via the umbilical cord (after it has been severed or clamped off from the neonate) and then stored frozen. In addition to the usual quality control testing of the cord blood, HLA Class I and II typing is performed as well as ABO/Rh typing.

TABLE 12-8   Categories of Indications for Therapeutic Apheresis

Category	Use of Therapeutic Apheresis
Category I	Disorders for which apheresis is accepted as first-line therapy, either as a primary standalone treatment or in conjunction with other modes of treatment.
Category II	Disorders for which apheresis is accepted as second-line therapy, either as a standalone treatment or in conjunction with other modes of treatment.
Category III	Optimum role of apheresis therapy is not established. Decision making should be individualized.
Category IV	Disorders in which published evidence demonstrates or suggests apheresis to be ineffective or harmful. Institutional review board approval is desirable if apheresis treatment is undertaken in these circumstances.

Information from Schwartz J, Padmanabhan A, Aqui N, et al. Guidelines on the use of therapeutic apheresis in clinical practice—evidence-based approach from the Writing Committee of the American Society for Apheresis: the seventh special issue. *J Clin Apheresis*. 2016;31:149–162.

Over 5000 related and unrelated (but HLA matched) cord blood transplants have been performed since the technique was first developed in 1988. Cord blood HPCs home readily to the host bone marrow and do not seem to be as alloreactive to recipient antigen-presenting cells as HPCs from adults. In addition, the large numbers of HLA-typed cord blood samples may improve the chances of finding unrelated matches. Cord transplants are also less likely to be complicated by GVHD or to transmit CMV. However, the total number of HPCs in each cord blood sample is small and engraftment is slower. This has led to the use of double cord transplants that accelerate engraftment, even though eventually one of the donor's HPCs dominates.

THERAPEUTIC APHERESIS

Therapeutic apheresis is the process of withdrawing blood from the body, selectively removing one particular element (i.e., plasma, leukocytes, platelets, or RBCs), and returning the remaining elements along with a replacement solution (crystalloid and/or colloid) to maintain isovolemia. There are several different therapeutic apheresis procedures that are designed to remove, or treat, specific components of the blood. These are described below.

Indications for Therapeutic Apheresis

An evidence-based approach has been taken to categorize the indications for therapeutic apheresis (**Table 12–8**) and a grade assigned based on the strength of the recommendation and the quality of the evidence. The specific disorders for which therapeutic apheresis has been evaluated as a treatment are shown in **Table 12–9**.

Therapeutic apheresis has been used as a treatment for numerous disorders. While it is clearly effective in some diseases, such as thrombotic thrombocytopenic purpura, the therapeutic benefit of apheresis in many other disorders is much less clear, because many of them are uncommon, and therefore it is extremely difficult to obtain information about efficacy based on large-scale, prospective, randomized clinical trials.

Plasmapheresis

In plasmapheresis (plasma exchange; see the figure in Chapter 2), blood is withdrawn from a patient and the plasma is separated from the cellular components by centrifugation or, less commonly, by filtration, in an apheresis instrument. The plasma is discarded and the cellular components are returned to the patient. Liters of abnormal plasma can be removed from the patient and replaced by saline, albumin, starch solutions, FFP, or combinations of these. This technique is used to remove autoantibodies, immune complexes, paraproteins, and protein-bound toxins.

TABLE 12–9   Selected Indications for Therapeutic Apheresis[a]

Disorders	Category I	Category II	Category III	Category IV
Solid organ transplantation	Antibody mediated rejection allograft (renal) (1) Desensitization LD allograft (renal) (1) Desensitization LD ABOi allograft (renal, liver) (1)	Antibody mediated rejection allograft (ABOi renal) (1) Bronchiolitis obliterans syndrome (lung allograft) (2) Cellular rejection (and prophylaxis) cardiac allograft (2) Desensitization (cardiac allograft) (1)	Antibody mediated rejection allograft (cardiac, lung, ABOi, and HLA liver) (1) Desensitization DD allograft (renal, lung) (1) Desensitization ABOi DD allograft (liver) (1)	
Renal	Goodpasture syndrome (1) Rapidly progressive glomerulonephritis with ANCA (DAH, dialysis dependent) (1) Focal segmental glomerulosclerosis (1)	Cryoglobulinemia (1) Myeloma cast nephropathy (1)	Goodpasture syndrome (dialysis independent) (1) Rapidly progressive glomerulonephritis with ANCA (dialysis independent) (1) IgA nephropathy (1)	
Neurologic	Acute Guillain–Barré syndrome (1) CIDP (1) Myasthenia gravis (1) N-methyl D-aspartate receptor antibody encephalitis (1) Paraproteinemic peripheral neuropathy (IgA/IgG, IgM) (1)	Acute CNS multiple sclerosis (1) Acute disseminated encephalomyelitis (1) Lambert–Eaton myasthenic syndrome (1) Neuromyelitis optica—acute (Devic syndrome) (1) PANDAS (1)	Chronic focal (Rasmussen's) encephalitis (1) Chronic, progressive multiple sclerosis (1) Hashimoto encephalopathy (1) Paraneoplastic syndromes (1) Paraproteinemic peripheral neuropathy (anti-MAG, multiple myeloma) (1) Stiff person syndrome (1) Sydenham chorea (1)	Multifocal motor neuropathy (1)
Metabolic	Familial hypercholesterolemia (homozygous) (5) Wilson disease—fulminant (1)	Familial hypercholesterolemia (heterozygotes) (1) Lipoprotein hyperlipidemia (a) Mushroom poisoning (1) Refsum disease (1)	Acute liver failure (1) Hereditary hemachromatosis (4) Non-mushroom poisoning/overdose (1) Pancreatitis with hypertriglyceridemia (1) Sepsis with multi-organ failure (1) Thyrotoxicosis (1)	
Hematologic and oncologic	Erythrodermic cutaneous lymphoma (2) Erythrocytosis—polycythemia vera (4) Hyperviscosity/paraproteinemia—symptomatic (1) Leukocytosis/leukostasis (3) Sickle cell disease—stroke, acute or prophylaxis (4) Thrombotic thrombocytopenic purpura (1) Thrombotic microangiopathy—Factor H autoantibodies; ticlopidine-induced (1)	ABO-incompatible HPC transplant (1) Babesiosis severe (4) Cold autoimmune hemolytic anemia (1) Graft versus host disease (2) HPC transplant—ABOi (1) Maternal alloimmunization (1) Sickle cell disease—acute chest syndrome (4) Thrombocytosis (symptomatic) (3)	Aplastic anemia, pure red cell aplasia (1) Erythrocytosis—secondary (4) HELLP syndrome—postpartum (1) Heparin induced thrombocytopenia and thrombosis (1) Malaria—severe (4) Nonerythrodermic cutaneous lymphoma (2) Posttransfusion purpura (1) Sickle cell disease—multi-organ failure, recurrent vaso-occlusion, preanesthesia, pregnancy, priapism, splenic/hepatic sequestration (4) Thrombotic microangiopathy—mutations in THBD, complement, or MCP genes; clopidogrel, calcineurin inhibitors; Shiga-toxin (1) Warm autoimmune hemolytic anemia (1)	Amyloidosis (1) Coagulation factor inhibitors—autoantibody (1) HELLP syndrome—prepartum (1) Immune thrombocytopenia (1) Medication-associated thrombotic microangiopathy—gemcitabine, quinine (1)
Autoimmune		Catastrophic antiphospholipid antibody syndrome (1) Severe systemic lupus (1)	Behcet's syndrome (1) Pemphigus vulgaris (2) Progressive systemic scleroderma (1) Psoriasis (1)	Dermatomyositis polymyositis (1, 3) Polyarteritis nodosa—idiopathic (1) Progressive systemic scleroderma (2) Systemic lupus nephritis (1)

ABOi, ABO incompatible; ANCA, antineutrophil cytoplasmic antibody; CIDP, chronic inflammatory demyelinating polyneuropathy; CNS, central nervous system; DAH, diffuse alveolar hemorrhage; DD, deceased donor; LD, living donor; MCP, membrane cofactor protein (a complement regulatory protein); PANDAS, pediatric autoimmune neuropsychiatric disorders associated with streptococcal infections; THBD, genes coding for thrombomodulin.

[a]Number in parentheses refers to specific apheresis procedure as follows: (1) therapeutic plasma exchange; (2) photopheresis; (3) cytapheresis; (4) red cell exchange; (5) selective column adsorption.

Information on the categorization from Schwartz J, Padmanabhan A, Aqui N, et al. Guidelines on the use of therapeutic apheresis in clinical practice—evidence-based approach from the Writing Committee of the American Society for Apheresis: the seventh special issue. *J Clin Apheresis*. 2016;31:149–162. This reference also includes the grading for each indication which is based on strength of the recommendation and the quality of the evidence.

Cytapheresis

Cytapheresis is the removal of one of the cellular elements of the blood. *Leukapheresis* is occasionally indicated for patients with acute myelogenous leukemia or chronic myelogenous leukemia in the accelerated phase with a high level of circulating blasts and evidence of leukostasis with pulmonary or CNS involvement. Myeloid blast forms adhere to the vascular endothelium and can impede blood flow in the lungs and the brain. The collection of peripheral HPCs and granulocytes is a variation of leukapheresis.

Plateletpheresis may be indicated in patients with myeloproliferative disorders, such as essential thrombocytosis, who develop platelet counts that exceed $1 \times 10^6/\mu L$ and also show signs of hemorrhage or thrombosis.

Erythrocytapheresis (RBC Exchange)

Although most sickle crises are managed with hydration, pain medication, and supplemental oxygen, RBC exchange is occasionally performed for patients who are experiencing a severe infarctive crisis complicated by stroke, acute chest syndrome, retinal infarction, or priapism. Exchange is performed less commonly to prepare patients for surgery. In the exchange replacement of sickle RBCs with normal RBCs, the usual goals are to reduce the hemoglobin S concentration to less than 30% of total hemoglobin, and to increase the hematocrit to 30%. Red cells chosen for exchange are often screened for hemoglobin S (since donors with sickle trait may be unaware of it and have a normal hemoglobin level) and may be partially phenotype matched (e.g., for Kell and the Rh antigens) to prevent alloimmunization. Red cell exchange also has been used to treat patients with malaria or babesiosis who have a high percentage (e.g., >10%) of RBCs infected with organisms despite adequate medical therapy, and signs of decompensation such as marked hemolysis, pulmonary involvement, CNS involvement, renal failure, or disseminated intravascular coagulation. Patients who are immunosuppressed, asplenic, or elderly seem to be particularly at risk to develop complications from infection with *Babesia*.

Photopheresis

In this apheresis procedure, the patient's leukocytes are separated from whole blood and exposed to psoralen and ultraviolet light, ex-vivo. The psoralen/ultraviolet light-treated leukocytes are then returned to the patient. Photopheresis has been used to treat cutaneous T-cell lymphoma and has been shown to increase patient survival when compared with conventional chemotherapy. Photopheresis has also been used to treat GVHD and cardiac allograft rejection.

SELF-ASSESSMENT QUESTIONS

1. After a unit of whole blood is collected from a normal donor for transfusion, which step in the processing of the whole blood happens next?
   A. Testing of blood for infectious disease
   B. Blood component preparation
   C. Assessment of donor–recipient compatibility
   D. Treatment of the blood product to minimize potential adverse effects

2. One unit of which of the following blood component restores the largest number and amount of plasma proteins?
   A. Packed red blood cells
   B. Fresh frozen plasma
   C. Cryoprecipitate
   D. Platelet concentrate (whole blood derived)

3. Which of the following blood components is stored at room temperature?
   A. Packed red blood cells
   B. Fresh frozen plasma
   C. Platelets—both concentrates from whole blood and apheresis
   D. Cryoprecipitate

4. Which of the following blood components can be used to increase the circulating concentration of coagulation factors in the recipient?
   A. Packed red blood cells
   B. Fresh frozen plasma
   C. Platelets—both random donor and single donor
   D. Cryoprecipitate

5. Which of the following recombinant coagulation factors is used clinically to a much lower extent than the other choices?
   A. Recombinant VIIa
   B. Recombinant VIII
   C. Recombinant IX
   D. Recombinant IIa

6. Mandatory infectious disease testing of donated blood includes testing for all but one of the following. Identify the one infectious agent or infectious disease below that is not considered.
   A. Human immunodeficiency virus (HIV)
   B. Ebola virus
   C. Hepatitis C virus
   D. Syphilis

7. Which of the following represents an incompatibility between donor and recipient for red blood cells?
   A. Donor is type O/Recipient is type A
   B. Donor is type A/Recipient is type AB
   C. Donor is type B/Recipient is type A
   D. Donor is type O/Recipient is type AB

8. Which one of the following tests detects IgG or complement bound to the red blood cell surface in vivo?
   A. Indirect antiglobulin test
   B. Red blood cell crossmatch
   C. Direct antiglobulin test
   D. Test to identify antibodies directed at specific red blood cell antigens

9. Which of the following would not be considered an appropriate indication for transfusion?
   A. A hemoglobin value less than 7 g/dL with uncompromised cardiovascular function
   B. Bleeding in a patient with an INR greater than 2.0
   C. Prophylaxis against bleeding for a platelet count less than 10,000/μL for an adult
   D. Fresh frozen plasma to treat an INR value of 1.3 in a nonbleeding patient

10. Which of the following statements characterizes a delayed hemolytic transfusion reaction that appears 5 to 7 days, with a range of 3 to 21 days, after the transfusion? This is in contrast to an acute hemolytic transfusion reaction occurring within 24 hours of transfusion.
    A. The hemolytic transfusion reaction typically presents with a temperature elevation.
    B. These hemolytic transfusion reactions occur in patients who already have antibodies to red blood cell antigens, and the hemolysis ensues when they are transfused with red blood cells bearing those target antigens.
    C. Hemolysis is generally intravascular in this type of hemolytic transfusion reaction.
    D. These hemolytic transfusion reactions are usually more severe.

11. Which of the following major red blood cell antigen systems is not associated with hemolytic disease of the newborn and not commonly implicated in hemolytic transfusion reactions?
    A. Lewis
    B. Duffy
    C. Kidd
    D. Rh

12. After ABO red blood cell antigens, what is the second most important antigen system with regard to transfusion safety of red blood cells?
    A. Kell
    B. Kidd
    C. Duffy
    D. Rh

13. A febrile nonhemolytic transfusion reaction is mediated by which of the following?
    A. A reaction involving red blood cells
    B. A reaction involving white blood cells
    C. A reaction involving platelets
    D. A reaction involving plasma blood components

14. The transfusion complication known as transfusion-related acute lung injury (TRALI) is attributed to which of the following?

    A. Antileukocyte antibodies in the donor's plasma
    B. Antiplatelet antibodies in the donor's plasma
    C. Anti-red blood cell antibodies in the donor's plasma
    D. Antileukocyte antibodies in the recipient's plasma

15. Which one of the following pairings of complications of blood transfusion and their proposed cause is incorrect?

    A. Iron overload/Elimination of excess iron from red blood cell transfusions is insufficient
    B. Potassium toxicity/Transfusion of free potassium that leaked out of red blood cells during storage
    C. Citrate toxicity/Products are anticoagulated with citrate, and large amounts of citrate are transfused into patients during massive transfusion
    D. Depletion of 2,3 diphosphoglycerate (2,3 DPG) in red blood cells/Active transfer of 2,3 DPG from red blood cells to platelets

16. Which of the following tests is not part of a transfusion reaction evaluation in the blood bank?

    A. A clerical check to determine if the product intended for the recipient was administered.
    B. A visual check of the posttransfusion specimen in comparison to the pretransfusion specimen for hemolysis and hyperbilirubinemia.
    C. The Kell and Duffy antigen types of the posttransfusion specimen are determined to confirm that the unit transfused was appropriate.
    D. A direct antiglobulin test is performed on the posttransfusion specimen to identify any antibody-coated red blood cells.

17. Which of the following is not a category I indication for therapeutic apheresis. A category I indication is a first-line treatment.

    A. Acute Guillain–Barré syndrome
    B. Sickle cell crisis with stroke
    C. Thrombotic thrombocytopenic purpura
    D. Immune thrombocytopenia

FURTHER READING

American Association of Blood Banks. *Circular of Information for the Use of Human Blood and Blood Components*. Bethesda, MD: American Association of Blood Banks; 2017.

Andrzejewski C, Davenport RD. Therapeutic apheresis. In: Fung MK, Eder AF, Spitalnik SL, Westhoff CM, eds. *Technical Manual*. 19th ed. Bethesda, MD: AABB Press; 2017:641–682.

Bowden RA, et al. A comparison of filtered leukocyte-reduced and cytomegalovirus (CMV) seronegative blood products for the prevention of transfusion-associated CMV infection after marrow transplant. *Blood*. 1995;86:3598–3603.

Denomme G, Flegel W. Applying molecular immunohematology discoveries to standards of practice in blood banks: now is the time. *Transfusion*. 2008;48:2461–2475.

Fresh-Frozen Plasma, Cryoprecipitate, and Platelets Administration Practice Guidelines Development Task Force of the College of American Pathologists. Practice parameter for the use of fresh-frozen plasma, cryoprecipitate, and platelets. *JAMA*. 1994;271:777.

Gassner C, et al. Matrix-assisted laser desorption/ionization, time-of-flight mass spectrometry-based blood group genotyping—the alternative approach. *Transfus Med Rev*. 2013;27:2–9.

Goldman M, et al. TRALI Consensus Panel. Proceedings of a consensus conference: towards an understanding of TRALI. *Transfus Med Rev*. 2005;19:2–31.

Harm SK, Dunbar NM. Transfusion service related activities. In: Fung MK, Eder AF, Spitalnik SL, Westhoff CM, eds. *Technical Manual*. 19th ed. Bethesda, MD: AABB Press; 2017:457–488.

Hébert PC, et al. A multicenter, randomized, controlled clinical trial of transfusion requirements in critical care. *N Engl J Med*. 1999;340:409.

Leger RM, Borge PD. The positive direct antiglobulin test and immune-mediated hemolysis. In: Fung MK, Eder AF, Spitalnik SL, Westhoff CM, eds. *Technical Manual*. 19th ed. Bethesda, MD: AABB Press; 2017:385–412.

McLeod BC, Weinstein R, Winters JL, Szczepiorkowski ZM, eds. *Apheresis: Principles and Practice*. 3rd ed. Bethesda, MD: AABB Press; 2010.

Mintz PD, ed. *Transfusion Therapy: Clinical Principles and Practice*. 3rd ed. Bethesda, MD: American AABB Press; 2010.

Ooley PW, ed. *Standards for Blood Banks and Transfusion Services*. 30th ed. Bethesda, MD: AABB Press; 2016.

Popovsky MA, ed. *Transfusion Reactions*. 4th ed. Bethesda, MD: AABB Press; 2012.

Practice guidelines for blood component therapy: a report by the American Society of Anesthesiologists' Task Force on Blood Component Therapy. *Anesthesiology*. 1996;84:732–747.

Rebulla P, et al. The threshold for prophylactic platelet transfusion in adults with acute myeloid leukemia. *N Engl J Med*. 1997;337:1870–1875.

Reid ME, Lomas-Francis C, Olsson ML. *The Blood Group Antigens. Factsbook*. 3rd ed. San Diego, CA: Academic Press; 2012.

Schwartz J, Padmanabhan A, Aqui N, et al. Guidelines on the use of therapeutic apheresis in clinical practice—evidence-based approach from the Writing Committee of the American Society for Apheresis: the seventh special issue. *J Clin Apheresis*. 2016;31:149–162.

Simon TL, McCullough J, Snyder EL, Solheim BG, Strauss RG, eds. *Rossi's Principles of Transfusion Medicine*. 5th ed. Bethesda, MD: AABB Press/Wiley-Blackwell; 2016.

Smith JW. Blood component collection by apheresis. In: Roback JD, Grossman BJ, Harris T, Hillyer CD, eds. *Technical Manual*. 17th ed. Bethesda, MD: AABB Press; 2011:227–238.

Trial to Reduce Alloimmunization to Platelets Study Group. Leukocyte reduction and ultraviolet B irradiation of platelets to prevent alloimmunization and refractoriness to platelet transfusions. *N Engl J Med*. 1997;337:1861–1869.

Uniform Donor Health Questionnaire. Available at: http://www.aabb.org/tm/questionnaires/Documents/dhq/v2/DHQ%20v2.0.pdf. Accessed November 17, 2017.

Wagner SJ. Whole blood and apheresis collections for components intended for transfusion. In: Fung MK, Eder AF, Spitalnik SL, Westhoff CM, eds. *Technical Manual*. 19th ed. Bethesda, MD: AABB Press; 2017:125–160.

Wong EC, Roseff S, eds. *Pediatric Transfusion Medicine: A Physician's Handbook*. 4th ed. Bethesda, MD: AABB Press; 2014.

Diseases of White Blood Cells, Lymph Nodes, and Spleen

Daniel E. Sabath

CHAPTER OUTLINE

Abnormalities in white blood cells (WBCs) are nearly always quantitative (e.g., too many or too few WBCs). These disorders may be neoplastic, as found in leukemia, or nonneoplastic. A qualitative or functional disorder of WBCs may accompany the quantitative disorder. Qualitative defects in WBC function with a normal WBC count occur, but they are uncommon. The approach to diagnosis of WBC disorders is shown in **Figure 13–1**.

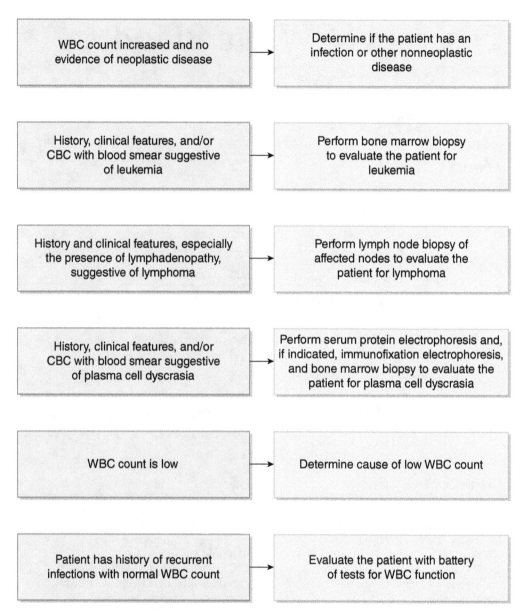

FIGURE 13–1 **An approach to the patient with a white blood cell disorder.**

LEUKOPENIA

Description and Diagnosis

A low WBC count can occur because of a decreased number of lymphocytes, granulocytes, or both.

A low WBC count can occur because of a decreased number of lymphocytes, granulocytes, or both. A number of the immunodeficiency diseases are associated with a lymphocytopenia (see Chapter 3). Granulocytopenia primarily reflects a reduction in the number of neutrophils (neutropenia) in the peripheral blood. When the number of neutrophils decreases below about 1000 neutrophils/μL, the neutropenic patient becomes susceptible to infections. These illnesses range from mild to severe, depending on the type of organism and the effectiveness of the antibiotics used to treat it. A classification of granulocytopenic disorders follows.

Defects in the production of granulocytes may be caused by:

- Diseases associated with marrow failure, such as aplastic anemia.
- Diseases in which the marrow is infiltrated by leukemic cells or by metastatic cancer cells originating from another site; the decreased neutrophil production in this setting is typically associated with defects in the production of other blood cells as well.

- Suppression of granulocyte production by exposure to certain drugs; the list of drugs that can produce neutropenia is extensive; noteworthy examples are chemotherapeutic agents used in cancer treatment and certain nonsteroidal anti-inflammatory drugs (NSAIDs).
- Vitamin B_{12} or folate deficiency; these disorders produce a megaloblastic anemia and defective DNA synthesis in granulocyte precursors.
- Suppression of granulocyte production by neoplastic cells, for example, large granular lymphocytic leukemia.

Accelerated removal of granulocytes may be caused by:

- Immunologically mediated injury to neutrophils following exposure to drugs, with the injury occurring from an immune response on the neutrophil surface.
- Immunologically mediated injury to neutrophils as part of an autoimmune disorder; for example, Felty syndrome is a variant of rheumatoid arthritis with neutropenia, splenomegaly, leg ulcers, and the joint lesions found in rheumatoid arthritis; the neutropenia can dominate the clinical course in patients with Felty syndrome.
- Immunologically mediated injury to neutrophils that is idiopathic and not associated with any identifiable abnormality.
- Excessive destruction of granulocytes from splenic sequestration of the neutrophils in an enlarged spleen or from overwhelming infection.

NONNEOPLASTIC PROLIFERATION OF WBCs

Description and Diagnosis

An elevated peripheral WBC count is commonly found in patients with infections and other inflammatory states, such as those associated with autoimmune disorders.

An elevated peripheral WBC count is commonly found in patients with infections and other inflammatory states, such as those associated with autoimmune disorders.

Lymphocytes

Patients can develop a lymphocytosis in a variety of different conditions such as tuberculosis, acute bowel infections, and infectious mononucleosis and other viral infections.

Eosinophils

An increase in circulating eosinophils is most commonly found in patients with allergic disorders and those with asthma. An increase in circulating eosinophils is also found in patients with certain parasitic infections and in patients with dermatologic disorders such as eczema. Increases in eosinophils can also be caused by some drugs and some autoimmune disorders. Increases in eosinophils can be seen in certain neoplastic conditions such as Hodgkin lymphoma and T-cell lymphomas. Finally, there is a set of hypereosinophilic syndromes in which there is overproduction of eosinophils, either due to neoplastic stem cells or other poorly defined causes.

Monocytes

The peripheral monocyte count is increased in a number of situations where the lymphocyte count is also increased, such as tuberculosis. Rheumatoid arthritis, systemic lupus erythematosus, and other connective tissue diseases also may be associated with a monocytosis.

Neutrophils

A mild increase in circulating neutrophils can occur without disease after strenuous exercise, during menstruation, and in the course of pregnancy. An increased neutrophil count is clinically significant when it is indicative of a bacterial infection, a neoplastic disorder, ischemia, an autoimmune disorder, or an effect of certain drugs, such as corticosteroids or epinephrine. The most frequently identified immature neutrophil in the blood when there is an increased WBC count is the neutrophilic band cell. The percentage of WBCs represented by band cells or more immature neutrophil precursors is a commonly used indicator of infection. However, band counts are poorly reproducible among medical technologists, so the current trend is to not report band counts. Other less mature neutrophil precursors can be seen in infections and other conditions where the bone marrow is attempting to produce granulocytes rapidly.

NEOPLASTIC PROLIFERATION OF WBCs

White cell neoplasms are broadly divided into two large categories, lymphoid (the lymphocyte lineage) and myeloid (the lineage including granulocytes, monocytes, megakaryocytes, and erythroid cells).

WBC neoplasms frequently involve the peripheral blood, and can result in leukocytosis. White cell neoplasms are broadly divided into two large categories, lymphoid (the lymphocyte lineage) and myeloid (the lineage including granulocytes, monocytes, megakaryocytes, and erythroid cells). Lymphoid disorders include acute precursor lymphoblastic leukemias (ALL) and mature B-, T-, and NK-cell neoplasms. Myeloid disorders include acute myeloid leukemias, myeloproliferative neoplasms, and myelodysplastic syndromes (MDS).

LYMPHOID MALIGNANCIES

Description and Diagnosis

The lymphoid malignancies are caused by neoplastic transformation of lymphocytes or their precursors. Lymphoid cells can be found in the lymph nodes, blood, bone marrow, spleen, and extranodal sites such as the skin, mucosae, and respiratory and gastrointestinal tracts. Lymphoid neoplasms can occur at any of these sites. Neoplasms that primarily involve the bone marrow and peripheral blood are referred to as leukemias, and those involving tissue sites are called lymphomas. However, many lymphoid malignancies can involve both tissues and the blood/bone marrow, so the leukemia/lymphoma distinction is somewhat arbitrary. A selection of entities in the 2017 World Health Organization (WHO) classification system for lymphoid malignancies is shown in **Table 13–1**.

Lymphoid leukemias can correspond to precursor B or T cells or mature lymphoid cells. Precursor lymphoid malignances are also called lymphoblastic leukemias/lymphomas. Relatively common B- and T-cell malignancies that frequently present in a leukemic phase include chronic lymphocytic leukemia (CLL)/small lymphocytic lymphoma, hairy cell leukemia, mantle cell lymphoma, Burkitt lymphoma/leukemia, T-cell prolymphocytic leukemia, T-cell large granular lymphocytic leukemia, and Sézary syndrome. Lymphoid leukemias generally present with elevated white counts (specifically lymphocytosis), and depending on the degree of bone marrow involvement, there can be decreased numbers of normal white cells, red cells, and/or platelets. Processes that involve the marrow extensively can result in the presence of myeloid and erythroid precursor cells in the peripheral blood. Leukemias are diagnosed by examination of the peripheral blood smear and bone marrow aspirates and biopsies. Additional studies such as immunophenotyping by flow cytometry, molecular diagnostic techniques, and cytogenetics are frequently used to establish a diagnosis.

When lymphoid malignancies are mostly tissue-based, they are referred to as lymphomas. Lymphomas are monoclonal, neoplastic proliferations of B, T, or NK cells. Most lymphomas are malignancies of mature lymphocytes, but precursor lymphocytic malignances can involve tissues, and thus be classified as lymphomas. Lymphomas are divided into two major groups, Hodgkin lymphoma and a much larger variety of lymphomas known generically as non-Hodgkin lymphomas. The patient with lymphoma often presents with an isolated, enlarged superficial lymph node, which may be discovered accidentally on physical exam. Alternatively, the patient may have generalized lymphadenopathy. If the enlarged lymph node develops in a site where it can produce signs and symptoms, it is more likely to be discovered early in the course of disease. An example is the enlargement of lymph nodes in the mediastinum, which can impair blood flow through the large vessels in the chest and produce symptoms on that basis. In some cases, organ involvement may be the first manifestation of a lymphoma. Non-Hodgkin lymphomas, for example, may become symptomatic when there is cellular proliferation in the orbit, the gastrointestinal tract, or the skin. Involvement of the bone marrow and peripheral blood also may be an initial indicator of the presence of a lymphoma.

Lymph node biopsy is the preferred method for diagnosis of lymphoma, since it allows the pathologist to determine the overall tissue architecture and get a large sample of the cells present.

TABLE 13-1   Major Entities of 2016 World Health Organization Classification of Lymphoid Neoplasms

B-cell neoplasms

Precursor B-cell neoplasms
B-cell lymphoblastic leukemia/lymphoma, unspecified
B lymphoblastic leukemia/lymphoma with specific cytogenetic/molecular abnormalities

Mature B-cell neoplasms
Chronic lymphocytic leukemia/small lymphocytic lymphoma
B-cell prolymphocytic leukemia
Splenic marginal zone lymphoma
Hairy cell leukemia
Monoclonal gammopathy of undetermined significance (MGUS)
Lymphoplasmacytic lymphoma/Waldenström macroglobulinemia
Heavy chain diseases (alpha, gamma, mu)
Plasma cell myeloma
Plasmacytoma (of bone or extraosseous)
Extranodal marginal zone lymphoma of mucosa-associated lymphoid tissue (MALT)
Nodal marginal zone B-cell lymphoma
Follicular lymphoma
Mantle cell lymphoma
Diffuse large B-cell lymphoma
Mediastinal (thymic) large B-cell lymphoma
Intravascular large B-cell lymphoma
ALK-positive large B-cell lymphoma
Plasmablastic lymphoma
Primary effusion lymphoma
Burkitt lymphoma/leukemia
High-grade B-cell lymphoma with rearrangements of *MYC* and *BCL2* and/or *BCL6* (see footnote)

T- and NK-cell neoplasms

Precursor T-cell neoplasms
Precursor T lymphoblastic leukemia/lymphoma
Blastic NK-cell lymphoma

Mature T- and NK-cell neoplasms
T-cell prolymphocytic leukemia
T-cell large granular lymphocytic leukemia
Adult T-cell leukemia/lymphoma
Extranodal NK/T-cell lymphoma, nasal type
Enteropathy-associated T-cell lymphoma
Hepatosplenic T-cell lymphoma
Subcutaneous panniculitis-like T-cell lymphoma
Mycosis fungoides
Sézary syndrome
Primary cutaneous anaplastic large cell lymphoma
Angioimmunoblastic T-cell lymphoma
Anaplastic large cell lymphoma

Hodgkin lymphoma

Nodular lymphocyte-predominant Hodgkin lymphoma
Classical Hodgkin lymphoma
Nodular sclerosis
Lymphocyte-rich
Mixed cellularity
Lymphocyte-depleted

Data from Swerdlow SH, Campo E, Harris NL, et al, eds. *WHO Classification of Tumours of Haematopoietic and Lymphoid Tissues.* Lyon, France: IARC Press; 2017.
MYC gene, a proto-oncogene that codes for a nuclear phosphoprotein; *BCL2* and *BCL6*, B-cell lymphoma genes 2 and 6.

Because the lymphoma may not be distributed evenly in all lymph nodes, it may be necessary to biopsy several lymph nodes to establish the diagnosis. In recent years, both fine needle aspiration and biopsy have been used more commonly to make diagnoses of lymphoma. Although fine needle aspiration does not allow optimal evaluation of tissue architecture, diagnostic procedures such as flow cytometry and/or molecular techniques can be used to render a diagnosis on minimal amounts of material.

Principal differentiating factors between Hodgkin and non-Hodgkin lymphomas are:

- Hodgkin lymphoma:
  (a) Proliferation of cells is typically localized to a single group of nodes such as the cervical or mediastinal nodes.
  (b) Proliferating cells spread by contiguity.
  (c) Mesenteric lymph nodes and extranodal sites are rarely involved.
- Non-Hodgkin lymphomas:
  (a) Frequent involvement of multiple groups of nodes.
  (b) Proliferating cells spread widely and noncontiguously.
  (c) Extranodal sites are commonly involved.

The Hodgkin and non-Hodgkin lymphomas are classified into clinical stages based on the distribution of the disease. These stages, with increased clinical severity associated with higher stage numbers, are as follows:

- Stage I—involvement of one group of lymph nodes or two contiguous lymph node clusters on the same side of the diaphragm.
- Stage II—involvement of two or more noncontiguous lymph node groups on the same side of the diaphragm.
- Stage III—lymph node involvement above and below the diaphragm.
- Stage IV—widespread disease, often involving the liver, bone marrow, lungs, bones, and skin.

In addition to the above staging scheme, the designation "B" is added for patients who have constitutional symptoms such as fever, night sweats, and weight loss. For example, a patient with involvement of two groups of lymph nodes on the same side of the diaphragm with fevers and night sweats would be considered stage IIB. In general, the presence of these "B symptoms" portends a more advanced stage of disease with worse prognosis. In addition, the designation "E" is used to designate lymphomas involving extranodal sites only (e.g., the gastrointestinal tract).

Lymphoma Classification

Historically the diagnosis of Hodgkin and non-Hodgkin lymphoma was primarily based on the histological appearance of the lymph nodes. For Hodgkin lymphoma, the Rye classification system was used for decades and has now been incorporated with relatively few changes into the current WHO classification system for hematologic malignancies. Classification of non-Hodgkin lymphomas has been more problematic. Non-Hodgkin lymphomas were organized in the Rappaport classification in 1966, the Lukes–Collins classification in 1973 to 1974, and in 1982 they were reclassified according to the Working Formulation of Clinical Usage by an international panel of experts.

By the early 1990s, significant progress was made in understanding the biology of lymphomas, so newer classification systems were developed based on typing lymphomas with antibodies specific for cytoplasmic and cell surface proteins (immunohistochemistry and flow cytometry) and by detecting specific molecular lesions. In 1994, the REAL classification was introduced by the International Lymphoma Study Group. The goal of the new classification was to integrate morphological, immunologic, and genetic information to better define the disease entities. The REAL classification system was modified somewhat to form the basis for the 2008 WHO classification system, which was revised in 2017 (**Table 13–1**).

The WHO classification system attempts to classify non-Hodgkin lymphomas according to the normal cell equivalent of the neoplastic cells. First, neoplastic cells are classified based on whether they are of B-cell or T-cell/NK-cell origin. Next, the cells are classified by the stage of differentiation to which they correspond. Most B- and T-cell neoplasms correspond to mature B and T cells.

In the end, lymphoma classification is determined by the architectural features observed under the microscope (e.g., follicular vs. diffuse growth pattern and the microscopic appearance of the malignant cells), the spectrum of proteins expressed on the surfaces and in the cytoplasm of the malignant cells (e.g., T- or B-cell markers and proteins not expressed in normal lymphocytes), the presence of clonal rearrangements of the immunoglobulin or T-cell receptor genes, and, in some

---

For Hodgkin lymphoma, the Rye classification system was used for decades and has now been incorporated with relatively few changes into the current WHO classification system for hematologic malignancies. Classification of non-Hodgkin lymphomas has been more problematic.

cases, the presence of specific genetic lesions in the malignant cells. The techniques used for lymphoma diagnosis include light microscopy, immunohistochemistry, flow cytometry, and molecular techniques including cytogenetics, fluorescence in situ hybridization (FISH), polymerase chain reaction (PCR), and newer techniques such as microarrays and next-generation sequencing.

Since it is beyond the scope of this chapter to discuss all the lymphoid malignancies in detail, the more common disorders have been selected for inclusion.

Precursor B- and T-cell Neoplasms

Neoplasms of immature B and T cells most commonly present as leukemias, with extensive blood and bone marrow involvement, but they can also involve the lymphoid tissues as lymphomas. For example, precursor T-cell leukemia/lymphoma often presents with a mediastinal mass and may not demonstrate blood or bone marrow involvement. ALL accounts for almost one-third of all childhood cancers and represents 75% of all pediatric leukemias. The median age at diagnosis is 10 years with a slight male predominance of 1.4:1. Pediatric leukemias are almost always (80% to 85%) of a precursor B-cell lineage, with the remainder being T-cell lineage.

> ALL accounts for almost one-third of all childhood cancers and represents 75% of all pediatric leukemias.

Diagnosis

- *Morphology*—Morphologically, the involved tissues show monomorphic collections of medium-sized cells with fine chromatin, high nuclear:cytoplasmic ratios, and inconspicuous nucleoli.
- *Immunophenotyping*—Depending on lineage, the cells will express B- or T-cell surface proteins. Both B- and T-cell precursor cells contain the enzyme terminal deoxynucleotidyl transferase.
- *Cytogenetics*—There are a number of recurrent chromosomal translocations associated with ALL that are associated with specific WHO classifications. Hyperdiploidy with 50 or more chromosomes is a favorable prognostic finding. The presence of the Philadelphia chromosome, t(9;22)(q43;q11), is one abnormality with an adverse prognostic finding.
- *Molecular genetics*—Cases of ALL will show clonal rearrangements of the immunoglobulin or T cell antigen receptor genes. Molecular methods can also be used to detect specific chromosomal translocations.

Chronic Lymphocytic Leukemia

Description

CLL is the most common of the non-Hodgkin lymphomas. The median age at diagnosis is 70 years with a slight male predominance of 1.7:1. The neoplastic cells in CLL are mature B cells. CLL is an indolent disease with a highly variable life expectancy. Transformation to aggressive disease occurs in 5% to 10% of cases at any time during the course of the illness, and is usually a terminal event.

> CLL is the most common of the non-Hodgkin lymphomas. CLL is an indolent disease with a highly variable life expectancy.

Diagnosis

- *Morphology*—The lymphocytes in CLL are usually small and well differentiated. They are sometimes difficult to distinguish from normal lymphocytes, but they can be identified by their somewhat larger size, coarsely clumped chromatin, and tendency to break apart on peripheral blood smears, forming "smudge cells." CLL can transform into a high-grade B-cell lymphoma known as Richter syndrome in approximately 3% of B-cell CLL cases. Another type of transformation is to the prolymphocytoid form, where patients can have a very high white count of characteristic prolymphocytes with prominent nucleoli.
- *Immunophenotyping*—The CLL tumor cells express low levels of monoclonal surface IgM and IgD in the majority of cases, surface IgM only in approximately 25% of the cases, and surface IgD, other immunoglobulin isotypes, or no surface immunoglobulin in a small percentage of cases. A characteristic finding in CLL is expression of CD5, which is normally a pan-T-cell antigen, but is expressed on a minor normal subset of B cells. CLL cells also express the B-cell antigens CD19, CD20 (low level), CD23, and CD200 . Immunophenotyping can also be used for prognosis: high-level expression of CD38 and ZAP-70 is associated with worse prognosis.

- *Cytogenetics*—Chromosomal abnormalities in CLL have prognostic significance. Deletions of 11q and 17p are associated with significantly shorter survival. Deletion of 13q is associated with better prognosis.
- *Molecular genetics*—The cells of CLL have clonally rearranged immunoglobulin genes. CLL with hypermutated immunoglobulin gene regions (compared with the baseline unmutated sequences) has a better prognosis. Unmutated immunoglobulin genes are associated with worse prognosis.

Hairy Cell Leukemia

Description

Hairy cell leukemia is an uncommon form of non-Hodgkin lymphoma. This disease generally occurs in men with a median age at diagnosis of 50 years. The male to female ratio is approximately 4:1. The clinical manifestations are primarily the result of infiltration of the tumor cells into the bone marrow, liver, and spleen. A significant clinical finding on physical examination is the often massive splenomegaly. The liver is also enlarged, but to a much lesser degree than the spleen. Marrow failure is common in this disease, resulting in pancytopenia and its associated complications. Patients generally present with splenomegaly, leukopenia with a relative decrease in monocytes, and an inaspirable bone marrow.

Diagnosis

> The diagnosis of hairy cell leukemia is supported by the identification of lymphocytes with bean-shaped nuclei and fairly abundant gray cytoplasm, giving the cells a somewhat monocytic appearance. Fine cytoplasmic projections that have a hair-like appearance on Wright–Giemsa-stained smears give this entity its name.

- *Morphology*—The diagnosis of hairy cell leukemia is supported by the identification of lymphocytes with bean-shaped nuclei and fairly abundant gray cytoplasm, giving the cells a somewhat monocytic appearance. Fine cytoplasmic projections that have a hair-like appearance on Wright–Giemsa-stained smears give this entity its name.
- *Cytochemistry*—The cells in hairy cell leukemia stain positively for acid phosphatase that is partially or completely resistant to removal on the addition of tartrate. This is known as TRAP, for **t**artrate-**r**esistant **a**cid **p**hosphatase. TRAP-positive lymphocytes with fine cytoplasmic projections are highly consistent with a diagnosis of hairy cell leukemia.
- *Immunophenotyping*—The hairy cells have a B-cell phenotype, with monoclonal surface immunoglobulin, CD19 (increased), and CD20 (increased). Antigens that are relatively specific for hairy cell leukemia include the interleukin 2 receptor alpha, CD25, as well as surface CD11c and CD103. Immunohistochemistry performed on bone marrow biopsies or spleen can be used to detect DBA44, which is relatively selective, although not specific, for hairy cell leukemia. These results are all consistent with the identification of hairy cell leukemia as a B-cell disorder.
- *Molecular genetics*—The neoplastic B cells of hairy cell leukemia have clonally rearranged immunoglobulin genes. In addition, virtually all hairy cell leukemias have a mutation of the *BRAF* gene (V600E) that was previously found in melanoma. This mutation is relatively specific for hairy cell leukemia and does not appear to affect disease prognosis.

Plasma Cell Neoplasms

The plasma cell neoplasms are disorders in which there is an expansion of a single clone of immunoglobulin-secreting cells. This results in the appearance of high levels of complete or incomplete immunoglobulin molecules in the serum or urine. The monoclonal immunoglobulin in the serum is known as an M-component because it is found in the prototype disorder in this group of diseases, *m*ultiple *m*yeloma. Incomplete immunoglobulins containing only light chains or only heavy chains may be produced in certain plasma cell neoplasms. The free light chains, which are known as Bence–Jones proteins, may be excreted into the urine. Disorders in this grouping of plasma cell neoplasms include plasma cell myeloma, smoldering myeloma, solitary plasmacytoma, Waldenström macroglobulinemia/lymphoplasmacytic leukemia, heavy chain disease, primary amyloidosis, and monoclonal gammopathy of unknown significance (MGUS). Amyloidosis is discussed in Chapter 3; the other entities are described below.

Plasma Cell Myeloma

Description

Plasma cell myeloma, also known as multiple myeloma, is a disorder resulting from proliferation of a single plasma cell clone that produces a monoclonal immunoglobulin. The median age for presentation is 62 years. The most frequent presenting symptom is bone pain resulting from osteolytic lesions produced by clusters of plasma cells infiltrating the bone. The bones most often affected are the skull, the ribs, the vertebrae, and the long bones of the extremities. Because patients with multiple myeloma are often anemic, fatigue and weakness are common presenting symptoms. Patients may also experience recurrent bacterial infections as a result of the leukopenia that occurs later in the disease. In addition, the passage of free light chains into the urine may result in "myeloma kidney" and lead to renal failure. The diagnosis of myeloma depends on the presence of a monoclonal protein in the serum or urine, and then the type of myeloma is further classified based on the severity of the disease (**Table 13–2**). A skeletal survey is included in the initial workup of myeloma to assess the extent of bone involvement.

> The diagnosis of myeloma depends on the presence of a monoclonal protein in the serum or urine, and then the type of myeloma is further classified based on the severity of the disease.

Diagnosis

- *Morphology*—The diagnosis of plasma cell neoplasm is made when increased numbers of plasma cells are observed in a bone marrow or tissue biopsy. In the bone marrow, plasma cell numbers will be increased, and they form small clusters to extensive sheets in bone marrow biopsies. Solitary tissue lesions, often involving bone, may also show sheets of abnormal plasma cells and are classified as plasmacytomas. Abnormal plasma cells are rarely seen in the peripheral blood, and "plasma cell leukemia" is considered an end-stage presentation of this disorder.
- *Immunophenotyping*—Abnormal plasma cells can be detected by flow cytometry based on abnormal loss of CD19 and CD45, expression of CD38 and CD138, and monoclonal immunoglobulin light chain in the cytoplasm. The abnormal cells may express CD56, which is absent on normal plasma cells. In tissue sections, the abnormal plasma cells are recognized by expression of CD138 and monoclonal cytoplasmic immunoglobulin light chain expression.
- *Cytogenetics*—Chromosomal abnormalities in myeloma have prognostic significance. Most commonly FISH is used to identify specific abnormalities. For FISH, fluorescent DNA probes for the genes of interest are used to localize these genes in chromosome preparations or in cell nuclei. These probes can determine if two separate genes are brought together in a translocation or if a gene is broken apart by a translocation. It is helpful to use some kind of enrichment technique, such as magnetic beads coated with antibodies that plasma cells express (e.g., CD138), to obtain enough plasma cells to study. Favorable risk cytogenetic abnormalities include hyperdiploidy, t(11;14) or t(6;14). Poor risk cytogenetic abnormalities include deletion of chromosome 13, t(4;14), t(14;16), t(14;20), deletion of 17p13, and hypodiploidy.
- *Molecular genetics*—Plasma cell neoplasms have clonal rearrangements of their immunoglobulin genes.
- *Protein electrophoresis*—The evaluation of a patient for multiple myeloma begins with protein electrophoresis of serum and urine to identify any monoclonal proteins (see Chapter 2 for protein electrophoresis and immunofixation). An M-component on an electrophoretic gel is a dense band of protein that is not usually present. It most often migrates in the gamma region of the gel, but occasionally appears in the beta or alpha-2 region. To increase the likelihood of M-component detection in the urine, the samples evaluated for M-components must be

TABLE 13–2 **Diagnostic Criteria for Plasma Cell Myeloma**

Plasma cell myeloma is divided into symptomatic and asymptomatic forms, depending on evidence of end-organ damage
Symptomatic plasma cell myeloma: • Plasmacytoma or >10% clonal plasma cells in bone marrow • Evidence of end-organ damage including hypercalcemia, renal insufficiency, and anemia or bone lesions or >60% clonal plasma cells in bone marrow or free light chain ratio >100
Smoldering (or asymptomatic) myeloma: • M-protein in serum >30 g/L and/or • 10–60% clonal plasma cells in the bone marrow

concentrated prior to electrophoresis. Confirmation that a band identified on serum or urine protein electrophoresis represents an M-component involves further analysis by immunofixation electrophoresis (see Chapter 2). These tests permit identification of the specific heavy chain and light chain of the M-component, if both are present. It is also necessary to quantify serum immunoglobulins to determine if the concentration of the M-component is greater than 30 g/L and if the free light chain ratio is greater than 100 (excess of one type of light chain, kappa or lambda, over the other).

- *Other chemistry tests*—Beta-2 microglobulin is the light chain of a class 1 major histocompatibility complex protein, and is present on the surface of all nucleated cells. Increased levels of the unbound beta-2 microglobulin in the plasma are found in multiple myeloma and are considered a reflection of tumor burden. Other tests used to evaluate myeloma include measurement of serum calcium and evaluation of renal function.

Waldenström Macroglobulinemia/Lymphoplasmacytic Lymphoma

Description

Waldenström macroglobulinemia is the clinical syndrome associated with lymphoplasmacytic lymphoma in the WHO classification. There is a diffuse infiltration of the bone marrow by small lymphocytes and plasma cells that synthesize an IgM immunoglobulin, which is referred to as a macroglobulin. It is similar to plasma cell myeloma in that both have an M-component. However, the M-component in Waldenström macroglobulinemia is always an IgM molecule, and unlike the relatively rare IgM myeloma patient, individuals with Waldenström macroglobulinemia do not have lytic bone lesions. The mean age for presentation is 63 years, with a slight male predominance. Patients frequently present with fatigue, weight loss, weakness, and bleeding from anemia and thrombocytopenia. When present in sufficient concentration, the large circulating IgM protein produces a hyperviscosity syndrome in the plasma and tissue deposition of IgM. Most patients with Waldenström macroglobulinemia have an elevated serum viscosity, but only 15% to 20% are symptomatic. The most common symptoms associated with slow blood flow from hyperviscosity are blurred vision, mucosal bleeding, dizziness, and, on funduscopic examination of the eye, papilledema, hemorrhage, and distention of the retinal veins.

> The M-component in Waldenström macroglobulinemia is always an IgM molecule, and unlike the relatively rare IgM myeloma patient, individuals with Waldenström macroglobulinemia do not have lytic bone lesions.

Diagnosis

- *Morphology*—The pathological correlate of Waldenström macroglobulinemia is lymphoplasmacytic lymphoma. The abnormal cells are small mature-appearing lymphocytes, some of which may resemble small plasma cells. The cells can be present in tissue biopsies, peripheral blood, or bone marrow.
- *Immunophenotyping*—The abnormal cells express the B cell markers CD19 and CD20 without coexpression of CD5 or CD10. The cells will have surface expression of monoclonal immunoglobulin. The abnormal cells may express plasma cell antigens such as CD38 or CD138.
- *Protein electrophoresis*—The diagnosis of Waldenström macroglobulinemia requires demonstration of an IgM serum protein concentration greater than 30 g/L. As with multiple myeloma, Waldenström macroglobulinemia must be differentiated from an IgM MGUS.
- *Molecular genetics*—The abnormal cells will demonstrate clonal immunoglobulin gene rearrangements. In addition, a mutation in the myeloid differentiation primary response (*MYD88*) gene (L265P) is specifically associated with Waldenström macroglobulinemia.

Heavy Chain Disease

Description

The heavy chain diseases are a group of lymphoproliferative disorders in which there is production of monoclonal immunoglobulins with only heavy chains. Each type of heavy chain disease is named for the abnormal heavy chain produced, resulting in:

- Alpha chain disease—a high serum concentration of the heavy chain present in IgA
- Gamma chain disease—a high serum concentration of the heavy chain present in IgG
- Mu chain disease—a high serum concentration of the heavy chain present in IgM

All the heavy chain diseases are rare, with alpha chain disease having the highest incidence of the related disorders. In all three disorders, the monoclonal heavy chain is defective with internal deletions of most of the variable region of the protein and some portion of the first constant region domain. Common clinical findings in patients with heavy chain disease are splenomegaly, hepatomegaly, and lymphadenopathy. Almost all cases of mu chain disease have been associated with CLL. Gamma chain disease has been found in the presence of a variety of autoimmune disorders and in lymphoplasmacytic lymphoma. Alpha chain disease is associated with extranodal marginal zone lymphoma of the MALT type, which usually involves the gastro-intestinal tract.

Diagnosis

The diagnosis of heavy chain disease is made primarily by demonstration of a monoclonal heavy chain by protein electrophoresis of serum, concentrated urine, or both. The diagnosis of heavy chain disease should prompt an investigation into the presence of lymphoma if that diagnosis has not already been made.

Monoclonal Gammopathies of Unknown Significance

Description

Patients with MGUS are asymptomatic but have a monoclonal protein in their serum and/or urine. There is an increasing incidence of MGUS with aging. Because the incidence of malignant monoclonal gammopathies also increases with age, it is essential to differentiate patients who have MGUS from those who have plasma cell myeloma or Waldenström macroglobulinemia. Most patients with MGUS remain clinically stable without therapy for many years. However, as many as 15% to 20% develop myeloma, macroglobulinemia, amyloidosis, or lymphoma. Indolent myeloma and smoldering myeloma, disorders with many features of multiple myeloma and Waldenström macroglobulinemia that do not meet the criteria for diagnosis, can be differentiated from MGUS because MGUS has a lower amount of immunoglobulin in the serum and a lower percentage of plasma cells in the bone marrow.

> Because the incidence of malignant monoclonal gammopathies also increases with age, it is essential to differentiate patients who have MGUS from those who have plasma cell myeloma or Waldenström macroglobulinemia.

Diagnosis

MGUS is diagnosed by the presence of a monoclonal serum or urine immunoglobulin at a concentration less than 30 g/L, less than 10% abnormal plasma cells in the bone marrow, no lytic bone lesions, and no symptoms suggestive of multiple myeloma.

Hodgkin Lymphoma

Description and Diagnosis

Hodgkin lymphoma is distinguished from non-Hodgkin lymphoma by the presence of large abnormal-appearing neoplastic cells known as Reed–Sternberg cells in the lymph node. For many years the lineage of the Reed–Sternberg cell was controversial, but it is clear now that the Reed–Sternberg cell is an abnormal malignant B cell. Hodgkin lymphoma is a common form of malignancy in young adults with a second peak incidence in older individuals. Unlike the multiple classification schemes for non-Hodgkin lymphomas, a classification of Hodgkin disease known as the Rye classification was accepted for decades. This classification system has now been incorporated with minor changes into the WHO classification system for hematologic malignancies. Hodgkin lymphoma is divided into two broad categories: classical Hodgkin lymphoma and nodular lymphocyte-predominant Hodgkin lymphoma. Classical Hodgkin lymphoma is characterized by infrequent Reed–Sternberg cells in a background of normal lymphocytes, plasma cells, eosinophils, and granulocytes. The Reed–Sternberg cells lack expression of the pan-hematopoietic marker CD45; they occasionally express the B-cell marker CD20, and they characteristically express CD30 and CD15. The different subtypes of classical Hodgkin lymphoma in the WHO classification are characterized primarily by differences in tissue architecture and the composition of the cellular background.

> Hodgkin lymphoma is distinguished from non-Hodgkin lymphoma by the presence of a neoplastic giant cell known as a Reed–Sternberg cell in the lymph node.

Nodular lymphocyte-predominant Hodgkin lymphoma also shows scattered large abnormal cells, but these do not have the appearance of Reed–Sternberg cells. The abnormal cells in nodular lymphocyte-predominant Hodgkin lymphoma have convoluted nuclei, leading to the term "popcorn cells." These abnormal cells express the pan-hematopoietic marker CD45 and the B-cell marker CD20; they variably express CD30 and do not express CD15. The abnormal cells are frequently ringed by normal T cells. Nodular lymphocyte-predominant Hodgkin lymphoma is best thought of as a low-grade B-cell lymphoma.

MYELOID DISORDERS

Acute Myeloid Leukemias

> Acute myeloid leukemia is a neoplasm of a hematopoietic stem cell that has lost its capacity to differentiate and regulate its own proliferation. The outcome of the expansion of the leukemic clone is an accumulation of poorly differentiated WBC precursors known as blasts in the bone marrow.

Acute myeloid leukemias (AML) are hematologic malignancies that primarily involve the peripheral blood and bone marrow. AML is a neoplasm of a hematopoietic stem cell that has lost its capacity to differentiate and regulate its own proliferation. The outcome of the expansion of the leukemic clone is an accumulation of poorly differentiated WBC precursors known as blasts in the bone marrow. There is a corresponding lack of production of normal blood cells. A diagnosis of AML requires that 20% or more of the bone marrow cells be blasts. The blasts commonly appear in the peripheral blood and permit preliminary diagnosis from review of the peripheral blood smear. However, it is frequently difficult to distinguish AML from precursor acute lymphocytic leukemias by morphology alone. Leukemia is usually rapidly progressive, and patients can die within days to weeks without therapeutic intervention. Acute leukemias of lymphoid cells are included in the B- and T-cell malignancy classification scheme and were discussed above. In this section, we will consider the AML, which are malignancies of myeloid stem and precursor cells.

Leukemias cannot generally be diagnosed by morphology alone. Special cytochemical stains can sometimes help identify the lineage of the leukemic cells, but definitive classification is best done by immunophenotyping using flow cytometry. It is also important to perform cytogenetic and/or molecular analysis of leukemias, to obtain prognostic information and, in some cases, information that can be used to design specific therapy.

A uniform classification for the acute leukemias was developed in 1976 by the French–American–British (FAB) cooperative group. The classification from the FAB cooperative group ultimately divided AML into seven types, M1 to M7. These types were based primarily on the morphology of the leukemic blasts and in some cases on cytochemical staining. In 1990, the National Cancer Institute established guidelines for an M0 type of AML that is not within the M1 to M7 classification. The distinction between AML and the MDS was clarified at that time (see the section "Myelodysplastic Syndromes"). As more has been learned about the molecular pathophysiology of AML, it has become clear that the FAB categories do not correspond to distinct biological entities. For example, the translocation t(8;21) can be found in several different FAB types. The one exception is FAB type M3, acute promyelocytic leukemia. This leukemia has a recurrent translocation t(15;17), and is unique among the myeloid leukemias in its response to treatment by all-*trans* retinoic acid and arsenic trioxide.

The WHO classification system recognizes some of the drawbacks of the FAB system. New features of the WHO system include defining specific leukemias by their molecular pathology for those with recurrent chromosomal abnormalities or specific gene mutations, and creating categories for leukemias evolving from previous MDS and from patients treated with leukemogenic chemotherapy for prior malignancies that do not fit neatly into the FAB categories (see **Table 13–3**). For the remaining myeloid leukemias ("not otherwise specified"), classification is similar to the FAB system.

Leukemias with Recurrent Genetic Abnormalities

Certain common chromosomal translocations are found in AML. These translocations usually result in the generation of an abnormal transcription factor that alters gene expression, leading to leukemia. The most common recurrent translocation is the t(8;21)(q22;q22) involving the genes Runt-related transcription factor 1 and RUNX1 translocation partner 1 (*RUNX1–RUNX1T1*). It is seen in several FAB types of AML and is associated with a relatively good prognosis. The inv(16) translocation involves the genes core binding factor subunit beta–myosin heavy chain 11 (*CBFB–MYH11*) and is associated with a type of myelomonocytic leukemia that has increased eosinophils in the bone marrow (FAB type AML M4-Eo). It is also associated with a relatively

TABLE 13-3   2016 World Health Organization Classification of Myeloid Neoplasms

Acute myeloid leukemias

Acute myeloid leukemias with recurrent genetic abnormalities
AML with t(8;21)(q22;q22), *RUNX1/RUNX1T1*
AML with inv(16) or t(16;16)(p13;q22), *CBFB/MYH11*
Acute promyelocytic leukemia (APL) with t(15;17)(q22;q12), *PML/RARA*
AML with t(9;11)(p22;q23), *MLLT3/KMT2A*
AML with t(6;9)(p32;q34), *DEK/NUP214*
AML with inv(3)(q21;q26.2) or t(3;3)(q21;q26.2)
AML (megakaryoblastic) with t(1;22)(p13;q13), *RBM15/MKL1*
AML with mutated *NPM1*
AML with biallelic mutations of *CEBPA*

Acute myeloid leukemia with myelodysplasia-related changes
Therapy-related myeloid neoplasms
Acute myeloid leukemia, not otherwise characterized
Acute leukemias of ambiguous lineage

Myeloproliferative neoplasms

Chronic myeloid leukemia
Chronic neutrophilic leukemia
Polycythemia vera
Primary myelofibrosis
Essential thrombocythemia
Chronic eosinophilic leukemia
Mastocytosis
Myeloid and lymphoid neoplasms with eosinophilia and abnormalities of PDGFRA, PDGFRB, or FGFR1
Myelodysplastic/myeloproliferative neoplasms
Chronic myelomonocytic leukemia
Atypical chronic myeloid leukemia
Juvenile myelomonocytic leukemia

Myelodysplastic syndromes
Refractory cytopenia with unilineage dysplasia (anemia, neutropenia, or thrombocytopenia)
Refractory anemia with ringed sideroblasts
Refractory cytopenia with multilineage dysplasia
Refractory anemia with excess blasts
MDS with isolated del(5q) chromosome abnormality

Data from Swerdlow SH, Campo E, Harris NL, et al, eds. *WHO Classification of Tumours of Haematopoietic and Lymphoid Tissues.* Lyon, France: IARC Press; 2008.

good prognosis. The t(15;17) translocation involves the genes *PML–RARA* and is uniquely associated with acute promyelocytic leukemia (FAB type M3). This translocation results in an abnormal form of the retinoic acid receptor α (*RARA*). Interestingly, acute promyelocytic leukemia can be treated with all-*trans* retinoic acid in addition to standard leukemia chemotherapy, and many patients have a good outcome. The all-*trans* retinoic acid presumably interacts with the abnormal product of the t(15;17) fusion gene and interferes with its leukemogenic function. This was the first acute leukemia therapy described that was directed at the molecular pathology of the leukemia. Another recurrent chromosomal abnormality associated with AML is the t(9;11) involving the genes *MLLT3* and lysine-specific methyltransferase 2A (*KMT2A*), the latter of which is at chromosome 11q23. In addition to mixed lineage leukemia translocated to chromosome 3 (*MLLT3*), *KMT2A* forms fusion genes with many different partner genes. It is found more commonly in pediatric AML and is associated with a somewhat worse clinical outcome. Rarer translocations that are defined entities in the WHO classification include t(6;9)/*DEK–NUP214* (a chimeric gene following a translocation), inv(3), and t(1;22)/*RBM15–MKL1* (a fusion product of two genes).

A number of recurrent gene mutations have been identified that have an important prognostic impact on AML, and two mutations are definitive of specific AML diagnoses. These include AML with mutations of the nucleophosmin gene (*NPM1*) and mutation in both copies (biallelic) of the CCAT/enhancer binding protein alpha (*CEBPA*) gene. Both of these types of AML have a relatively good prognosis. The availability of high-throughput (next-generation) DNA sequencing has led to detailed genetic characterization of AML, and numerous recurrent gene mutations

Acute promyelocytic leukemia can be treated with all-trans retinoic acid in addition to standard leukemia chemotherapy, and many patients have a good outcome.

have been discovered that are associated with prognosis, although none yet are indications for targeted therapies. This is a rapidly evolving area of discovery.

Secondary Acute Myeloid Leukemia

Unlike the leukemias with recurrent genetic abnormalities, which are thought to represent de novo events, there is a group of leukemias that evolve out of previously existing conditions. One set consists of the leukemias that develop from patients with stem cell disorders such as the MDS (see below). These leukemias are associated with morphological abnormalities in all hematopoietic lineages. The other secondary leukemias develop in patients who have had previous chemotherapy for other malignancies. These leukemias occur in patients who were treated with alkylating agents such as cyclophosphamide or nitrogen mustard or with topoisomerase inhibitors such as the epipodophyllotoxins or anthracyclines. Both sets of leukemias are associated with complex cytogenetic abnormalities and have poor prognoses. Next-generation sequencing is valuable in identifying recurrent genetic changes in these leukemias as well.

Other Acute Myeloid Leukemias

Leukemias that do not have characteristic genetic abnormalities or documented previous stem cell disorders or therapy are characterized by their putative lineage as determined by immunophenotyping, morphology, and cytochemical staining. Their classification is most similar to the FAB system used prior to the WHO classification.

Biphenotypic and Mixed Lineage Leukemias

There is a subset of acute leukemias that express both myeloid and lymphoid markers at the same time on the same blasts. These are called mixed lineage leukemias. These leukemias may reflect a lack of marker specificity or aberrant gene expression by a malignant hematopoietic stem cell. Biphenotypic leukemias have separate subpopulations of leukemic blasts with different immunophenotypes (e.g., myeloid on one set and lymphoid on another). Both types of leukemias generally have a relatively poor prognosis.

MPO identifies cells of myeloid lineage, which usually stain intensely positive for MPO. Monoblasts and promonocytes, which appear in acute myelomonocytic leukemia, can also react with MPO. NSE is confined mostly to cells of monocytic lineage, which predominate in acute monoblastic/monocytic leukemia.

Diagnostic Techniques for AML

- *Cytochemistry*—Two cytochemical stains are widely used in the diagnostic evaluation of an acute leukemia. These are myeloperoxidase (MPO) and nonspecific esterase (NSE). MPO identifies cells of myeloid lineage, which usually stain intensely positive for MPO. Monoblasts and promonocytes, which appear in acute myelomonocytic leukemia, can also react with MPO. NSE is confined mostly to cells of monocytic lineage, which predominate in acute monoblastic/monocytic leukemia.
- *Immunophenotyping*—Flow cytometry, which uses fluorescently labeled antibodies that bind to specific cell-surface proteins, is the standard method for distinguishing AML from ALL, and identifying the individual subtypes of AML. Immunophenotyping is particularly important in the identification of blasts that show no morphological features to indicate their lineage, as found in the minimally differentiated subtype of AML. Markers such as CD14 and CD64 can be useful in identification of monocytic cells in AML. The detection of hemoglobin or glycophorin A aids in the diagnosis of erythroleukemia. Identification of platelet glycoprotein antigens supports a diagnosis of acute megakaryoblastic leukemia.
- *Cytogenetics and FISH*—As described above, certain types of AML are defined by specific chromosomal rearrangements. Traditionally, chromosomal rearrangements are detected by cytogenetic studies, in which the chromosomes of dividing leukemic blasts are stained and examined under the microscope, which allows the different chromosomes to be identified, and where abnormal chromosome rearrangements can be detected. To look for specific gene rearrangements, FISH is used, which is the fastest and most sensitive method for detecting the specific rearrangements in leukemias with recurrent genetic abnormalities.
- *Molecular genetics*—Molecular genetic tests are also used to provide diagnostic and/or prognostic information not available from morphological analysis. For example, PCR gene amplification (in addition to FISH) can be used to detect the recurrent cytogenetic translocations of AML. Molecular analysis can also be used to detect mutations in specific genes

such as FMS-like tyrosine kinase 3 (*FLT3*), *NPM1*, and *CEBPA*, which frequently occur in AML with otherwise normal cytogenetics. Next-generation sequencing can be used to characterize genes important in AML prognosis. PCR to detect translocation-specific fusion RNAs can sensitively detect residual leukemic cells after chemotherapy or transplantation and thereby permit earlier intervention.

Laboratory Approaches for Determination of AML Prognosis

Acute myeloid leukemia is currently treated initially with one of a small number of chemotherapy regimens, all of which are quite toxic to the bone marrow and other organs. By studying large numbers of patients with AML, it has become clear that certain types of AML tend to respond well to standard chemotherapy, whereas others do poorly and require more intensive chemotherapy regimens and/or stem cell transplantation if a patient has a chance to be cured. This research has shown that cytogenetic and molecular abnormalities correlate well with prognosis, and thus the clinical laboratory has a critical role to play in determining the therapy for patients with AML: the goal is to identify those patients who need more aggressive treatment at the time of their diagnosis while sparing those with a better prognosis exposure to unnecessary and possibly life-threatening therapy.

The traditional way of determining AML prognosis has been to use cytogenetic studies to place patients into favorable, unfavorable, or intermediate risk groups (see **Table 13–4**). Favorable risk cytogenetics include AML with t(8;21), inv(16), or t(15;17). Unfavorable risk cytogenetics include AML lacking more than one chromosome, inv(3), *KMT2A* rearrangements, and AML with multiple cytogenetic abnormalities. Those meeting neither favorable risk nor unfavorable risk criteria are considered intermediate risk, including AML with no cytogenetic abnormalities.

Further information about AML prognosis has come from studying individual genes found to have an impact on a patient's likelihood of cure with standard chemotherapy. One of the most important genes for prognosis is the *FLT3* gene. When this gene is mutated in AML cells, it puts a patient into an unfavorable risk category, even if the AML has other more favorable risk characteristics. In contrast, mutation of the *NPM1* gene confers more favorable risk if there is no *FLT3* mutation. Similarly, if both copies of the *CEBPA* gene are mutated, the patient is considered favorable risk, again in the absence of a *FLT3* mutation. Mutations of *NPM1* and *CEPBA* now define specific types of AML. Mutation of the *KIT* gene confers a poor prognosis on the t(8;12) and inv(16) AMLs, which ordinarily have a good prognosis. Currently many more genes are being recognized as having an impact on AML prognosis, and genetic analysis is likely to

> The traditional way of determining AML prognosis has been to use cytogenetic studies to place patients into favorable, unfavorable, or intermediate risk groups. Further information about AML prognosis has come from studying individual genes found to have an impact on a patient's likelihood of cure with standard chemotherapy.

TABLE 13–4 Prognostic Markers in Acute Myeloid Leukemia

Good prognosis
AML with t(8;21)(q22;q22), *RUNX1/RUNX1T1*
AML with inv(16) or t(16;16)(p13;q22), *CBFB/MYH11*
Acute promyelocytic leukemia (AML) with t(15;17)(q22;q12), *PML/RARA*, and variants
NPM1 mutation without *FLT3* mutation
Biallelic *CEBPA* mutation without *FLT3* mutation

Intermediate prognosis
Normal karyotype
Neither good nor poor prognosis
FLT3 mutation with *NPM1* mutation
FLT3 mutation with *CEBPA* mutation

Poor prognosis
AML with t(9;11)(p22;q23), *MLLT3/MLL*, and other *MLL* translocations
AML with t(6;9)(p32;q34), *DEK/NUP214*
AML with inv(3)(q21;q26.2) or t(3;3)(q21;q26.2), *RPN1/EVI1*
AML with t(9;22)(q34;q11), *BCR/ABL1*
Monosomal karyotype (multiple chromosome losses)
Complex karyotype (more than 4 abnormalities)
FLT3 mutation without other modifying mutations
TP53 mutations

replace cytogenetics for determining AML prognosis. Next-generation sequencing technologies are rapidly evolving and will allow numerous genes, or even the entire genome, of AML cells to be determined, which will improve the ability to determine disease prognosis and hopefully lead to therapies that can target each individual's unique cancer cells.

MYELOPROLIFERATIVE NEOPLASMS

Disorders in which there is a clonal neoplastic proliferation of a multipotent myeloid stem cell are grouped together in the myeloproliferative disorders. The major disorders in this grouping include:

- Chronic myeloid leukemia, with cell proliferation in the granulocytic series
- Polycythemia vera, in which erythrocytic precursors dominate the picture (see the section "Erythrocytosis" in Chapter 10)
- Essential thrombocythemia in which megakaryocytes are the primary cytological feature (see the section "Bleeding Disorders" in Chapter 11)
- Primary myelofibrosis (see the following), a disorder in which the bone marrow is initially hypercellular in multiple cell lineages and then gradually becomes markedly hypocellular with the development of marrow fibrosis

> Disorders in which there is a clonal neoplastic proliferation of a multipotent myeloid stem cell are grouped together in the myeloproliferative disorders.

The myeloproliferative neoplasms have a fair amount of overlap in their clinical and hematologic findings, including increased numbers of red cells, platelets, and/or white cells, the presence of circulating immature cells, and the presence of marrow fibrosis. The fibrosis is a reactive response to the neoplastic elements of the bone marrow. Myeloproliferative neoplasms are differentiated from the myelodysplastic disorders because in the myeloproliferative neoplasms, there are few, if any, dysplastic changes in the blood cell precursors in the marrow. The prognosis of the myeloproliferative neoplasms varies depending on the diagnosis. Polycythemia vera and essential thrombocythemia tend to have very long survival and a low incidence of transformation to acute leukemia. Chronic myeloid leukemia and primary myelofibrosis have worse prognoses.

Chronic myeloid leukemia is distinct from the other myeloproliferative disorders in that it contains a specific chromosomal translocation, t(9;22)(q34;q11), also known as the Philadelphia chromosome. This will be discussed in detail below.

The other myeloproliferative disorders commonly contain a mutation in the *JAK2* tyrosine kinase gene. JAK2 is a tyrosine kinase involved in transmitting growth signals for several different hematopoietic growth factors. In approximately 80% to 90% of polycythemia and in approximately 40% to 50% of essential thrombocythemia and primary myelofibrosis, the valine at amino acid 617 is mutated to a phenylalanine (designated V617F). This mutation inactivates a domain of the JAK2 protein that normally inhibits its tyrosine kinase activity. The result is that the kinase becomes activated without growth factor stimulation, and this leads to uncontrolled proliferation of the cells. A significant fraction of essential thrombocythemia and primary myelofibrosis cases have mutations in the calreticulin (*CALR*) or thrombopoietin receptor gene (designated *MPL*). Molecular testing for the *V617F* mutation in the *JAK2* gene, and for the *CALR* and *MPL* mutations has become standard practice for patients suspected of having a myeloproliferative neoplasm.

Chronic Myeloid Leukemia

Description

CML represents approximately 15% of all leukemias in the United States. The median age at diagnosis is 65 years, and there is a slight male predominance, with a male to female ratio of 1.7:1. In CML, the disease begins with a chronic phase that usually lasts for 3 to 4 years after diagnosis. The chronic phase evolves into a more aggressive accelerated phase of the disease. This phase persists for 1 to 2 years in most cases. At least 25% of patients with CML die in this phase of the disease. The remainder progress to an acute leukemia, which is known as blast crisis. The blast crisis typically leads to death within 6 months because it is highly resistant to chemotherapy. Approximately 25% of the patients with CML advance rapidly from chronic phase to blast crisis, without a significant intervening period of acceleration. Hematopoietic stem cell transplantation in chronic phase for patients who can tolerate the procedure is highly effective at curing CML.

CML is characterized by a characteristic chromosomal translocation, t(9;22), also known as the Philadelphia chromosome. Discovered in 1960, this was the first genetic lesion associated with a human cancer. When molecular cloning techniques became available, the t(9;22) was found to produce an abnormal RNA and protein product, BCR–ABL1. BCR–ABL1 is a tyrosine kinase that is constitutively active and leads to uncontrolled proliferation of myeloid cells. In 1996, a drug, imatinib mesylate, was discovered that inhibits the tyrosine kinase activity of BCR–ABL1, and this has led to a revolution in the treatment of CML, which previously relied primarily on interferon-alpha and bone marrow transplantation. Long-term treatment with imatinib can lead to drug resistance however, so alternative BCR–ABL1 inhibitors can be tried as needed. The only curative treatment for CML is still bone marrow transplantation, although a small subset of patients seems to have been cured by inhibitor therapy alone.

> CML is characterized by a characteristic chromosomal translocation, t(9;22), also known as the Philadelphia chromosome.

Diagnosis

The diagnosis of CML is based on the morphological appearance of the bone marrow, peripheral blood cell morphology, and cytogenetic and molecular genetic studies. Cytochemistry and immunophenotyping are not particularly valuable in the diagnosis of CML in its chronic phase. This is the stage of the disease in which most CML patients first present.

- *Chronic-phase CML*—A significant hematologic finding in this phase of CML is a moderate to significant elevation of the neutrophil count, often with all stages of neutrophil maturation detectable in the peripheral blood smear. An increase in basophils is important to recognize, as modest basophilia is an early indication of CML. Approximately 50% of CML patients also have an elevation in their platelet count. The appearance of the bone marrow is hypercellular as the disease progresses in the chronic phase of CML, with an increase in the myeloid/erythroid ratio from 2:1-4:1 to 10:1-30:1. There is complete maturation of the granulocytes in CML.
- *Accelerated-phase CML*—There is no widely accepted definition for the accelerated phase of CML. The characteristic features of this phase of the disease include splenomegaly, an increase in the proportion of myeloblasts (10% to 19%) and promyelocytes in the bone marrow over that found in the chronic phase, basophilia to >20% of the total WBC count, and anemia or thrombocytopenia.
- *CML in blast crisis*—By definition, when the percentage of blasts is 20% or more in the blood or bone marrow, blast transformation of CML has occurred. The blasts can be of either myeloid or lymphoid lineage; this determination is made by flow cytometry immunophenotyping. Approximately 70% of blast crises are myeloid. CML transforms into ALL in approximately 30% of cases of blast crisis. The immunophenotype is most commonly precursor B-cell ALL.
- *Cytogenetics*—The Philadelphia chromosome, t(9;22), is present in essentially 100% of CML cases; if the Philadelphia chromosome cannot be demonstrated by cytogenetics, FISH, or molecular studies, another diagnosis should be considered. Blast crisis is usually accompanied by additional cytogenetic abnormalities that appear with clonal evolution.
- *Molecular genetics*—The diagnosis of CML is still possible in cases that are Philadelphia chromosome negative by using FISH or reverse transcriptase PCR to detect the *BCR–ABL1* fusion RNA. PCR can also be used to detect minimal residual disease in patients being treated for CML. Newer techniques are now available to quantify *BCR–ABL1* RNA in the peripheral blood or bone marrow. These are being used to assess clinical responses to imatinib and to detect early evidence of imatinib resistance.

Polycythemia Vera

Description

Polycythemia vera is diagnosed by an increase in red cell mass with no apparent cause such as chronic oxygen deprivation (living at high altitude or heavy smoker). Transformation to AML is rare, but patients with polycythemia vera are at increased risk for the development of leukemia

> Polycythemia vera is diagnosed by an increase in red cell mass with no apparent cause such as chronic oxygen deprivation (living at high altitude or heavy smoker).

(see Chapter 10 for additional information on polycythemia vera). There is also an increased risk of venous thrombosis.

Diagnosis

- *Cell counts and the peripheral blood smear*—By definition, the hemoglobin, hematocrit, and red cell count are all elevated. Patients often present with microcytosis and a normal hematocrit due to the iron deficiency that develops due to excessive red cell production. Because of this, these patients are sometimes initially thought to have thalassemia trait. The WBC count and platelet count are also often moderately elevated.
- *Bone marrow morphology*—The bone marrow can appear normal, but is often hypercellular with an increase in red cell precursors. With progressive disease, the bone marrow can become fibrotic.
- *Cytogenetics and molecular pathology*—Cytogenetic findings are usually normal. Definitive diagnosis is made by demonstrating a point mutation in the *JAK2* gene.

Essential Thrombocythemia
Description

Essential thrombocythemia is diagnosed by an increase in platelet count with no other explanation. Platelet counts can frequently exceed 1 million/μL. Patients with essential thrombocythemia can manifest abnormal bleeding or blood clotting, although these complications are not very common. Transformation to AML is rare (see Chapter 11 for additional information on essential thrombocythemia).

Diagnosis

- *Cell counts and the peripheral blood smear*—Diagnosis is made by demonstrating a chronically elevated platelet count. The WBC count and hematocrit may also be moderately elevated.
- *Bone marrow morphology*—The bone marrow demonstrates an increase in megakaryocytes and an overall increase in cellularity. With progressive disease, the bone marrow can become fibrotic.
- *Cytogenetics and molecular pathology*—Cytogenetic findings are usually normal. Definitive diagnosis is made by demonstrating a point mutation in the *JAK2* gene, which occurs in about 50% of cases. Another 40% of patients have mutations in the *CALR* gene. Activating mutations in the thrombopoietin receptor gene, *MPL*, have also been described in 5% to 10% of cases.

Primary Myelofibrosis
Description

Patients with primary myelofibrosis typically present with marked splenomegaly and some degree of hepatomegaly. The disease affects primarily older individuals. As the marrow becomes fibrotic and cytopenias in the peripheral blood develop, the complications associated with the cytopenias appear. Bleeding from low platelet counts and infections from low WBC counts may be lethal. A minority of patients with primary myelofibrosis (less than 10%) progress to acute leukemia, with a higher incidence in those who are treated with radioactive phosphorus or alkylating agents in the highly proliferative phase of their disease.

Diagnosis

- *Cell counts and the peripheral blood smear*—The peripheral blood frequently demonstrates a "leukoerythroblastic" picture, with leukocytosis, immature granulocytes including blasts, thrombocytosis, and the presence of immature erythroid cells including reticulocytes and nucleated red cells. The cell counts decline with disease progression.
- *Bone marrow morphology*—Initially, the bone marrow shows trilineage hypercellularity with megakaryocyte hyperplasia and reticulin fibrosis. With disease progression, there is replacement of the bone marrow by extensive fibrosis allowing little space for hematopoiesis.

- *Cytogenetics and molecular pathology*—Cytogenetic abnormalities are present in 30% to 60% of patients. Approximately 40% to 50% of patients with idiopathic myelofibrosis have the *JAK2* V617F mutation. Like essential thrombocythemia, another 40% have mutations in *CALR* and 5% to 10% have mutations in *MPL*.

MYELODYSPLASTIC SYNDROMES

Description

MDS include a group of bone marrow disorders with dysplastic (not normal, but not neoplastic) changes of the cells of the myeloid series. In myelodysplasia, the myeloblasts in the bone marrow must represent less than 20% of all nucleated marrow cells, because if there are 20% or more blasts, a diagnosis of AML is made. Because the myelodysplastic cells originate from an abnormal stem cell clone that is genetically unstable, there is a tendency for myelodysplasia to evolve into acute leukemia.

MDS can occur as a primary disease or as a secondary disorder following exposure to chemotherapeutic agents or radiotherapy. Most cases of primary MDS are found in individuals over the age of 50 years. Many names have been applied to what is now called MDS, including preleukemia, refractory anemia (RA), and smoldering leukemia.

Diagnosis

Peripheral blood cytopenias are a hallmark of the MDS. As a result of ineffective hematopoiesis, myelodysplasia patients present with the complications of reduced blood cell counts in one or more cell lines. The complications include infections from low WBC counts, hemorrhage from low platelet counts, and weakness from anemia. In all forms of MDS, the bone marrow biopsy reveals hypercellularity.

A cytogenetic abnormality is found in 40% to 80% of the cases of primary myelodysplasia and 90% to 97% of patients with secondary myelodysplasia. These abnormalities may be useful as prognostic indicators. The most common changes are an interstitial deletion of the long arm of chromosome 5 (5q–) and deletions of chromosome 7 (–7, 7p–, or 7q–).

WHO Classification of the Myelodysplastic Syndrome

The MDS include a heterogeneous, but definable group of disorders. A brief description of each the disorders in the MDS is provided as follows:

- *MDS with single lineage dysplasia*—This is defined as an anemia refractory to therapy. Dysplastic changes are only seen in one of the erythroid, megakaryocytic, or myeloid lineages. There are less than 5% bone marrow blasts, and ring sideroblasts are less than 15% of the erythroid precursors.
- *MDS with multilineage dysplasia*—This disorder is like MDS with single lineage dysplasia except that dysplasia is present in two or more lineages (lineages being myeloid, erythroid, and megakaryocytic). Auer rods (abnormal inclusions in myeloid blasts) are absent.
- *MDS with ring sideroblasts (MDS-RS)*—This disorder is like MDS with single or multilineage dysplasia except that 15% or more of the nucleated RBCs in the marrow are ring sideroblasts. A ring sideroblast, as noted in the section "Sideroblastic Anemia" (Chapter 10), is a cell in which at least 30% of the circumference of the nuclear membrane is covered by mitochondria containing iron granules.
- *MDS with excess blasts-1 (MDS-EB-1)*—The major criterion for RAEB-1 is the presence of 5% to 9% of total nucleated cells in the bone marrow or 2% to 4% in the peripheral blood as blasts. There can be unilineage or multilineage dysplasia. In addition, the percentage of WBC blasts in the peripheral blood must be less than 5% of nucleated cells. Auer rods are absent.
- *MDS with excess blasts-2 (MDS-EB-2)*—This disease is present if there are 10% to 19% blasts in the bone marrow, 5% to 19% blasts in the blood, or Auer rods in myeloblasts or other neutrophilic precursors. There can be unilineage or multilineage dysplasia.

Myelodysplastic syndromes include a group of bone marrow disorders with dysplastic (not normal, but not neoplastic) changes of the cells of the myeloid series. In myelodysplasia, the myeloblasts in the bone marrow must represent less than 20% of all nucleated marrow cells, because if there are 20% or more blasts, a diagnosis of acute myeloid leukemia is made.

Many names have been applied to what is now called myelodysplastic syndrome, including preleukemia, refractory anemia (RA), and smoldering leukemia.

- *MDS with isolated del(5q)*—Also known as "5q- syndrome," there are normal to increased megakaryocytes with hypolobated nuclei, less than 5% blasts, no Auer rods, and the sole cytogenetic abnormality of del(5q).

MYELODYSPLASTIC/MYELOPROLIFERATIVE NEOPLASMS

The myelodysplastic/myeloproliferative neoplasm (MDS/MPN) category is for clonal stem cell disorders that do not fit well into either the myelodysplastic or myeloproliferative disorders. The most common of these disorders is chronic myelomonocytic leukemia (CMML). Other rare disorders in this category include atypical chronic myeloid leukemia, juvenile myelomonocytic leukemia, MDS/MPN with ring sideroblasts and thrombocytosis, and an unclassifiable category.

- *CMML*—This disorder is a chronic leukemia with dysplastic changes in the bone marrow that are indicative of an increased risk for transformation into acute myeloblastic leukemia. Patients with CMML have an absolute peripheral monocytosis greater than 1000 monocytes/μL, less than 20% blasts in the bone marrow, and dysplasia of one or more myeloid lineages.
- *MDS/MPN with ring sideroblasts and thrombocytosis*—As its name suggests, this disorder features dysplastic morphological changes, ring sideroblasts, and increased numbers of platelets. Mutations of *JAK2* are frequently detected in this disorder.

DISORDERS ASSOCIATED WITH IMPAIRED WBC FUNCTION

Many WBC qualitative disorders result in functional impairment and no increased risk for infections. However, other WBC functional abnormalities may be clinically significant and predispose to life-threatening infections.

WBCs must be present in appropriate numbers and also function normally. The disorders previously discussed in this chapter are associated with alterations in WBC number, and in some cases, impaired function as well. The three disorders presented in the following sections represent examples of WBC functional disorders with no alteration in WBC number. It is for this reason that they are also known as qualitative (as opposed to quantitative) WBC disorders. Many WBC qualitative disorders result in functional impairment and no increased risk for infections. However, other WBC functional abnormalities may be clinically significant and predispose to life-threatening infections.

Chediak–Higashi Syndrome
Description
This disorder is due to a mutation in a lysosomal trafficking regulator. The disorder is characterized by functional defects associated with azurophilic granules in the cells that have these granules. They are particularly prominent in neutrophils and melanocytes. Most patients with Chediak–Higashi syndrome are subject to recurrent infections. Chediak–Higashi patients also have partial albinism because they have defective melanosomes (which provide skin coloration). The platelets from these patients have a defect in storage granules. This platelet granule deficiency may produce a bleeding tendency because release of the granule contents is necessary for the platelets to aggregate and form platelet plugs.

Diagnosis
A personal and family history consistent with Chediak–Higashi syndrome, along with abnormal granules in all granulated hematopoietic cells and lymphocytes, strongly suggests the diagnosis. The disease appears to be associated with mutations in the lysosomal trafficking regulator (*LYST*) gene on chromosome 1q.

Chronic Granulomatous Disease
Description
Chronic granulomatous disease (CGD) comprises a heterogeneous group of disorders in which recurrent bacterial infections can lead to an early death. The WBCs in CGD do not exhibit obvious

morphological differences from normal WBCs. However, there are multiple biochemical defects in neutrophil function in CGD that limit their ability to produce peroxide and superoxides that destroy bacteria.

Diagnosis

Patients with CGD have a negative nitroblue tetrazolium (NBT) dye test. In this assay, a yellow dye is oxidized by the oxidative enzymes in the normal granules of neutrophils to form an insoluble blue-black compound detectable by light microscopy. CGD can be caused by mutations in a number of different genes.

Myeloperoxidase Deficiency

Description

This disorder results from a defect in the pathway required for generation of free radicals, which are important in the destruction of invading microorganisms, similar to CGD. Although individuals with MPO deficiency may experience recurrent infections, the disorder is benign in most cases. The absence of MPO may be congenital or acquired.

Diagnosis

In patients with MPO deficiency, MPO staining of freshly prepared blood smears will produce only faint staining of the granules in neutrophils.

SELF-ASSESSMENT QUESTIONS

1. For which of the following is a bone marrow biopsy most important as part of the initial evaluation?

    A. Leukemia evaluation
    B. Lymphoma evaluation
    C. Evaluation for an autoimmune disorder
    D. Recurrent infections in the presence of a normal white blood cell count

2. In which of the following disorders is an increase in circulating eosinophils not commonly found?

    A. Allergic disorders
    B. Selected parasitic infections
    C. Eczema
    D. Acute lymphocytic leukemia

3. Which of the following is a differentiating feature for Hodgkin and against non-Hodgkin lymphoma?

    A. There is a much larger variety of lymphoma types
    B. Proliferating cells spread widely and noncontiguously
    C. Mesenteric lymph nodes commonly involved
    D. Typically, involvement of a single group of lymph nodes only, such as the mediastinal lymph nodes

4. Which of the following leukemias is most common in young children?

    A. Chronic lymphocytic leukemia
    B. Acute myelocytic leukemia
    C. Chronic myelocytic leukemia
    D. Acute lymphocytic leukemia

5. Which of the following has a median age at diagnosis of approximately 70 years?

    A. Chronic lymphocytic leukemia
    B. Acute myelocytic leukemia
    C. Chronic myelocytic leukemia
    D. Acute lymphocytic leukemia

6. Which of the following is not a plasma cell neoplasm?

    A. Plasma cell myeloma
    B. Hairy cell leukemia
    C. Waldenström macroglobulinemia
    D. Heavy chain disease

7. Which of the following is a description of a Bence–Jones protein?
   A. Intact IgM
   B. Free light chains
   C. Free heavy chains
   D. Intact IgG

8. The M component in Waldenström macroglobulinemia is always which type of immunoglobulin?
   A. IgG
   B. IgM
   C. IgA
   D. IgE

9. Patients with monoclonal gammopathy of unknown significance (MGUS) have a monoclonal protein in their serum and/or urine. Approximately what percentage of patients with MGUS develops plasma cell neoplasms with advancing age?
   A. 1
   B. 15
   C. 50
   D. 75

10. A Reed–Sternberg cell in a lymph node is an indicator of Hodgkin lymphoma. What is the cell type of the Reed–Sternberg cell?
   A. Abnormal malignant B cell
   B. Nonneoplastic T cell
   C. Nonneoplastic B cell
   D. Neoplastic plasma cell

11. In the World Health Organization (WHO) classification of leukemias, what is the basis of the different classifications?
   A. By morphology of the leukemic blast cells
   B. According to the cell of origin
   C. According to the cytochemical staining
   D. According to the cell type that has an increased count

12. Myelodysplasia with ring sideroblasts and Myelodysplasia with excess blasts are two disorders in which of the following categories?
   A. Acute myeloid leukemia
   B. Myelodysplastic syndrome
   C. Acute lymphocytic leukemia
   D. Primary myelofibrosis

13. Which of the following is least commonly used as a test to establish a diagnosis of acute myeloid leukemia?
   A. Cytochemistry
   B. Immunophenotyping
   C. Cytogenetics and FISH
   D. Serum protein electrophoresis

14. Which of the following is not classified as a myeloproliferative neoplasm?
   A. Primary myelofibrosis
   B. Essential thrombocythemia
   C. Polycythemia vera
   D. Multiple myeloma

15. Which of the following is primarily a disorder of white blood cell function with a normal white blood cell count?
   A. Chediak–Higashi syndrome
   B. Myeloperoxidase deficiency
   C. Chronic granulomatous disease
   D. Chronic myeloid leukemia

FURTHER READING

Bejar R, Steensma DP. Recent developments in myelodysplastic syndromes. *Blood*. 2014;124:2793.

Bennett JM, et al. Proposed revised criteria for the classification of acute myeloid leukemia. *Ann Intern Med*. 1985;103:620.

Brunning RD. Acute leukemias. In: Rosai J, ed. *Tumors of the Bone Marrow. Atlas of Tumor Pathology*. Washington, DC: Armed Forces Institute of Pathology; 1994. Series 3, Fascicle 9.

Cheson BD, et al. National Cancer Institute-sponsored working group guidelines for chronic lymphocytic leukemia: revised guidelines for diagnosis and treatment. *Blood*. 1996;87:4990.

Dickstein JI, Vardiman JW. Hematopathologic findings in the myeloproliferative disorders. *Semin Oncol*. 1995;22:355.

Ferry JA, Harris NL. *Atlas of Lymphoid Hyperplasia and Lymphoma*. Philadelphia, PA: WB Saunders; 1997.

Foucar K. Myelodysplastic/myeloproliferative neoplasms. *Am J Clin Pathol*. 2009;132:281.

Grossmann V, et al. A novel hierarchical prognostic model of AML solely based on molecular mutations. *Blood*. 2012;120:2963.

Heaney ML, Golde DW. Myelodysplasia. *N Engl J Med*. 1999;340:1649.

Hunger SP, Mullighan CG. Redefining ALL classification: toward detecting high-risk ALL and implementing precision medicine. *Blood*. 2015;125:3977.

Kjeldsberg C, et al. *Practical Diagnosis of Hematologic Disorders*. 5th ed. Chicago, IL: ASCP Press; 2010.

Kyle RA, Rajkumar SV. Multiple myeloma. *Blood*. 2008;111:2962.

Lorsbach RB, et al. Plasma cell myeloma and related neoplasms. *Am J Clin Pathol*. 2011;136:168.

Quintas-Cardama A, Cortes J. Molecular biology of bcr–abl1-positive chronic myeloid leukemia. *Blood*. 2009:113:1619.

Radich JP. How I monitor residual disease in chronic myeloid leukemia. *Blood*. 2009;114:3376.

Rajkumar SV, Dimopoulos MA, Palumbo A, et al. International Myeloma Working Group updated criteria for the diagnosis of multiple myeloma. *Lancet Oncol*. 2014;15:e538.

Rowley JD. Chromosomal translocations: revisited yet again. *Blood*. 2008;112:2183.

Siddon AJ, Rinder HM. Pathology consultation on evaluating prognosis in incidental monoclonal lymphocytosis and chronic lymphocytic leukemia. *Am J Clin Pathol*. 2013;139:708.

Swerdlow SH, Campo E, Harris NL, et al., eds. *WHO Classification of Tumours of Haematopoietic and Lymphoid Tissues*. Lyon, France: IARC Press; 2017.

Taylor J, Xiao W, Abdel-Wahab O. Diagnosis and classification of hematologic malignancies on the basis of genetics. *Blood*. 2017;130:410.

Vijay A, Gertz MA. Waldenstrom macroglobulinemia. *Blood*. 2007;109:5096.

Wood B. 9-Color and 10-color flow cytometry in the clinical laboratory. *Arch Pathol Lab Med*. 2006;130:680.

The Respiratory System

Alison Woodworth and Erin Schuler

APPROACH TO THE PATIENT WITH PULMONARY DISEASE

Impaired exchange of gases is the unifying theme of respiratory disorders (**Figure 14–1**). Although they do not play a significant role in the diagnosis of specific pulmonary diseases, blood gas and electrolyte measurements (see Chapter 2 for blood gas determinations) are commonly used to assess the severity of different pulmonary abnormalities. The analysis of fluid located in the pleural space, which collects with certain abnormalities, constitutes another battery of tests often useful in the evaluation of pulmonary diseases. Careful analysis of respiratory secretions along with accompanying white blood cells, immune mediators, and foreign pathogens through bronchoalveolar lavage (BAL) aids in the diagnosis and management of lung disease. Infections in the respiratory tract are a major cause of pulmonary disorders. These are nearly always diagnosed using clinical laboratory tests (respiratory infections are discussed in Chapter 5). This chapter begins with a discussion of laboratory tests utilized in the diagnosis and monitoring of respiratory diseases and is followed by a section describing the most common lung diseases—asthma, respiratory distress syndrome (RDS) in adults and neonates, chronic obstructive pulmonary disease (COPD), sepsis, and lung cancer.

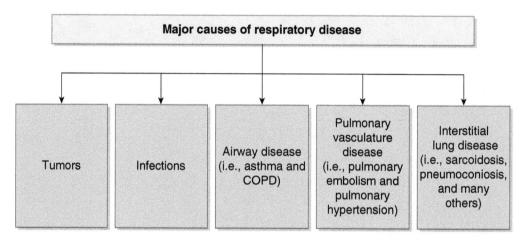

FIGURE 14-1 An overview of the major causes of respiratory disease.

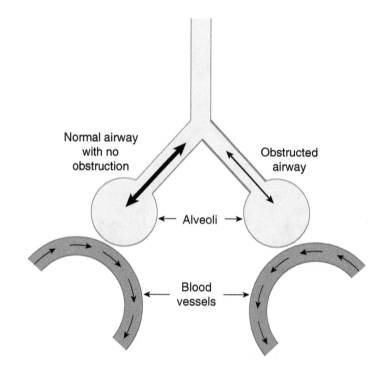

FIGURE 14-2 Diagram of diseases of the airway resulting in impaired ventilation.

Pulmonary disorders other than infections and tumors can be classified into three major groups. One group of disorders includes emphysema, bronchitis, asthma, and RDS. These are airway-based (bronchial) diseases. Inflammation or damage to the bronchi results in impaired ventilation of alveoli (**Figure 14-2**). Another group of disorders affects the blood vessels, and, thereby, blood flow in the lung. Pulmonary vascular diseases are associated with reduced blood flow, resulting in nonuniform perfusion of the lungs (**Figure 14-3**). The third major group of pulmonary diseases is the interstitial lung disorders, which affect the tissue and space around the alveoli. These are a heterogeneous group of disorders associated with lung tissue damage due to scarring or inflammation. Damaged lung tissue is unable to fully expand, leading to thickening of the interface between alveoli and adjacent capillaries resulting in impaired diffusion of gases (**Figure 14-4**).

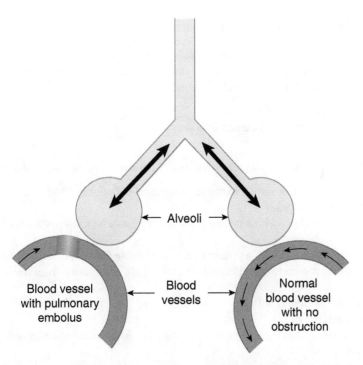

FIGURE 14–3 Diagram of diseases with reduced blood flow, resulting in impaired perfusion of the lung.

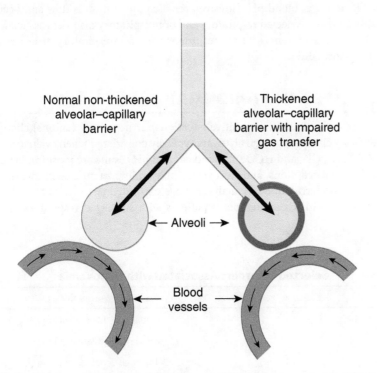

FIGURE 14–4 Diagram of diseases with a thickened interface between alveoli and adjacent capillaries, resulting in impaired diffusion of gases.

Clinical progression of pulmonary disease can lead to life-threatening respiratory failure. Acute RDS is a rapid-onset disease associated with severe breathing problems resulting from multiple insults to the lung (see more information below). It is distinct from "end-stage lung," which is the result of a chronic pulmonary disorder.

BLOOD GASES AND BLOOD pH

Many disorders are associated with abnormalities in arterial blood pO_2, pCO_2, and pH. While these tests are not themselves diagnostic, they are valuable in assessment of the severity of respiratory diseases. The blood gas test panel includes:

- pO_2 or partial pressure of oxygen
- pCO_2 or partial pressure of carbon dioxide
- pH

The functional abnormalities most commonly detected with this battery of tests are:

- Low pO_2 (hypoxemia or low O_2 in blood, as opposed to hypoxia, which is reduced O_2 in tissues)
- High pCO_2 (hypercapnia)
- Low arterial blood pH with a primary respiratory cause (respiratory acidosis from an increased arterial pCO_2)
- Low arterial blood pH with a primary metabolic cause (metabolic acidosis, usually from increased acid production and/or impaired renal H^+ elimination, resulting in a decreased arterial HCO_3^-)
- High arterial blood pH with a primary respiratory cause (respiratory alkalosis from a decreased arterial pCO_2)
- High arterial blood pH with a primary metabolic cause (metabolic alkalosis from an increased arterial HCO_3^-)

The lungs respond within minutes to acid–base disturbances by (1) eliminating CO_2 (hyperventilation) to increase blood pH or (2) retaining CO_2 (hypoventilation) to decrease the pH. The kidney has the ability to (1) excrete H^+ and retain HCO_3^- to increase pH or (2) retain H^+ and excrete HCO_3^- to lower blood pH. However, renal compensation is slow and occurs over hours to days. **Table 14–1** lists selected respiratory and nonrespiratory disorders associated with hypoxemia, and **Table 14–2** presents selected respiratory and nonrespiratory disorders that can result in acid–base abnormalities.

> The lungs respond within minutes to acid–base disturbances by (1) eliminating CO_2 (hyperventilation) to increase blood pH or (2) retaining CO_2 (hypoventilation) to decrease the pH.

ELECTROLYTES AND ANION GAP

Electrolytes are defined as either positively (cations) or negatively (anions) charged ions in the blood. Four freely circulating electrolytes are typically considered when evaluating acid–base disturbances (Na^+, K^+, Cl^-, and HCO_3^-). Blood gas and pH results are most important when investigating acid–base disruptions, and electrolytes play an important role in identifying the nature of the problem. Modern blood gas analyzers have expanded test menus to include electrolytes, facilitating their use in the evaluation of patients with suspected respiratory and/or metabolic disorders.

TABLE 14–1   Selected Disorders Associated with Hypoxemia

Disorder	Basis of Abnormality
Chronic bronchitis	Impaired ventilation of lung
Emphysema	Impaired ventilation of lung
Asthma	Impaired ventilation of lung
Pneumoconioses	Impaired ventilation of lung
Central or peripheral neuromuscular disorders	Impaired ventilation of lung
Right-to-left shunts of great vessels	Impaired perfusion of blood into lungs
Pulmonary embolism and pulmonary infarction	Impaired perfusion of blood into lungs
Sarcoidosis	Impaired diffusion of gases into blood
Selected lung cancers	Impaired diffusion of gases into blood

The anion gap refers to the difference between the major free cations (Na^+ and K^+) and free anions (Cl^- and HCO_3^-). The calculation of the anion gap from measured electrolyte concentrations is critical for evaluation of acidosis. An elevated anion gap occurs when acid anions (such as lactate or ketones) are present. The amount of the increase in anion gap is equal to the amount of acid present because an increase in acid results in a proportional decrease in bicarbonate. **Table 14–2** presents selected metabolic acidoses associated with an elevated anion gap.

PLEURAL FLUID ANALYSIS

There are a number of disorders associated with the accumulation of fluid in the pleural space (**Table 14–3**). A pleural tap, also known as thoracentesis, is used to collect pleural fluid. An initial evaluation of color, physical characteristics, and odor of the fluid may help identify the source. Next, the fluid is classified as an exudate or a transudate to limit the differential diagnosis and

> The anion gap refers to the difference between the major free cations (Na^+ and K^+) and free anions (Cl^- and HCO_3^-). The calculation of the anion gap from measured electrolyte concentrations is critical for evaluation of acidosis.

TABLE 14–2   Selected Disorders Associated with Acid–Base Abnormalities[a]

Disorder	Metabolic Alterations
Selected causes of metabolic acidosis: Arterial pH decreased with arterial HCO_3^- decreased (often from increased acid production associated with an elevated anion gap or impaired renal elimination) as a primary change and arterial pCO_2 decreased as a compensatory change	
Uncontrolled diabetes	Increased ketoacids, increased anion gap
Methanol intoxication	Increased formic acid, increased anion gap; increased osmolal gap
Tissue hypoxia	Increased lactic acid, increased anion gap
Renal failure from a variety of causes	Impaired H^+ excretion and/or HCO_3^- absorption
Gastrointestinal HCO_3^- loss from diarrhea	Decrease in HCO_3^- results in a relative increase in acidity, normal anion gap, increased Cl^-, decreased Na^+ and K^+
Selected causes of respiratory acidosis: Arterial pH decreased with arterial pCO_2 increased as a primary change and arterial HCO_3^- increased as a compensatory change	
Neuromuscular disorders that decrease breathing such as brain stem injury, myasthenia gravis, and poliomyelitis	Decreased pCO_2 excretion results in increased carbonic acid (H_2CO_3)
Severe pulmonary emboli, infections, lung cancers, asthma, COPD, and respiratory distress syndrome with impaired ventilation, perfusion, and/or diffusion	Decreased pCO_2 excretion results in increased carbonic acid (H_2CO_3)
Selected causes of metabolic alkalosis: Arterial pH increased with arterial HCO_3^- increased as a primary change and arterial pCO_2 increased as a compensatory change	
Vomiting or nasogastric suction	Loss of stomach acids (HCl); decreased Cl^-; increased HCO_3^- reabsorption by the kidneys
Diuretic (ab)use	Decreased H^+ and K^+ from increased renal excretion; increased HCO_3^- reabsorption by the kidneys
Cushing syndrome and hyperaldosteronism	Decreased K^+ from increased renal excretion; leads to increased H^+ excretion and HCO_3^- reabsorption by the kidneys
Selected causes of respiratory alkalosis: Arterial pH increased with arterial pCO_2 decreased as a primary change and arterial HCO_3^- decreased as a compensatory change	
Hyperventilation in response to hypoxemia from a variety of causes	Increased pCO_2 excretion results in decreased carbonic acid (H_2CO_3)
Hyperventilation without hypoxemia as a stimulus, as in anxiety and central nervous system disorders that increase the respiratory rate	Increased pCO_2 excretion results in decreased carbonic acid (H_2CO_3)

[a]Blood pH = 6.1 + (log[arterial HCO_3^- concentration]/[0.03 × pCO_2]) is the equation that associates the measured parameters in this table.

TABLE 14-3   Selected Disorders with Transudate or Exudate Formation

	Basis of Abnormality
Disorders associated with transudate formation	
Heart failure	An increased systemic venous pressure and pulmonary capillary pressure, due to the decreased effectiveness of the heart as a pump, results in leakage of fluid into the pleural space
Hypoalbuminemia	Decreased albumin results in a low vascular osmotic pressure and fluid accumulation in body tissues and cavities, including the pleural space
Disorders associated with exudate formation	
Pulmonary embolism and pulmonary infarction	Blockage of blood vessels results in tissue damage and leakage of fluid, or in some cases whole blood, into the pleural space
Pulmonary infections	Tissue damage results in leakage of fluid into the pleural space
Lung tumors	Tissue damage results in leakage of fluid into the pleural space
Autoimmune diseases with pulmonary involvement	Tissue damage results in leakage of fluid into the pleural space
Trauma to the lung or chest wall	Tissue damage results in leakage of fluid into the pleural space

help identify the cause of its accumulation. Exudates and transudates are defined by the following criteria:

- Exudate—A filtrate of plasma out of the blood vessel, resulting from capillary damage or lymphatic obstruction (i.e., significant loss of the blood/tissue barrier), with a relatively high concentration of protein (>3.0 g/dL). Light's criteria describe a pleural effusion as likely exudative if one of the following exists:

  (a) $\dfrac{\text{Pleural fluid total protein}}{\text{Serum total protein}} > 0.5$

  (b) Pleural fluid lactate dehydrogenase (LDH) > 2/3 times the upper limit of normal serum LDH

  (c) $\dfrac{\text{Pleural fluid LDH}}{\text{Serum LDH}} > 0.6$

- Transudate—An ultrafiltrate of plasma with a relatively low protein concentration (<3.0 g/dL) and values for ([pleural fluid total protein]/[serum total protein]), pleural fluid LDH, and ([pleural fluid LDH]/[serum LDH]) below what is required to define the fluid as an exudate.

  (a) $\dfrac{\text{Pleural fluid total protein}}{\text{Serum total protein}} < 0.5$

  (b) $\dfrac{\text{Pleural fluid LDH}}{\text{Serum LDH}} < 0.6$

Other laboratory testing on pleural fluid, while not diagnostic, may provide useful information in identifying the source of the fluid accumulation. These include total cell counts and differential, Gram stain, pH, glucose, lactate, amylase, triglycerides, and tumor markers. The section "Infections of the Lung and Pleurae" in Chapter 5 contains information on pleural fluid testing that is specific for infections.

TABLE 14–4   Selected Respiratory Diseases and Laboratory Tests Useful in Their Diagnosis or Management

Disorder	Results/Comment
Sarcoidosis	Elevated serum angiotensin-converting enzyme is found in 30%–80% of sarcoidosis cases and may be a surrogate marker of disease burden; in BAL fluid CD4/CD8 ratio >3.5
Pulmonary embolism	A diagnostic algorithm based on a clinical significance score combined with radiography and laboratory testing is most accurate in predicting an embolism. A negative test result for D-dimer (a fibrin degradation product) in a patient with low-to-moderate clinical probability effectively rules out PE. A pulmonary embolism is confirmed with a multidetector CT pulmonary angiogram in patients with a high clinical probability or a positive D-dimer test; elevated BNP and troponin measurements are associated with a poor prognosis in patients with PE (see Chapter 8 for a related discussion in the section "Deep Vein Thrombosis and Pulmonary Embolism"; thrombosis is also reviewed in Chapter 11)
Alpha-1 antitrypsin deficiency	Decreased serum alpha-1 antitrypsin; AAT phenotype assay to identify protein variants; molecular testing of the SERPINA1 gene to identify allelic variants associated with reduced activity in adults with early onset COPD or emphysema; (see Chapter 16 for a discussion of alpha-1 antitrypsin deficiency)
Goodpasture syndrome	Increased concentrations of serum glomerular basement membrane (GBM) antibody IgG are found in Goodpasture syndrome; ANCA antibody testing helps classify disease and rule out other syndromes; blood cell counts are important to monitor anemia; and renal function tests are useful for detection of renal failure; CRP to identify inflammation; and urinalysis to detect blood in urine
Pulmonary vasculitis	Discussed in the section "Vasculitis" of Chapter 8 (such as Granulomatous polyangiitis and Eosinophilic granulomatous polyangiitis)
Cystic fibrosis	Discussed in Chapter 7
Autoimmune-related	Discussed in Chapter 3

BRONCHOALVEOLAR LAVAGE FLUID ANALYSIS

Analysis of the components of BAL fluid is an important diagnostic tool in assessment of numerous respiratory disorders. BAL analysis is most helpful when used in conjunction with clinical data and imaging results to aid in the diagnosis of pulmonary infections, particularly ventilator-acquired pneumonia, interstitial lung diseases, and lung cancers, and for monitoring of the allograft post lung transplant. Several aliquots of warmed saline are instilled in different areas of the lungs. At least 30% of the instilled fluid is carefully aspirated. BAL fluid is collected with the aid of a bronchoscope.

Bacterial cultures of the pooled fluid sample help identify an infectious cause of respiratory disease. Analysis of physical characteristics of the BAL collections also aids in the differentiation of disease. Bloody BAL fluid may indicate a diffuse alveolar hemorrhage, while cloudy BAL fluid suggests a diagnosis of pulmonary alveolar proteinosis. BAL fluid can also be processed to allow analysis of soluble biomarkers and cells. Studies of the BAL cell pellet include bacterial cultures, WBC count and differential, and Gram stain.

LABORATORY TESTS USEFUL IN THE DIAGNOSIS OR MANAGEMENT OF PULMONARY DISEASES

There are a number of pulmonary diseases for which laboratory tests (other than blood gases, BAL, and exudate/transudate determination discussed above) are useful in establishing a diagnosis. The most common of these are described below, while the rarer disorders are listed in **Table 14–4** with their accompanying clinical laboratory test results. The infectious diseases of the respiratory tract and pleurae are presented in Chapter 5. Pulmonary function tests provide information on airflow and lung volumes. Spirometry assesses pulmonary mechanics by quantitating the volume of air moved in different inspiratory and expiratory maneuvers, and the rate at which the air moves. In addition, the uptake of a gas can be measured as an indicator of an impaired alveolar–capillary interface. These tests on airflow and gas exchange often do not identify a specific respiratory disorder, but they can suggest a category of diseases that may account for the airflow abnormalities. Because pulmonary function tests are performed outside the clinical laboratory, they are not discussed further in this text. However, in patients presenting with lung disease where underlying genetic or autoimmune causes are suspected, laboratory-based diagnostic testing may be employed in addition to pulmonary function tests. As an example, patients presenting with severe pulmonary disease that cannot be attributed to an underlying cause may be tested for alpha-1 antitrypsin (AAT) deficiency. Similarly, patients affected by autoimmune disorders resulting in pulmonary disease may be screened for the presence of relevant serum antibodies, such as antiglomerular basement membrane antibodies associated with Goodpasture syndrome.

Radiologic studies, particularly plain chest radiographs, computed tomographic (CT) scans, magnetic resonance imaging (MRI), positron emission tomography (PET) scans, and nuclear medicine studies such as ventilation/perfusion scanning, play a prominent role in the diagnosis of pulmonary disorders.

COMMON LUNG DISORDERS

Asthma

Asthma is a chronic disease associated with reversible inflammation of the bronchial walls leading to narrowing of the airways. It is among the most common chronic diseases, and its prevalence is rising particularly in children. Acute onset of bronchial inflammation can lead to an asthma attack, with severe forms being life threatening. While the exact cause of bronchial inflammation is unknown, there are numerous triggers including environmental allergens (pollen, dust, and others), chemical allergens (cleaning agents, smoke, and others), exercise, stress, cold air, and medications.

Diagnosis and Management

The diagnosis of asthma is challenging because the clinical signs and symptoms overlap with many other respiratory diseases. Laboratory testing to rule out diseases such as cystic fibrosis (see Chapter 7) and infections (see Chapter 5) is important for the evaluation. Diagnosis begins with assessment of airway obstruction with spirometry and chest x-ray. The diagnostic evaluation for asthma must involve identification of inflammatory triggers. Detection of elevated concentrations of IgE in the plasma indicates a generalized allergic response. Antigen-specific IgE testing identifies immune responses to specific allergens and is useful in young children and patients with a contraindication to skin testing.

Initial diagnosis and monitoring of patients with an acute asthmatic reaction involves assessment of oxygenation for disease severity and pulmonary function. Evaluation of arterial blood gases also assesses oxygenation status. Evaluation of electrolytes, pH, and anion gap is helpful in evaluating acid–base status, pulmonary function, and tissue hypoxia (**Table 14–2**).

Chronic Obstructive Pulmonary Disease

Like asthma, COPD is a chronic inflammatory lung disease associated with airway obstruction. Inflammation leads to thickening of the airway wall and decreased airflow, as well as destruction of the alveoli and increased airspace. Patients with COPD have two main conditions, emphysema or chronic bronchitis. The biggest risk factor for both is cigarette smoking, followed by exposure to pollution. Currently, COPD is a major cause of morbidity and mortality worldwide, because it can lead to respiratory failure.

Diagnosis and Monitoring

A diagnosis of COPD is confirmed by the presence of clinical symptoms such as chronic cough, wheezing, and/or respiratory failure, combined with airflow obstruction determined by spirometry. Patients with COPD are followed by measuring arterial blood gases to assess oxygen status and monitor the benefit of long-term oxygen therapy. Exacerbations and increased disease severity are commonly monitored by measuring a complete blood count (CBC) to assess the level of inflammation, testing for respiratory infections (Chapter 5), and measurement of electrolytes, pH, and anion gap to assess acid–base status, pulmonary function, and tissue hypoxia (**Table 14–2**). A report from the Global Initiative on Chronic Obstructive Lung Disease (GOLD) recommends categorizing the severity of COPD by both spirometric grade and assessment of symptoms/risk of exacerbations (ABCD grouping). This categorization system may aid in directing therapeutic options and evaluating prognosis. The WHO also recommends patients with COPD to be evaluated for AAT deficiency as an underlying cause of COPD. AAT is a glycoprotein produced in the liver that functions to protect tissue from neutrophil elastase. As in emphysema and COPD, AAT deficiency results in degradation of elastin in the alveoli. Confirmation of AAT deficiency can direct the use of AAT replacement therapy.

Respiratory Distress Syndrome

Acute Respiratory Distress Syndrome (ARDS)

ARDS is the rapid onset of respiratory failure due to systemic inflammation, trauma, or severe pulmonary infection in anyone over 1 year of age. It is associated with significant morbidity and mortality primarily due to oxygen deprivation and multisystem organ dysfunction that results from pulmonary failure. A consensus group published the Berlin definition of ARDS as hypoxemia with bilateral lung infiltrates and/or respiratory failure within 1 week of a clinical insult, with new or worsening respiratory symptoms in the absence of cardiovascular insult or left pulmonary hypertension.

Diagnosis and Treatment

The diagnosis of ARDS requires a careful clinical history to identify a recent clinical insult and/or the timing of new-onset respiratory symptoms. Chest x-ray or CT scan should be performed to visualize bilateral opacities. Cardiovascular ischemia and fluid overload should be ruled out by echocardiogram and/or cardiac biomarker analysis. Hypoxemia is classified by measuring arterial blood gases and calculating the ratio of arterial partial pressure of oxygen to the fraction of inspired oxygen (PaO_2/F_{IO_2}). The Berlin definition divides hypoxemia into mild (PaO_2/F_{IO_2} between 200 and 300 mm Hg), moderate (PaO_2/F_{IO_2} between 100 and 200 mm Hg), and severe ($PaO_2/F_{IO_2} < 100$ mm Hg). ARDS is treated with oxygen supplementation, IV fluids, and medications to treat etiology of disease, such as antibiotics to treat infection.

Neonatal Respiratory Distress Syndrome

RDS of the newborn is most commonly associated with incomplete development of the fetal lungs. The pulmonary system is one of the last to completely develop, and as a result, RDS is a common cause of morbidity and mortality in preterm infants. In fact, as noted in Chapter 7, if there is a medical need to deliver a preterm fetus, that delivery will proceed regardless of a lung maturity result. Symptoms of RDS begin within a few hours of birth due to a deficiency of pulmonary surfactant. Surfactant, a mixture of phospholipids and proteins, coats the alveolar surfaces and separates alveolar airspace from liquid-coated lung epithelial cells, preventing lung collapse during exhalation. RDS patients suffer both lung collapse and hyperextension of alveoli leading to fibrosis, or hyaline membrane disease. The alveoli in an RDS lung are perfused, but not ventilated, resulting in hypoxia, hypercapnia, and respiratory acidosis.

RDS can be addressed by preventing preterm births or by administration of corticosteroids for high-risk women within 7 days of delivery and/or at least 48 hours prior to a premature birth. Corticosteroids induce surfactant production, significantly reducing neonatal morbidity and mortality due to RDS. Infants with RDS may be treated with intratracheal injection of surfactant. Therefore, evaluation of FLM status is not essential for clinical decisions for women with symptoms of preterm labor and for those whose labor is induced prior to 39 weeks gestation. Advances in ultrasound technology have eliminated a large percentage of lung maturity assays.

> Respiratory distress syndrome of the newborn is most commonly associated with incomplete development of the fetal lungs. The pulmonary system is one of the last to completely develop, and as a result, RDS is a common cause of morbidity and mortality in preterm infants.

Selected Laboratory Tests for Assessment of Fetal Lung Maturity (FLM)

Though much less commonly evaluated than it has in the past, FLM is assessed by estimating the amount of surfactant in the amniotic fluid in women after 30 weeks gestation. The diagnostic test most commonly used to assess FLM is the lamellar body count (LBC) assay. Surfactant is packaged into storage granules called lamellar bodies that pass into amniotic fluid in the third trimester of pregnancy. LBCs >50,000/μL suggest maturity. Lamellar bodies are similar in size to platelets and can be counted on a standard whole blood counter.

Another method to assess FLM is through calculation of the surfactant–albumin (S/A) ratio. The S/A ratio increases throughout gestation proportionally with lung maturity. Surfactant-based phospholipids, particularly lecithin (phosphatidylcholine) and phosphatidylglycerol (PG), also increase in the amniotic fluid during fetal lung maturation. Qualitative detection of PG in amniotic fluid is a rapid and sensitive alternative for predicting FLM in late pregnancy. PG measurements are particularly useful in blood and meconium-contaminated amniotic fluid specimens as all other tests described above are affected by these contaminants.

Sepsis

Sepsis is a disorder associated with a severe physiological and biochemical response to a global infection. This syndrome affects over 1.5 million Americans, is conservatively the cause of >250,000 deaths, and accounts for over $20 billion in US healthcare expenses per year. As the population ages and comorbidities are more common, the incidence of sepsis has increased significantly, representing up to 40% of the patients in Critical Care Units. Lung infections, like pneumonia, are among the most common causes of sepsis.

Sepsis pathobiology begins with a host's response to an infecting agent. A normal host response first localizes and controls the infectious agent and then initiates repair of injured tissue. Proinflammatory and anti-inflammatory mediators work in parallel to kill the infectious agent and restore homeostasis. Sepsis begins when a host's response is no longer localized. During globalized inflammation, also known as systemic inflammatory response syndrome (SIRS), proinflammatory cytokines act directly or indirectly through secondary mediators to induce fever, leukocytosis, and activation of endothelial cell function and coagulation. If untreated, widespread cell damage, mitochondrial dysfunction and tissue injury ensue. In later stages of disease, tissue injury leads to organ dysfunction, failure, and ultimately death. Advanced forms of sepsis are associated with significant mortality, up to 70% in shock patients. Early identification and treatment with antimicrobial therapy significantly reduces sepsis-related mortality.

The definition of sepsis has evolved over time. In the 1990s, the initial consensus group defined sepsis as systemic inflammatory response syndrome (SIRS) secondary to a documented infection. SIRS was diagnosed in patients with two out of four of the following:

- Temperature >38°C or <36°C
- White blood cells >12 or <4 ×10^3 cells/μL
- Respiratory rate >20/min
- Heart rate >90 beats/min

Septic shock was defined as sepsis plus organ failure and hypotension. Experts currently favor a clinical definition that now describes sepsis as a "life-threatening organ dysfunction caused by a dysregulated host response to infection." They further define septic shock as that found in septic patients with advanced disease characterized by hypotension and organ failure.

Diagnosis and Monitoring of Sepsis

While rapid diagnosis and treatment of sepsis is a priority for healthcare teams, there is currently no single biomarker with sufficient diagnostic strength to differentiate patients with early stages of sepsis from those with noninfectious sources of inflammation. Several laboratory and clinical parameters are used to predict prognosis and/or monitor therapy in patients confirmed to have sepsis. Lactate, procalcitonin (PCT), C-reactive protein (CRP), and inflammatory hematological parameters are routinely assessed in septic patients.

Lactate, an end product of anaerobic glycolysis, is increased when oxygen supply in blood and subsequently in tissues is depleted (i.e., in hypoperfusion associated with septic shock). Patients with established septic shock usually have elevated blood lactate concentrations, while those early in the septic pathobiological process may not. Therefore, the clinical utility of lactate measurements is in the management of known septic patients. Current guidelines recommend a lactate measurement within 6 hours of presentation. An elevated lactate is an indicator of severe sepsis, septic shock, and increased mortality, and it prompts caregivers to initiate fluid resuscitation. Lactate clearance, defined by the percent decrease in lactate after 6 hours of therapy, is a measure of treatment response and predicts overall survival. If the initial lactate is elevated, a second lactate is measured within 6 hours of presentation. A clearance of >10% within 6 hours is associated with a better prognosis and a positive response to therapy. Lactate is measured enzymatically, utilizing LDH or lactate oxidase assays on a standard chemistry analyzer or amperometrically using a blood gas analyzer (see Chapter 2).

Two other biomarkers, PCT and CRP, may be elevated in septic patients. PCT expression is upregulated by proinflammatory mediators. When synthesized in the thyroidal C-cells, the N-terminal signal sequence is proteolytically cleaved to form calcitonin. Non-thyroidal cells lack enzymes to cleave the PCT signal sequence, and therefore PCT is secreted unprocessed into circulation. Interferon-γ which counteracts viral infections, inhibits PCT synthesis. As a result, PCT secretion is much less in response to viral infections. Because PCT is upregulated by proinflammatory cytokines, it is elevated in both sepsis and noninfectious causes of inflammation, and is therefore not a specific diagnostic marker for sepsis. When measured over time, changes in PCT concentrations may predict prognosis. When PCT concentrations are low or decreasing with time, the patient's chance of survival is significantly higher than if PCT concentrations are steady or increasing. As a result, PCT assays are FDA approved to guide antibiotic therapy. In septic adults, decreasing PCT concentrations, in combination with other clinical and laboratory parameters, may be used to recommend antibiotic cessation, but high PCT concentrations should NOT be used to increase or change the antibiotic regimen.

CRP is an acute phase reactant that is upregulated in response to a proinflammatory stimulus. Like PCT, an initial value for CRP is not useful in identifying infectious SIRS (sepsis). This is due to its long half-life and its lack of specificity for bacterial causes of inflammation. Because of its long half-life, there is no role for CRP in monitoring the success of antibiotic therapy over time. However, CRP may have a role in predicting prognosis in patients already on antimicrobial therapy.

Inflammatory hematological parameters, such as an elevated white blood cell (WBC) count, and in particular, a neutrophil count, are commonly followed in septic patients. During an infection, neutrophils regulate the immune response by releasing cytokines that attract macrophages which phagocytize cell debris. For this reason, an increased absolute neutrophil count (ANC) is a common finding in patients with an infection or an inflammatory condition. During systemic inflammation, the bone marrow sustains hyperproliferation of neutrophils, resulting in release of immature granulocytes into the peripheral blood. The presence of immature myelocytic cells outside of the bone marrow, commonly termed a "left shift," is one indicator of infection. Taken together, it is the combination of the presence of >10% immature granulocytic cells, along with a positive blood culture if present, and the other diagnostic parameters described above, that are used to make a diagnosis of sepsis—in the absence of a single specific biomarker for sepsis.

Lung Cancer

Lung cancer, defined as any tumor of the respiratory epithelium or pneumocytes, is the leading cause of cancer-related mortality worldwide. The leading risk factor for lung cancer is cigarette smoking, accounting for up to 90% of cases. Exposure to environmental carcinogens, irradiation, and genetic disorders are also risk factors for developing lung cancer. There are two main types of lung cancers: small cell lung carcinoma (SCLC) and non-small cell lung carcinoma (NSCLC). Among NSCLCs, the most common lung tumor type is adenocarcinoma. Most lung cancers are caused by acquired mutations, amplifications, or rearrangements in oncogenes, including epidermal growth factor receptor (EGFR), fibroblast growth factor receptor type 1 (FGFR1), anaplastic lymphoma kinase (ALK), Kirsten rat sarcoma viral oncogene (KRAS), neuroblastoma rat sarcoma viral oncogene (NRAS), proto-oncogene B-RAF (BRAF), human epidermal growth factor receptor 2 (HER2), phosphatase and tensin homolog (PTEN), and mesenchymal-epithelial transition factor (MET), among others. Although some lung cancers are discovered in asymptomatic patients, the most common clinical signs include coughing up blood, wheezing, and shortness of breath.

Diagnosis and Monitoring

The diagnostic workup for lung cancer begins with discovery of a new pulmonary mass by chest x-ray, CT scan, or MRI. A definitive diagnosis of lung cancer and type is determined through histological and immunohistochemical analysis of tumor tissue. Small cell lung cancer (SCLC) represents 14% of lung cancers. Diagnosis of SCLC is complicated by the lack of screening methods capable of detecting early-stage disease. Chemotherapy is recommended for patients with SCLC. Additional stage and performance status specific therapies (i.e., radiotherapy) may also be utilized. Guidelines recommend combination therapy for patients with limited-stage SCLC and a good performance status.

Molecular testing of advanced-stage adenocarcinoma type (NSCLC) is required to direct therapy. In particular, patients with EGFR mutations are more likely to respond to tyrosine kinase inhibitor (TKI) therapy and have longer progression-free survival. Patients with a KRAS gene mutation with or without an EGFR mutation do not respond to TKI therapy and should be treated alternatively. Advanced-stage NSCLC should also be tested for rearrangements in the ALK gene. About 5% to 10% of all NSCLC patients carry this rearrangement, which can be treated with an ALK inhibitor. Presently, guidelines recommend a minimum initial testing strategy to include screening for rearrangements in ALK, EGFR, and ROS1 to determine eligibility for targeted therapies such as TKI. Immunohistochemistry (IHC) testing for PD-L1 expression in patients with metastatic non-squamous NSCLC is recommended to predict therapeutic responsiveness to PD-1 inhibitors. Other tumor-specific targeted therapy options may be identified through mutation detection via multiplex or next-generation sequencing.

Prior to initiating therapy, baseline CBC and liver function panel should be measured to screen for metastases. Response to therapy and tumor recurrence can be monitored by performing regular chest x-rays and/or CT scans, as well as a CBC and liver function tests. Measurement of cytokeratin 19 fragments (CYFRA 21-1) in serum is useful for assessing prognosis in early and late stages, and in monitoring therapy in advanced stages of NSCLC. Serum neuron-specific enolase (NSE) may be useful in monitoring therapy and tumor recurrence in both NSCLC and SCLC. Other indicators of prognosis may include identification of circulating tumor cells (CTC) in the peripheral blood.

SELF-ASSESSMENT QUESTIONS

1. Which of the following lung disorders named on the left side of the dash is a mismatch with the anatomical portion of the lung affected by the disease that is listed on the right side of the dash?
   A. Pulmonary embolism—Pulmonary vasculature
   B. Asthma—Airways
   C. Sarcoidosis—Lung interstitium
   D. Chronic obstructive pulmonary disease—Pulmonary vasculature

2. Which of the following tests is not part of a traditional blood gas panel?
   A. Partial pressure of oxygen
   B. Partial pressure of nitrogen
   C. Partial pressure of carbon dioxide
   D. pH

3. Which of the following items is not part of the anion gap calculation?
   A. Sodium
   B. Potassium
   C. Chloride
   D. Calcium

4. For patients with uncontrolled diabetes, which of the following is likely to be present?
   A. Metabolic acidosis
   B. Respiratory acidosis
   C. Metabolic alkalosis
   D. Respiratory alkalosis

5. For patients with severe chronic obstructive pulmonary disease, which of the following is likely to be present?

   A. Metabolic acidosis
   B. Respiratory acidosis
   C. Metabolic alkalosis
   D. Respiratory alkalosis

6. For patients with severe chronic vomiting, which of the following is likely to be present?

   A. Metabolic acidosis
   B. Respiratory acidosis
   C. Metabolic alkalosis
   D. Respiratory alkalosis

7. For patients with hyperventilation as a result of severe anxiety, which of the following is likely to be present?

   A. Metabolic acidosis
   B. Respiratory acidosis
   C. Metabolic alkalosis
   D. Respiratory alkalosis

8. Which one of the following parameters is likely to be associated with a transudate rather than an exudate?

   A. A low protein concentration of less than 3.0 g/dL
   B. Pleural fluid lactate dehydrogenase (LDH) greater than 20 IU/dL
   C. Pleural fluid total protein divided by serum total protein greater than 0.5
   D. Pleural fluid LDH divided by serum LDH greater than 0.6

9. Which one of the following disorders is more likely to be associated with the formation of a transudate rather than an exudate?

   A. Pulmonary infections
   B. Pulmonary embolism
   C. Lung tumors
   D. Congestive heart failure

10. Which of the following tests is not commonly ordered for diagnosis or monitoring of a patient with chronic obstructive pulmonary disease?

    A. Arterial blood gas
    B. Electrolytes with calculation of anion gap
    C. Pulmonary function tests (spirometry)
    D. Hemoglobin AIc

11. Which one of the following tests is not a test for fetal lung maturity using an amniotic fluid specimen from a woman after 30 weeks of gestation?

    A. Lamellar body count
    B. Qualitative detection of phosphatidylcholine
    C. Surfactant/Albumin ratio
    D. Lecithin/Sphingomyelin ratio

12. Which one of the following acquired mutations, amplifications, or rearrangements in the genes for the proteins listed below is not known to be causative for lung cancer?

    A. Epidermal growth factor receptor (EGFR)
    B. Anaplastic lymphoma kinase (ALK)
    C. KRAS (Kirsten rat sarcoma viral oncogene homolog)
    D. Cystathionine β-synthase

FURTHER READING

American College of Obstetricians and Gynecologists. ACOG Practice Bulletin No. 97: fetal lung maturity. *Obstet Gynecol*. 2008;112:717–726.

Ball JA, Young KR Jr. Pulmonary manifestations of Goodpasture's syndrome. Antiglomerular basement membrane disease and related disorders. *Clin Chest Med*. 1998;19:777–791, ix.

Carlsson A, Nair VS, Luttgen MS, et al. Circulating tumor microemboli diagnostics for patients with non–small-cell lung cancer. *J Thorac Oncol*. 2014;9:1111–1119.

Carmona EM, Kalra S, Ryu JH. Pulmonary Sarcoidosis: diagnosis and treatment. *Mayo Clin Proc*. 2016;91:946–954.

Cheng S, Schindler EI, Scott MG. Disorders of water, electrolyte, and acid–base metabolism. In: Rifai N, et al, eds. *Tietz Textbook of Clinical Chemistry and Molecular Diagnostics*. 6th ed. St. Louis, MO: Elsevier Saunders; 2018:1324–1347.

Dellinger RP, Levy MM, Rhodes A, et al. Surviving sepsis campaign: international guidelines for management of severe sepsis and septic shock, 2012. *Intensive Care Med*. 2013;39:165–228.

Froudarakis ME. Diagnostic work-up of pleural effusions. *Respiration*. 2008;75:4–13.

Gal AA, Staton GW Jr. Current concepts in the classification of interstitial lung disease. *Am J Clin Pathol*. 2005;123(suppl):S67–S81.

Grenache DG, Gronowski AM. Fetal lung maturity. *Clin Biochem*. 2006;39:1–10.

Hellmark T, Segelmark M. Diagnosis and classification of Goodpasture's disease (anti-GBM). *J Autoimmun*. 2014;48-49:108–112.

Herbst RS, et al. Lung cancer. *N Engl J Med*. 2008;359:1367–1380.

Homburger HA. Allergic diseases. In: McPherson RA, Pincus MR, eds. *Henry's Clinical Diagnosis and Management by Laboratory Methods*. Philadelphia, PA: Saunders Elsevier; 2007:961–971.

Hughes JM. Assessing gas exchange. *Chron Respir Dis*. 2007;4:205–214.

Hunt JM, Bull TM. Clinical review of pulmonary embolism: diagnosis, prognosis, and treatment. *Med Clin North Am*. 2011;95:1203–1222.

Kahnert K, Alter P, Young D, et al. The revised GOLD 2017 COPD categorization in relation to comorbidities. *Respir Med*. 2018;134:79–85.

Kohnlein T, Welte T. Alpha-1 antitrypsin deficiency: pathogenesis, clinical presentation, diagnosis, and treatment. *Am J Med*. 2008;121:3–9.

Konstantinides S. Clinical practice. Acute pulmonary embolism. *N Engl J Med*. 2008;359:2804–2813.

Korpanty GJ, Graham DM, Vincent MD, Leighl NB. Biomarkers that currently affect clinical practice in lung cancer: EGFR, ALK, MET, ROS-1, and KRAS. *Front Oncol*. 2014;4:204.

Leighl NB, Rekhtman N, Biermann WA, et al. Molecular testing for selection of patients with lung cancer for epidermal growth factor receptor and anaplastic lymphoma kinase tyrosine kinase inhibitors: American Society of Clinical Oncology Endorsement of the College of American Pathologists/International Association for the Study of Lung Cancer/Association for Molecular Pathology Guideline. *J Clin Oncol*. 2014;32:3673–3679.

Lindeman NI, et al. Molecular testing guideline for selection of lung cancer patients for EGFR and ALK tyrosine kinase inhibitors. *J Mol Diagn*. 2013;15:1–39.

Lynch JP 3rd, Ma YL, Koss MN, et al. Pulmonary sarcoidosis. *Semin Respir Crit Care Med*. 2007;28:53–74.

Marshall WJ. Hydrogen ion homeostasis and blood gases. In: *Clinical Chemistry*. Philadelphia, PA: Mosby; 2008:45–68.

McGrath EE, Anderson PB. Diagnosis of pleural effusion: a systematic approach. *Am J Crit Care*. 2011;20:119–127.

Meyer KC. Bronchoalveolar lavage as a diagnostic tool. *Semin Respir Crit Care Med*. 2007;28:546–560.

Moyer VA, U.S. Preventive Services Task Force. Screening for lung cancer: U.S. Preventive Services Task Force recommendation statement. *Ann Intern Med*. 2014;160:330–338.

National Asthma Education and Prevention Program. Expert Panel Report 3 (EPR-3): guidelines for the diagnosis and management of asthma—summary report. *J Allergy Clin Immunol*. 2007;120:S94–S138.

NCCN Clinical Practice Guidelines in Oncology, Lung Cancer Screening. National Comprehensive Cancer Network. Fort Washington, PA. Accessed February 2018.

NCCN Clinical Practice Guidelines in Oncology, Non-Small Cell Lung Cancer. National Comprehensive Cancer Network. Fort Washington, PA. Accessed February 2018.

NCCN Clinical Practice Guidelines in Oncology, Small Cell Lung Cancer. National Comprehensive Cancer Network. Fort Washington, PA Accessed February 2018.

Normanno N, Rossi A, Morabito A, et al. Prognostic value of circulating tumor cells' reduction in patients with extensive small-cell lung cancer. *Lung Cancer*. 2014;85:314–319.

Olson AL, et al. Interstitial lung disease. In: Schraufnagel DE, et al, eds. *Breathing in America: Diseases, Progress and Hope*. New York, NY: American Thoracic Society; 2010.

Qaseem A, et al. Diagnosis and management of stable chronic obstructive pulmonary disease: a clinical practice guideline update. *Ann Intern Med*. 2011;155:179–191.

Ranieri VM, et al. Acute respiratory distress syndrome: the Berlin definition. *JAMA*. 2012;307:2526–2533.

Sahn SA. The value of pleural fluid analysis. *Am J Med Sci*. 2008;335:7–15.

Sandhaus RA, Turino G, Brantly ML, et al. The diagnosis and management of alpha-1 antitrypsin deficiency in the adult. *J COPD Foundation*. 2016;3:668–682.

Sepsis. Centers for Disease Control and Prevention. August 25, 2017. Available at: https://www.cdc.gov/sepsis/datareports/index.html. Accessed February 9, 2018.

Singer M, Deutschman CS, Seymour C, et al. The third international consensus definitions for sepsis and septic shock (sepsis-3). *JAMA*. 2016;315:801–810.

Tan DS, Yom SS, Tsao MS, et al. The International Association for the Study of Lung Cancer Consensus Statement on optimizing management of EGFR mutation-positive non-small cell lung cancer: status in 2016. *J Thorac Oncol.* 2016;11:946–963.

Tang BMP, Eslick GD, Craig JC, McLean AS. Accuracy of procalcitonin for sepsis diagnosis in critically ill patients: systematic review and meta-analysis. *Lancet Infect Dis.* 2007;7:210–217.

Vogelmeier CF, Criner GJ, Martinez FJ, et al. Global strategy for the diagnosis, management, and prevention of chronic obstructive lung disease 2017 report. GOLD executive summary. *Am J Respir Crit Care Med.* 2017;195:557–582.

Women's Health Care Physicians. Antenatal corticosteroid therapy for fetal maturation—ACOG. Available at: https://www.acog.org/Clinical-Guidance-and-Publications/Committee-Opinions/Committee-on-Obstetric-Practice/Antenatal-Corticosteroid-Therapy-for-Fetal-Maturation#45. Accessed February 10, 2018.

The Gastrointestinal Tract

Michael Laposata

LEARNING OBJECTIVES

1. Understand the relative contributions of clinical laboratory tests and other diagnostic studies in the evaluation of the patient for a disorder of the gastrointestinal tract.

2. Learn the appropriate selection of diagnostic tests required to establish a diagnosis of ulcer disease from *Helicobacter pylori* infection.

3. Select the most appropriate tests for evaluation of suspected celiac disease, and learn the situations where results may be misleading.

4. Understand the causes of both upper and lower gastrointestinal bleeding.

5. Describe the recommended approaches to screening for colon cancer, and the benefits and limitations of laboratory tests for this purpose.

CHAPTER OUTLINE

Most diseases of the gastrointestinal tract can be directly visualized by endoscopy or from a histopathologic review of a biopsy obtained during the endoscopic procedure. In addition, many gastrointestinal tract disorders can be identified with various imaging studies. This accessibility of lesions for direct examination and biopsy, and the availability of imaging studies, has limited the need for clinical laboratory tests in identifying most gastrointestinal disorders. However, imaging studies are often expensive, and endoscopic procedures are both expensive and invasive. Laboratory tests aid in the diagnosis and management of patients with a number of gastrointestinal disorders. Infectious diseases involving the gastrointestinal tract are numerous, and are discussed in Chapter 5. The clinical laboratory plays an important role in identifying pathogenic microorganisms of the gastrointestinal tract.

The clinical laboratory also plays a role in the evaluation of dyspepsia (abdominal discomfort caused by acid), and/or ulcer disease, particularly that induced by *Helicobacter pylori* infection; in the recognition and monitoring of celiac disease; identification of gastrointestinal bleeding and the causes for it; and in the detection and genetic profiling of colorectal cancer. Laboratory tests for these disorders are presented in this chapter.

DYSPEPSIA, ULCER DISEASE, AND *H. PYLORI*

Description

According to the American Gastroenterological Association (AGA), dyspepsia is defined as chronic or recurrent pain or discomfort centered in the upper abdomen. There are several common causes of pain the upper abdomen. Reflux of acid into the esophagus, referred to as gastroesophageal reflux disease [GERD] can cause abdominal discomfort. There is great variability in incidence between countries among those with upper abdominal symptoms who are found to have peptic ulcers. Other causes for abdominal pain include gastritis related to use of nonsteroidal anti-inflammatory agents, and functional dyspepsia, in which no obvious pathology is present in the stomach.

The major cause of peptic ulcer disease is infection with *H. pylori*. The infection is most likely to occur in childhood, especially if the children are living in low socioeconomic conditions. In developed countries, *H. pylori* infection prevalence increases with age. Not all patients with *H. pylori* infection develop ulcer disease, as many suffer from dyspepsia without ulcers. The infection initially produces an acute gastritis that lasts 1 to 4 weeks. Once infected, however, chronic active gastritis occurs in the majority of individuals and may lead to more serious outcomes. Especially when infected in early childhood, individuals are at risk for the development of multifocal atrophic gastritis and over time, subsequently, have an increased risk for gastric adenocarcinoma.

> The major cause of peptic ulcer disease is infection with *H. pylori*. Not all patients with *H. pylori* infection develop ulcer disease, as many suffer from dyspepsia without ulcers.

Diagnosis

The evaluation of individuals with dyspepsia depends on age and the severity of symptoms. According to guidelines, direct visualization of the upper gastrointestinal tract by endoscopy is the preferred initial step in persons over age 55 years, in younger patients who have a family history of gastric cancer, those or who also have more worrisome symptoms such as weight loss, difficulty swallowing food, recurrent vomiting, or gastrointestinal bleeding. In younger patients without these symptoms, the recommended approach is to test for the presence of active *H. pylori* infection and treat infected individuals. Those without evidence of infection are treated with drugs that inhibit acid production.

Conventional upper endoscopic examination is commonly performed to diagnose *H. pylori* associated diseases. These include peptic ulcer disease, atrophic gastritis, and gastric cancer. The biopsy obtained from the stomach can show negative results in an infected patient due to a sampling error because of the uneven distribution of *H. pylori* in the stomach. The biopsy can be used for multiple diagnostic procedures. A portion of the sample can be processed for histology, which is the gold standard for the direct detection of *H. pylori* infection and is usually the first method used for detection of *H. pylori*. Routine hematoxylin and eosin staining is usually sufficient for the diagnosis of *H. pylori* infection, although immunohistochemical stains are also commonly used for microscopic detection of *H. pylori*. The biopsy can also be used to test for the activity of the *H. pylori* urease enzyme. *H. pylori*, if present in the biopsy, converts the urea test reagent to carbon dioxide and ammonia, and that increases the pH and changes the color on a pH monitor. The biopsy can also be cultured with the understanding that *H. pylori* is a fastidious organism and that if the specimen is of poor quality or transport is delayed, there may be a failure of growth of the organisms in culture. Another diagnostic option for the biopsy is using a polymerase chain reaction-based test for the diagnosis of *H. pylori* in the specimen. This testing can also be performed on saliva, stool, and gastric juice. A number of genes in the *H. pylori* organism can be used as target genes to identify the organism using this molecular method (**Table 15–1**).

The invasiveness of endoscopy and biopsy is avoided with the urea breath test which is still a popular and accurate noninvasive test for the diagnosis of *H. pylori* infection. This test involves ingestion of food products containing urea labeled with a small amount of radioactive carbon. If urease is present, the urea will be split into ammonia and radioactive carbon dioxide. The amount of radioactive carbon dioxide in the breath is proportional to the amount of urease activity. Use of drugs that suppress acid production may result in false-negative values for the urea breath test. The urea breath test is also recommended for test and treat strategies and for the confirmation of *H. pylori* eradication.

Another noninvasive test involves the use of a stool specimen to identify the *H. pylori* antigens. *H. pylori* has a unique surface antigen that can be detected in the stool of infected individuals, but

TABLE 15-1   **Summary of Diagnostic Recommendations for *H. pylori* Studies**

To establish the diagnosis of *H. pylori* infection	A biopsy positive for *H. pylori*
	A positive test for urease using the biopsy
	Molecular tests for *H. pylori* genes in the biopsy
	A culture positive from the biopsy for *H. Pylori*
	A positive urea breath test for urease activity
To assess the success of eradication of *H. pylori*	A negative urea breath test for urease activity
To assess for resistance to clarithromycin	Molecular tests for *H. pylori* genes that confer resistance to clarithromycin

not in those with inactive infection. Stool antigen testing with kits using monoclonal antibodies to the antigen is sensitive and specific. These kits have a high accuracy for both initial diagnosis of *H. pylori* and post-treatment follow-up testing. Like the urea breath test, the stool antigen test can be used to evaluate the success of antibiotic treatment to eradicate *H. pylori*. Successful treatment using this test is indicated by the loss of stool antigen after several weeks. *H. pylori* antigens can be identified by conventional immunoassays. The use of serum to assess *H. pylori* infection involves an assessment for circulating anti-*H. pylori* IgG antibodies. Serologic tests for IgG antibodies to *H. pylori* indicate past or current infection. Unlike the stool antigen and urease test, serologic tests remain positive for years after successful treatment, and because of that they are of no use to monitor the effective treatment.

To summarize the diagnostic methods, the reference tests to identify *H. pylori* require endoscopy with biopsy and microscopic review, rapid urease testing, molecular testing, and culture. The urea breath test can be used to diagnose an infection, and to monitor the progress of an infection or the success of treatment to eradicate the organism. Antibiotic resistance to clarithromycin can be diagnosed with molecular methods using a tissue sample obtained from endoscopy.

CELIAC DISEASE

Description

Celiac disease is a systemic immune-mediated disorder. In genetically susceptible individuals, it is triggered by dietary gluten. Gluten is a complex of proteins that are found in wheat, rye, and barley. Gliadin is the water-soluble component in gluten. Celiac disease is extremely common, affecting 0.6% to 1% of the worldwide population. However, only a small percentage of cases of celiac disease are recognized. Its prevalence is higher in women, with increased incidence in individuals with an affected first-degree relative, or a relative with type 1 diabetes, Hashimoto thyroiditis, or other autoimmune disease. Importantly, genetic background greatly influences the predisposition to celiac disease. In 90% of patients with celiac disease, the HLA-DQ2 haplotype is expressed (which is present in only approximately one-third of the general population). The HLA-DQ8 haplotype is expressed in 5% of the patients with celiac disease. This genetic predisposition occurs because the HLA-DQ2 and HLA-DQ8 haplotypes are expressed on the surface of antigen-presenting cells that bind activated (deamidated) gluten peptides. The HLA-DQ2 and HLA-DQ8 haplotypes are necessary, but their presence alone is not sufficient for the development of celiac disease. There are dozens of non-HLA genes that confer predisposition to celiac disease, and most of these are involved in the inflammatory and immune response.

Patients with celiac disease have chronic inflammation of the proximal small intestinal mucosa. The inflammation can heal when foods containing gluten are excluded from the diet. The inflammation returns if foods containing gluten are reintroduced. Gluten-associated storage proteins derived from wheat, barley, and rye undergo partial digestion in the upper gastrointestinal tract. The partial digestion results in the generation of derivatives of the native peptides, and these specific peptides can elicit an immune response. The enzyme transglutaminase deamidates glutamine to negatively charged glutamic acid residues in gliadin peptides, which then stimulate the immune response and the subsequent intestinal injury.

Celiac disease is an immunologic disorder caused by immune reactions triggered by gluten and related proteins that are components of wheat, barley, and rye grain products.

Mildly affected individuals may have symptoms such as bloating, irregular bowel movements, and cramps (often referred to as irritable bowel syndrome). Celiac disease patients may present with malabsorption of certain essential nutrients, including iron. About 5% of iron deficiency in adults is thought to be due to celiac disease. Malabsorption of folate and vitamin D, which may present clinically as osteoporosis, can also occur. Patients with celiac disease can be differentiated from patients with simple gluten sensitivity and patients with wheat allergy because the antibodies found in celiac disease are absent in those with gluten sensitivity or wheat allergy. In addition, for celiac disease, the interval between exposure to gluten and onset of symptoms is weeks to years. This is in contrast to simple gluten sensitivity where the interval between exposure and onset of symptoms is hours to days, and to wheat allergy where the interval is minutes to hours.

Diagnosis

Laboratory testing for celiac disease is summarized in **Table 15–2**. Patients who merit testing for celiac disease include those with evidence of malabsorption, those with a first-degree family member with a confirmed diagnosis of celiac disease, patients with an elevated aminotransferase level with no other etiology, and a type 1 diabetes mellitus patient with digestive symptoms.

Serologic Tests

For celiac disease, a serologic test for IgA anti-tissue transglutaminase (tTG) antibodies is recommended as the initial testing for individuals who do not have a concomitant IgA deficiency.

A serologic test for IgA antitissue transglutaminase (tTG) antibodies is recommended as the initial testing for individuals who do not have a concomitant IgA deficiency. This is the most widely used test and has a sensitivity and a specificity over 98%, especially now that human tTG is used in the test as a reagent. As many as 3% of those with classic celiac disease have a deficiency of IgA, which results in a falsely negative test result. In a person with a high suspicion for celiac disease and a negative anti-tTG result, measurement of IgA to determine if the patient is IgA deficient is recommended. In persons with IgA deficiency, IgG, instead of IgA, anti-tTG antibodies can be measured. Another alternative for IgA-deficient patients is the measurement of the IgG deamidated gliadin peptide antibodies. Tests for antibodies to deamidated gliadin peptides are less sensitive and less specific in adults for diagnosis of celiac disease, but they are more sensitive than anti-tTG assays in children. Antibody tests to gliadin are less likely to be positive in milder cases, and, like the other serologic tests, often become negative when gluten is eliminated from the diet. Some patients may be monitored with antibody levels to gliadin to monitor compliance with treatment.

The endomysium is a connective tissue that ensheaths each individual muscle fiber. Antiendomysial antibodies are present in patients with celiac disease. They are useful in the diagnosis of the disease, but do not cause any direct symptoms associated with muscles. The presence of antiendomysial antibodies is nearly 100% specific for active celiac disease, but these antibodies are

TABLE 15–2   Commonly Used Diagnostic Tests for Celiac Disease

Test	Advantages	Disadvantages
Tissue transglutaminase (tTG) IgA antibodies	Most reliable noninvasive test and first-level screening test	Falsely negative with IgA deficiency (3% of patients with celiac disease)
	High sensitivity and specificity	May be negative if on low-gluten diet
tTG IgG antibodies	Useful in patients with IgA deficiency	Widely variable sensitivity and specificity
IgG deamidated gliadin peptide antibodies	Useful in patients with IgA deficiency and in young children	Not as sensitive or specific as tTG IgA antibodies
Small bowel biopsy	Reliable test, considered gold standard	Requires endoscopy and biopsy
	Reflects response to treatment	Very expensive
HLA-DQ2 or HLA-DQ8	High negative predictive value for celiac disease	Test is complex and expensive
IgA antiendomysial antibodies	May be useful in patients with borderline results for tTG antibodies	Sensitivity for celiac disease less than IgA anti-transglutaminase antibody test

found in other autoimmune diseases, and for that reason this antibody measurement should only be used as a confirmatory test for borderline cases initially tested with an anti-tTG antibody assay.

Biopsy

The diagnosis of celiac disease currently requires endoscopy with biopsy of the duodenum. In severe cases, there is atrophy of villi and flattening of the mucosa, but milder cases may show only lymphocytes infiltrating the mucosa. In children, recent guidelines suggest that a biopsy may not be required if there are typical symptoms and a high titer of anti-tTG antibodies, along with HLA-DQ2 and/or HLA-DQ8 genotypes.

In summary, the recommendations for diagnosis of celiac disease are as follows. IgA anti-tTG antibody is the preferred single test for detection of celiac disease. If there is a high possibility of IgA deficiency, total IgA should be measured. IgG deamidated gliadin peptides may be measured when IgA deficiency is present. Serologic testing should be done when patients are on a gluten-free diet. Upper endoscopy with small bowel biopsy is highly informative for the diagnostic evaluation for celiac disease and is recommended to confirm the diagnosis. Intestinal biopsy should be pursued in patients with a high suspicion of celiac disease, even if the serologic tests are negative. Multiple biopsies of the duodenum may be required. There are a number of histological mimics of celiac disease in patients who are seronegative. These include a variety of autoimmune diseases, and non-celiac gluten sensitivity, to name just two.

When screening children younger than 2 years of age for celiac disease, the IgA tTG test should be combined with IgG deamidated gliadin peptide antibody assay. Human leukocyte antigen DQ2/DQ8 testing is not routinely used in the initial diagnosis of celiac disease, but can be used to effectively rule out the disease in selected clinical situations that include those with equivocal small bowel histologic findings and in patients with discrepant serology and histology results.

GASTROINTESTINAL BLEEDING

Description
Upper Gastrointestinal Bleeding

There are many causes for upper gastrointestinal bleeding. The most common causes in both men and women of upper gastrointestinal bleeding are esophageal varices, typically as a result of liver disease from one cause or another; peptic ulcer disease; GERD; gastritis; and duodenitis. Less common causes include cancer of the esophagus and stomach.

Lower Gastrointestinal Bleeding

A major cause of lower gastrointestinal bleeding is colorectal cancer (discussed in detail below). Other causes include hemorrhoids, which is the most frequent cause of visible blood in the lower digestive tract. Anal fissures, which are tears in the lining of the anus, can also cause bleeding and are very painful. Two common inflammatory bowel diseases, ulcerative colitis and Crohn disease, result in bleeding from the lower intestinal tract. The bleeding arises from the surface of the bowel wall because of inflammation and tiny ulcerations in the wall of the intestine. Diverticula, small "pouches" that extend out of the colon wall, can rupture and lead to significant bleeding acutely.

Diagnosis

Upper and lower gastrointestinal endoscopy, with or without a biopsy and histologic examination, most often identifies the cause for the bleeding. However, tests not involving endoscopy may be performed to establish a diagnosis following visual inspection of the gastrointestinal tract. Taken together, however, the diagnosis of most of the underlying causes for both upper gastrointestinal and lower gastrointestinal bleeding requires a biopsy with microscopic review.

The loss of blood from the gastrointestinal tract can result in anemia if the blood loss is significant, either acutely, or persistent with small amounts of blood loss over time. The presence of blood in stool or in vomit is detected using methods described below under colorectal cancer. The stool in patients with lower gastrointestinal bleeding can show bright red blood, dark blood,

Upper and lower gastrointestinal endoscopy, with or without a biopsy and histologic examination, most often identifies the cause for the bleeding.

or have a black or tarry appearance. Similarly for upper gastrointestinal bleeding, the vomitus may contain bright red blood or it may have a "coffee grounds" appearance. A number of medications and foods can give the stool a red or black appearance that resembles blood but is not.

COLORECTAL CANCER

Description

Colon cancer is currently the second leading cause of cancer death in developed countries. It is one of the most preventable cancers when the appropriate colorectal cancer screening is performed (**Table 15–3**). The goal of the screening is to detect early-stage colorectal cancer and precancerous lesions in asymptomatic individuals who do not have a prior history of cancer. Screening for colorectal cancer should begin at age 50 or at age 45 for those of African descent. Panels of expert gastroenterologists representing multiple gastroenterological societies have provided consensus recommendations for colorectal cancer screening. Increased screening has resulted in a decline in mortality from colorectal cancer in all races and in both sexes. In addition, the decreased use of tobacco and the wide use of aspirin for cardioprotection have also contributed to the lower incidence of colorectal cancer. Individuals who have higher risk are those who have a personal history of colorectal cancer or adenomatous polyps, those with a history of ulcerative colitis or Crohn disease involving the colon, and those with first-degree relatives with colorectal cancer at or before age 60.

Diagnosis

Numerous tests have been developed for colorectal cancer screening. Each of the tests will be described, and then the recommendations from the expert panels on the use of the test in screening for colorectal cancer will follow.

The most important screening test is colonoscopy because it has the highest sensitivity for cancer and all classes of precancerous lesions. In this study, a flexible endoscope is inserted through the rectum, and the entire colon is visually examined. A bowel preparation is required along with sedation. The process allows polyps, if present, to be removed and examined for cancer. Expert panels recommend repeat testing every 10 years after a normal study. There is a relatively high initial cost associated with performing the procedure.

Another screening test in common use is the fecal immunochemical test (FIT) for human hemoglobin in stool. This is a home-based test in which a single stool sample is smeared on a test card which is mailed to a laboratory for analysis. The test is noninvasive, and its sensitivity for cancer is 79%. Thus, colorectal cancer may be missed in 20% to 30% of patients who have colorectal cancer along with a negative test result. It has a low initial cost, and it is recommended for repeat testing annually. A repeat test may detect colorectal cancer missed in an earlier study.

The related fecal occult blood test, which has been available for decades, has a much lower sensitivity for detection of colorectal cancer than FIT, identifying only 20% to 50% of the colorectal cancers. FIT has several advantages when compared to the fecal occult blood test. The guaiac

TABLE 15–3   **Screening for Colorectal Cancer: Recommendations for Physicians and Patients from the 2017 US Multi-Society Task Force on Colorectal Cancer**

First-tier tests	Colonoscopy every 10 years
	FIT annually
If first-tier tests not chosen	
Second-tier tests	CT colonography every 5 years
	FIT—fecal DNA test every 3 years
	Flexible sigmoidoscopy every 5–10 years
If second-tier tests not chosen	
Third-tier tests	Capsule colonoscopy every 5 years

reagent in the fecal occult blood test relies on the detection of peroxidase in human blood. However, peroxidase is also present in dietary constituents such as rare red meat, certain vegetables and fruits, and its presence leads to false positive test results in individuals who have eaten these foods. In addition, unlike the guaiac test, FIT is not subject to false-negative results in patients who take high-dose vitamin C which blocks the peroxidase reaction. FIT is also more specific for lower gastrointestinal bleeding. Because the guaiac test is routinely performed at the bedside, it is still a favored option for rapid identification of bleeding from the large intestine, that occurs in an emergency setting. The guaiac test requires three stool samples for colorectal cancer screening, and 50% to 80% of patients with colorectal cancer still have a negative test using this assay.

Another colorectal screening test is a combination of the FIT along with tests for DNA found in colorectal cancers that has been delivered into the stool. Tumor cells in the large intestine can exfoliate into the stool to allow detection of certain mutations and methylated DNA markers. This test has been approved in the United States for the screening of asymptomatic average risk individuals. This test has a one-time sensitivity for colorectal cancer of 92%. Several driver mutations have been identified, such as APC (adenomatous polyposis coli) and TGFBR2/SMAD4 (transforming growth factor-beta receptor type 2/SMA- and MAD-related protein 4), and for some subclasses of colorectal cancer, BRAF mutations. A number of other mutations have also been detected in the stool of colorectal cancer patients that are informative in the genetic analysis for colorectal cancer. The FIT component in this test detects human hemoglobin in the stool. Performance of this test needs one sample with no special diet requirement. It is a home-based test, with the stool sample mailed to a reference laboratory for analysis. Although there is still uncertainty regarding the interval for repeat testing, expert panels in gastroenterology recommend a 1- or a 3-year interval.

Other tests for screening are also available. CT colonography has replaced double contrast barium enema for colorectal imaging for nearly all indications. It is more effective and better tolerated by the patient. The test requires a bowel preparation and a visit to an imaging center, and if this test is used for screening, a 5-year interval for repeat testing is recommended. It has a high initial cost. Flexible sigmoidoscopy requires a limited bowel preparation. A flexible endoscope is inserted into the lower colon to a distance of approximately 60 cm. It can be performed in an office visit without sedation. The disadvantages include limited protection against right-sided colon cancer. The concept of examining only a part of the colon has made the test unpopular in the United States, and it is not commonly used for colorectal cancer screening. Capsule colonoscopy for imaging the proximal colon in patients with previous incomplete colonoscopies is available. However, the bowel preparation is more extensive than that for colonoscopy, and for this reason, it has limited appeal over standard colonoscopy. There is a serum test for colorectal screening, involving the detection of Septin9. This is a blood test which has a sensitivity of only 48% for the detection of colorectal cancer, and it is unable to detect precancerous polyps. The true clinical utility of this blood test for colon cancer remains uncertain at this time.

In summary, the US guidelines for colorectal cancer screening in individuals at average risk for colorectal cancer include an annual test for fecal occult blood, with a preference for FIT over the guaiac-based text. Colonoscopy is recommended every 10 years. The combined test for DNA mutation analysis and FIT in a stool sample may be included, to be performed at 1- to 3-year intervals. If this approach to screening is not pursued by the patient, it is recommended that CT colonography be performed every 5 years along with the DNA-FIT test every 3 years, and flexible sigmoidoscopy every 5 to 10 years. If this option is not accepted, capsule colonoscopy every 5 years is a third option. Individuals at high risk for colorectal cancer by one criteria or another are evaluated using the same tests but more frequently, and the frequency is dependent upon the specific cause of the increased risk. For example, patients with ulcerative colitis or Crohn colitis should undergo colonoscopy every 2 years, while those with a first-degree relative under 60 years of age with colorectal cancer should undergo colonoscopy every 5 years.

> Colonoscopy needs to be repeated infrequently, every 10 years if no adenomas are found, although more frequently in those with adenomas or with a strong family history of colon cancer.

Genetic Profiling for Colorectal Cancer

Histologically, the most common subtype of colorectal cancer is adenocarcinoma. Colorectal adenocarcinomas can arise upon acquisition of a variety of mutations over many years. These genetic alterations can lead to the conversion of normal colonic epithelium first to adenoma, and then to carcinoma, and this carcinoma frequently metastasizes. There has been increasing recognition that some of the genetic alterations can be used as prognostic markers for outcome and can be useful in the selection of specific therapies for the patient with colorectal cancer. As an example, one genetic profile for colon cancer involves the analysis of 63 mutations in the following seven genes—KRAS, BRAF, PIK3CA, AKT1, SMAD4, PTEN, and NRAS.

SELF-ASSESSMENT QUESTIONS

1. Dyspepsia is chronic or recurrent pain/discomfort in the upper abdomen. Which of the following conditions is not associated with dyspepsia?

   A. Asthma
   B. Peptic ulcer disease
   C. Chronic use of nonsteroidal anti-inflammatory agents
   D. Gastroesophageal reflux disease

2. Which of the following choices is not true about peptic ulcer disease associated with infection by *Helicobacter pylori*?

   A. Infection with *H. pylori* is the major cause of peptic ulcer disease.
   B. The infection is more common in individuals living in higher socioeconomic conditions.
   C. Not all patients with *H. pylori* infection develop ulcer disease.
   D. Infected individuals have an increased risk for gastric adenocarcinoma.

3. The laboratory tests for *H. pylori* infection can be divided into the tests that identify exposure to *H. pylori* and the tests that detect active infection by *H. pylori*. Which of the following tests indicates exposure without providing information about whether the infection is active?

   A. Urea breath test
   B. Serologic tests for IgG antibodies to *H. pylori*
   C. Rapid urease test using biopsy material
   D. Molecular tests for *H. pylori*

4. Which of the following is not a commonly used diagnostic test for celiac disease?

   A. Tissue transglutaminase IgA antibodies
   B. IgA antiendomysial antibodies
   C. Fecal immunochemical test
   D. Small bowel biopsy

5. Celiac disease is an immune-mediated disorder, and in genetically susceptible individuals it is triggered by a dietary compound. Which of the following choices is unrelated to the dietary compound that triggers this immune-mediated disorder?

   A. Gluten proteins found in wheat, rye, and barley
   B. Gliadin, the water-soluble component in gluten
   C. Gluten-associated storage proteins that have undergone partial digestion in the upper gastrointestinal tract
   D. Glycine, delivered as a dietary supplement

6. What is the reason to evaluate a patient for celiac disease using the test for IgG, rather than IgA, tissue transglutaminase antibodies?

   A. The test involving IgA antibodies has widely variable sensitivity and specificity.
   B. As many as 3% of patients with celiac disease are IgA deficient and produce a false-negative result.
   C. The test for IgA antibodies is more complex and expensive than the test for IgG antibodies.
   D. IgG antibodies are in much greater concentration in the circulation than IgA antibodies.

7. Which of the following choices is not a reason why the fecal immunochemical test is preferred as a screening test for colon cancer over the guaiac fecal occult blood test?

   A. The guaiac test reacts with animal hemoglobin, which necessitates a restriction on meat intake for several days before stool samples are collected for analysis.
   B. The guaiac test has a sensitivity of less than 50% for detection of colorectal carcinoma.
   C. The fecal immunochemical test is significantly less expensive than the guaiac test.
   D. The fecal immunochemical test uses antibodies to human hemoglobin.

8. Colorectal adenocarcinomas can arise with the acquisition of different genetic mutations over decades. Some of the genetic alterations found in patients with colorectal cancer can be used as prognostic markers for outcome or in the selection of therapies. Which one of the following choices is commonly included in a genetic profile for colon cancer?

   A. EGFR (Epidermal growth factor receptor)
   B. ALK (Anaplastic lymphoma kinase)
   C. BRAF (Proto-oncogene B-RaF)
   D. Cystathionine β-synthase

FURTHER READING

Dyspepsia and *Helicobacter pylori*:

Lopes AI, et al. *Helicobacter pylori* infection—recent developments in diagnosis. *World J Gastroenterol.* 2014;20:9299–9313.

Parsonnet J. *Helicobacter pylori* in the stomach: a paradox unmasked. *N Engl J Med.* 1996;335:278.

Wang Y-K, et al. Diagnosis of *Helicobacter pylori* infection—current options and developments. *World J Gastroenterol.* 2015;21:11221–11235.

Celiac Disease:

Boettcher E, Crowe SE. Dietary proteins and functional gastrointestinal disorders. *Am J Gastroenterol.* 2013;108:728–736.

Fasano A, Catassi C. Celiac disease. *N Engl J Med.* 2012;367:2419–2426.

Kelly CP, et al. Advances in diagnosis and management of celiac disease. *Gastroenterology.* 2015;148:1175–1186.

Ludvigsson JF, et al. Diagnosis and management of adult coeliac disease: guidelines from the British Society of Gastroenterology. *Gut.* 2014;63:1210–1228.

Rubio-Tapia A, et al. American College of Gastroenterology clinical guideline: diagnosis and management of celiac disease. *Am J Gastroenterol.* 2013;108:656–677.

Gastrointestinal Bleeding:

Elrazek A, et al. The value of U/S to determine priority for upper gastrointestinal endoscopy in the emergency room. *Medicine.* 2015;94:e2241.

Colon Cancer

Ahlquist DA, et al. Next-generation stool DNA test accurately detects colorectal cancer and large adenomas. *Gastroenterology.* 2012;142:248–256.

Dickinson BT, et al. Molecular markers for colorectal cancer screening. *Gut.* 2015;64:1485–1494.

Lee JK, et al. Accuracy of fecal immunochemical tests for colorectal cancer: systematic review and meta-analysis. *Ann Intern Med.* 2014;160:171–181.

Rex DK, et al. Colorectal cancer screening: recommendations for physicians and patients from the U.S. Multi-Society Task Force on Colorectal Cancer. *Am J Gastroenterol.* 2017;112:1016–1030.

Schoen RE, et al. Colorectal-cancer incidence and mortality with screening flexible sigmoidoscopy. *N Engl J Med.* 2012;366:2345–2357.

The Liver and Biliary Tract

William E. Winter

LEARNING OBJECTIVES

1. Identify the laboratory tests useful in the evaluation of liver function, and the pathophysiology that results in the generation of these abnormal test results.

2. Understand the clinical laboratory evaluation of the patient for viral hepatitis.

3. Associate specific disorders of the liver with the laboratory test results expected for those clinical diagnoses.

CHAPTER OUTLINE

INTRODUCTION

Laboratory evaluation of the hepatobiliary system centers on measurements of (1) hepatocyte plasma membrane integrity, (2) measurements of the detoxifying and excretory functions of the hepatobiliary system, and (3) measurements of the synthetic capacity of hepatocytes.

PLASMA MEMBRANE INTEGRITY AND DISORDERS PREDOMINANTLY ASSOCIATED WITH ELEVATED CONCENTRATIONS OF LIVER-DERIVED ENZYMES IN THE BLOOD

With hepatocyte or biliary tract disease, many cellular enzymes are released that enter the circulation. Enzymes indicative of hepatocyte disease are alanine aminotransferase (ALT) and aspartate aminotransferase (AST). Alkaline phosphatase (ALP) elevations relate to biliary tract disease (**Table 16–1**). Note that ALP is also derived from other sources such as bone.

Enzyme concentrations are usually measured by determining the enzyme activity in serum or plasma. Such measurements are reported as units per liter or international units per liter, where the unit is an activity measurement (e.g., the rate of appearance of product or disappearance of substrate per unit time).

> Enzymes indicative of hepatocyte disease are alanine aminotransferase (ALT) and aspartate aminotransferase (AST). Alkaline phosphatase (ALP) elevations relate to biliary tract disease.

Normally, the healthy plasma membrane and various organelles contain (e.g., "hold") enzymes within the cell. An elevated enzyme level in the blood suggests organ dysfunction because of a functional or anatomic disruption in the plasma membrane. One way to assess the degree of elevation of an enzyme is to calculate the ratio of the patient's enzyme concentration relative to the upper limit of the reference interval. For example, if the upper limit of the reference interval for ALT were 40 U/L and the patient's ALT was 120 U/L, the patient's ALT would be said to be "three times above the upper limit of normal."

While not specific for hepatocytes, elevations of ALT and AST are characteristic of hepatocellular disease. The major sources of ALT include the liver and the kidney. Lesser amounts are released from skeletal and cardiac muscle. AST is also found in these organs. ALT is exclusively localized in the cell cytoplasm. AST is located in the cytoplasm and mitochondria. However, AST derived from the cytoplasm and mitochondria cannot be distinguished through currently available clinical laboratory testing. ALT is more specific for the liver than AST. Usually ALT and AST rise in tandem in liver disease states. Although there is more AST in hepatocytes than ALT, ALT is metabolized more slowly than AST, accounting for similar concentrations of these enzymes in the patient's plasma as released from the liver.

One condition where AST is often elevated to a greater extent than ALT is in chronic liver disease resulting from chronic alcohol abuse. People with alcoholism are at higher risk for pyridoxine deficiency because of deficient dietary intake of this vitamin. While both AST and ALT are pyridoxine dependent for their biochemical activity, ALT is more dependent on pyridoxine than AST. Thus, a rise in the measured ALT may not be as great as the rise in measured AST because ALT activity suffers more from pyridoxine deficiency than does AST. If the AST to ALT ratio is greater than 2 in the setting of chronic liver disease, alcoholic liver disease is strongly suggested. With cirrhosis of any etiology, enzyme elevations may be modest, or their concentrations may be surprisingly normal, reflecting a marked loss in hepatocyte mass and, thereby, a loss of enzymes within the liver. However, a characteristic finding in advanced cirrhosis is that the AST exceeds the ALT. Thus, the etiology of the increased AST/ALT ratio in advanced cirrhosis is believed to be a result of the synthesis of enzymatically inactive ALT.

TABLE 16–1   Enzymes Indicative of Liver Plasma Membrane Integrity

Indicative of hepatocellular disease
Alanine aminotransferase (ALT)
Aspartate aminotransferase (AST)
Lactate dehydrogenase (LD)
Indicative of biliary tract disease
Alkaline phosphatase (ALP)
Gamma-glutamyltransferase (GGT)
5′-Nucleotidase (5′-NT)

In the past, lactate dehydrogenase (LD) was also regularly employed as a marker of hepatocellular disease. (*Note*: The older abbreviation for lactate dehydrogenase was "LDH, and LD and LDH are used interchangeably in this book.") However, LD is not favored for routine evaluation of the hepatocyte integrity currently because LD is released with injury of many different tissues (including red blood cell hemolysis). Both ALT and AST are more specific for liver disease or injury than LD.

Measurement of LD isoenzymes is possible, but there are more informative tests that can be ordered to evaluate specific organ dysfunction. LD is composed of four subunits. The subunits are H (for heart) and M (for muscle). Different combinations of H and M subunits produce five types of LD isoenzymes (types 1 through 5). If required, LD isoenzymes can be determined by electrophoresis. The subunit composition and major sources of each of the five isoenzymes are listed in **Table 16–2**. The LD4 isoenzyme provides no specific clinically useful information.

If the total LD is increased in a patient with suspected liver disease, and the patient lacks skeletal muscle and prostate disease, it is expected that LD5 will be elevated because of the liver disease. The enzyme marker of choice for the evaluation of skeletal muscle injury or disease is creatine kinase (CK; archaically abbreviated "CPK"). If the CK is within the reference interval in the setting of an elevated LD5, skeletal muscle is not likely to be the source of the elevated LD5. Presently, LD measurements are most useful for the assessment of hemolysis where LD is greatly elevated, and, in the absence of liver disease, AST and ALT are not elevated. Elevated LD is recognized in a variety of recently described disorders, such as SARS-associated coronavirus (SARS-CoV) infection and Middle East respiratory syndrome (MERS) which is also caused by a human coronavirus.

Biliary tract disease produces relatively greater increases in ALP than increases in ALT, AST, or LD. ALP is associated with the plasma membrane of hepatocytes adjacent to the biliary canaliculus. Obstruction or inflammation of the biliary tract results in an increased concentration of the ALP in the circulation. Similar to ALT and AST, ALP is not specific for biliary tract disease. ALP is released by osteoblasts, the ileum, and the placenta. ALP is elevated (1) in children two to threefold over adults because the child's skeleton is growing, (2) with bone disease involving osteoblasts (e.g., metastatic cancer, following a fracture or in Paget disease of the bone), (3) in hyperparathyroidism where parathyroid hormone stimulates osteoblasts that, through a series of steps, enhance bone resorption (e.g., parathyroid adenoma, hyperplasia, or secondary hyperparathyroidism from vitamin D deficiency or renal disease), (4) in cases of ileal disease, and (5) during the third trimester of pregnancy because the placental ALP isoenzyme is elevated.

> Biliary tract disease produces relatively greater increases in ALP than increases in ALT, AST, or LD. ALP is associated with the plasma membrane of hepatocytes adjacent to the biliary canaliculus.

When the etiology of the elevated ALP is unclear, the diagnostic challenge is greater. In the past ALP isoenzymes were determined. However, there are many technical problems with these assays. Today it has proven more pragmatic to measure other biliary tract enzyme markers such as gamma-glutamyl transpeptidase (GGT; aka gamma-glutamyltransferase) or 5'-nucleotidase (5'-NT). If bone is thought to be the source of the excess ALP, bone ALP (aka BAP) can be measured by immunoassay. It is beyond the scope of this chapter on liver disease to discuss other markers of bone turnover such as osteocalcin, hydroxyproline, N-telopeptides, C-telopeptides, pyridinoline, and deoxypyridinoline.

Regarding GGT, the proximal convoluted tubule of the kidney, the liver, the pancreas, and the intestine are sources of GGT, in decreasing order of tissue concentration. Within the cell, GGT

TABLE 16–2   Lactate Dehydrogenase (LD) Isoenzymes: Subunit Composition and Distribution

Isoenzyme	Subunits	Distribution
LD1	H4	Heart, red blood cell, renal cortex
LD2	H3M	Heart, red blood cell, renal cortex
LD3	H2M2	Pancreas, lung, lymphocyte, platelet
LD4	HM3	No specific distribution
LD5	M4	Hepatocyte, skeletal muscle, prostate

H, the heart subunit; M, the muscle subunit.

is located in microsomes and along the biliary tract plasma membrane; GGT is more commonly measured than 5′-NT because GGT testing is widely available on a variety of laboratory instruments. GGT is typically not elevated with bone disease. Combined elevations of ALP and GGT are compatible with biliary tract disease. However, if the ALP is elevated to a far greater extent than the GGT (or the GGT is within the reference interval), ALP sources other than the biliary tract, such as bone, must be investigated. GGT elevations occur in response to alcohol use and anticonvulsants, as GGT is induced by such agents.

While there is no specific biochemical test to prove that a patient suffers from alcohol abuse, carbohydrate-deficient transferrin levels can be elevated in patients suffering from alcoholism. Under investigation are many potential markers of alcohol exposure, including ethyl glucuronide, ethyl sulfate, acetaldehyde, acetaldehyde adducts, anti-adduct antibodies, fatty acid ethyl esters, phosphatidylethanol, β-hexosaminidase, the plasma sialic acid index of apolipoprotein J, total serum sialic acid, cholesteryl ester transfer protein, 5-hydroxytryptophol, 5-hydroxyindole-3-acetic acid, salsolinol, and dolichol. However, at the present time, none of these markers are recommended for clinical use.

Using the information presented, one can interpret liver enzyme elevations in patients with suspected liver disease. If the relative increase in ALT or AST over the upper limit of normal exceeds the relative increase in ALP over the upper limit of normal, the liver disease is predominantly hepatocellular as opposed to biliary tract.

Causes of acute hepatocellular disease include (**Table 16–3**) viral hepatitis (e.g., hepatitis A, B, or C), alcoholic hepatitis, toxic injury (e.g., acetaminophen poisoning), and ischemic injury (e.g., hypotension). In cases of ischemic injury or toxic injury following an acute toxic ingestion, the ALT and AST levels can rise and peak within 24 hours of the precipitating event. Less common causes of acute liver disease include hepatitis due to hepatitis D, hepatitis E, cytomegalovirus (CMV), Epstein–Barr virus (EBV), and herpes virus; autoimmune hepatitis (marked by positivity for antinuclear antibodies [ANA], smooth muscle autoantibodies [ASMA], and/or liver–kidney microsome autoantibodies [anti-LKM$_1$ autoantibodies] and negative antimitochondrial autoantibodies [AMA]); Wilson disease; and liver disease of pregnancy. Three forms of liver disease in pregnancy include (1) fatty liver, (2) intrahepatic cholestasis, and (3) hepatic dysfunction associated with toxemia (e.g., part of the HELLP syndrome: *h*emolysis, *e*levated *L*FTs [e.g., enzymes], and *l*ow *p*latelets).

Chronic hepatocellular disease is diagnosed when liver disease is present for more than 6 months (**Table 16–3**). Causes of chronic hepatocellular disease include hepatitis B or C, drug toxicity (e.g., statins, sulfonamides, or INH), alcoholic liver disease, nonalcoholic fatty liver (NAFL),

---

TABLE 16–3   Causes of Hepatocellular Disease^a

Acute: present for less than 6 months

Common
Viral hepatitis (hepatitis A, B, or C)
Alcoholic hepatitis
Toxic injury
Ischemic injury

Less common
Viral hepatitis that is not hepatitis A, B, or C (includes hepatitis D, hepatitis E, cytomegalovirus [CMV],
    Epstein–Barr virus [EBV], and herpes virus)
Autoimmune hepatitis
Wilson disease
Liver disease of pregnancy

Chronic: present for more than 6 months

Viral hepatitis B or C
Drug toxicity
Alcoholic liver disease
Nonalcoholic fatty liver (NAFL)
Inborn errors (include hemochromatosis, alpha-1 antitrypsin deficiency, Wilson disease,
    glycogen storage disease, and Gaucher disease)
Autoimmune hepatitis

^{a}The relative elevations in ALT and AST exceed the relative elevation in ALP.

inborn errors of metabolism, and autoimmune hepatitis. NAFL is one of the most common causes of nonviral and nonalcoholic liver disease. NAFL is part of the spectrum of disorders characterized as the "metabolic syndrome." NAFL can progress to nonalcoholic steatohepatitis (NASH), cirrhosis, liver failure, and even hepatocellular carcinoma in some cases. Inborn errors causing chronic liver disease encompass hemochromatosis, alpha-1 antitrypsin deficiency, Wilson disease, glycogen storage disease (GSD), and Gaucher disease.

The AST to ALT ratio can be used to suggest alcoholic liver disease. One can argue that, excluding the setting of alcoholism, hepatocellular disease can be adequately assessed with the measurement of ALT alone. However, it is common medical practice to measure both enzymes, and the enzyme measurements are rapidly available and can be performed at low cost in modern automated laboratories.

If the relative increase in ALP over the upper limit of normal exceeds the relative increase in ALT or AST over the upper limit of normal, the liver disease predominantly involves the biliary tract (**Table 16–4**). A major manifestation of obstructive biliary tract disease is an elevated bilirubin concentration. Clinical jaundice results when the total bilirubin exceeds 2 to 3 mg/dL.

> Bilirubin is predominantly derived from hemoglobin in the normal turnover of red blood cells, and to a lesser extent, from myoglobin in muscle.

DETOXIFYING AND EXCRETORY FUNCTIONS OF THE HEPATOBILIARY SYSTEM AND DISORDERS ASSOCIATED PREDOMINANTLY WITH AN ELEVATED BILIRUBIN CONCENTRATION

A major biochemical responsibility of the liver is to metabolize toxins, drugs, and biologic end products and excrete many of the resulting metabolites into the bile. The easiest endogenous end product to assess is the bilirubin concentration in the plasma. Bilirubin is predominantly derived from hemoglobin in the normal turnover of red blood cells, and to a lesser extent, from myoglobin from muscle, and from cellular cytochromes. Red blood cells normally circulate for approximately 120 days. Red blood cell senescence and destruction in monocytes/macrophages, primarily in the spleen, releases hemoglobin from red blood cells. Within the phagocyte, hemoglobin is then metabolized to biliverdin and finally to bilirubin. The bilirubin then enters the circulation. This form of bilirubin (i.e., "unconjugated" bilirubin) is relatively insoluble in water and is transported to the hepatocyte bound to albumin. It is not excreted in the urine. Unconjugated bilirubin is normally taken up into hepatocytes via a transport system (the organic anion transport protein [OATP]). Inside the hepatocyte via the action of UDP-glucuronyl transferase, either one or two glucuronide molecules are conjugated to bilirubin, making the bilirubin water soluble. Conjugated bilirubin is bilirubin monoglucuronide or bilirubin diglucuronide. Conjugated bilirubin is then transported across the plasma membrane into the bile canaliculi along with bile via multiple drug resistance (MDR) transporter proteins. If the concentration of either

TABLE 16–4   **Causes of Biliary Tract Disease**[a]

Failure of formation of the bile ducts
Biliary atresia
Obstruction or obliteration of the bile ducts
Cholelithiasis
Cholangitis
Primary biliary cirrhosis
Primary sclerosing cholangitis
Postsurgical strictures
Parasitic infection
Compression of the bile ducts
Pancreatic cancer
Pancreatitis
Hepatic cancers

[a]The relative elevation in ALP exceeds the relative elevations in ALT and AST.

If the concentration of either conjugated or unconjugated bilirubin rises pathologically, the skin and sclera can develop a yellowish color, termed jaundice.

conjugated or unconjugated bilirubin rises pathologically, the skin and sclera can develop a yellowish color, termed jaundice. Icterus is another term for jaundice. With marked elevations in bilirubin, patients may acquire a green hue. Pathologic elevations in water-soluble bilirubin (e.g., conjugated bilirubin) can lead to bilirubin excretion in the urine (bilirubinuria), causing the urine to develop a yellow-brown or green-brown color. Normally, bilirubin is absent from the urine.

Bilirubin is most often measured by reacting the patient's serum or plasma with Ehrlich reagent that includes a diazo compound. The conjugated fraction reacts most rapidly with the reagent because the conjugated fraction is water soluble. This is termed "direct acting," or more commonly, "direct" bilirubin. To measure total bilirubin, solubilizing agents must be added to the serum or plasma to enhance the reaction of the water-insoluble bilirubin (i.e., unconjugated bilirubin) with the reagents. Caffeine or benzoate can be used for this purpose. Because only direct and total bilirubin can be measured, indirect (unconjugated bilirubin) is calculated as the difference between the total and the direct bilirubin. While the terms "direct" and "conjugated" are used synonymously just as the terms "indirect" and "unconjugated" bilirubin are used synonymously, it should be noted that these are approximations. In fact, direct bilirubin measures 70% to 90% of the conjugated bilirubin, delta bilirubin (biliprotein, see below), and 5% to 10% of the unconjugated bilirubin.

While the chemical measurement of bilirubin using Ehrlich reagent is the scheme used in the majority of automated chemistry analyzers, it is necessary to review how bilirubin is measured using dry slide technology that was originally developed by Kodak. The unique feature of dry slide technology (as provided in the present Vitros series of analyzers) is the ability to spectrophotometrically determine the unconjugated (BU: bilirubin unconjugated) and conjugated bilirubin (BC: bilirubin conjugated) fractions. The difference between the sum of the BU and BC and the total bilirubin measured via the Ehrlich reaction is the delta bilirubin (aka biliprotein). Delta bilirubin is bilirubin that is covalently bound to albumin. Elevated levels of delta bilirubin are consistent with chronic elevations in bilirubin. However, only one analytical system is able to estimate delta bilirubin (i.e., dry slide technology) and the calculation of the delta bilirubin has not yet been shown to be clinically informative in the usual diagnosis or management of liver disease.

In most cases involving hepatocellular dysfunction (notably, acute viral hepatitis), the major relative increase in bilirubin is an increased conjugated bilirubin fraction because transport of conjugated bilirubin into the bile canaliculus is typically the rate-limiting step in bilirubin excretion. With the failure of transport of conjugated bilirubin into the bile canaliculus, the conjugated bilirubin refluxes into the systemic circulation. However, with severe hepatocellular dysfunction, as might occur in cases of end-stage liver disease, there can be defective conjugation in addition to defective canalicular transport.

It is useful to classify hyperbilirubinemia as predominantly unconjugated or conjugated. When the ratio of conjugated to total bilirubin is 0.4 or greater, predominantly a conjugated hyperbilirubinemia is present.

It is useful to classify hyperbilirubinemia as predominantly unconjugated or conjugated. This assists in the development of an appropriate differential diagnosis. If the ratio of the conjugated bilirubin to total bilirubin is less than 0.4, an unconjugated hyperbilirubinemia is present. When the ratio of conjugated to total bilirubin is 0.4 or greater, predominantly a conjugated hyperbilirubinemia is present. In neonates, the cutoff ratio is near 0.2 because unconjugated bilirubin is normally much higher in neonates than in children or adults. In neonates, transcutaneous bilirubinometry can be used to estimate total bilirubin levels. However, a 2009 review cautioned that transcutaneous bilirubinometry underestimates total bilirubin levels above 12 to 14 mg/dL, suggesting that a serum measurement of total bilirubin is more reflective of the true value at such levels.

Causes of unconjugated hyperbilirubinemia involve three basic mechanisms: (1) increased red blood cell destruction ("prehepatic"), (2) defects in the transport of unconjugated bilirubin into the hepatocyte, and (3) defective conjugation. Major causes of increased red blood cell destruction include intramarrow hemolysis (e.g., vitamin B_{12} deficiency causing ineffective erythropoiesis), intravascular or extravascular hemolysis (e.g., microangiopathic hemolytic anemia, hemolysis from an artificial heart valve, and autoimmune hemolytic anemia ["warm," IgG-mediated and "cold," IgM-mediated]), intrinsic membrane defects in red blood cells (e.g., congenital spherocytosis or elliptocytosis), red blood cell enzyme defects (e.g., glucose-6-phosphate dehydrogenase [G6PD] deficiency or pyruvate kinase [PK] deficiency), and hemoglobinopathies (e.g., sickle cell anemia) (**Table 16–5**).

TABLE 16–5   Unconjugated Hyperbilirubinemia with Hemolysis

	Comment
Schistocytes present	
Microangiopathic hemolytic anemia	Rule out DIC, TTP, and HUS
Artificial heart valve	History of valve replacement
Autoimmune hemolytic anemia	Perform Coombs testing
Schistocytes absent	
Intramarrow hemolysis	Rule out vitamin B$_{12}$ deficiency
Red blood cell membrane defects	Review peripheral smear for spherocytes, elliptocytes
Red blood cell enzyme defects	Review peripheral smear for bite cells, measure G6PD
Hemoglobinopathies	Perform hemoglobin analysis

DIC, disseminated intravascular coagulation; G6PD, glucose-6-phosphate dehydrogenase; HUS, hemolytic uremic syndrome; TTP, thrombotic thrombocytopenic purpura.

TABLE 16–6   Unconjugated Hyperbilirubinemia without Hemolysis

Newborn
Mild-to-moderate and transient unconjugated hyperbilirubinemia Physiological jaundice Breast milk jaundice
Persistent unconjugated hyperbilirubinemia Crigler–Najjar syndrome types I (severe) and II (mild)
Child or adult
Gilbert syndrome

A variety of nonhemolytic conditions can cause an unconjugated hyperbilirubinemia (**Table 16–6**). Gilbert syndrome is a benign autosomal dominant disorder in which there is a mild defect in the uptake of bilirubin by the hepatocyte, combined with a mild defect in conjugation. Clinical jaundice does not usually occur in the absence of concurrent disease (e.g., gastroenteritis or other mild conditions). Liver enzyme concentrations and hepatic synthetic ability are normal, and, therefore, Gilbert syndrome is best considered a variation of normal and not a disease. An additional dinucleotide repeat in the UDP-glucuronyl transferase promoter region [A(TA)7TAA instead of the normal A(TA)6TAA] is the most common cause of Gilbert syndrome in Caucasians. On the other hand, a congenital deficiency of UDP-glucuronyl transferase is a very serious condition. Absolute deficiency of UDP-glucuronyl transferase, which results in Crigler–Najjar syndrome type I, will cause marked elevations in unconjugated bilirubin that will result in kernicterus in infants in the absence of treatment. The treatment of this disease is liver transplantation. A milder deficiency of UDP-glucuronyl transferase, Crigler–Najjar syndrome type II, may be treated with barbiturates to stimulate production of the deficient enzyme. A transient, mild, self-limited deficiency of UDP-glucuronyl transferase activity is common in newborns (e.g., neonatal jaundice; aka icterus neonatorum). However, if the bilirubin rises above ~5 to 10 mg/dL in a neonate, phototherapy is used to reduce the bilirubin concentration. One recommendation is to begin phototherapy when the bilirubin is five times the birth weight. An unconjugated, transient hyperbilirubinemia occurs in 2% to 10% of breastfed infants (i.e., breast milk jaundice). In these infants, it is believed that a constituent in the breast milk interferes with bilirubin conjugation, thereby elevating unconjugated bilirubin.

The etiologies of conjugated hyperbilirubinemia involve two basic mechanisms: (1) hepatocellular disorders with decreased transport of conjugated bilirubin into the bile canaliculus (**Table 16–3**) or (2) anatomic biliary tract obstruction (**Table 16–4**). Moderate-to-severe acute or chronic hepatocellular disease can produce a conjugated hyperbilirubinemia. Hepatocellular disorders associated with impaired plasma membrane integrity and release of enzymes into the circulation were discussed earlier.

Of note are two disorders in which there is a conjugated hyperbilirubinemia with otherwise normal hepatic function. These are Dubin–Johnson syndrome and Rotor syndrome. Dubin–Johnson syndrome results from dysfunction of the multidrug resistance protein 2 (MRP2) that is a canalicular multispecific organic anion transporter (cMOAT), the gene product of *ABCC2* (ATP-binding cassette subfamily C member 2). The liver is stained black in this condition. Rotor syndrome is a consequence of decreased hepatic glutathione-*S*-transferase levels (hGSTA1-1). In the absence of a liver biopsy, Dubin–Johnson and Rotor syndromes have been distinguished by urine testing for coproporphyrins and coproporphyrin I that are abnormal in Dubin–Johnson syndrome. DNA testing is being increasingly used to distinguish these disorders.

> **Biliary tract obstruction can be intrahepatic or extrahepatic. The most common cause of extrahepatic biliary tract obstruction after the neonatal period is cholelithiasis.**

Anatomic biliary tract obstruction can be intrahepatic or extrahepatic. Infants with a persistent conjugated hyperbilirubinemia most commonly suffer from biliary atresia or neonatal hepatitis. The most common cause of extrahepatic biliary tract obstruction after the neonatal period is cholelithiasis. This can be accompanied by inflammation of the gall bladder (e.g., cholecystitis). Rupture of the gall bladder will produce peritonitis that can be life-threatening. Other causes of biliary tract obstruction include inflammation (e.g., cholangitis or pancreatitis), neoplasia (e.g., pancreatic adenocarcinoma or a hepatic cancer with compression of the bile duct), postsurgical strictures, autoimmunity (e.g., primary sclerosing cholangitis [PSC]), and parasites (e.g., helminths or their ova).

Compared with the timing of elevations in the enzymes of hepatic origin following a liver insult, elevations in bilirubin occur later. Also, while the degree of increase in the concentration of the hepatic enzymes correlates poorly with the degree of liver injury or disease, greater elevations in the level of conjugated bilirubin do correlate with more severe degrees of liver disease. In end-stage liver disease as found in alcoholic cirrhosis, for example, ALT and AST may only be modestly elevated, yet the patient may exhibit intense jaundice. In such cases, portal hypertension is frequent with ascites and esophageal varices, hemorrhoids, and splenomegaly is also observed.

SYNTHETIC FUNCTION OF THE LIVER AND DISORDERS ASSOCIATED WITH LOW CIRCULATING CONCENTRATIONS OF ALBUMIN, TRANSTHYRETIN, RETINOL-BINDING PROTEIN, AND COAGULATION FACTORS

Excluding immunoglobulins, which are the products of B lymphocytes and plasma cells, the liver is the major source of circulating plasma proteins. On a strictly quantitative basis, albumin is a better measure of synthetic ability than total protein. A substantial degree of hypoalbuminemia can exist, yet the total protein may be normal or elevated because of a coexistent polyclonal or monoclonal hypergammaglobulinemia. Besides liver disease, there are several other causes of hypoalbuminemia. They include malnutrition and malabsorption (insufficient nutritional substrate for albumin synthesis), acute inflammation where protein synthesis is redirected from albumin to acute-phase reactants (e.g., complement proteins, C-reactive protein, mannose-binding lectin, and serum amyloid A; **Table 16–7**), increased protein catabolism (as in pregnancy and hyperthyroidism), protein loss from nephrotic syndrome, and protein-losing enteropathy.

> **An increase in the prothrombin time (PT), or the international normalized ratio (INR) derived from it, can be a sign of serious liver dysfunction.**

In nutritionally deficient patients, nutritional replenishment can be assessed by measurement of retinol-binding protein, or, more commonly, transthyretin (thyroxine-binding prealbumin). While transthyretin is commonly referred to as "prealbumin," strictly speaking, prealbumin is a region on a serum protein electrophoresis gel that precedes (e.g., is anodal to) albumin. In contrast to albumin, transthyretin and retinol-binding protein are not usually measured as indices of hepatic dysfunction.

Assessment of clotting factor proteins through measurement of clotting factor activity tests (such as the prothrombin time [PT]) is a useful assessment of liver synthetic function. An increase in the PT, or the international normalized ratio (INR) derived from it, can be a sign of serious liver dysfunction. Because the half-life of many clotting factors is much shorter than the half-life of albumin, in cases of acute liver dysfunction, measurement of the PT can provide a more sensitive index of decreased liver protein synthesis than albumin. The PT involves factors VII, X, V, II

TABLE 16–7   Acute-phase Reactants Synthesized in the Liver

Positive acute-phase reactants (concentrations increase with acute inflammation)

Immune-related
Complement (C′)
Mannose-binding lectin (MBL)
C-reactive protein (CRP)
Orosomucoid (alpha-1 acid glycoprotein)
Serum amyloid A (SAA)

Antiproteases (antienzymes)
Alpha-1 antitrypsin (A1-AT)
Alpha-2 macroglobulin (A2M)

Antioxidants
Ceruloplasmin

Coagulation factors
Fibrinogen
Factor VIII

Others
Haptoglobin
Plasma fibronectin
Lipopolysaccharide-binding protein (LBP)
Ferritin

Negative acute-phase reactants (concentrations decrease with acute inflammation)

Retinol-binding protein (RBP)
Transthyretin (TBPA)
Albumin
Transferrin

(prothrombin), and I (fibrinogen). The half-life of factor VII is the shortest of any clotting factor and is only 4 to 5 hours.

The INR calculation was initially developed to assist in the comparison of PT results among different laboratories when patients are treated with warfarin (a drug that reduces vitamin K-dependent factor synthesis and activity) as an anticoagulant. However, currently, INR is additionally used together with two other factors (creatinine and bilirubin) in predicting the risk of death over a 3-month period of time after patients with cirrhosis are listed for liver transplant. This is termed the MELD (model for end-stage liver disease) score. The degree to which the MELD score predicts death is somewhat controversial.

Despite the hepatic synthetic information provided by a prolonged PT, the severity of the coagulopathy in cases of liver disease may not correlate closely with the degree of prolongation of the PT because anticoagulant factor production may also be reduced with severe liver disease (e.g., reduced synthesis of antithrombin, protein S, and protein C). This means that the degree of bleeding in cases of liver disease may actually be less than expected based on the degree of prolongation of the PT.

Moderate-to-serious liver disease can lead to bleeding for many reasons. Vitamin K malabsorption, decreased clotting factor concentrations and activity (the vitamin K-dependent factors are II, VII, IX, and X), and impaired clearance of fibrin-split products can all occur with liver dysfunction. Fragments of fibrin can interfere with the formation of a stable and firm thrombus. With cirrhosis, increased portal pressure can produce esophageal varices that are easily traumatized, resulting in bleeding. Increased portal pressure can produce splenomegaly, leading to platelet sequestration. Thrombocytopenia is not uncommon in severe liver disease. Thrombopoietin is produced by the liver, and the role of thrombopoietin is to stimulate platelet production from bone marrow megakaryocytes.

THE DIAGNOSIS OF VIRAL HEPATITIS

Hepatitis serologic tests are used to diagnose viral hepatitis or recognize past exposure or immunization to a virus that can cause hepatitis. The hepatitis A virus (HAV) is an RNA virus that commonly causes acute hepatitis and is transmitted through the fecal–oral route. Fulminant hepatic

Hepatitis serologic tests are used to diagnose viral hepatitis or recognize past exposure or immunization to a virus that can cause hepatitis.

necrosis is possible but very rare, and chronic liver disease does not result from HAV infection. Total antibody to HAV can be measured, and when it is positive, there are elevations of IgM and/or IgG antibodies to HAV. Positivity for the IgM antibody to HAV indicates acute or recent infection, or immunization. Positivity for the HAV total antibody test does not distinguish patients with acute infection from those with a past infection who have recovered or from immunized individuals (**Table 16–8**).

Acute hepatitis B virus (HBV; a DNA virus) infection is serologically first noted by the appearance of HBV surface antigen (HBsAg). This is followed by HBV e antigen (HBeAg) and then HBV IgM core antibody (HBc IgM antibody). The e antigen is derived from the same gene as the core (c) antigen, but the e antigen is not required for acute infection or replication. During recovery, the HBsAg and HBeAg disappear from the circulation, HBc IgM antibody converts to negative, and HBc total antibody appears, followed by HBe antibody (HBeAb), and then HBs antibody (HBsAb). The detection of nucleic acid from HBV DNA polymerase can be used as evidence of HBV infection.

In cases of chronic HBV infection, HBsAg remains positive. HBeAg positivity is variable, and its presence indicates increased infectivity. HBeAb positivity is also highly variable. Sometimes HBc IgM antibody may reappear in cases where chronic HBV infection undergoes reactivation.

Immunization results in positivity for HBsAb, but not HBcAb, as the immunogen used for immunization is recombinant-DNA derived HBsAg. There are rare HBsAg variants that may not be detected by immunoassay. These give rise to "HBsAg-negative" cases of HBV infection.

The HBV carrier state is a chronic condition that is established when the HBsAg is positive without evidence of active clinical disease. Such individuals should be considered potentially infectious.

TABLE 16–8   Tests for Viral Hepatitis and Selected Liver Disorders

	Importance in Liver Disease
HAV total antibody	Positivity indicates present or past infection with HAV or immunization against HAV infection
HAV IgM antibody	Positivity indicates acute infection with HAV
HBV surface antigen (HBsAg)	Positivity indicates acute or chronic HBV infection
HBV e antigen (HBeAg)	Positivity indicates acute or chronic HBV infection and increased infectivity
HBV core IgM antibody	Positivity indicates acute infection with HBV or infection activation in chronic HBV infection
HBV core total antibody	Positivity indicates present or past infection with HBV
HBV e antibody	Positivity indicates chronic or past infection with HBV
HBV surface antibody	Positivity indicates chronic or past infection with HBV or immunization against HBV infection
HCV antibody	Positivity indicates present or past infection with HCV
HDV IgM antibody	Positivity indicates acute infection with HDV
HDV antibody	Positivity indicates present or past infection with HDV
Antinuclear autoantibodies	Can be positive in autoimmune hepatitis
Antismooth muscle autoantibodies	Can be positive in autoimmune hepatitis
Anti-LKM1 autoantibodies	Can be positive in autoimmune hepatitis
Antimitochondrial autoantibodies	Can be positive in primary biliary cirrhosis
Alpha-fetoprotein	Marker of hepatocellular carcinoma
Ammonia	Can be elevated in cases of end-stage liver disease
Serum bile acids	Can be elevated in many forms of hepatocellular disease; sometimes ordered to support the diagnosis of cholestasis of pregnancy

Hepatitis C virus (HCV; an RNA virus) is the most common viral cause of chronic hepatitis with 40% to 80% of acute infections leading to chronic hepatitis (e.g., hepatic disease exceeding 6 months duration). A positive HCV antibody test does not distinguish acute from chronic infection, and it does not distinguish patients with active infection from those who have recovered. HCV antibody positivity was previously confirmed by the recombinant immunoblot assay (RIBA). This has now been replaced by nucleic acid testing for HCV RNA in plasma. Evidence of active HCV infection is provided by elevations in transaminases, an abnormal liver biopsy, or detection of HCV RNA. Normal levels of AST and ALT do not exclude chronic HCV infection (see Chapter 2 for illustrations of molecular methods).

Hepatitis D virus (HDV; an RNA virus) is a defective virus that requires coinfection of the host with HBV for the expression of HDV hepatitis. HBV and HDV infection can occur concurrently or HDV infection can be superimposed on chronic HBV infection. HDV uses the surface antigen of HBV to form a virion. IgM antibody to HDV indicates acute infection. HDV total antibody has the same diagnostic limitations as HCV antibody; notably, active infection is not differentiated from recovery, and acute and chronic infections are not distinguished.

SELECTED ADDITIONAL LIVER DISEASES WITH LABORATORY TESTS USED IN THE EVALUATION OF LIVER FUNCTION

Alpha-1 Antitrypsin Deficiency

In individuals with unexplained and/or early onset emphysema or liver disease, alpha-1 antitrypsin deficiency should be considered. Alpha-1 antitrypsin is an antiprotease that protects the lungs from endogenous elastases, collagenases, and proteases. Deficiency of alpha-1 antitrypsin can produce early onset panlobular emphysema. The liver disease of alpha-1 antitrypsin deficiency results from the inability to release a mutated alpha-1 antitrypsin protein from the hepatocyte.

Mutations in the *Pi* (protease inhibitor) gene *SERPINA1* (on chromosome 14q32.13) result in alpha-1 antitrypsin deficiency. The normal allele is denoted as "M." The common abnormal allele is "Z." Homozygosity for Z (e.g., Z/Z) causes alpha-1 antitrypsin deficiency. In some forms of alpha-1 antitrypsin deficiency where the enzyme is not synthesized at all within the hepatocyte (aka "null" alleles), emphysema can develop without liver disease as the defective enzyme is not present in the liver and does not accumulate.

Glycogen Storage Diseases (GSDs)

GSDs are disorders of glycogen production (GSD type 0) or glycogen breakdown. They are a group of heterogenous disorders affecting the liver, skeletal muscle, and/or myocardium. GSD types I, III, and VI can produce fasting hypoglycemia. GSD type I (von Gierke disease) results from a deficiency of glucose-6-phosphatase (type 1a). However, variants exist as type Ib: T1 transporter defects; type 1aSP: glucose-6-phosphatase stabilizing protein deficiency; type 1c: T2 beta transporter deficiency; and type 1d: GLUT7 glucose transporter deficiency. GSD type III (Cori or Forbes disease) is a deficiency of amylo-1,6 glucosidase. GSD type VI (Hers disease) results from a deficiency of liver phosphorylase or phosphorylase b kinase.

Hemochromatosis

Iron overload in the absence of chronic transfusion therapy most commonly results from hemochromatosis type 1 (HH1) that is inherited as an autosomal recessive disorder. HH1 results from mutations in the *HFE* gene that is encoded within the major histocompatibility complex located on the short arm of chromosome 6. Two possible genotypes cause HH1: C282Y/C282Y or C282Y/H63D. Homozygosity for H63D (H63D/H63D) does not cause clinical disease. HFE mutations (*HFE* gene; on chromosome 6p22.2) lead to deficient hepatic secretion of hepcidin. In turn, hepcidin deficiency permits excessive expression of ferroportin with consequent hyperabsorption of iron from the GI tract, leading to iron overload.

Iron overload in the absence of chronic transfusion therapy most commonly results from hemochromatosis type 1 (HH1) that is inherited as an autosomal recessive disorder.

Increased transferrin saturation is the earliest biochemical marker of hemochromatosis. Elevations in ferritin follow. Percent transferrin saturation is the recommended screening test for iron overload. Elevated ferritin is not specific for iron overload. Ferritin is elevated as an acute-phase reactant. In states of chronic inflammation, such as anemia of chronic disease, ferritin is released from the liver with disease or injury. It is elevated in patients with the metabolic syndrome, and in those with the hemophagocytic syndrome. Ferritin enters the circulation through a nonclassical lysosomal secretory pathway.

HH1 has a population frequency of ~1 in 300, with a 5:1 to 7:1 excess of affected males over females. The onset of symptoms is typically between 40 and 50 years of age. Iron deposition occurs in the heart (potentially causing cardiac failure), liver (producing liver disease including cirrhosis), endocrine organs (causing diabetes, hypopituitarism, hypothyroidism, and/or hypogonadism), and skin. Arthropathy is another feature of HH1.

There are several other types of hemochromatosis in addition to HH1. HH2a results from hemojuvelin (*HFE2*; on chromosome 1q21.1) mutations, while HH2b is caused by primary hepcidin deficiency. Hepcidin is encoded by the *HAMP* (hepcidin antimicrobial peptide; on chromosome 19q13.12) gene. HH2a and HH2b present in childhood. Mutations in the transferrin receptor 2 (*TfR2*; on chromosome 7q22.1) gene cause HH3. HH4a is a consequence of loss-of-function mutations in ferroportin encoded by the *SLC40A1* (solute carrier family 40 member 1; on chromosome 2q32.2) gene. Aceruloplasminemia causes HH4b. Aceruloplasminemia (*CP* gene; on chromosome 3q25.1) causes HH4b, and this is a different condition from Wilson disease (see below). HH4a and HH4b cause greater iron deposition in the reticuloendothelial system than in the solid organs and liver. Hyperabsorption of iron from the gastrointestinal tract can occur in various forms of anemia with ineffective erythropoiesis (e.g., in cases of thalassemia or sideroblastic anemia). Hemochromatosis can be differentiated from transfusion-related iron overload by noting whether the patient has a history of repeated transfusions. Whereas total body iron in a healthy adult is 3.5 to 5.0 g, each transfusion of a unit of blood administers 250 mg of iron parenterally. Fifteen to 20 g of iron can be present in the body in cases of iron overload causing toxicity. Iron overload from transfusion and hemochromatosis rarely coexist.

Wilson Disease

Wilson disease is a rare autosomal recessive disorder estimated to affect 1 in 200,000 persons. Mutations leading to alterations in *ATP7B* result in copper overload with consequent copper deposition in the brain, liver, kidneys, and cornea (the Kayser–Fleischer ring). The ATP7B protein is the product of the copper-transporting ATPase gene on chromosome 13q. ATP7B normally moves copper into the bile. In >90% of patients with Wilson disease, the ceruloplasmin level is decreased. Copper excretion is increased in the urine, and therefore urinary copper is a useful noninvasive test in the investigation of possible Wilson disease. Liver biopsy can provide a quantitative measure of the degree of copper overload, as elevated hepatic copper is highly supportive of the diagnosis of Wilson disease. The most common presentation of Wilson disease is chronic liver disease (including cirrhosis), but it can present as acute, fulminant hepatitis that may require liver transplantation for survival.

Hepatocellular Carcinoma and Alpha-fetoprotein (AFP)

AFP is the major plasma protein produced by the fetal liver early in gestation. In adults, in contrast, AFP concentrations are normally very low. AFP may be elevated in many pathologic circumstances. It may be transiently increased with acute liver disease or persistently increased in chronic liver disease and cirrhosis. In patients with chronic liver disease or cirrhosis, an elevated AFP should trigger evaluation of the patient for hepatocellular carcinoma. For this cancer, elevated AFP levels serve as a tumor marker with a 40% to 80% sensitivity.

Hepatic Encephalopathy and Ammonia

Ammonia is an end product that results from amino acid deamination. The urea cycle captures ammonia (and thus nitrogen) in the form of urea for excretion by the kidney. Significant impairments in liver function produce hyperammonemia. Inborn errors of the Krebs urea cycle can cause hyperammonemia. The most common of these defects is ornithine transcarbamylase (OTC) deficiency, which is inherited as an X-linked recessive trait. Of interest, respiratory alkalosis can be observed in persons with inborn errors in urea production. In contrast, inborn errors that affect acid/base balance more often cause acidosis.

Hyperammonemia is associated with hepatic encephalopathy. A characteristic physical finding in patients with a toxic or metabolic encephalopathy is asterixis (e.g., unintended jerking movements particularly of the hands when they are dorsiflexed). To prevent ammonia being generated from protein deamination in a blood sample, immediately after collection, the blood sample should be placed on ice. During phlebotomy, the tourniquet should be left on for as short a time as possible to also avoid protein deamination. Refrigerated centrifugation should be accomplished at 4°C. While continuing to keep the sample cold (e.g., "on ice"), plasma should be aliquoted into a screw-top plastic tube and frozen within 2 hours of phlebotomy. Because smoking tobacco products produces ammonia gas, technologists must not wear their laboratory coats if they smoke, as both cloth-bound and liberated ammonia can be detected by analyzers. Ammonia is also present in some floor cleaning products, and enough ammonia can be generated in the atmosphere to interfere with measurement of ammonia by the laboratory instrument.

> Acute (fulminant) hepatic failure can result from a wide variety of insults, but the most common causes are acute viral hepatitis, toxins (e.g., *Amanita phalloides* mushrooms), and poisonings (e.g., acetaminophen).

Cholestasis of Pregnancy and Serum Bile Acid

Serum bile acid concentrations reflect the ability of the liver to remove bile acids from the circulation and excrete them back into the bile as part of the normal bile enterohepatic recirculation. Impaired hepatocyte uptake or secretion of bile acids, and portosystemic shunting, can elevate serum bile acid levels. Serum bile acids are often measured in women with cholestasis of pregnancy; otherwise, serum bile acids are rarely measured as they add little valuable information to the standard tests of hepatic function thus far discussed. Many argue that the diagnosis of cholestasis of pregnancy can be readily established without the measurement of serum bile acids.

Acute (Fulminant) Hepatic Failure

Acute (fulminant) hepatic failure can result from a wide variety of insults, but the most common causes are acute viral hepatitis (e.g., HBV and less commonly HAV), toxins (e.g., *Amanita phalloides* mushrooms), and poisonings (e.g., acetaminophen). Other causes of acute hepatic failure include adenovirus infection, varicella-zoster virus (VZV) infection, acute fatty liver of pregnancy, Wilson disease, Reye syndrome, and portal vein thrombosis.

With the recognition that aspirin use was associated with Reye syndrome and that aspirin should, therefore, not be used in children, Reye syndrome has become a rare disease compared to its peak incidence in the late 1970s. Reye syndrome is characterized by hyperammonemic encephalopathy and possible cerebral edema due to severely impaired liver function from fatty infiltration of the liver and presumed mitochondrial dysfunction. Other organs such as the kidney, gastrointestinal tract, and the heart can also become impaired in Reye syndrome.

In acute liver failure, the clinical course is rapid. Unless spontaneous recovery takes place or liver transplantation is performed, the outcome is fatal. Acute and chronic liver failure share many potential characteristics (**Table 16–9**): profound hyperbilirubinemia, coagulopathy (e.g., bleeding with a prolonged PT and thrombocytopenia), hypoproteinemia (e.g., hypoalbuminemia with edema), hypoglycemia, hyperammonemia with encephalopathy, and oliguric renal failure (the hepatorenal syndrome resulting from, in part, splanchnic vasodilation and hypovolemia). Chronic liver failure is also associated with intrapulmonary shunting leading to hypoxia and clubbing of the digits (e.g., the hepatopulmonary syndrome). Liver failure that occurs after 6 months of recognized liver disease is chronic liver failure.

Cirrhosis

Cirrhosis is the outcome of any chronic disorder of the liver parenchyma or intrahepatic biliary tract that causes continuous or repeated episodes of cellular necrosis and inflammation, followed by subsequent episodes of repair with fibrosis. At some point, recurrent injury to the liver can

TABLE 16–9   Commonly Observed Laboratory Findings in Hepatic Failure

	Comment(s)
Elevated conjugated and unconjugated bilirubin	Defects in conjugation and excretion of bilirubin
Hypoalbuminemia	Decreased albumin synthesis although there are many causes of hypoalbuminemia
Elevated ALT and AST	Elevations of ~100-fold with acute liver failure; rapid decline to normal can indicate permanent loss of hepatocytes; in chronic liver disease, ALT and AST can be normal
Hyperammonemia	Impaired urea cycle; late manifestation of a failing liver
Hypoglycemia	Impaired gluconeogenesis in the fasting state after glycogenolysis has exhausted liver glycogen stores
Prolonged PT	Decreased production of clotting factors, malabsorption of vitamin K, and decreased clearance of fibrin-split products
Thrombocytopenia	As a result of DIC or thrombopoietin deficiency
Anemia	Bone marrow suppression leads to chronic anemia; blood loss from esophageal varices
Elevated creatinine and BUN	Decreased urine output; the hepatorenal syndrome may be present; elevated BUN and a normal creatinine can indicate a GI bleed

DIC, disseminated intravascular coagulation; GI, gastrointestinal; PT, prothrombin time.

destroy the connective tissue architecture that is the reticular structure of the liver. This results in scarring with the deposition of increasing amounts of collagen. Bridging fibrosis can disturb intrahepatic blood flow, leading to portal hypertension, with the consequent development of ascites and esophageal varices. The liver becomes small and firm from fibrosis, yet on physical examination the abdomen is distended because of ascites. In some patients, reopening of the umbilical vein occurs and produces periumbilical varices termed "caput medusa" (after the mythical Greek character Medusa). Cirrhosis can predispose to hepatocellular carcinoma. Histologically, proliferating hepatocytes appear as regenerating nodules among the fibrotic bands. Nodules can be small (<3 mm—micronodular) or large (>3 mm—macronodular).

> **Ethanol abuse is the most common cause of cirrhosis in Westernized countries, accounting for 60% to 70% of cases.**

Ethanol abuse is the most common cause of cirrhosis in Westernized countries, accounting for 60% to 70% of cases. Other causes include chronic viral hepatitis (~10%), biliary tract diseases (~5% to 10%), and hereditary hemochromatosis (~5%). NAFL is increasingly being recognized as a cause of cryptogenic cirrhosis, that is, cirrhosis of otherwise unknown origin.

Patients with cirrhosis can experience severe functional liver impairment, also called "end-stage liver disease." Such patients can have a mixed unconjugated and conjugated hyperbilirubinemia, profound hypoalbuminemia, hypoglycemia, coagulopathy (from decreased clotting factor production, decreased clearance of fibrin-split products, and thrombocytopenia), and hyperammonemia.

Laboratory data can indicate the degree of liver dysfunction. However, cirrhosis remains a clinical diagnosis until the definitive diagnosis is established by the results of a liver biopsy. Researchers have attempted to develop biomarker panels that can diagnose cirrhosis. Over 10 models have been proposed. One of these "tools" is the FibroSure test that creates a score based upon ALT, α2-macroglobulin, apolipoprotein A1, total bilirubin, GGT, haptoglobin, and the patient's age and sex. A 2014 review concluded that this test could exclude cirrhosis caused by chronic hepatitis B infection, but that it is otherwise suboptimal for the identification of significant cirrhosis or fibrosis in chronically infected patients.

Primary Biliary Cirrhosis

> **Primary biliary cirrhosis (PBC) affects the interlobular bile ducts and is a chronic autoimmune biliary tract disease causing obstructive jaundice.**

Primary biliary cirrhosis (PBC; aka primary biliary cholangitis) affects the interlobular bile ducts and is a chronic autoimmune biliary tract disease causing obstructive jaundice. Thus, patients with PBC show a conjugated hyperbilirubinemia and relative elevations in ALP exceeding the ALT and AST elevations. Indeed, ALT and AST can be normal.

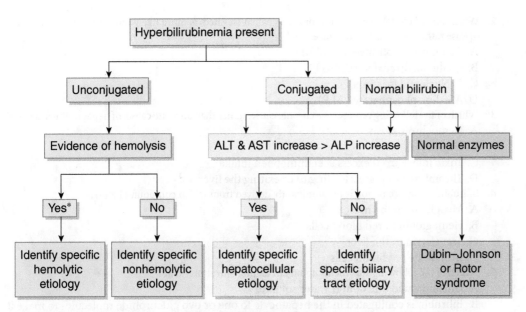

FIGURE 16–1   One approach to the evaluation of liver function. (*) Increased LD, decreased haptoglobin; with or without an abnormal peripheral smear.

Approximately 95% of patients with PBC are positive for anti-mitochondrial antibodies (AMA). Portal inflammation and progressive scarring can progress to liver failure requiring liver transplantation. The condition most often affects women between the ages of 40 and 50 years.

Primary Sclerosing Cholangitis

PSC affects the larger bile ducts. Men are more commonly affected than women (70:30 ratio), with a mean age at onset near 40 years. Tests for AMA are negative in patients with PSC. Inflammatory bowel disease, such as Crohn disease or ulcerative colitis, is identified in about 75% of patients with PSC. The definitive diagnosis of PSC is established by liver biopsy.

APPROACH TO THE PATIENT WITH LIVER DISEASE

One reasonable approach to the evaluation of liver function is to first consider the bilirubin concentration (**Figure 16–1** and **Tables 16–3 to 16–6**). If there is an unconjugated hyperbilirubinemia, possible hemolysis should be investigated. If this is absent, other causes of an unconjugated hyperbilirubinemia need to be considered, such as neonatal jaundice, Gilbert syndrome, and Crigler–Najjar syndrome.

If there is a conjugated hyperbilirubinemia, the liver enzymes can be used to separate hepatocellular disease (e.g., predominant elevations in ALT and AST) from biliary tract disease (e.g., predominant elevations in ALP, or if measured, GGT and 5'-NT). Disorders are then investigated based on their relative frequency and whether the disease is acute or chronic. Not noted in **Figure 16–1** is end-stage liver disease in which there can be significant elevations in both the conjugated and unconjugated fractions. In the absence of hyperbilirubinemia, the focus on liver dysfunction becomes the pattern of enzyme elevation.

SELF-ASSESSMENT QUESTIONS

1. Which one of the following laboratory tests, when elevated, is more likely indicative of biliary tract disease rather than hepatocellular disease?
   A. Aspartate aminotransferase (AST)
   B. Lactate dehydrogenase (LD)
   C. Alkaline phosphatase (ALP)
   D. Alanine aminotransferase (ALT)

2. Which one of the following laboratory tests, when elevated, is more likely indicative of hepatocellular disease rather than biliary tract disease?
   A. Alanine aminotransferase (ALT)
   B. γ-Glutamyltransferase (GGT)
   C. 5'-Nucleotidase (5'-NT)
   D. Alkaline phosphatase (ALP)

3. Which of the following represents a chronic cause, rather than an acute cause, of hepatocellular disease?
   A. Hemochromatosis
   B. Hepatitis A
   C. Toxic injury from excess acetaminophen intake
   D. Thrombosis in vessels leading to or exiting the liver

4. Bilirubin in the circulation is predominantly derived from which compound below?
   A. Myoglobin in the muscle
   B. Hemoglobin in red blood cells
   C. Transferrin in the liver
   D. Iron in the red blood cells

5. Which of the following statements about circulating bilirubin is true?
   A. Unconjugated bilirubin is water soluble.
   B. Bilirubin is conjugated in the hepatocyte to one or two glucuronide molecules to make it water soluble.
   C. If the concentration of circulated bilirubin, conjugated or unconjugated, rises significantly, the skin and sclerae can develop a pinkish color termed jaundice.
   D. Conjugated bilirubin is transported into the urine via the bile canaliculi.

6. In patients with acute viral hepatitis, primarily involving hepatocellular dysfunction, the increase in the conjugated bilirubin fraction in the circulation is because of which one of the following choices?
   A. Decreased transport of conjugated bilirubin into the bile canaliculi
   B. Impaired conversion of hemoglobin to bilirubin
   C. Increased conjugation of bilirubin to bilirubin glucuronide
   D. Decreased excretion of conjugated bilirubin into the urine

7. Which of the following choices below represents hyperbilirubinemia that is primarily unconjugated?
   A. The ratio of conjugated to total bilirubin is 0.7 in an adult.
   B. The ratio of conjugated to total bilirubin is 0.3 in a neonate.
   C. The ratio of conjugated to total bilirubin is 0.6 in a 3-year-old child.
   D. The ratio of conjugated to total bilirubin is 0.3 in an adult.

8. Which of the following is not a cause of unconjugated hyperbilirubinemia?
   A. Red blood cell destruction as a result of autoimmune hemolytic anemia
   B. Defective transport of unconjugated bilirubin into the hepatocyte
   C. Defective conjugation of bilirubin to glucuronide in the hepatocyte
   D. Impaired transport of conjugated bilirubin into the bile ducts

9. Which of the following choices represents a condition associated with extravascular, rather than intravascular, hemolysis?
   A. Microangiopathic hemolytic anemia
   B. Hemolysis from an artificial heart
   C. Sickle cell anemia
   D. Vitamin B_{12} deficiency causing ineffective erythropoiesis

10. Which of the following represents an unconjugated hyperbilirubinemia without hemolysis?
    A. Red blood cell enzyme defects such as pyruvate kinase deficiency
    B. Red blood cell membrane defects such as hereditary spherocytosis
    C. Crigler–Najjar syndromes
    D. Thrombotic thrombocytopenic purpura

11. Obstruction of the biliary tract can occur inside the liver (intrahepatic) or extrahepatic. Which of the following is the most common cause of extrahepatic biliary tract obstruction in adults?
    A. Biliary atresia
    B. Cholelithiasis
    C. Pancreatic adenocarcinoma
    D. Parasitic infection

12. Which of the following proteins, synthesized in the liver, has the highest concentration of all the plasma proteins?
    A. Immunoglobulins
    B. Fibrinogen
    C. Complement component C3
    D. Albumin

13. The half-life of many clotting factors is much shorter than the half-life of albumin. Therefore, measurement of a parameter of coagulation may provide a more sensitive index of decreased liver protein synthesis than the concentration of albumin in the plasma. Which of the following coagulation tests is commonly used to assess the patient for serious liver dysfunction?
    A. PTT
    B. PT/INR
    C. Fibrinogen
    D. Factor VII

14. Serious long-standing liver disease can lead to bleeding for all except one of the choices below. Identify the choice which is not a cause of bleeding in a patient with severe liver disease.
    A. Decreased synthesis of coagulation factors by the liver
    B. Impaired clearance of fibrin-split products by the liver, which leads to inhibition of clotting by a high concentration of fibrin-split products
    C. Increased synthesis of coagulation factor VIII outside the liver
    D. Presence of esophageal varices that are easily traumatized

15. Which of the following tests indicates, when positive, the presence of an acute or chronic hepatitis B virus infection with increased infectivity?
    A. Hepatitis B virus surface antigen
    B. Hepatitis B virus e antigen
    C. Hepatitis A virus IgM antibody
    D. Hepatitis D virus antibody

16. Which of the following tests is most likely to be positive or elevated in patients with primary biliary cirrhosis?
    A. α-Fetoprotein
    B. Antismooth muscle autoantibodies
    C. Antimitochondrial antibodies
    D. α_1-Antitrypsin

17. Which of the following liver diseases is associated with iron overload in the absence of chronic transfusion therapy?
    A. Wilson disease
    B. Hepatocellular carcinoma
    C. Glycogen storage disease
    D. Hemochromatosis

18. Which one of the following laboratory test abnormalities or conditions is not likely to be present in a patient with hemochromatosis?
    A. Increased transferrin saturation
    B. Decreased plasma or serum ferritin
    C. Iron deposition in the liver
    D. Cardiac failure from iron deposition in the heart

19. Which one of the following is not likely to be present in a patient with Wilson disease?
    A. Liver disease, either chronic or acute
    B. Kayser–Fleischer rings in the cornea
    C. Increased ceruloplasmin in the serum or plasma
    D. Increased excretion of copper into the urine

20. Which one of the following is not commonly observed in patients with fulminant hepatic failure?
    A. Elevated ammonia concentration in the circulation
    B. Decreased blood glucose concentration
    C. Prolonged prothrombin time (PT)
    D. Decreased conjugated and unconjugated bilirubin

21. Of the following choices, which is the most common cause of cirrhosis in Westernized countries, accounting for 60% to 70% of cases?

A. Ethanol abuse

B. Chronic viral hepatitis

C. Biliary tract diseases

D. Hereditary hemochromatosis

22. Which of the following disorders affects the interlobular bile ducts and is a chronic autoimmune biliary tract disease associated with obstructive jaundice?

A. Primary sclerosing cholangitis

B. Primary biliary cirrhosis

C. Hepatic encephalopathy

D. Cholestasis of pregnancy

FURTHER READING

American Academy of Pediatrics Subcommittee on Hyperbilirubinemia. Management of hyperbilirubinemia in the newborn infant 35 or more weeks of gestation. *Pediatrics*. 2004;114:297–316.

Castera L. Noninvasive methods to assess liver disease in patients with hepatitis B or C. *Gastroenterology*. 2012;142:1293–1302.e4.

Cohen LA, Gutierrez L, Weiss A, et al. Serum ferritin is derived primarily from macrophages through a nonclassical secretory pathway. *Blood*. 2010;116:1574–1584.

Dufour DR, et al. Diagnosis and monitoring of hepatic injury. I. Performance characteristics of laboratory tests. *Clin Chem*. 2000;46:2027–2049.

Dufour DR, et al. Diagnosis and monitoring of hepatic injury. II. Recommendations for use of laboratory tests in screening, diagnosis, and monitoring. *Clin Chem*. 2000;46:2050–2068.

El-Beshbishi SN, Shattuck KE, Mohammad AA, Petersen JR. Hyperbilirubinemia and transcutaneous bilirubinometry. *Clin Chem*. 2009;55:1280–1287.

Fix OK, Kowdley KV. Hereditary hemochromatosis. Minerva Med. 2008;99(December):605–617.

Hogarth DK, Rachelefsky G. Screening and familial testing of patients for alpha 1-antitrypsin deficiency. *Chest*. 2008;133:981–988.

Jastrzębska I, Zwolak A, Szczyrek M, Wawryniuk A, Skrzydło-Radomańska B, Daniluk J. Biomarkers of alcohol misuse: recent advances and future prospects. *Prz Gastroenterol*. 2016;11:78–89.

Klein KB, Stafinski TD, Menon D. Predicting survival after liver transplantation based on pre-transplant MELD score: a systematic review of the literature. *PLoS One*. 2013;8:e80661.

Langner C, Denk H. Wilson disease. *Virchows Arch*. 2004;445:111–118.

Limdi JK, Hyde GM. Evaluation of abnormal liver function tests. *Postgrad Med J*. 2003;79(June):307–312.

Mallory MA, et al. Abnormal liver test results on routine screening. How to evaluate, when to refer for a biopsy. *Postgrad Med*. 2004;115:53–56, 59–62, 66.

Milich D, Liang TJ. Exploring the biological basis of hepatitis B e antigen in hepatitis B virus infection. *Hepatology*. 2003;38:1075–1086.

Salkic NN, Jovanovic P, Hauser G, Brcic M. FibroTest/Fibrosure for significant liver fibrosis and cirrhosis in chronic hepatitis B: a meta-analysis. *Am J Gastroenterol*. 2014;109:796–809.

Pancreatic Disorders

David N. Alter and Michael Laposata

INTRODUCTION

The pancreas is an endocrine/exocrine organ transversely oriented in the retroperitoneum with its "head" nestled in the duodenum and its "tail" approaching the spleen, measuring approximately 20 cm long by 2 to 3 cm in thickness. Eighty-five percent of the organ is exocrine in function, consisting of cells that secrete digestion-related enzymes (many in their inactive "pro" form) into the gastrointestinal tract (**Table 17-1**), whereas the endocrine portion consists of hormone-producing cell clusters (islets of Langerhans) histologically interspersed throughout the exocrine cellular component. There are four major cell types that produce their respective hormone, as listed in **Table 17-2**.

Pancreatitis is the most common exocrine disorder and diabetes is the most common endocrine disorder. In terms of malignancy, exocrine tumors (95%) tend to be adenocarcinomas arising from pancreatic ductal epithelium with the much less common endocrine tumors arising from the islets of Langerhans characterized by their "progenitor" cell (insulinoma, gluconoma, etc.) type.

TABLE 17–1   **Exocrine Pancreas**

Enzyme	Function
Amylase	Catalyzes breakdown of complex carbohydrates into individual glucose residues
Lipase	Catalyzes hydrolysis of triglycerides into monoglyceride and free fatty acids
Trypsin (storage form—trypsinogen)	Cleaves digested proteins (protease) at carboxyl groups on lysine and arginine amino acids
Chymotrypsin (storage form—chymotrypsinogen)	Cleaves digested proteins (protease) at peptide bonds of tryptophan, leucine, tyrosine, and phenylalanine
Elastase	Cleaves digested proteins (protease) at carboxyl groups on glycine, alanine, and valine

TABLE 17–2   **Endocrine Pancreas**

Cell Type	Hormone	Major Functions
Alpha	Glucagon	Increases blood glucose
Beta	Insulin	Decreases blood glucose
Delta	Somatostatin	Inhibits insulin and glucagon release
Gamma	Pancreatic polypeptide	Regulates pancreatic function

ACUTE PANCREATITIS

Description

Acute pancreatitis is an acute inflammatory disorder of the pancreas clinically characterized by acute to chronic epigastric pain with nausea, vomiting and, if severe enough, fever, hypotension, and tachycardia. The top three causes of acute pancreatitis are biliary tract obstruction (40% to 70%), alcohol abuse (25% to 35%), and idiopathic causes (20%). Other less frequent etiologies include hypercalcemia, hypertriglyceridemia, infection, mechanical (post procedure), and medication related. The latter cause is usually due to toxic metabolites or hypersensitivity reactions (e.g., asparaginase, azathioprine, estrogens, furosemide, sulfonamides, tetracycline, and thiazides). Hereditary forms of acute pancreatitis have also been described due to mutations in the trypsinogen gene or the trypsin inhibitor gene. Underlying all of these disorders is activation of intra-pancreatic digestive pro-enzymes that act on the pancreas itself (auto-digestion), triggering an inflammatory response causing edema, necrosis, and hemorrhage. These changes cause, or exacerbate, ductal obstruction, aggravating the initial inflammatory response. Of all possible pancreatic enzymes, amylase and lipase have been historically characterized as pathognomonic markers of acute pancreatitis. In fact, if amylase and/or lipase are elevated in the appropriate clinical situation, acute pancreatitis is the diagnosis until proven otherwise.

> Acute pancreatitis is a potentially lethal disorder associated with intracellular activation of digestive enzymes in the pancreas. This results in autodigestion of the pancreatic tissue by the powerful enzymes normally secreted into the gastrointestinal tract to degrade ingested foods.

Diagnosis

Diagnosis of acute pancreatitis requires two out of the three following criteria: (a) abdominal pain, (b) characteristic radiologic findings, and (c) elevated lipase and/or amylase. Additional laboratory findings include, but are not limited to, leukocytosis, hypocalcemia, hypoglycemia, and an elevated C-reactive protein.

An amylase or lipase elevation greater than $3\times$ the upper limit of normal satisfies the biochemical criteria for the diagnosis of acute pancreatitis, with amylase having a sensitivity from 67% to 83% and specificity from 85% to 98%. In contrast, both sensitivity/specificity of lipase for diagnosing acute pancreatitis is greater than 95%. Amylase/lipase elevations are not solely associated with pancreatitis and should be interpreted in light of the patient's clinical presentation. **Tables 17–3** and **17–4** list causes of non-pancreatitis etiologies of hyperamylasemia and lipasemia, respectively.

TABLE 17-3   Hyperamylasemia Not Associated with Acute Pancreatitis

Abdominal and thoracic malignancies
Biliary disease
Dissecting aortic aneurysm
Gastrointestinal viscus perforation
Head trauma with intracranial bleeding
Intestinal obstruction
Liver disease
Macroamylasemia
Mesenteric infarction
Myocardial infarction
Pancreatic pseudocyst
Pancreatic disease not otherwise specified
Pulmonary embolism
Renal insufficiency
Ruptured ectopic pregnancy
Salivary gland disease

TABLE 17-4   Hyperlipasemia Not Associated with Acute Pancreatitis

Biliary disease
Diabetic ketoacidosis
HIV infection
Intestinal obstruction
Pancreatic carcinoma
Pancreatic disease not otherwise specified
Pancreatic pseudocyst
Renal failure

Lipase has better test characteristics because it is more organ specific than amylase as well as peaking sooner and declining later in comparison to amylase. Amylase levels rise within 6 to 12 hours and normalize within 3 to 5 days, whereas lipase levels will increase within 4 to 8 hours and normalize over 8 to 14 days. As a result, timing is everything and an isolated normal amylase level may be falsely decreased due to either being collected too late or too early. Of interest, studies have noted that there is no increased diagnostic power by combining both assays.

A number of laboratory tests and computed tomography may be useful to assess prognosis in patients with acute pancreatitis. One system to assign prognosis in acute pancreatitis is the simplified Glasgow criteria. Features associated with a worse prognosis include age >55 years, white blood cell count >15,000/uL, LD >600 U/L, glucose >180 mg/dL, albumin >3.2 g/dL, calcium >8 mg/dL, arterial PO_2 >60 mm Hg, and BUN >45 mg/dL.

Macro-amylasemia is an important but infrequent and often neglected cause of a persistently elevated amylase level. Macro-amylase is a complex of amylase and immunoglobulin (typically IgA but IgG is possible) too big to be filtered at the glomerulus, resulting in a persistent hyperamylasemia. Advanced testing using electrophoresis, immunofixation, and carbohydrate staining is necessary to make this diagnosis in this situation. Of note, several other analytes can present with falsely elevated results due to "macro" complex formation. They are creatinine kinase (macro-CK), prolactin (macro-PRL), aspartate aminotransferase (macro-AST), and thyroid stimulating hormone (macro-TSH).

CHRONIC PANCREATITIS

Description

Following an attack of acute pancreatitis, the patient may experience a complete recovery, exhibit recurrence without permanent pancreatic damage, or suffer multiple recurrences leading to chronic pancreatitis. Chronic pancreatitis is characterized by cellular destruction, with scar tissue replacement leading to pancreatic duct obstruction. Chronic pancreatitis has a variety of etiologies. However, in industrialized countries prolonged excessive alcohol consumption is the primary cause, and in developing countries it is more likely to arise from malnutrition. Cystic fibrosis is the most common cause in children (see Chapter 7).

Following an attack of acute pancreatitis, the patient may experience a complete recovery, have an additional recurrence without permanent damage to the pancreas, or suffer multiple recurrences leading to chronic pancreatitis and significant damage to the organ.

Diagnosis

Patients with chronic pancreatitis often have impaired glucose tolerance (IGT) or diabetes. Additional manifestations include abdominal pain, weight loss, pancreatic calcifications on x-ray, and steatorrhea. The sensitivity of laboratory tests to diagnose chronic pancreatitis depends on the extent of pancreatic tissue destruction and the length of time over which the damage has occurred. In these cases, amylase and lipase may be less informative, and the diagnosis depends on clinical history and imaging studies.

Duodenal intubation using endoscopic retrograde cholangiopancreatography (ERCP), with injection of x-ray contrast medium into the common bile duct and pancreatic ducts, is the most sensitive test, but the test itself may induce pancreatitis and should therefore be reserved for selected cases. More recently, endoscopic ultrasound has gained favor, and it is equally sensitive and specific for chronic pancreatitis as ERCP.

PANCREATIC TUMORS

Exocrine Pancreas Neoplasms

Description

> Pancreatic cancer affects more than 30,000 adults in the United States annually and is usually rapidly fatal.

Most (95%) pancreatic cancers are histologically adenocarcinoma (which can be cystic, or not, with multiple histologic subtypes not relevant for this discussion) arising in the exocrine pancreas. Pancreatic cancer affects more than 30,000 adults in the United States annually and is usually fatal with a 5-year survival rate of less than 5%.

Diagnosis

Pancreatic carcinoma's high fatality rate is due to the fact that there are no available screening tests and that the tumor is clinically silent until adjacent structure infiltration (metastasis) occurs. At that stage, symptoms present with pain, jaundice, and weight loss as the top three. Because of the late stage at identification, only 15% to 20% of the patients are candidates for surgical resection. These patients have slightly better 5-year survival rates than nonsurgical candidates but not by much (10% for node positive and 30% for node negative disease).

CA 19-9 is available as a tumor marker for pancreatic cancer. However, its use is limited to diagnosis (in the appropriate clinical situation) and monitoring of treatment. It is normally present in the adult and fetal pancreas, esophagus, stomach, small intestine, gallbladder, bile duct, and salivary glands. For the diagnosis of pancreatic cancer, its reported sensitivity increases with tumor size, ranging from 70% to 92% with a specificity that ranges from 68% to 92%. Therefore, the more advanced the tumor, the higher the CA 19-9 and the greater its diagnostic power. However, CA 19-9 is not specific to pancreatic cancer and may be elevated in other types of gastrointestinal cancers and in some nonneoplastic disorders as well. Importantly, CA 19-9 requires the presence of the Lewis blood group antigen for its expression, and if absent, CA 19-9 will be undetectable (5% to 7% of the general population).

In the last 10 years, pancreatic cyst fluid analysis has entered clinical practice. Endoscopic ultrasound guided fine needle aspiration of pancreatic fluid to test for CEA, CA 19-9, CA 125, and CA 15-3 is being used at some institutions to distinguish mucinous from nonmucinous pancreatic neoplasms with reported sensitivities and specificities in the high 80% range. At this time, however, none of those assays have been FDA approved for clinical use.

Endocrine Pancreas Neoplasms

Islet Cell Tumors (Pancreatic Neuroendocrine Tumors [Pancreatic NETs])

Description and Diagnosis

Islet cell tumors may be nonfunctional, hypofunctional, or hyperfunctional with respect to their progenitor specific hormone-secreting cells (beta, alpha, and delta). If nonfunctional, they may only present with symptoms of a mass lesion, sometimes only discovered incidentally. Functional islet cell tumors secrete a variety of hormones; in descending order of frequency, they are the

TABLE 17–5   American Diabetes Association Classification of Diabetes Mellitus

Classification	Pathogenesis
Type 1 diabetes	Absolute deficiency of insulin secretion, usually due to immune-mediated beta-cell destruction
Type 2 diabetes	Varying degrees of insulin resistance; even if there is increased plasma insulin, it is insufficient to compensate for the resistance
Other specific types of diabetes	Heterogenous causes, subclassified as: genetic defects of beta-cell function, genetic defects in insulin receptors, exocrine pancreatic disease, drugs or chemicals toxic to islet cells or that antagonize insulin, infectious destruction of islet cells, uncommon forms of immune-mediated diabetes, or other endocrine diseases that impair glucose regulation
Gestational diabetes	Various causes, including unrecognized type 1 diabetes and subclinical incipient type 2 diabetes

following: gastrin, insulin, serotonin, and vasoactive intestinal peptide (VIP). The cell types and their respective hormones are summarized below:

- **Beta cell tumors (insulinoma)** are clinically significant when they produce enough insulin to induce hypoglycemia (discussed below). Laboratory studies include blood glucose, C-peptide, insulin, and the insulin to glucose ratio.
- **Alpha cell tumors (glucagonoma)** are associated with elevated serum levels of glucagon. These tumors can be associated with a characteristic migratory erythema, as well as glucose intolerance, weight loss, deep vein thrombosis, and depression.
- **Delta cell tumors (somatostatinoma)** are typically associated with diabetes-related symptoms, diarrhea, steatorrhea, cholelithiasis, and weight loss. These tumors are most often located in the duodenum or jejunum, rather than in the pancreas.
- Tumors of the pancreatic islets that secrete gastrin **(gastrinoma)** are found in both pancreas and duodenum with a higher incidence in the pancreas (60% to 85% depending on source reviewed) with 90% of them occurring in the "gastrinoma triangle," a triangle with its base parallel to the cystic duct and its apex pointing toward the tail. Gastrin elevations are associated with increased gastric acid secretion, diarrhea, and malabsorption (Zollinger–Ellison syndrome). Patients with peptic ulcer disease without *Helicobacter pylori* infection or a history of nonsteroidal anti-inflammatory drug use may have Zollinger–Ellison syndrome and should be evaluated for a gastrinoma.
- Lastly, VIP-secreting tumors are known as **VIPomas**. VIPomas induce a syndrome of watery diarrhea, hypokalemia, hypochlorhydria, and acidosis.

DIABETES MELLITUS

Description

Diabetes mellitus (DM) represents a heterogeneous group of glucose regulatory disorders with the common feature of hyperglycemia due to defects in insulin secretion, insulin action, or a combination of these two factors. The classification of diabetes according to the American Diabetes Association (ADA) are listed in **Table 17–5** with the majority of patients (90% to 95%) having type 2 diabetes. Disease sequelae are not directly related to the degree of hyperglycemia as much as they are related to the acute and chronic effects of hyperglycemia on end-organ processes. Chronic hyperglycemia has been strongly associated with the development of polyneuropathy, nephropathy, and retinopathy, as well as a reduced ability to fight infections. Almost 13% of Americans have DM, of which 40% are unaware of their disorder and a significant fraction will already have some degree of nephropathy, neuropathy, and/or retinopathy upon diagnosis. Importantly, many of the complications of diabetes can be avoided through early diagnosis and aggressive management. The ADA has advocated screening everyone over 45 years old with a fasting plasma glucose (FPG) (*"plasma" is synonymous with "blood" and is the verbiage used in the guidelines*) test, with a repeat test every

Almost 13% of Americans have DM, of which 40% are unaware of their disorder. A significant fraction will already have some degree of nephropathy, neuropathy, and/or retinopathy when they are first diagnosed with DM.

3 years if the results are negative. Screening of groups with high risk for DM (**Table 17–6**) has been proposed for individuals 45 years old or greater.

For the acute inpatient population, abrupt hyperglycemic excursions have been associated with increased morbidities and poorer prognoses, leading hospitals to develop "tight glycemic control" policies and procedures to minimize hyperglycemic episodes for both the diabetic and nondiabetic patient.

Diagnosis

The ADA Expert Committee on the Classification and Diagnosis of Diabetes Mellitus and the World Health Organization (WHO) have developed, over time, guidelines and criteria for the diagnosis of diabetes. Both have also refined the diagnostic criteria for gestational diabetes. The diagnosis of any type of diabetes involves measurement of blood glucose in fasting and nonfasting states as well as the timing of response to a measured oral dose of glucose. Specific diagnostic criteria for DM, prediabetes (increased risk of diabetes), and gestational DM (GDM) are given in **Tables 17-7**, **17-8**, and **17-9**, respectively.

TABLE 17–6   High-risk Individuals for Whom Diabetes Mellitus Screening Is Recommended by the American Diabetes Association

Individuals of the following ancestry: African, Asian, Hispanic, Native American, and Pacific Islander
Mothers with newborns ≥9 lb or history of gestational diabetes mellitus
Individuals with hypertension >140/90, HDL cholesterol ≤35 mg/dL, or triglycerides ≥250 mg/dL
Individuals with a history of impaired fasting glucose or impaired glucose tolerance; HbA1c >5.7%
Obese individuals weighing ≥120% of ideal body weight
Individuals with first-degree relatives with diabetes mellitus

HDL, high-density lipoprotein.

TABLE 17–7   Criteria for Diagnosis of Diabetes Mellitus (Nongestational)

Hemoglobin A1c (HbA1c) greater than or equal to 6.5%. The method used should be certified and standardized to the diabetes control and complications trial (DCCT) assay.
Or
Fasting plasma glucose greater than or equal to 126 mg/dL (7.0 mmol/L). Fasting is defined as no caloric intake for at least 8 h.
Or
A 2-h plasma glucose value greater than 200 mg/dL (11.1 mmol/L) during an oral glucose tolerance test (OGTT). The tests should be performed using a glucose load containing the equivalent of 75 g of anhydrous glucose dissolved in water.
Or
A patient with classic symptoms of hyperglycemia or hyperglycemic crisis, a random plasma glucose value greater than 200 mg/dL (11.1 mmol/L).

In the absence of unequivocal hyperglycemia, results should be confirmed by repeat testing.

TABLE 17–8   Criteria for Prediabetes (Increased Diabetes Risk)

Fasting plasma glucose 100 mg/dL (5.6 mmol/L) to 125 mg/dL (6.9 mmol/L)—Impaired fasting glucose (IFG)
Or
A 2-h plasma glucose in the 75 g oral glucose tolerance test (OGTT) 140 mg/dL (7.8 mmol/L) to 199 mg/dL (11.0 mmol/L)—Impaired glucose tolerance (IGT)
Or
Hemoglobin A1c (HbA1c) 5.7 to 6.4% (39–47 mmol/mol)

DIABETES

Random Plasma Glucose

A random fasting (at least 8 hours) plasma glucose level of 200 mg/dL, combined with symptoms of DM (polyuria, polydipsia, and unexplained weight loss), can be used to establish a diagnosis of DM. These criteria do not depend on the time since the last meal, but the test should not be done when the patient is acutely ill.

Fasting Plasma Glucose

An FPG can be used to diagnose diabetes. The patient can drink water while fasting, but should abstain from eating, smoking, or taking medications. Acute illness, surgery, and hospitalization within the previous 8 weeks are relative contraindications to testing, as false-positive results can arise in these situations. FPG greater than or equal to 126 mg/dL is considered diagnostic for diabetes.

Oral Glucose Tolerance Test

If the clinical picture merits further testing despite normal or impaired findings (see section on prediabetes), an oral glucose tolerance test (OGTT) is indicated. The OGTT is a stimulation test that assesses an individual's glycemic response after administration of a standard dose of glucose under standardized conditions. Prior (3 days) to the test, the patient should have a regular diet, with a carbohydrate intake of at least 100 g per day. The patient's activity should be unrestricted, and only severe illness or hospitalization represents relative contraindications. Minor illnesses with gastrointestinal manifestations are not significant. The glucose bolus for nonpregnant adults

TABLE 17–9   Laboratory Evaluation for Gestational Diabetes Mellitus (GDM)

One-Step Strategy

75 g OGTT with glucose measurements at fasting, 1 and 2 hours at 24–28 weeks gestation in women without previous diagnosis of diabetes after an overnight fast of at least 8 h.

The diagnosis of GDM is made when any ONE of the following criteria are exceeded.

GDM One-Step Strategy Diagnostic Criteria

Fasting	92 mg/dL (5.1 mmol/L)
1 hour	180 mg/dL (10.0 mmol/L)
2 hour	153 mg/dL (8.5 mmol/)

Two-Step Strategy

Step 1
50 g OGTT (nonfasting) at 1 h 24–28 weeks gestation women without previous diagnosis of diabetes.

If the glucose level at 1 h is ≥130 mg/dL, 135 mg/dL, or 140 mg/dL (7.2 mmol/L, 7.5 mmol/L, or 7.8 mmol/L) proceed to the 100 g OGTT. *The multiple criteria reflects debate as to which cutoff has the best diagnostic power. (See Donovan L et al. Screening tests for gestational diabetes mellitus: a systematic review for the U.S. Preventive Services Task Force. Ann Intern Med. 2013;159:115–122.)*

Step 2
100 g OGTT with glucose measurements at fasting, 1, 2, and 3 hours after an overnight fast of at least 8 h.

The diagnosis of GDM is made when 2 of the following 4 plasma glucose levels are met or exceeded.

Time	Carpenter/Coustan	National Diabetes Data Group (NDDG)
Fasting	95 mg/dL (5.3 mmol/L)	105 mg/dL (5.8 mmol/L)
1 hour	180 mg/dL (10.0 mmol/L)	190 mg/dL (10.6 mmol/L)
2 hour	155 mg/dL (8.6 mmol/L)	165 mg/dL (9.2 mmol/L)
3 hour	140 mg/dL (7.8 mmol/L)	140 mg/dL (8.0 mmol/L)

is 75 g of anhydrous glucose dissolved in 10 to 12 oz of water consumed over 5 minutes. The testing protocol has been simplified from previous versions to include only two specimens: a fasting specimen and one at 2 hours after the bolus. A 2-hour postbolus FPG level of 200 mg/dL is diagnostic of DM.

Hemoglobin A1c

In 2009, hemoglobin A1c (HbA1c) was added as a diagnostic marker for diabetes (prior to that it was only recommended for monitoring treatment). HbA1c is formed by the nonenzymatic linkage of glucose to hemoglobin within the red blood cell to form a stable ketoamine, which persists for the life span of the red blood cell (typically 120 days). This complex is immune to short-term FPG fluctuations such that HbA1c formation is directly proportional to blood glucose concentration in the blood and reflects a time-weighted average of glucose values over the preceding 8 to 12 weeks. HbA1c had been primarily used for monitoring long-term glycemic status/metabolic control in diabetic patients and as a marker of chronic hyperglycosylation. However, in 2009, the International Expert Committee on the Role of HbA1c in the Diagnosis of Diabetes concluded that the HbA1c assay can also be used in diagnosis because the reproducibility of assay methods had vastly improved. The committee recommended that a diagnosis of diabetes can be made if the HbA1c level is >6.5%.

In diabetic patients, retinopathy incidence increases substantially at HbA1c values between 6.0% and 7.0%. ADA recommendations state to keep the HbA1c less than 7.0% or lower to minimize diabetes-related complications. The ADA recommends measurement of HbA1c at least twice per year in all persons with DM.

Prediabetes

Although not meeting criteria for diabetes, an intermediate group of subjects exist whose glucose levels are too high to be considered normal but not high enough to be classified as diabetic. Individuals with an impaired fasting glucose (IFG) have an FPG ranging from 100 to 125 mg/dL and those with an IGT post OGTT have glucose results in the range 140 to 199 mg/dL. These patients (IFG, IGT) are considered to be "prediabetic," and therefore, with a higher risk of developing diabetes and diabetes-related complications. They are not clinical entities in their own right, but instead identify patients at risk for DM and its cardiovascular complications. Loss of 5% to 10% of body weight, exercise, and treatment with appropriate medications can prevent or delay the onset of DM in these patients. "Impaired criteria" have changed over time as more data has become available and probably will continue to change over time, thereby shifting formerly "prediabetic" individuals into the "diabetic" category or vice versa.

GESTATIONAL DIABETES MELLITUS

Description

Gestational diabetes mellitus (GDM) represents any level of glucose intolerance initially identified during pregnancy, even if unrecognized before the pregnancy. When hyperglycemia occurs for the first time during pregnancy, it usually develops late in the second or in the third trimester. Most of these patients will revert to normoglycemia after pregnancy. Among the complications of untreated gestational DM are macrosomia (birth weight >4000 g or 8.82 lb), intrauterine fetal demise, and pulmonary immaturity. Approximately 1 in 25 pregnancies in the United States is complicated by gestational DM, with a higher incidence in some ethnic groups (up to one in seven in Native Americans).

Diagnosis

Screening for GDM was previously recommended for all pregnant women; however, some experts suggest that screening women at low risk for diabetes is not cost-effective. Low-risk women are of Caucasian or Middle-Eastern ancestry, less than 25 years old, of normal weight, have no first-degree relatives with DM, and have no history of abnormal glucose metabolism. Women with a high risk for GDM should be evaluated as soon as feasible into the pregnancy. All other women should be screened between 24 and 28 weeks gestation, with the exception of women with clinical symptoms consistent with gestational DM before 24 weeks, who should be tested when symptoms appear. There are different approaches and criteria that are used in the diagnosis of GDM. They are summarized in **Table 17–9**.

Six weeks after the end of a pregnancy complicated by GDM, the woman should be retested. Normoglycemic women with a history of GDM should be rescreened at 3-year intervals, and women with IFG or IGT should be screened more frequently. Blood glucose assessment of the newborn infant is not part of the follow-up for patients with GDM.

Diabetes—Testing Issues

For the most accurate glucose results, specimens should be collected in tubes containing a sodium fluoride additive (gray-top tube typically). Sodium fluoride inhibits glycolysis which can be a source of falsely lowered results due to white blood cell glycolysis (5% to 7% per hour). However, if the "plasma" component is quickly separated from the "cellular" component, metabolic loss will be minimal.

Point-of-care glucose testing is widely available in inpatient, outpatient, and home use populations. It is a very convenient and a simple modality for monitoring FPG levels before meals, assessing potential bouts of hypoglycemia or hyperglycemia, and for monitoring compliance with personalized diabetic regimens. However, fasting capillary (fingerstick) glucose levels are approximately 10 mg/dL lower than venous blood levels and are equal to or higher after a glucose bolus. For those and other reasons, these devices are not recommended nor FDA validated for the diagnosis of diabetes. Point-of-care HbA1c devices are also available for monitoring disease but have not been approved for the diagnosis of diabetes.

Other Markers

Trace excretion of urinary albumin, termed "microalbuminuria," is routinely measured in patients with DM as an early marker of nephropathy. This test is not usually a part of routine urinalysis, and must therefore be ordered as a microalbumin test, along with a creatinine level, on a random urine specimen (see Chapter 18).

Considerable attention is now focused on the detection of autoantibodies as a screening tool for asymptomatic individuals with a strong family history of type 1 DM. The presence of autoantibodies to two or more of the following—glutamic acid decarboxylase (GAD65), islet tyrosine phosphatase (ICA512), or insulin—is a strong predictor of progression to type 1 DM (greater than 50%). It remains to be shown, however, whether early intervention can slow or prevent the subsequent onset of disease. Therefore, the ADA does not currently advocate screening for diabetes with these tests.

An important aspect of the ADA classification system is the prognosis for the patients based upon the etiology of DM in a given patient. DM from certain causes such as drug use or endocrine tumors may be completely reversible. DM from other causes such as insulin receptor defects are not reversible, and are often difficult to manage. DM categorized as "other specific types of diabetes" in **Table 17–6** are much rarer than type 1 or type 2 DM. Additional tests that can be helpful in the evaluation of these patients are listed in **Table 17–10**.

TABLE 17–10   Laboratory Evaluation for Selected Other Causes of Diabetes Mellitus

Etiology	Test(s) for Evaluation
Exocrine pancreatic disease	Amylase, lipase
Cushing syndrome	24-h urine-free cortisol
Glucagonoma	Plasma glucagon
Hyperthyroidism	Thyroid-stimulating hormone (TSH)
Hemochromatosis	Iron, ferritin, total iron-binding capacity

HYPOGLYCEMIA

Description

The fasting plasma glucose level in hypoglycemic patients decreases well below the reference range, often to less than 40 mg/dL. Hypoglycemia is most commonly observed in patients being treated for diabetes.

Hypoglycemia is a low FPG state. Symptoms result from activation of the autonomic pathways and from inadequate glucose delivery to the central nervous system. This explains the clinical features of hypoglycemia that are, in the acute form, intermittent episodes of sweating, tachycardia, anxiety, dizziness, slurred speech, double vision, and confusion, with complete recovery on restoration of FPG to normal levels.

The FPG level in hypoglycemic patients decreases well below the reference range, often to less than 40 mg/dL. Hypoglycemia can be divided into reactive postprandial hypoglycemia and fasting hypoglycemia. Overall, hypoglycemia is most commonly observed in patients being treated for diabetes.

- *Reactive hypoglycemia*: Reactive hypoglycemia may occur in patients who have had gastric surgery, in children with inborn errors in enzymes leading to fructose intolerance, or following ethanol consumption. Normally, the ingestion of a high-carbohydrate meal increases the FPG level and stimulates the release of an appropriate amount of insulin. In reactive hypoglycemia, the peak concentration of insulin is inappropriately high and causes the FPG level to decrease below the reference range. Reactive hypoglycemia is diagnosed if there are hypoglycemic symptoms, and an FPG level below 50 mg/dL following a high-carbohydrate meal, with resolution of symptoms after administration of glucose.
- *Fasting hypoglycemia*: Fasting hypoglycemia may result from a variety of causes including drugs (ethanol, sulfonamides, salicylate, and pentamidine), insulinoma and other islet cell tumors, autoantibodies to insulin or its receptor, malignancy (such as sarcoma and hematopoietic tumors), various inborn errors of metabolism, critical illness, and selected endocrine disorders, among other causes. In general, fasting hypoglycemia can be classified into hyperinsulinemic (insulinoma related) and nonhyperinsulinemic types. In addition, patients with insulinomas have high levels of insulin and C-peptide (formed during the conversion of proinsulin to insulin) in equimolar concentrations, providing a reliable indication of insulin synthesis by the beta cells of the pancreas.
- *Surreptitious insulin injection*: Patients who inject themselves with insulin to produce a hypoglycemic state will have the same hypoglycemic symptoms as patients with hypoglycemia from other causes. These patients can be differentiated from patients with insulinomas based on C-peptide level testing, as C-peptide is not present in injectable insulin formulations.
- *Excess administration of sulfonylureas*: As with insulin, patients who have purposely taken sulfonylureas (an oral antidiabetic medication) in greater than prescribed doses suffer from hypoglycemia. Because oral antidiabetic medications are not naturally occurring compounds, a high serum concentration of these medications can reveal excess intake.
- *Impaired liver function*: Hypoglycemia can also occur in the presence of liver disease, often when it is associated with excess alcohol intake or ingestion of certain medications.

Diagnosis

To diagnose hypoglycemia, the following three criteria (known as Whipple's triad) must be met:

- Characteristic signs and symptoms of hypoglycemia
- FPG level below 45 to 50 mg/dL coincident with symptoms
- Symptom reversal within 15 to 45 minutes of the administration of glucose, in the absence of cerebral edema

Providers should be recommended to write their patients suspicious for hypoglycemia, a random glucose test request that they carry around with them as to have a specimen collected when symptomatic.

The 5-hour glucose tolerance test for the diagnosis of hypoglycemia has been disavowed for the last 20 years.

A portion of this chapter appeared previously in Clinical Laboratory Reviews (a publication for the Massachusetts General Hospital physicians) 2000;8:2 and 1999;7:4. It has been included with permission.

SELF-ASSESSMENT QUESTIONS

1. Which one of the following is not a commonly encountered cause for acute pancreatitis?
   A. Ethanol abuse
   B. Gallstones
   C. Hypertriglyceridemia
   D. Hypercholesterolemia

2. Which one of the following choices is least likely to be contributory to a diagnosis of acute pancreatitis?
   A. Serum amylase elevation
   B. Serum lipase elevation
   C. Serum calcium elevation
   D. Amylase/creatinine clearance

3. Which of the following is not a clinical or laboratory manifestation of chronic pancreatitis?
   A. Recurrence of an earlier bout of acute pancreatitis
   B. Impaired glucose tolerance or, in severe cases, diabetes mellitus
   C. A serum amylase level that is significantly higher than in cases of acute pancreatitis
   D. Abdominal x-ray films showing calcifications within the pancreas

4. Which of the following is not true about the pancreatic tumor marker, CA 19-9 antigen?
   A. The sensitivity of the marker for diagnosis of pancreatic neoplasm is proportional to the size of the tumor.
   B. The marker is of little value as a screening test because patients with early-stage tumors have normal levels of CA 19-9.
   C. CA 19-9 is most useful to monitor patient response to therapy.
   D. CA 19-9 is specific for the diagnosis of pancreatic cancer and is normal in other types of cancers.

5. Which of the following pairs is not a correct match?
   A. Tumors of the delta cells of the endocrine pancreas/Glucagonoma
   B. Beta cell tumors of the endocrine pancreas/Insulinoma
   C. Gastrin-secreting tumors of the pancreatic islets/Zollinger–Ellison syndrome
   D. VIP-secreting islet cell tumors/Watery diarrhea, hypokalemia, and achlorhydria (WDHA) syndrome

6. Which one of the following is not a criterion for diagnosis of diabetes mellitus?
   A. Hemoglobin A1C greater than or equal to 6.5%
   B. Fasting plasma glucose greater than or equal to 126 mg/dL
   C. Classic symptoms of hyperglycemia and a random plasma glucose value >150 mg/dL
   D. A 2-hour plasma glucose value >200 mg/dL during an oral glucose tolerance test with the glucose load containing 75 g of glucose dissolved in water

7. The classification of diabetes mellitus established by the American Diabetes Association is based on which of the following?
   A. Whether the patient requires insulin to maintain blood glucose levels
   B. According to the etiology—that is, absolute deficiency of insulin secretion versus varying degrees of insulin resistance
   C. Whether the patient can be managed with oral medications to control blood glucose levels
   D. Whether the patient has developed complications of diabetes such as neuropathy, nephropathy, and retinopathy

8. Among the choices below, which is not a high-risk group that requires screening for diabetes mellitus?
   A. Mothers with newborns >9 lb
   B. Individuals with first-degree relatives with diabetes mellitus
   C. Healthy individuals with a hemoglobin A1C 3% to 5%
   D. Obese individuals weighing more than 120% of ideal body weight

9. Which of the following statements is not true about the requirements for fasting to obtain a fasting blood glucose level?
   A. The patient must have no food intake for 8 to 12 hours before the sample is collected.
   B. The patient cannot drink water while fasting.
   C. The patient must abstain from smoking and taking medications.
   D. An acute illness within the previous 8 weeks is a relative contraindication to performing a fasting blood glucose test.

10. One of the statements below about the oral glucose tolerance test is incorrect. Identify the incorrect statement.
    A. The glucose bolus for nonpregnant adults is 75 g of anhydrous glucose dissolved in 10 to 12 oz of water.
    B. Only two specimens are required—a fasting specimen and a sample collected 2 hours after the bolus of glucose.

C. A 2-hour postbolus plasma glucose level of >200 mg/dL is diagnostic of diabetes mellitus.

D. A 2-hour postbolus plasma glucose level of >80 mg/dL but <200 mg/dL defines a patient with impaired glucose tolerance.

11. The hemoglobin A1C concentration is a reflection of glucose values over which of the preceding periods of time prior to sample collection?

A. 1 to 2 weeks

B. 2 to 4 weeks

C. 8 to 12 weeks

D. 12 to 16 weeks

12. What value for hemoglobin A1C below represents tight glycemic control in type 1 diabetic patients and is associated with lowering the risk for the development and progression of microvascular disease?

A. <6.5%

B. <8.5%

C. <10.5%

D. <12.5%

13. Which of the following statements below regarding gestational diabetes mellitus is not true?

A. Glucose intolerance unrecognized before pregnancy, but initially recognized during pregnancy, qualifies for a diagnosis of gestational diabetes mellitus.

B. Complications of untreated gestational diabetes mellitus include macrosomia, intrauterine fetal demise, and pulmonary immaturity.

C. Approximately 1 in 1000 pregnancies in the United States is complicated by gestational diabetes mellitus.

D. Gestational diabetes mellitus usually develops late in the second or in the third trimester when it occurs for the first time during a pregnancy.

14. All but one of the following choices is part of the laboratory evaluation for gestational diabetes mellitus. Identify the choice which is not part of the evaluation.

A. A screening oral glucose tolerance test during pregnancy with a 50 g glucose bolus.

B. A confirmatory oral glucose tolerance test during pregnancy with a 100 g glucose load for patients with an abnormal screening oral glucose tolerance test.

C. A follow-up postpartum fasting plasma glucose test for patients who have had gestational diabetes mellitus, performed at 6 months after delivery and every 3 years postpartum.

D. A fasting plasma glucose level for the neonate before the age of 6 months.

15. Which of the following is an unlikely cause for hypoglycemia?

A. A reaction to a high carbohydrate meal, with blood glucose values <50 mg/dL, and resolution of symptoms after administration of glucose

B. Insulinoma and other islet cell tumors

C. Inadequate insulin administration for patient with diabetes mellitus

D. Surreptitious insulin injection with decreased levels of C-peptide

16. To diagnose hypoglycemia, three criteria, known as Whipple triad, must be met. Which one of the following choices is not part of Whipple triad?

A. A value for hemoglobin A1C <6.5%

B. Characteristic signs and symptoms of hypoglycemia

C. Coincident with symptoms of hypoglycemia, a blood glucose level <45 mg/dL

D. In the absence of cerebral edema, reversal of symptoms within 15 to 45 minutes of the administration of glucose

FURTHER READING

Alter D, Deines G. Tight glycemic control and point-of-care testing. *Clin Lab Med.* 2009;29:511–512.

American Diabetes Association. Diagnosis and classification of diabetes mellitus. *Diabetes Care.* 2013;36:S11–S66.

American Diabetes Association. 2. Classification and diagnosis of diabetes. *Diabetes Care.* 2017;40:S11–S24.

Ballehaninna UK, Chamberlain RS. The clinical utility of serum CA 19-9 in the diagnosis, prognosis and management of pancreatic adenocarcinoma: an evidence based appraisal. *J Gastrointest Oncol.* 2012;3:105–119.

Cowie CC. Full accounting of diabetes and pre-diabetes in the U.S. population in 1988–1994 and 2005–2006. *Diabetes Care.* 2009;33:S287–S294.

Diabetes Control and Complications Trial Research Group. The effect of intensive treatment of diabetes on the development and progression of long-term complications in insulin-dependent diabetes mellitus. *N Engl J Med.* 1993;329:977.

Forsmark CE, Vege SS, Wilcox CM. Acute pancreatitis. *N Engl J Med.* 2016;375:1972–1981.

Galli C, Basso D, Plebani M. CA 19-9: handle with care. *Clin Chem Lab Med*. 2013;51:1369–1383.

Haffner SM. Management of dyslipidemia in adults with diabetes. *Diabetes Care*. 1998;21:160.

Kazmierczak SC, et al. Diagnostic accuracy of pancreatic enzymes evaluated by use of multivariate data analysis. *Clin Chem*. 1993;39:1960.

Malesci A, et al. Clinical utility of CA 19-9 test for diagnosing pancreatic carcinoma in patients: a prospective study. *Pancreas*. 1992;7:497.

Meko JB, Norton JA. Management of patients with Zollinger–Ellison syndrome. *Annu Rev Med*. 1995;46:395.

Metzger BE. Summary and recommendations of the fifth international workshop-conference on gestational diabetes mellitus. *Diabetes Care*. 2007;30:S251–S260.

Mounzer R, Whitcomb DC. Genetics of acute and chronic pancreatitis. *Curr Opin Gastroenterol*. 2013;29(5):544-551.

Nathan DM, et al. Translating the A1C assay into estimated average glucose values. *Diabetes Care*. 2008;31:S1473–S1478.

Palmer-Toy DE, Godine J. The role of the laboratory in the diagnosis of diabetes mellitus. *Clin Lab Rev*. 1999;7:4.

Parker SL, et al. Cancer statistics. *CA Cancer J Clin*. 1997;47:5.

Ritts RF, Pitt HA. CA 19-9 in pancreatic cancer. *Surg Oncol Clin North Am*. 1998;7:93.

Rompianesi G, Hann A, Komolafe O, Pereira SP, Davidson BR, Gurusamy KS. Serum amylase and lipase and urinary trypsinogen and amylase for diagnosis of acute pancreatitis. *Cochrane Database Syst Rev*. 2017;21.

Service FJ, Vella A. Hypoglycemia in adults without diabetes mellitus: diagnostic approach. *UpToDate*. Accessed on November 1, 2017.

Service FJ, Vella A, Cryer P. Hypoglycemia in adults: clinical manifestations, definition, and causes. *UpToDate*. Accessed on November 1, 2017.

Shepherd PR, Kahn BB. Glucose transporters and insulin action. *N Engl J Med*. 1999;341:248–257.

Stapleton RD, Heyland DK. Glycemic control and intensive insulin therapy in critical illness. *UpToDate*. Accessed on November 1, 2017.

Staubli SM, Oertli D, Nebiker CA. Laboratory markers predicting severity of acute pancreatitis. *Crit Rev Clin Lab Sci*. 2015; 273-283.

The International Expert Committee. International Expert Committee report on the role of the A1C assay in the diagnosis of diabetes. *Diabetes Care*. 2008;32:1–8.

UK Prospective Diabetes Study Group. Intensive blood-glucose control with sulphonylureas or insulin compared with conventional treatment and risk of complications in patients with type 2 diabetes (UKPDS 33). *Lancet*. 1998;352:837.

The Kidney

William E. Winter

CHAPTER OUTLINE

OVERVIEW OF RENAL DISEASE

The homeostatic roles of the kidney include maintenance and regulation of fluid balance, acid/base and electrolyte balance (e.g., sodium, potassium, chloride, bicarbonate, calcium, phosphate, and magnesium), conservation of glucose, amino acids, and proteins, the excretion of wastes, and the production of hormones such as erythropoietin and 1,25-dihydroxyvitamin D. The renal blood vessels provide blood to the glomerulus and the tubules for the generation of urine. The glomerulus filters blood to create a plasma ultrafiltrate by retaining cells and proteins, whereas the tubules "process" the plasma ultrafiltrate to urine, thereby concentrating wastes such as urea, creatinine, nitrogenous wastes, and hydrogen ions.

Renal disease is suggested by any of the following findings:

1. Nonspecific symptoms of malaise, headache, visual disturbances, nausea, or vomiting (e.g., many of these findings suggest uremia or hypertension [see below]).
2. Flank pain (e.g., from pyelonephritis), pain that radiates to the groin from the flank (e.g., from ureteral colic as a result of nephrolithiasis), or simple dysuria (e.g., from a lower urinary tract infection).
3. A reduction in the volume of urine output. In adults, oliguria, a pathologically reduced urine output, is defined as less than 500 mL of urine produced per day. Anuria, which is essentially absent urine production, is defined in adults as less than 100 mL of urine produced per day. In infants, oliguria can be defined as urine output of less than 1 mL/kg/h, and in children older than infants, oliguria is defined as urine output of less than 0.5 mL/kg/h.

4. Hematuria, red blood cell casts, white blood cell casts, proteinuria, proteinaceous casts, pyuria, or other abnormalities on urinalysis.
5. Discolored or malodorous urine (e.g., from a urinary tract infection).
6. Elevations in the plasma or serum concentrations of creatinine or blood urea nitrogen (BUN).
7. Malar rash (e.g., from systemic lupus erythematosus).
8. Hypertension.
9. Otherwise unexplained hypokalemia or hyperkalemia, hypocalcemia, hypophosphatemia or hyperphosphatemia, pathologic fractures, hypomagnesemia, acidosis, anemia, edema, or bleeding.

Renal function should be evaluated when patients are taking drugs that can damage the kidney (e.g., gentamicin) or drugs whose metabolism and/or excretion is dependent on the kidney (e.g., low molecular weight heparin).

Nitrogen retention, as shown by an elevated BUN concentration, is termed "azotemia." Azotemia can be classified as prerenal, renal, or postrenal. Prerenal azotemia refers to conditions with reduced blood flow to the kidney, thereby reducing urine output and causing the retention of waste products. Examples of prerenal causes of azotemia are congestive heart failure, GI hemorrhage, renal artery stenosis, and severe dehydration.

> Renal azotemia indicates that the kidney itself is dysfunctional. Renal azotemia results from diseases of the renal blood vessels, glomerulus, tubules, or mesangium.

Renal azotemia indicates that the kidney itself is dysfunctional. The number of individual causes of intrinsic renal disease is large. In the broad view, however, renal azotemia results from diseases of the renal blood vessels, glomerulus, tubules, or mesangium. Glomerulonephridites may be the result of a primary process in the kidney (e.g., autoantibodies against the phospholipase A2 receptor causing membranous nephropathy) or a secondary disorder leading to glomerulonephritis (e.g., anti-basement membrane autoantibodies causing Goodpasture syndrome). A biopsy is often necessary to identify the type of glomerulonephritis (e.g., lupus nephritis, acute postinfectious [poststreptococcal] glomerulonephritis, IgA nephropathy, hereditary nephritis, or rapidly progressive glomerulonephritis). The histopathologic characteristics of the different glomerulonephridites and nephropathies are described in textbooks of anatomic pathology (e.g., podocyte effacement in minimal change, "tram-tracks" in membranoproliferative glomerulonephritis, IgA deposition in IgA nephropathy, and "basket weaving" in Alport syndrome). It is worth noting that IgA nephropathy can produce nephritis or nephrotic syndrome. Acute tubular necrosis (aka acute kidney injury) can cause renal failure. This may occur as a result of exposure to a toxin or as a result of ischemic damage to the tubules.

Postrenal azotemia results from an anatomic obstruction to urine flow out of the kidney. The ureter, bladder outlet, or urethra may be obstructed by a stone (e.g., nephrolithiasis), congenital anomaly, inflammatory lesion, or neoplasm.

Among prerenal, intrinsic renal, and postrenal-induced renal failure, the dominant etiology is prerenal.

"Uremia," unlike azotemia, is a clinical term that describes the patient's signs and symptoms when symptomatic end-stage renal failure is present. Findings in uremia include fatigue, headache, restlessness, depression, altered sensorium, nausea, vomiting, diarrhea, hiccups, bleeding, edema, shortness of breath, and pulmonary edema. Left untreated, uremia progresses to coma and death. Renal failure produces a wide variety of adverse clinical and metabolic consequences (**Table 18–1**).

Chronic renal failure is a deterioration or pathological alternation in renal structure or function that persists for more than 3 months. It occurs with progressive renal damage, and is independent of the cause of kidney disease. It is the ultimate consequence of the loss of functioning nephrons. The dominant etiologies of chronic renal failure in adults are multifactorial including diabetes mellitus, hypertension, glomerulonephritis, pyelonephritis/interstitial nephritis, cystic kidney disease, and toxicity from drugs. A significant percentage of patients with chronic renal failure have no known etiology for their disease.

Renal function can be assessed using a variety of clinical laboratory analyses. Acid/base and electrolyte balance is initially assessed by ordering a profile of tests that includes serum or plasma sodium, potassium, chloride, total serum CO_2 (bicarbonate), BUN, creatinine, calcium, and glucose.

A more detailed analysis of acid/base balance would also include a measurement of arterial blood gases (pH, pCO_2, pO_2, and calculated bicarbonate) and urine pH. The effect of erythropoietin is assessed by measuring the patient's hemoglobin, hematocrit, and red blood cell indices.

TABLE 18–1   Selected Consequences of Untreated Renal Failure

Pathophysiology	Immediate Consequences	Later Possible Consequences
Salt and water retention	Hypertension	Heart failure, pulmonary edema
Potassium retention	Hyperkalemia	Cardiac arrhythmias
Phosphate retention	Hypocalcemia Hyperphosphatemia	Secondary hyperparathyroidism with renal osteodystrophy causing osteitis fibrosa cystica
Decreased synthesis of 1,25-dihydroxyvitamin D	Hypocalcemia	Secondary hyperparathyroidism with renal osteodystrophy causing osteitis fibrosa cystica
Decreased production of erythropoietin	Anemia	Reduced delivery of oxygen to the tissues; heart failure
Decreased waste excretion	Azotemia, acidosis	Uremia
Decreased waste excretion	Platelet dysfunction	Bleeding tendency

The kidney's role in producing active vitamin D, that is, 1,25-dihydroxyvitamin D, and controlling phosphate excretion is evaluated, in part, through measurements of serum or plasma calcium and albumin (or ionized calcium), phosphate, and parathyroid hormone (PTH). Measurements of 25-hydroxy vitamin D assess vitamin D stores. 1,25-Dihydroxyvitamin D levels reflect the most active form of vitamin D in the body. However, measurements of 1,25-dihydroxyvitamin D are rarely clinically required.

Urinary tract infections are especially common in females. Females are more prone to urinary tract infections than men because in females the urethra is shorter, and the distance from the urethra to the anus is shorter than in males. Discussion of pathogenic organisms resulting in bacterial infections of the kidney and urinary tract appears in Chapter 5.

CLINICAL LABORATORY PARAMETERS

Creatinine

Creatinine is a breakdown product of creatine and phosphocreatine, also known as creatine phosphate. Creatine is produced in skeletal muscle, the kidney, and the pancreas and is then transported to the tissues, especially the skeletal muscle and brain, via the bloodstream. Within cells, creatine is phosphorylated to phosphocreatine via the enzymatic action of creatine kinase (CK). Phosphocreatine provides a ready, rapid source of energy. For example, phosphocreatine is used as a short-term energy source as required during a sprint.

With an approximate 1% to 2% daily turnover rate, creatine and phosphocreatine are metabolized to creatinine at a fairly constant rate. Therefore, the plasma concentration of creatinine is usually stable day to day. Creatinine can be measured in the clinical laboratory by its ability to form an orange-red-colored product in a chemical reaction with alkaline picric acid. This is the classic Jaffe reaction. Creatinine can also be measured enzymatically using creatininase. Modern alkaline picric acid methods have been improved to minimize interferences by other substances. Nonetheless, at this time creatinine measurements using the picric acid method can be falsely elevated by a number of substances including ketones, glucose, and various drugs, such as cephalosporins and sulfonamides. Using creatininase to measure creatinine, interferences are less common but do occur.

Creatinine is freely filtered. However, 10% of the total excreted creatinine is secreted by the tubules. Negligible amounts of creatinine are reabsorbed. The alkaline picric acid method overestimates serum creatinine by at least 10% because of endogenous positive interferences. Creatininase methods are calibrated to report a creatinine concentration comparable to creatinine measured by the alkaline picric acid method. Therefore, the creatininase methods used to measure serum or plasma creatinine also display a positive bias. Standardization of creatinine measurements among analyzers has become an important goal for laboratory medicine.

The glomerulus is investigated by determining the GFR. GFR is the number of milliliters of body fluid cleared by the kidneys per unit time reported in mL/min.

The creatinine concentration in blood is inversely related to glomerular filtration rate (GFR; see below). If the GFR declines by 50%, the plasma creatinine approximately doubles. The creatinine concentration is directly related to skeletal muscle mass. Creatinine is higher in men than in women, and increases with protein intake and with creatine intake. Creatine is sometimes used as a "nutritional" supplement by body builders or athletes. The clearance of creatinine by the kidney is a suitable estimate of GFR that is universally used by physicians. In the research laboratory, inulin clearance is an accurate method for measuring GFR. Iothalamate may also be used as a bolus or continuous infusion. However, neither inulin nor iothalamate studies are applicable to routine clinical medicine. Also in the research laboratory, renal plasma flow (RPF) can be estimated by measuring *para*-aminohippurate (PAH) clearance. Both the RPF and GFR allow the filtration fraction to be calculated (e.g., the fraction [or percent] of the plasma volume that passes through the kidney per unit time which crosses the glomerular capillary barrier to enter the Bowman space).

The Glomerular Filtration Rate and Creatinine Clearance

Laboratory evaluation of the kidney as discussed in this chapter centers on assessments of glomerular and tubular function. The glomerulus is investigated by determining the GFR. GFR is the number of milliliters of body fluid cleared by the kidneys per unit time reported in mL/min. Ideally, GFR is measured using a substance that is produced by the body at a constant rate that is freely filtered by the glomerulus and is neither secreted nor reabsorbed by the tubules (i.e., inulin). As GFR is reduced, waste retention occurs. Measurable waste products excreted by the kidney include creatinine, urea, and uric acid. With a decline in the GFR, these waste products are retained and their circulating concentrations rise. Measurement of the GFR is a very important assessment of renal function. A steady decline in GFR can serve as a harbinger of eventual end-stage renal disease.

GFR measurements are most commonly based on the clearance of creatinine by the kidney. This entails a serum or plasma creatinine measurement and a concurrent timed urine collection for the measurement of excreted urinary creatinine and urine volume. In individuals aged 18 years and above, an estimate of the GFR (eGFR) can be calculated solely from the serum creatinine and various patient parameters such as age, sex, and ethnicity.

A complete urine collection is essential for an accurate determination of the creatinine clearance because the equation contains a measurement of urine volume. The blood sample for serum creatinine is usually collected at the beginning of the timed urine collection. The clearance is expressed in terms of volume of fluid cleared per unit time (e.g., mL/min).

The basic formula for creatinine clearance is as follows (serum creatinine and plasma creatinine are used interchangeably in the formulae):

> GFR measurements are most commonly based on the clearance of creatinine by the kidney. This entails a serum or plasma creatinine measurement and a concurrent timed urine collection for the measurement of excreted urinary creatinine and urine volume.

$$\frac{\text{Urine creatinine}}{\text{Serum creatinine}} \times \frac{\text{Urine volume (mL)}}{\text{Collection time (minute)}}$$

The clearance can be corrected for the patient's body surface area to be compared with a standard body surface area of 1.73 m².

When corrected for body surface area, the formula for creatinine clearance is as follows:

$$\frac{\text{Urine creatinine}}{\text{Serum creatinine}} \times \frac{\text{Urine volume (mL)}}{\text{Collection time (minute)}} \times \frac{1.73}{\text{Body surface area (m}^2)}$$

For creatinine clearance (see the above formula), a 12- or 24-hour urine specimen is collected.

The GFR in persons aged 18 years and above can be reliably estimated (also known as the eGFR [estimated GFR]) solely from the patient's serum creatinine, age, gender, and ethnicity (e.g., African American or non-African American). The use of the modification of diet in renal disease (MDRD) equation, which is:

$$eGFR = 186(S_{Cr})^{-1.154} \times (Age)^{-0.203} \times F$$

TABLE 18–2   National Kidney Foundation Definitions of Kidney Damage Relative to the Glomerular Filtration Rate (GFR)

Stage	GFR	Comment
0	≥90	Normal kidney function and no proteinuria
1	≥90	Kidney damage despite a normal or increased GFR
2	60–89	Mildly decreased GFR with evidence of kidney damage
3	30–59	Moderately decreased GFR
4	15–29	Severely decreased GFR
5	<15	Renal failure and dialysis or transplant needed

GFR is reported in mL/min/1.73 m².

where $F = 0.742$ for females and $F = 1.210$ for African Americans, provides GFR estimates comparable to measured creatinine clearance when the GFR is less than 60 mL/min/1.73 m². Because of difficulties in obtaining a complete timed urine collection, the National Kidney Foundation (NKF) advises that eGFR be used in place of creatinine clearance measurements when the GFR is between 15 and 60 mL/min/1.73 m². It is not presently advised that eGFR be calculated in children because pediatric equations are not as well validated, unlike the MDRD equation that has been well validated in adults.

The MDRD equation provides eGFR determinations that are reliable between 15 and 60 mL/min/1.73 m². However, below 15 mL/min/1.73 m² and above 60 mL/min/1.73 m², GFR should be estimated using the traditional creatinine clearance measurement. The lower limit of the reference range for GFR is 90 mL/min/1.73 m². However, the upper limit of the reportable eGFR is 60 mL/min/1.73 m². Therefore, there is a "gray" zone between the upper limit of the reportable eGFR and the lower limit of the reference interval (90 mL/min/1.73 m²). Therefore, it is practical to report eGFR values greater than 60 mL/min/1.73 m² as simply "greater than 60 mL/min/1.73 m²" with a comment that "the lower limit of the reference interval is 90 mL/min/1.73 m²." Concerning drug dosing based on renal function, clinicians should be aware that the eGFR value cannot be substituted for the Cockcroft and Gault equation-calculated renal clearance in determining drug dosages as the two formulas do not give identical results. Some authors suggest that the Chronic Kidney Disease Epidemiology Collaborative formula (CKD-EPI) is superior for estimating renal clearance and possibly in the future the CKD-EPI calculation will replace the Cockcroft and Gault equation.

Many pathologic renal and systemic conditions can reduce the GFR. As GFR declines, creatinine clearance can, however, begin to overestimate GFR. This is because the fraction of the creatinine that is secreted by the tubules becomes a proportionately higher percentage of the urine creatinine excreted as GFR declines. However, since clinical practice is almost always based on assessment of the creatinine clearance, the difference between the "true" GFR and the creatinine clearance as a reflection of the GFR is usually not problematic when making clinical judgments.

The development of renal impairment is frequently unrecognized until late in its course, when intervention is less likely to be successful. Screening for reductions in GFR is championed by the NKF. The NKF provides guidelines for the interpretation of the GFR result (**Table 18–2**). It defines kidney damage as any pathologic kidney abnormality reflected by a marker of damage, as shown in a blood, urine, or imaging study. Kidney damage that is present for more than 3 months is termed "chronic" kidney damage.

The NKF stresses that the creatinine clearance (unlike the eGFR) does provide useful information in estimating the GFR in individuals who have exceptional dietary intakes (such as those on vegetarian diets or those taking creatine supplements) or muscle mass changes (such as people with amputations, malnutrition, or wasting conditions). Creatinine clearance measurements are also valuable when deciding on the initiation of dialysis. This decision is made when the GFR is <15 mL/min/1.73 m² where the eGFR is not reliable at this very low range.

Urea and the Blood Urea Nitrogen

Urea is produced by the liver to create a metabolite of ammonia (nitrogen) that can be excreted in the urine. The nitrogen in ammonia is derived from the deamination of amino acids.

Modern laboratory methods actually measure urea in serum or plasma (and not in whole blood) with back-calculation of the nitrogen content, yet the term "BUN" has persisted.

The initially developed laboratory measurements of urea depended on liberating nitrogen from urea in whole blood. Therefore, the term "BUN" was created. However, modern laboratory methods actually measure urea in serum or plasma (and not whole blood) and back-calculate the nitrogen content, but the term "BUN" has persisted.

Urea is freely filtered by the glomerulus. However, because ~50% of urea is reabsorbed by the tubules, urea clearance greatly underestimates GFR and, therefore, urea clearance is not usually determined. Furthermore, although creatinine production by the body occurs at a fairly constant rate, providing stable serum creatinine concentrations over time (assuming there is no acute disease affecting the kidneys such as acute tubular necrosis), BUN levels can vary considerably. BUN is affected by the patient's state of hydration, protein intake, and the presence of large amounts of blood in the gastrointestinal tract. If a large gastrointestinal hemorrhage occurs, the metabolism of this additional protein originating from red blood cells in the gastrointestinal tract leads to urea production. With a decline in the GFR, BUN rises. Lastly, BUN can decline if there is liver failure, leading to decreased urea production, or when there is malnutrition and amino acids are "conserved" for protein synthesis.

The 24-hour urea excretion in the urine can be used as an assessment of nutritional replacement in malnourished patients. If sufficient nitrogen is present in the diet and utilized by the body, normal levels of urea are excreted in the urine.

The Blood Urea Nitrogen/Creatinine Ratio

If either the creatinine or BUN concentrations are above the upper limit of the reference interval, it is advised that the BUN to creatinine ratio (BUN/Cr) be calculated (**Table 18–3**). The normal BUN/Cr ratio is between 10:1 and 20:1. The ratio is helpful in determining the cause of renal impairment. However, the ratio, by itself, is rather uninformative, without the corresponding measurements of creatinine and BUN, and the assessment of whether these analytes are within or outside their reference intervals.

If the BUN alone or the BUN and creatinine are both elevated, and if the BUN/Cr ratio is 20:1 or higher, prerenal azotemia is likely to be present. Prerenal azotemia results from a reduction in the GFR while the kidney tubules are functioning. The causes of prerenal azotemia include hypovolemia, as from dehydration or hemorrhage, heart failure, or hypoalbuminemia.

The explanation why the BUN rises to a greater extent than creatinine involves two observations: (1) renal tubular secretion of creatinine persists even as GFR declines, opposing what would otherwise be a rise in serum creatinine, and (2) with decreased renal blood flow, the rate of capillary blood flow around the renal tubules is reduced, providing more time for the reabsorption of urea out of the urine into the tubules (returning urea to the circulation), raising the serum or plasma BUN concentration.

When the BUN/Cr ratio is near 10:1 and creatinine and/or BUN are elevated, renal azotemia is likely, assuming that a chronic urinary tract obstruction has been excluded. In cases of renal azotemia, the BUN and creatinine rise proportionate to one another because, in part, tubular dysfunction will not maintain the tubular secretion of creatinine.

In the early phase of postrenal obstruction, the BUN/Cr ratio is ~20:1 because urea is reabsorbed from urine that is "stagnant" in the excretory system because of the anatomic obstruction. Therefore, if the BUN/Cr ratio is elevated at the time of patient presentation, the treating physician is obligated to consider the possibility of an anatomic obstruction to urine flow, as well as prerenal azotemia. If there is persistent urinary tract obstruction, postrenal azotemia can evolve into renal azotemia from damage to the kidneys. Obstruction appears to trigger inflammation in the glomerulus. If renal impairment then supervenes, the BUN/Cr ratio would fall to 10:1, similar to other conditions associated with intrinsic renal disease.

In adults, proteinuria greater than 1 g per day is considered to be very significant clinically. Levels of protein excretion of 3.5 g per day or greater are consistent with the nephrotic syndrome.

TABLE 18–3   Clinical Use of the BUN/Creatinine (Cr) Ratio

	Action
Both BUN and creatinine within the reference range	Do not calculate the BUN/Cr ratio
BUN and/or creatinine above the reference range	Calculate the BUN/Cr ratio (reference range: 10:1–20:1) • ≥20:1 suggests prerenal azotemia or early postrenal azotemia • ≤10:1 suggests renal azotemia or late postrenal azotemia

Urine Protein Quantitation

The general health of the kidney is assessed in part by the measurement of urinary protein excretion. In normal adults, 24-hour urinary protein excretion does not exceed 150 mg. If one assumes that a normal adult urine output is 1500 mL per day and a maximum of 150 mg of protein is excreted per day, the urine protein concentration should not exceed approximately 10 mg/dL. Elevated concentrations of protein in the urine can result from glomerular disease, tubular disease, overflow from elevated concentrations of plasma proteins, such as immunoglobulins or immunoglobulin light chains in patients with myeloma, urinary tract inflammation, as found in interstitial nephritis or urinary tract infection, trauma, or neoplasia.

In adults, proteinuria greater than 1 g per day is considered to be very significant clinically. Levels of protein excretion of 3.5 g per day or greater are consistent with the nephrotic syndrome. The nephrotic syndrome is the clinical syndrome of massive proteinuria ($\geq$3.5 g/day in adults), hypoalbuminemia, edema, and hyperlipidemia. Primary renal diseases causing the nephrotic syndrome include minimal-change disease, focal segmental glomerulosclerosis, membranous nephropathy, membranoproliferative glomerulonephritis, and IgA nephropathy. Secondary causes of nephrosis include diabetes mellitus, amyloidosis, lupus, drugs (e.g., gold, penicillamine, heroin), infections (e.g., malaria, syphilis, HBV, HIV), and malignancy (e.g., carcinoma, melanoma). Nephritis is the clinical syndrome of hypertension, mild edema, mild proteinuria, hematuria, and red blood cell casts (see discussion of casts below).

In children, an elevated level of urinary protein excretion is >4 mg/m^2/h (normal: $\leq$4 mg/m^2/h). Nephrotic range proteinuria in children can be defined as >40 mg/m^2/h. Per day, an elevated urinary protein excretion is >100 mg/m^2 (normal: $\leq$100 mg/m^2) while nephrotic range proteinuria is >1000 mg/m^2. In newborns who normally reabsorb lower quantities of filtered protein, an increased urinary protein excretion is >300 mg/m^2/day (normal: $\leq$300 mg/m^2/day).

The most cost-effective way to initially screen for proteinuria is urine protein dipstick testing. In this semiquantitative system, proteinuria is reported as negative, trace (10–20 mg/dL), 1+ (30 mg/dL), 2+ (100 mg/dL), 3+ (300 mg/dL), or 4+ (1000–2000 mg/dL). Urine dipsticks for protein measurements are relatively insensitive to immunoglobulin light chains and, thus, a negative dipstick does not exclude Bence-Jones (monoclonal light chain) proteinuria. A more accurate measure of proteinuria can be made using a 24-hour urine sample. The urine protein concentration in milligrams per deciliter is multiplied by the urine volume in milliliters per 24 hours yielding milligrams of protein excreted per 24 hours.

Minimal but persistent amounts of albumin excretion in the urine (e.g., microalbuminuria) are associated with diabetic nephropathy and with hypertensive renal damage. For this reason, people with diabetes mellitus are screened for minimal albumin excretion, also known as microalbuminuria. The albumin measurement is carried out using an immunoassay to provide analytical sensitivity, accuracy, and reproducibility. Microalbuminuria can be reported as the albumin-to-creatinine ratio obtained on a random urine sample, the albumin excretion in milligrams per minute on a timed urine sample collection (e.g., a 4-, 6-, or 12-hour collection), or the albumin excretion per 24 hours when a 24-hour urine sample is collected. **Table 18–4** provides an interpretation of microalbumin results.

> Minimal but persistent amounts of albumin in the urine are associated with diabetic nephropathy and with hypertensive renal damage. For this reason, people with diabetes mellitus are screened for minimal albumin excretion, also known as microalbuminuria.

It is recommended that all patients with type 2 diabetes mellitus be tested yearly for microalbuminuria from the time of diagnosis. For type 1 diabetes mellitus patients, testing is recommended to be performed annually beginning 5 years after the diagnosis of diabetes mellitus. Screening can begin with protein dipstick testing. If the dipstick is positive, microalbumin testing can be bypassed and testing should proceed to a 24-hour urine collection for the measurement of urine protein excretion. For patients with a negative dipstick result for proteinuria,

TABLE 18–4   Interpretation of Albumin Excretion in the Urine

	Units	Normal	Microalbuminuria	Clinical Albuminuria
Spot collection	µg/mg Cr	<30	30–299	$\geq$300
Timed urine	µg/min	<20	20–199	$\geq$200
24-Hour urine	mg/24 h	<30	30–299	$\geq$300

Cr, creatinine.

TABLE 18–5   Laboratory and Blood Pressure Findings in Type 1 Diabetic Nephropathy

Stage	GFR	UAE	Dipstick Proteinuria	Blood Pressure
1	Increased	Normal	Transient	Normal
2	Normal	Normal	Negative	Normal
3	Normal	Increased	Negative	± Increased
4	Decreased	Increased	Positive	Increased
5	Severely decreased	Increased	Positive	Severely increased

GFR, glomerular filtration rate; UAE, urinary albumin excretion.

microalbuminuria testing should be performed. If microalbuminuria is detected, a second sample should be obtained within 3 months. If the second sample does not display microalbuminuria, a third, "tie-breaker" sample is obtained. Thus, microalbuminuria must be present in two of two or in two of three samples to classify the patient as having persistent microalbuminuria.

With persistent microalbuminuria, the patient with type 1 diabetes is diagnosed with stage 3 (e.g., incipient) diabetic nephropathy (**Table 18–5**). Stage 1 nephropathy immediately follows the diagnosis of type 1 diabetes mellitus and is characterized by renal hypertrophy and hyperfiltration. These patients have an elevated GFR from the expanded plasma volume induced by hyperosmolality caused by hyperglycemia. With the initiation of insulin treatment, stage 1 resolves but clinically silent histologic changes subsequently occur in the glomerulus with mesangial hypertrophy and thickening of the glomerular basement membrane as observed on electron microscopy. This is stage 2 diabetic nephropathy. With the recognition of incipient nephropathy (stage 3) and intervention with improved glycemic control, as evidenced by a reduction in hemoglobin A1c level, and the administration of antihypertensive drugs (e.g., angiotensin-converting enzyme inhibitors or angiotensin II receptor blockers), further progression to frank diabetic nephropathy can be averted or at least delayed. Proteinuria by dipstick, a falling GFR, and persistent hypertension identify stage 4 diabetic nephropathy. Stage 5 nephropathy is characterized by the development of end-stage renal failure requiring either dialysis or transplantation. Systems for the histologic description of diabetic nephropathy applicable to types 1 and 2 diabetes have been proposed.

Patterns of Proteinuria

When proteinuria is diagnosed, the subsequent diagnostic issues concern the cause of the proteinuria and the structural portion of the kidney that is functionally impaired. The glomerulus normally retains all plasma proteins with a molecular weight of greater than ~100,000 Da (**Table 18–6**). Variable amounts of plasma proteins with molecular weights between ~10,000 and ~100,000 Da are excreted into the urine. This includes albumin with a molecular weight of ~69,000 Da and free immunoglobulin light chains with a molecular weight of ~25,000 Da. Plasma proteins below ~10,000 Da, such as insulin (~5800 Da), are essentially freely filtered by the kidney.

Urine protein electrophoresis (UPE) can identify the following patterns of protein loss: glomerular, tubular, overflow, and nonselective proteinuria. Glomerular proteinuria is characterized by albuminuria and the excretion of beta globulins, notably transferrin. Tubular proteinuria is recognized in UPE by an alpha-2 doublet in addition to increased albumin excretion. Isoforms of alpha-2 microglobulin (a member of the lipocalin family) produce the alpha-2 doublet.

Overflow proteinuria can result from a monoclonal immunoglobulin in high concentration in the plasma that "spills over" into the urine. For example, free monoclonal light chains are visualized on UPE as a band of restricted mobility. Immunofixation electrophoresis (IFE) would then confirm the identity of the "M-spike" as being monoclonal kappa or monoclonal lambda light chains. The light chain loss occurs because the ability of the proximal convoluted tubules to reabsorb filtered protein is exceeded at high levels of proteinuria. With extensive renal injury, intact monoclonal immunoglobulins can be lost. Persistent glomerular proteinuria can injure the

TABLE 18–6   Approximate Molecular Weights of Selected Plasma Proteins

Location on Serum Protein Electrophoresis Gel	Approximate Molecular Weight (kDa)
Prealbumin zone	
Retinol-binding protein (RBP)	21
Transthyretin (aka thyroxine binding prealbumin; TBPA)	54
Albumin zone	
Albumin	69
Alpha-1 globulin zone	
Alpha-1 antitrypsin (A1AT)	54
High-density lipoprotein (HDL)	200–400
Thyroxine-binding globulin (TBG)	54
Alpha-1-acid glycoprotein	40
Prothrombin	72
Alpha fetoprotein (AFP)	69
Alpha-2 globulin zone	
Alpha-2 macroglobulin (A2M)	800
Haptoglobin	86
Ceruloplasmin	160
Antithrombin	58
Erythropoietin (Epo)	38
Beta globulin zone	
Transferrin (Tf)	77
C-reactive protein (CRP)	115–140
Complement component 3 (C3)	185
Beta$_2$-microglobulin (B2M)	12
IgA	170
Gamma globulin zone	
IgM	900
IgG	160

Also see serum protein electrophoresis in Chapters 2 and 3.

tubule, later resulting in a combined glomerular and tubular proteinuria. The excretion of multiple low-molecular-weight proteins that arise as part of the inflammatory acute-phase response can also produce overflow proteinuria where the IFE is negative for monoclonal immunoglobulins in the urine. Nonselective proteinuria, which can occur with various degrees of renal dysfunction, is identified when the UPE pattern is similar to that of serum lacking a prominent alpha-2 doublet, beta peak, or band-of-restricted mobility.

The Fractional Excretion of Sodium as an Indicator of Tubular Function

Tubular dysfunction can result in many abnormalities: glycosuria, amino aciduria, renal tubular acidosis (bicarbonate wasting or failure to generate new bicarbonate), electrolyte wasting (e.g., hyponatremia, hypokalemia, and hypophosphatemia), and tubular proteinuria (see above). A readily available test of the resorptive function of the tubules is the "fractional excretion of sodium (FENa)."

A readily available test of the resorptive function of the tubules is the "fractional excretion of sodium (FENa)." FENa is calculated using creatinine and sodium measurements in serum or plasma and a simultaneously collected "spot" urine.

FENa is calculated using creatinine and sodium measurements in serum or plasma and a simultaneously collected "spot" urine ("spot" = a random urine sample). The equation for the FENa is given as follows (where S_{Na+} = serum sodium and S_{Cr} = serum creatinine, but plasma can be substituted for serum):

$$FENa = \frac{[U_{Na^+}]\,[S_{Cr}]}{[S_{Na^+}]\,[U_{Cr}]} \times 100$$

The unit is percent sodium excreted (%). Normally the FENa is less than 1%. If there is acute tubular disease or injury, such as acute tubular necrosis, sodium wasting will occur and the FENa can exceed 1%. Tubular reabsorption of sodium is 100% minus the FENa. FENa calculations are not valid when patients are treated with diuretics because the diuretic will induce urinary sodium loss. Likewise, FENa is not used in cases of chronic kidney disease.

Urinalysis

> Examination of the physical, chemical, and microscopic contents of urine constitutes urinalysis testing. A urinalysis should complement BUN and creatinine testing in any patient undergoing a renal evaluation.

Examination of the physical, chemical, and microscopic contents of urine constitutes urinalysis testing. The physical characteristics of the urine include its color, clarity, and specific gravity. Chemical analyses of urine include pH and detection of glucose, protein, blood, ketones, bilirubin, urobilinogen, nitrite, and leukocyte esterase. The microscopic examination is an assessment for cells, bacteria, crystals, casts, lipids, and contaminants.

A urinalysis should complement BUN and creatinine testing in any patient undergoing a renal evaluation. If the urine dipstick is completely normal, some laboratories will not perform the microscopic examination.

The clinical significance of positive findings in urinalysis studies is briefly detailed below.

Urine Color and Clarity

> Normal urine is straw-colored. With dehydration, the color intensifies. With higher levels of fluid intake, the straw color is less intense. The color of normal urine is produced largely by urobilin (an intestinal metabolite of bilirubin; aka urochrome) and pigments present in the diet, such as the pigments in vegetables.

Normal urine is straw-colored. With dehydration, the color intensifies. With higher levels of fluid intake, the straw color is less intense. The color of normal urine is produced largely by urobilin (aka urochrome; an intestinal metabolite of bilirubin that undergoes enterohepatic recirculation with renal excretion) and pigments present in the diet, such as the pigments in vegetables. Patients with elevated urine bilirubin or urobilinogen can have urine that is darkly colored, brown, or even green in color. Red urine can be caused by blood (including menstrual blood), beets, various medications (e.g., pyridium; phenolphthalein), or porphobilinogen. Smokey or cloudy red brown urine can result from intact red blood cells in the urine. Pyridinium, bilirubin, or rifampin can cause orange urine. Alkaptonuria (i.e., homogentisic acid excretion in the urine) can produce black urine when the sample is exposed to air.

Unusual urine colors have occasionally been reported. Green urine can result from propofol or from methylene blue which is used to stain lymphatics or to search for fistulae. Indocyanine green and isosulfan blue can also cause green urine. Urinary tract infections from *Pesudomonas aeruginosa*, *Escherichia coli*, *Klebsiella pneumoniae*, *Providencia stuartii*, and enterococcus species can rarely cause purple urine when the urine is alkaline.

Cloudy urine can reflect the presence of crystals, phosphates (e.g., amorphous phosphates present in a cooled normal urine at an alkaline pH), urates (e.g., urates present in a normal cooled urine at an acidic pH), red blood cells, pyuria (white blood cells in the urine), bacteriuria, or lymph (chyluria). Chyluria (e.g., a milky white fluid appearance) results from lymphatic leakage into the kidneys. Infection with *Wuchereria bancrofti* and various noninfectious etiologies (e.g., renal trauma, tumors, congenital lymphatic malformations [e.g., lymphangiomatosis], genetic syndromes [e.g., Turner or Noonan syndrome], and fistulae [e.g., lymphatic to vesical]) can cause chyluria.

Urine pH

Urine pH can be altered by conditions associated with metabolic acidosis or alkalosis. Freshly collected urine specimens should have a pH between 5.0 and 6.5. A urine pH greater than 8.0 suggests delayed analysis or bacterial contamination. Upon standing, an uncapped urine sample loses CO_2, raising the pH ($H^+ + HCO_3^- \leftarrow H_2O + CO_2$). Urease-producing microorganisms can cleave urea liberating ammonia (NH_3) that will form ammonium hydroxide, raising the urine pH ($NH_3 + H_2O \rightarrow NH_4^+ + OH^-$).

A decreased urine pH is the physiological and appropriate renal response to systemic acidosis. Failure to adequately excrete acids into the urine in the setting of a systemic acidosis defines the pathologic condition termed "renal tubular acidosis." An increased urine pH occurs in the presence of systemic alkalosis.

Urine Specific Gravity

Urine specific gravity is defined as the ratio of the weight of urine to the weight of an equal volume of water. It provides an assessment of the capacity of renal tubules to concentrate or to dilute urine. The specific gravity of urine should range between 1.003 and 1.035. The presence of glucose, protein, or blood in the urine can raise the urine specific gravity and invalidate the assessment of urine specific gravity as a marker of urine concentrating ability. In such cases, urine osmolality should be assessed.

Failure to concentrate the urine can indicate tubular disease, central diabetes insipidus (e.g., antidiuretic hormone [ADH] deficiency), or nephrogenic diabetes insipidus (e.g., ADH resistance) that can result from drugs (e.g., lithium), chronic hypokalemia, or chronic hypercalcemia. A urine specific gravity of 1.000 is not physiologically possible and suggests that water was submitted instead of urine. This may be the intention of the person being tested if they wish to avoid drug detection during urine drug screening. The temperature of a fresh "urine" sample and creatinine concentration also help identify diluted urine, or water in place of urine. A very high specific gravity or unphysiological urine pH can suggest that a urine sample was adulterated through the addition of salt or bleach.

Dipstick Testing

The *dipstick for blood* reacts with heme. Heme is detected whenever red blood cells, hemoglobin, and/or myoglobin are present in urine. Therefore, dipstick positivity for blood does not identify whether red blood cells, hemoglobin, or myoglobin are present singly or in combination.

Hematuria refers to blood in the urine. It may be plainly visible (gross hematuria) or red blood cells may only be visible microscopically (microscopic hematuria). On a fresh urine sample, microscopic examination can reveal the presence of red blood cells and/or red blood cell casts. If red blood cell casts are present, nephritis or severe tubular injury is likely. In a fresh urine sample, red blood cells in the absence of casts indicate bleeding into the urinary tract or the presence of a hemorrhagic coagulopathy. Such bleeding can result from infection, inflammation, trauma, tumor, or a stone. Casts are fragile, and therefore they are most likely to be found in a fresh, early morning urine specimen. If red blood cells are present in the urine but sample analysis is delayed, casts can fall apart and cells can lyse. Therefore, immediate analysis of a recently collected urine is best.

In a fresh urine sample lacking red blood cells that tests positive for blood, either hemoglobin or myoglobin is present. Free hemoglobin can enter the urine in cases of intravascular hemolysis. Myoglobin is released with muscle disease or injury. Indeed, trauma can release large amounts of myoglobin into the blood. Both hemoglobin and myoglobin are toxic to the renal tubules.

Hemoglobin and myoglobin can be distinguished by precipitation methods and via centrifugation. In the precipitation methods, saturated ammonium sulfate is added, which precipitates hemoglobin but not myoglobin. Therefore, after precipitation if the dipstick of the supernatant for blood is positive, myoglobin is present. In centrifugation methods, the urine sample is centrifuged after application over a filter that retains hemoglobin but permits myoglobin to enter the infranate. If the infranate is dipstick positive for blood, myoglobin is present. In women of reproductive age, it is important to ensure that urine has not been contaminated with menstrual blood.

Proteinuria was discussed earlier in this chapter. Trace proteinuria can be observed in otherwise normal pregnancies. Trace proteinuria can also be seen with fever, exercise, and prolonged upright posture (aka "orthostatic" proteinuria). Such benign conditions define nonpathologic or "functional" proteinuria. Hemoglobin or myoglobin in urine can produce a positive protein dipstick.

Bacteriuria may be detected by a nitrite test on a urinalysis reagent strip, which is sensitive to the presence of clinically significant urinary bacteria concentrations. However, not all bacteria convert nitrates to nitrites. Also the urine must be retained in the bladder for some hours (approximately 4 hours or more) for this conversion to occur. Bacteriuria is often asymptomatic but a positive test result may reflect bacterial infection nonetheless. It is frequently accompanied by pyuria.

Urine *glucose* is generally not useful to diagnose diabetes mellitus or monitor patients with diabetes mellitus. There is only an approximate association between the level of plasma glucose and urinary glucose, as the renal threshold for glucose varies considerably among different individuals. Normally, glycosuria does not develop until the plasma glucose exceeds 150 to 180 mg/dL. This being said, if glycosuria is detected on a routine urinalysis, diabetes mellitus should be considered as a possible explanation. Trace glycosuria can be observed in normal pregnancies in the absence of diabetes mellitus because there is a reduction in the tubular threshold for the reabsorption of glucose. Glycosuria in the absence of hyperglycemia can indicate a renal tubular disorder including isolated defects in glucose reabsorption (i.e., renal glycosuria resulting from mutations in the sodium-glucose linked transporter 2 [SGLT2 protein encoded by the *SLC5A2* gene; aka solute carrier family 5 member 2; on chromosome 16p11.2]). Many institutions will routinely test urines from children under age 2 using the Benedict's copper reduction reaction in search of non-glucose inborn errors of metabolism such as galactosemia or hereditary fructose intolerance. In these cases, the Benedict's copper reduction reaction is positive and the glucose dipstick is negative.

Bilirubin should not be present in the urine, and when it is detected, it is indicative of extensive hemolysis, liver dysfunction, or biliary obstruction. Bilirubin present in the urine is conjugated, water-soluble bilirubin. See the liver chapter for a further discussion (Chapter 16).

Urinary *urobilinogen* is derived from bilirubin that is degraded by bacteria in the gastrointestinal tract. Urobilinogen then undergoes enterohepatic recirculation to then be excreted in the urine. Therefore, urobilinogen is normally present in urine. Conditions in which there is an elevated urinary urobilinogen include liver disease, because of failure of the liver to remove the urobilinogen from the blood, and hemolytic anemia in which bilirubin production increases the generation of urobilinogen. Complete obstruction of the biliary tract will cause urobilinogen to be absent from the urine. Acholic stools (gray colored) due to the absence of stercobilin (a breakdown product of bilirubin) in the stool also support the diagnosis of a complete obstruction of the biliary tract.

Ketones can appear in the urine of patients who have poorly controlled diabetes mellitus (including diabetic ketoacidosis), although ketones can also appear in stressed hospitalized patients who do not have diabetes mellitus, and in fasting or starving patients.

Urine Microscopy

Urinary casts are formed in the distal convoluted tubules and may be indicators of renal disease. Cellular casts can be formed by red blood cells, white blood cells, or renal tubular (epithelial) cells. Granular casts, which do not contain intact cells, and waxy casts (both derived from degenerating tubular cells) can also be found in patients with kidney disease. Renal tubular cell casts can be observed in cases of acute tubular necrosis (note: abundant squamous cells in the urine suggest that the urine was not a clean-catch sample). Hyaline casts are composed of protein. They can be observed in the absence of disease. Red blood cell casts indicate glomerulonephritis.

Pyuria refers to increased numbers of white blood cells in the microscopic urine sediment. This is often considered to be at least five white blood cells per high-powered field. A test for leukocyte esterase enzyme activity, found in neutrophils, is included on most urinalysis strips and can detect this activity whether the neutrophil is intact or disrupted. White blood cell casts originate in the tubules similar to red blood cell casts. White blood cell casts are consistent with pyelonephritis or noninfectious interstitial inflammation.

Stones and Crystals Found in Urine

Kidney stones are also referred to as nephrolithiasis or urolithiasis. The presence of a kidney stone is often associated with severe pain radiating from the back and/or flank into the groin. Although most stones pass spontaneously, some do not. The size of the stone, among other factors, determines whether the stone will be passed or retained. Stones can form when there is increased excretion of the components found in stones or the urinary volume is decreased, leading to elevated concentrations of urinary components. Calcium, phosphate, and oxalate are the most commonly found chemical constituents in renal stones, and less commonly identified are urate and cysteine stones.

If there is a sufficient amount of stone material for analysis, the composition of the stone can be determined. The value of knowing the composition of the stone is that information may be derived about the contributing factors to its formation and potential future prevention.

If there is a sufficient amount of stone material for analysis, the composition of the stone can be determined. The value of knowing the composition of the stone is that information may be derived about the contributing factors to its formation. This can lead to treatment, sometimes involving dietary modification.

An elevated concentration of calcium in the urine can lead to the generation of calcium oxalate and calcium phosphate stones. An increased concentration of oxalate in the urine can occur in patients who have an excess absorption of dietary oxalate. In Crohn disease, there is increased absorption of oxalate from the ileum. Ethylene glycol poisoning can produce urinary oxalate crystals. Also producing oxalate stones, oxalosis is an inborn error of metabolism that is additionally characterized by renal tubular acidosis, pediatric growth failure, recurrent fractures, progressive renal failure, cardiac arrhythmias, and death before age 20.

Cystine can accumulate in the urine when there is defective transport of cystine out of the urine by the proximal tubules, allowing cystine to reach a concentration at which it becomes insoluble in the urine. Cystinuria also involves defective reabsorption of the dibasic amino acids arginine, ornithine, and lysine. Defects in the *SLC3A1* gene (on chromosome 2p21) encoding solute carrier family 3 member 1 cause cystinuria.

High concentrations of urinary uric acid are found in patients with gout, and such patients are predisposed to form urate stones, particularly when the urine has a pH below 5.4. Stones consisting of calcium carbonate and struvite ($MgNH_4PO_4$) can occur in patients with urinary tract infections, particularly those caused by *Proteus*. Many patients presenting with a kidney stone have no identifiable underlying cause for its formation.

Crystals are frequently observed in a microscopic urine examination, and the majority are normal urinary components. However, in patients predisposed to forming kidney stones, the crystals may provide information that suggests the composition of the stone.

Selected Additional Tests to Evaluate Renal Function

Cystatin C

Cystatin C is a low-molecular-weight protein of ~13,000 Da that is produced by the body at a constant rate. Because cystatin C appears to be cleared solely by the kidney, elevated cystatin C levels are inversely proportional to the GFR. Epidemiologic data demonstrate that increased cystatin C levels are positively correlated with mortality. Because creatinine measurements are readily available (and inexpensive), cystatin C is unlikely to replace creatinine clearance measurements in the near term.

> Many patients presenting with a kidney stone have no identifiable underlying cause for its formation.

Uric Acid

While it is true that uric acid concentrations rise as the GFR declines, uric acid is not a very helpful indicator of GFR. This is because serum uric acid levels vary widely according to diet. High-protein diets elevate uric acid, as does high cellular turnover. Neoplasias with high cellular turnover rates elevate uric acid as does cell death from chemotherapy. Uric acid levels are markedly affected by variation in the rates of production and reabsorption of uric acid, as found in patients with gout.

Calcium, Phosphate, and Parathyroid Hormone

Calcium, phosphate, and bone metabolism are impaired in patients with renal failure. PTH normally stimulates a net decrease in calcium excretion in the urine, as it stimulates calcium reabsorption in the distal tubule. PTH increases phosphate excretion into the urine, as it decreases the loss of calcium into urine. See Chapter 22 for additional information on this topic.

Novel Biomarkers of Acute Kidney Injury

Presently a major goal of nephrology is to identify an early marker of acute kidney injury that will predict the development of acute renal failure. Such marker(s) would be analogous to markers of myocardial necrosis (e.g., cardiac troponin T or cardiac troponin I). Many markers are under investigation including lipocalins (e.g., neutrophil gelatinase-associated lipocalin-2; NGAL), heat shock proteins (e.g., HSP72), interleukins (e.g., IL-18), and a variety of other proteins (e.g., kidney injury molecule-1, cystatin C (as noted above), *N*-acetyl-β-D-glucosaminidase, and liver fatty acid-binding protein). One diagnostics company offers an assay for urinary NGAL on their automated immunoassay platform.

A recent test that has attracted attention is the "Nephrocheck" test for the prediction of acute kidney injury. The Nephrocheck result reflects TIMP-2 (tissue inhibitor of metalloproteinases 2) and IGFBP-7 (insulin-like growth factor-binding protein 7) in the urine. There are no outcome data as of yet to demonstrate that such testing improves patient outcome. Presently, none of these markers are used routinely, and their diagnostic and prognostic values are still under investigation.

SELF-ASSESSMENT QUESTIONS

1. A urine output in adults of <100 mL/d would be classified as which of the following?

    A. Oliguria
    B. Anuria
    C. Dysuria
    D. Hematuria

2. Nitrogen retention results in an elevated blood urea nitrogen concentration and is termed "azotemia." Azotemia can be classified as prerenal, renal, and postrenal. Which one of the following is a cause of prerenal azotemia?

    A. Reduced blood flow to the kidney as a result of renal artery stenosis
    B. Poststreptococcal glomerulonephritis
    C. Nephrolithiasis with obstruction of urinary outflow
    D. Acute tubular necrosis as a result of exposure to a toxin

3. Which of the following descriptions most accurately describes uremia?

    A. A deterioration in renal function that persists for >3 months
    B. Nitrogen retention as a result of kidney dysfunction
    C. A clinical term to describe the patient's signs and symptoms when symptomatic end-stage renal failure is present
    D. A reduction in the volume of urine output

4. Which of the following pairs regarding the consequences of untreated renal failure is an incorrect match?

    A. Hyperkalemia from potassium retention/Cardiac arrhythmias
    B. Decreased production of erythropoietin/Thrombocytopenia
    C. Decreased synthesis of 1,25-dihydroxyvitamin D/Hypocalcemia with hyperparathyroidism
    D. Salt and water retention/Hypertension

5. Which of the following statements about creatinine is not true?

    A. The creatinine concentration in blood is inversely related to the glomerular filtration rate.
    B. Creatinine is higher in females than males.
    C. The creatinine concentration is directly related to skeletal muscle mass.
    D. A suitable estimate of glomerular filtration rate (GFR) is the clearance of creatinine by the kidney.

6. All but one of the following measurements must be made to determine the creatinine clearance. Which of the choices below is not required for the basic formula for creatinine clearance?

    A. Urine creatinine
    B. Serum creatinine
    C. Blood urea nitrogen (BUN)
    D. Collection time in minutes—a 12- or 24-hour urine specimen is collected

7. The glomerular filtration rate (GFR) in persons above the age of 18 years can be reliably estimated. This is known as the eGFR. One of the following choices is not included in the formula to calculate the eGFR. Identify the choice not included in the eGFR formula.

    A. Urine creatinine
    B. Age and gender
    C. Serum creatinine
    D. Ethnicity (African American or non-African American)

8. The determination of eGFR is reliable between 15 and 60 mL/min/1.73 m². However, the lower limit of the reference range for eGFR is 90 mL/min/1.73 m². Which of the following statements is not true with regard to the values for the eGFR?

A. There is a "gray zone" between the upper limit of the reportable eGFR and the lower limit of the reference interval.

B. It is common to report eGFR values as ">60 mL/min/1.73 m²."

C. Values between 60 and 89 mL/min/1.73 m² are not associated with kidney damage.

D. Values for the eGFR less than 15 mL/min/1.73 m² indicate significant renal failure requiring dialysis or transplant.

9. Microalbuminuria is best described by which of the following choices?

A. Minimal albumin excretion, in amounts less than clinical albuminuria

B. Albumin excretion in the urine not associated with renal damage

C. Excretion of albumin over a brief urine collection period

D. Amount of albumin excreted by patients with nephrosis

10. Urine protein electrophoresis can identify patterns of protein loss from glomerular disease, tubular disease, protein overflow, and nonselective proteinuria. Each one has a different group of protein bands on a urine electrophoresis gel. Which one of these four patterns of protein bands is most likely to be present when a urine protein electrophoresis shows a band of restricted mobility, which is confirmed by immunofixation electrophoresis to be an immunoglobulin?

A. Glomerular pattern

B. Tubular pattern

C. Overflow pattern in a multiple myeloma patient

D. Nonselective proteinuria

11. The results of a urinalysis include the following: markedly positive for heme but negative for hematuria. In addition, the dipstick was still positive for blood after the addition of sodium ammonium sulfate. Which of the following clinical scenarios is most compatible with this set of results?

A. Infection in the kidney

B. Trauma from an auto accident with no apparent damage to the kidney

C. Advanced bladder cancer

D. Severe liver disease

12. The results of a urinalysis include the following: markedly positive for leukocyte esterase. On microscopic examination of the urine, white blood cell casts are present in the urine. In addition, the nitrite test on the urine dipstick is positive. Which of the following clinical scenarios is most compatible with this set of results?

A. Infection in the kidney

B. Trauma from an auto accident with no apparent damage to the kidney

C. Advanced bladder cancer

D. Severe liver disease

13. The results of a urinalysis include the following: a positive test for urine bilirubin and a markedly positive result for urinary urobilinogen. In addition, the urine appears to have a dark yellow color. Which of the following clinical scenarios is most compatible with this set of results?

A. Infection in the kidney

B. Trauma from an auto accident with no apparent damage to the kidney

C. Poorly controlled diabetes mellitus

D. Severe liver disease

14. The results of a urinalysis include the following: a positive test for urine protein by dipstick; a positive dipstick test for urine glucose; and a positive dipstick test for urinary ketones. Which of the following clinical scenarios is most compatible with this set of results?

A. Infection in the kidney

B. Trauma from an auto accident with no apparent damage to the kidney

C. Poorly controlled diabetes mellitus

D. Severe liver disease

15. Which one of the following compounds in high concentrations in the urine is least likely to contribute to the formation of urinary stones?

A. Calcium

B. Oxalate

C. Uric acid

D. Lactate

FURTHER READING

Barrera-Chimal J, Bobadilla NA. Are recently reported biomarkers helpful for early and accurate diagnosis of acute kidney injury? *Biomarkers*. 2012;17:385–393.

Beck LH Jr, Bonegio RG, Lambeau G, et al. M-type phospholipase A2 receptor as target antigen in idiopathic membranous nephropathy. *N Engl J Med*. 2009;361:11–21.

Boyer OG. Evaluation of proteinuria in children. Available at: https://www.uptodate.com/contents/evaluation-of-proteinuria-in-children. Accessed December 5, 2017.

Connolly JO, Woolfson RG. A critique of clinical guidelines for detection of individuals with chronic kidney disease. *Nephron Clin Pract*. 2009;111:c69–c73.

Jones GRD. Estimating renal function for drug dosing decisions. *Clin Biochem Rev*. 2011;32:81–88.

Kraut JA, Kurtz I. Metabolic acidosis of CKD: diagnosis, clinical characteristics, and treatment. *Am J Kidney Dis*. 2005;45:978–993.

Lameire N, Vanmassenhove J, Van Biesen W, Vanholder R. The cell cycle biomarkers: promising research, but do not oversell them. *Clin Kidney J*. 2016;9:353–358.

Levey AS, et al. *KDOQI clinical practice guidelines for chronic kidney disease: evaluation, classification, and stratification*. Available at: http://www.kidney.org/professionals/KDOQI/guidelines_ckd/toc.htm. Accessed December 7, 2017.

Miller WG. Reporting estimated GFR: a laboratory perspective. *Am J Kidney Dis*. 2008;52:645–648.

Myers GL, Miller WG, Coresh J, et al. Recommendations for improving serum creatinine measurement: a report from the Laboratory Working Group of the National Kidney Disease Education. *Clin Chem*. 2006;52:5–18.

Polkinghorne KR. Detection and measurement of urinary protein. *Curr Opin Nephrol Hypertens*. 2006;15:625–630.

Prigent A. Monitoring renal function and limitations of renal function tests. *Semin Nucl Med*. 2008;38:32–46.

Tervaert TW, Mooyaart AL, Amann K, et al. Renal Pathology Society. Pathologic classification of diabetic nephropathy. *J Am Soc Nephrol*. 2010;21:556–563.

Thomas L, Huber AR. Renal function—estimation of glomerular filtration rate. *Clin Chem Lab Med*. 2006;44:1295–1302.

Vassalotti JA, et al. Testing for chronic kidney disease: a position statement from the National Kidney Foundation. *Am J Kidney Dis*. 2007;50:169–180.

Zahran A, El-Husseini A, Shoker A. Can cystatin C replace creatinine to estimate glomerular filtration rate? A literature review. *Am J Nephrol*. 2007;27:197–205.

Male Genital Tract[*]

Mark H. Wener and Charles H. Muller

INTRODUCTION

The penis, testes, epididymis, vas deferens, seminal vesicles, and the prostate comprise the male genital tract, and disorders of the urethra and urinary bladder also are a consideration in patients presenting with genital tract symptoms. Circulating markers have been identified for prostate cancer and testicular cancer, and urine biomarkers have been proposed for bladder cancers. A discussion of these tumors and their serum and urine markers is presented in this chapter. Also, laboratory tests are often used in evaluating men with gonadal dysfunction and men who may be

---

*Acknowledgments to Dr. D. Robert Dufour for contribution to earlier versions of this chapter.

subfertile, infertile, or sterile. A summary of these tests and their usage is also provided. The male genital tract is the site of many infectious diseases, a significant proportion of which are sexually transmitted. These are discussed in Chapter 5.

Development of new tumor markers is an active area of research, in part because of ongoing clinical need, and in part because of scientific and technological changes that allow measurement of new biomarkers. Tumor markers most used in clinical practice have consisted of proteins (including glycoproteins) and hormones measured by various immunoassays. Results from measurement of more than one analyte can be combined using various algorithms and formulas to improve clinical associations and predictions. Emerging technologies and basic scientific advancements have led to assays for nucleic acids, including mutated DNA; DNA methylation and other epigenetic changes in DNA associated with malignancy; messenger RNAs that are enriched in tumors; and microRNAs (either free or associated with vesicles) associated with malignancy. Improvement in tumor marker assays has the potential to improve screening, diagnosis, prognostication, treatment selection, and monitoring of malignancy.

PROSTATE CANCER

Description

Cancer of the prostate (CaP) is second only to non-melanoma skin cancer as the most commonly diagnosed cancer in men (over 120 cases/100,000 men), and second only to lung cancer as the most common cause of cancer death in males, with a lifetime risk of 2.5% for a man to die from CaP. The incidence is higher in African American men (about 200/100,000) and the mortality rate is also higher (44/100,000 vs. 19/100,000 in whites). However, most CaP cases are slowly progressive and do not cause major morbidity or lead to death. A major unresolved challenge is differentiating the rapidly progressive and fatal forms of CaP from the indolent forms that do not cause death. Mortality associated with the disease has been decreasing. This has been attributed by some to early detection, although a systematic review of published studies has shown no convincing difference in CaP mortality between those populations that have and those that have not been screened for the disease. Measurement of the serum prostate-specific antigen (PSA) concentration, however, has had substantial impact on increased detection of this cancer.

Prostate-Specific Antigen—Increased in Prostate Cancer and BPH

PSA is a serine protease enzyme (also called human kallikrein 3) synthesized almost exclusively by the prostate and secreted into the seminal fluid. A small amount is also found in the blood. In the blood, PSA is largely bound covalently to enzyme inhibitor proteins such as alpha$_1$-antichymotrypsin and alpha$_2$-macroglobulin, with the bound forms referred to as "complexed PSA." A small fraction of circulating PSA is free (unbound), and remains unbound because free PSA in circulation is largely enzymatically inactive and therefore does not bind to the enzyme inhibitors. The ratio of free PSA/total PSA can be used in the setting of borderline elevated total PSA concentrations as a diagnostic marker for CaP, since a lower proportion of free PSA is generally found in patients with CaP (**Table 19–1**).

PSA levels in blood generally correlate with the size of the prostate: the larger the gland, the higher the PSA concentration. PSA may also increase transiently after a vigorous rectal examination, and after prostate biopsy or surgery. Inflammation and infarction of the prostate can also cause increased PSA, which returns to normal gradually. It is therefore often recommended that elevated PSA levels should be confirmed by repeat measurement (at least 2–3 months apart) before any other action is taken, to exclude one of these insignificant and transient causes of high PSA.

Prostate disease is common in men after the age of 50 years, and by age 70 years the majority of men have some component of prostate disease. The two major diseases of the aging prostate are prostate carcinoma and benign prostatic hyperplasia (BPH). Both CaP and BPH contribute to elevations in serum PSA and increased prostate size. A number of factors have been evaluated to try to distinguish between these causes of increased prostate size and/or increased PSA levels.

TABLE 19–1   Clinical Utility of Serum Tumor Markers for Prostate Cancer and Testicular Cancer

Cancer Purpose	Prostate Cancer: Prostate-specific Antigen (PSA)	Testicular Germ Cell Tumors (LD, AFP, hCG)
Screening	Controversial for men older than 50 years	Not useful
Establishing a diagnosis	Not useful	Can suggest histologic type(s) present, especially for small clusters of one tumor type that may be missed by histology
Indicator of disease extent	If PSA <20 ng/mL, bone metastasis unlikely	Of use in identifying clinically undetectable metastatic disease
Monitoring response to treatment	Useful to monitor success of treatment	Useful; markers should fall to undetectable with successful treatment
Monitoring for recurrence	Useful	Useful

In most laboratories, the PSA threshold considered positive for cancer screening is 4 ng/mL; above that threshold concentration, the positive predictive value for CaP (the likelihood that cancer will be found in a biopsied prostate gland) is about 30%. In general, PSA is increased to a greater extent in CaP than in BPH. The concentration of PSA is rarely >20 ng/mL in BPH, and in only about 10% of cases it is >10 ng/mL, whereas PSA concentrations at those levels are not unusual in the setting of CaP, especially with metastatic disease. A high PSA in a man with a small prostate gland on rectal examination is more worrisome for cancer than a similar PSA value in a person with a very large gland.

PSA has been used for several purposes related to CaP: screening (testing in persons without symptoms or signs of disease), prediction of the course of disease, prediction of the stage of disease, and follow-up after treatment. It is widely used and accepted as a tumor marker following radical prostatectomy, after which a detectable and rising serum PSA indicates recurrence of CaP from metastatic cells. The controversial use of PSA measurements is in screening. The topic has been reviewed recently in preparation of recommendations from the United States Preventive Services Task Force (USPSTF). Two large randomized trials have been published with long-term outcomes of CaP screening, and three large randomized trials have evaluated the effect of active treatment of CaP with radical prostatectomy or irradiation, versus watchful waiting or active surveillance for cancer. The US Prostate, Lung, Colorectal, and Ovarian Cancer Screening Trial showed no effect on prostate cancer-specific or all-cause mortality after a median follow-up of 14.8 years. The European Randomized Study of Screening for Prostate Cancer found that screening was associated with statistically significant reduced cancer-specific mortality in men aged 55 to 69 years; after a median follow-up of 13 years, mortality was 4.3 per 10,000 person-years in the screened group versus 5.4 in the usual care group. A study based in the United Kingdom found that active treatment with radical prostatectomy or irradiation, in comparison with active surveillance of screened patients, did not change mortality after 10 years. A Scandinavian study found a statistically significant effect of treatment on prostate cancer-specific mortality and all-cause mortality after 13 years of follow-up. A US-based randomized treatment trial showed no effect on overall mortality after 10 years. In summary, if there are benefits of PSA screening and early treatment of CaP, the benefits are relatively small and take over a decade to be significant.

Because of the side effects of diagnostic biopsy and complications of treatment of prostate cancer and the minimal, if any, survival benefit from CaP screening, in 2012, the USPSTF recommended that men *not* be screened for CaP with PSA testing. The updated and revised 2015 draft guideline from the USPSTF changed the recommendation: men ages 55 to 69 should individualize the decision to undergo CaP screening, via shared decision making between providers and patients. The current USPSTF draft guidelines for CaP screening are in accord with guidelines from most other professional groups, including the American Urological Association (AUA) and the American College of Physicians (ACP), which recommend individualized decision making with information provided to the patient about both potential risks and benefits, and that screening might be reasonably offered to men between ages 50 (for the ACP) or 55 (for the AUA) and age 69.

PSA has been used for several purposes related to prostate cancer: screening (testing in persons without symptoms or signs of disease), prediction of the course of disease, prediction of the stage of disease, and follow-up after treatment. The most controversial use of PSA measurements is in screening.

It should be noted that PSA is not highly sensitive for detecting cancer. It is estimated that only about 50% to 60% of those with localized and potentially curable cancer have increased PSA, and recent studies have found that many patients with less well-differentiated prostate cancers actually have PSA values as low as 1 ng/mL. Unfortunately, PSA also is not specific for cancer, so the majority of patients with positive tests in a typical screened population will not have cancer. Data analysis and synthesis by the USPSTF indicates that an estimated 28 to 88 men would need to be invited for screening to detect one additional case of CaP, and between 140 and 390 would need to be screened to avoid one death from CaP. It is estimated that 20% to 50% of men diagnosed with cancer via PSA screening would be "overdiagnosed"; that is, their cancers would not be symptomatic during their lifetime, and significant numbers would have side effects from the biopsy or the prostatectomy.

Limited evidence suggests that the rate of rise in PSA (termed PSA velocity) can predict more aggressive cancers. A review of published studies found that men with more rapid rises in PSA (an increase of more than 0.35 ng/mL per year 10 years before a definitive diagnosis, or a rise >2 ng/mL in the year before a definitive diagnosis) were far more likely to have recurrence after surgery and to die from cancer than those with more slowly rising PSA. In men who have decided to not have surgery, the rate of rise of PSA was also found to be predictive; if the PSA doubling time was less than 3 years, the likelihood of locally progressive disease was high, while it was very low for those whose PSA increased less than twofold over 10 years. More studies will be needed to confirm these findings and to determine whether this information can be useful in determining treatment.

PSA measurement is of some use in the initial staging of a patient with CaP. In general, the higher the PSA, the less likely that cancer is localized to the prostate and the more likely that it has spread. Distant metastases are rare in persons with PSA <20 ng/mL, so performance of imaging studies of bone (the most common site of metastasis) for preoperative staging of cancer has little benefit in those with lower PSA values, unless clinical features such as bone pain suggest otherwise. Guidelines from the National Comprehensive Cancer Network (NCCN) include PSA concentrations as one of the factors used to assign risk groups in newly diagnosed CaP, with PSA <10 ng/mL having low or very low risk for metastatic disease, >20 ng/mL as high risk, and PSA 10 to 20 ng/mL as intermediate risk.

PSA concentrations are also used as part of active surveillance in patients who elect not to have definitive therapy after the initial diagnosis of localized CaP. NCCN guidelines include measurement of PSA concentrations as frequently as every 6 months as a component of active surveillance. The most widely accepted use of PSA is to monitor patients after treatment. Since about 99% of prostate cancers produce PSA, and since PSA is made almost solely in the prostate, successful surgical removal of the gland (and cancer) should result in a serum PSA less than 0.1 ng/mL by 3 months after surgery. Failure of PSA to become <0.1 ng/mL following prostatectomy indicates residual cancer that was not removed by surgery. With recurrence of cancer, PSA levels increase up to a year and a half before clinical evidence of recurrent cancer, allowing treatment of persons with rising PSA before their clinical condition deteriorates. With radiation therapy, PSA typically will fall to normal (usually to <1 ng/mL by 1 year after completion of radiation) with successful treatment, but will usually not be undetectable. Because CaP responds to androgens, removal of the testes and the use of drugs that block androgen production are widely used to treat metastatic CaP. The production of PSA is androgen dependent. Rarely, PSA levels will fall dramatically with androgen deprivation even though there is little or no change in the amount of tumor. In most cases, though, PSA is a reliable marker of tumor response to androgen deprivation as a treatment for CaP.

Other biomarkers and combinations of biomarkers have been proposed to improve ability to diagnose CaP and to distinguish more aggressive CaP from CaP that is likely to run a more indolent course. Some laboratories perform tests for free PSA (fPSA, a circulating PSA form detected by PSA reagents and not bound to another protein), since the ratio of free PSA to total PSA is lower in the setting of CaP than in patients with elevated PSA due to benign disease. For example, if the total PSA is 4 to 10 ng/mL and the free PSA is <10% of the total PSA, a biopsy would be indicated, whereas cancer would be less likely if the fPSA is >25%. Among other markers that have been proposed includes the 4K score, which involves a calculated score based on measurement of four kallikrein proteins markers: immunoassay-detected total PSA (tPSA, kallikrein-3), fPSA, intact PSA, and kallikrein-related peptidase 2 (another member of the kallikrein protein family). The Prostate Health Index (PHI) test involves measurement of tPSA, fPSA, and (-2) proPSA (a PSA precursor protein) in a proprietary algorithm. Another proposed CaP biomarker known as CaP antigen 3 (PCA3) is a form of noncoding messenger RNA that is over-expressed in CaP cells. After digital rectal exam, PCA3 can be measured in the urine and typically reported as a ratio of PCA3 to PSA mRNA. None of these biomarkers or panels are recommended in standard guidelines advising approaches to screen or monitor CaP, although occasionally the tests may be ordered in situations in which the decision for prostate biopsy is more challenging.

There is an unmet clinical need to find a reliable noninvasive method to screen for those prostate cancers that are likely to cause metastatic disease and death, in contrast to the majority of cancers that run an indolent course. Ongoing investigations are underway in hopes of finding such markers.

"Liquid Biopsy" and Circulating Tumor DNA (ctDNA)

Increasingly, the choices of medical therapy of cancers may depend on finding the driver DNA mutations that are associated with a given case and that may be associated with sensitivity or resistance to particular treatments. Usually that analysis is performed on tissue specimens. In CaP, this kind of analysis is most likely to be useful in patients with metastatic castration-resistant prostate cancer, that is, after usual therapies of metastatic disease have failed.

Obtaining biopsies for analysis is invasive and may be challenging, especially if metastases are small, are located in inaccessible locations, or are unsafe to biopsy. A promising approach to avoid the need for tissue biopsy is to determine the DNA sequence of ctDNA, which is contained within the cell-free DNA (cfDNA) within plasma. Recent data from retrospective studies suggests that there is good concordance between ctDNA and matched metastatic tissue biopsy in patients with metastatic CaP, suggesting that this form of "liquid biopsy" may be appropriate in patients with CaP. Furthermore, detection of ctDNA in some instances may be more sensitive than tissue biopsy analyses because of tumor site heterogeneity: mutations from multiple sites may be detectable using ctDNA, whereas only mutations at the site biopsied are detectable using conventional tissue.

Several methods of DNA amplification have been employed successfully to detect ctDNA. In evaluation of non-small cell lung cancers, assay of ctDNA has become available with an FDA-approved assay and is increasingly being used. It is likely that assays for ctDNA will be applied in patients with CaP, to search for actionable mutations that can help guide targeted, individualized treatment for patients with metastatic disease.

TESTICULAR CANCER

Description

The two major categories of testicular tumors are germ cell tumors (which include seminomas and nonseminomatous germ cell tumors [NSGCT]) and sex cord or stromal tumors (mainly Leydig cell and Sertoli cell tumors). Seminomas and NSGCT comprise more than 90% of testicular cancers. Most persons with germ cell tumors have a mixture of histologic varieties. Testicular germ cell tumors have a peak incidence in 15- to 34-year-old males, and are the most common type of tumor found in men of that age group. Testicular cancer is most commonly identified by finding an enlarged testicle during a routine physical exam or by a man on self-examination. If an ultrasound examination confirms the presence of an intratesticular mass, surgery is usually performed quickly to remove the testicle, its adnexa, and a long segment of the spermatic cord (radical orchiectomy). The diagnosis of testicular cancer, like most other cancers, is made by histopathologic examination of the testicle.

More than 90% of testicular cancers arise from germ cell tumors. Germ cell tumors often produce substances that can be used as tumor markers to evaluate the patient for complete removal of the tumor, detect recurrent cancer, and monitor treatment for any residual or recurrent tumor.

Diagnosis

Germ cell tumors often produce proteins that can be used as tumor markers to evaluate the patient for complete removal of the tumor, detect recurrent cancer, and monitor treatment for any residual or recurrent tumor. The three important serum tumor markers for testicular cancers are human chorionic gonadotropin (hCG), alpha-fetoprotein (AFP), and lactate dehydrogenase (LD). LD elevation, while present in about 50% of seminomas and 10% of NSGCT, is not specific, since damage to erythrocytes, muscle, liver, cardiac, and other tissues can raise LD levels in the blood. Elevation of the LD-1 isoenzyme is characteristic of testicular tumors, but LD-1 is also elevated after myocardial infarction. Seminoma is associated with increased levels of hCG, but the increased levels are seen in only about 15% of seminoma cases. Pure seminomas do not produce AFP, but mixed tumors that contain predominantly seminomatous components may produce AFP. In NSGCT, approximately 85% to 90% of cases have at least one of the three tumor markers elevated. Yolk sac tumors produce AFP, a normal product of the fetal liver and yolk sac, in about 90% of cases. Choriocarcinoma, a malignant tumor resembling the placental cells, produces hCG in close to 100% of cases. As is generally true for circulating tumor markers, measurement of these proteins is most useful for monitoring recurrence of disease or as a measure of response to therapy. Neither hCG nor AFP is useful in screening patients for testicular tumors, and they have a limited but helpful role in establishing the diagnosis. Higher levels of hCG and LD-1 at the time of diagnosis are associated with more aggressive cancers and, overall, a less favorable outcome, and are therefore included in staging classifications for testicular cancer cases. In order to determine whether a testicular tumor is associated with elevated tumor marker levels, it is recommended that baseline levels of these three markers be measured prior to surgery, since levels may fall quickly after surgery.

hCG, LD, and AFP are significantly affected by diseases in other organs. LD is found in all cells. Therefore, damage to any cell can cause increased LD. Since red blood cells contain LD, a sample collected for LD measurement in which there is red blood cell hemolysis will show an elevated LD, with much of the LD originating from red blood cells. This is also particularly problematic in the setting of chemotherapy, where transient LD increases occur from the cell damage expected from chemotherapy treatment. AFP is also produced by hepatocytes, as discussed in Chapter 16. Injury to the liver, as occurs with acute or chronic hepatitis, also commonly causes mild-to-moderate increases in AFP that can lead to suspicion of recurrent testicular carcinoma.

BLADDER CANCER

Cancer of the urinary bladder has an overall incidence of about 20/100,000 in the United States, with mortality approximately 4.4 per 100,000. More common in an aging population, strongly associated with tobacco use and other environmental exposures, and more common in men than women, it is the fourth most frequent non-skin cancer in men, and is the eighth most common cause of cancer deaths in men. Worldwide, it is the ninth most common form of carcinoma. For unclear reasons, it is more common and has a higher death rate in Americans of European origin than in African Americans. Patients typically present with painless hematuria, and cystoscopy with biopsy typically leads to diagnosis. In North America and Europe, the most common histologic form of bladder cancer is urothelial/transitional cell carcinoma, but squamous cell carcinoma also exits and is more common in some parts of the world.

Urine specimens offer the hope to screen for bladder cancer or to detect recurrence. The traditional approach is to use cytology to detect sloughed cancer cells in urine, which has an overall sensitivity of about 20% for low-grade cancer, and 80% to 90% for high-grade cancers. A variety of other biomarkers have been investigated (**Table 19–2**). None of the available methods has been recommended in standard guidelines for diagnosis of bladder cancer or detection of recurrence because of limited sensitivity and/or specificity. All of the markers are more likely to be useful in the setting of more aggressive, high-grade bladder tumors, rather than more indolent forms of malignancy.

MALE GONADAL DYSFUNCTION

Description

While complete gonadal failure in men is rare (and is discussed more fully in Chapter 22), partial androgen deficiency is common with advancing age in men. This has also sometimes been referred to as "andropause," and considered by some to be analogous to menopause, the age-related gonadal failure in women. There are a number of differences between age-related

TABLE 19-2   **Potential Bladder Cancer Markers**

Urine Analyte	Method Example	Sensitivity	Specificity
Tumor cells in urine	Cytology	Overall High grade (53–90%) Low-grade (7–17%)	Overall High-grade (90–98%) Low-grade (50–75%)
Soluble uroepithelial cell protein antigen	BTA (bladder tumor antigen, Polymedco); complement factor H or Factor H-related proteins	Overall 64–65% 50–80%	Overall 74–77%
Soluble nuclear protein from tumor	NMP-22 (nuclear mitotic apparatus protein 22, Alere, Matritech), marker of urothelial cell death	Overall 58–69% Invasive disease 90% Noninvasive 50%	Overall 77–88%
Aneuploidy in exfoliated cancer cells	FISH, UroVysion (Abbott), aneuploidy for chromosome 3, 7, 17; and 9p21 loss	Overall 63% Low-grade cancer: 41%	Overall 87%
Protein antigens in exfoliated tumor cell	Immunohistochemistry, ImmunoCyt (Scimedx), glycosylated CEA, other mucins	Overall 78%	Overall 78%
Cancer-related mRNA in urine	CxBladder (Pacific Edge), 4 mRNA markers	Overall 82%	Overall 85%

Sensitivities and specificities adapted from Chou R, et al. *Ann Int Med.* 2015;163:922–931, and other sources.

declines in gonadal function in men and women, however. While gonadal failure in aging is inevitable in women, not all men develop low levels of testosterone. Menopause typically occurs between the mid-40s and mid-50s, whereas relative androgen deficiency develops over a much broader age range in men. Estrogen and progesterone levels fall to extremely low levels in women and are accompanied by high gonadotropin (FSH and LH) levels. However, partial androgen deficiency in men is associated with mildly decreased testosterone levels and is usually not associated with abnormally high gonadotropin levels. According to the Endocrine Society consensus guidelines based on testosterone levels in a reference population of healthy young men, only 7% of men in their 40s have low androgen levels. However, the figure rises to 30% of men in their 50s, almost half of men in their 60s, and to 90% of men in their 80s. Current guidelines indicate that the reference ("normal") range of testosterone should be based on the values found in healthy young men, despite some concerns that classifying such a large proportion of testosterone values seen in older men as abnormal might encourage inappropriate or unneeded supplemental androgen therapy.

As in women, routine use of hormone replacement in men is controversial. Androgens increase muscle and bone mass, and may protect against falls and bone fractures. Androgen deficiency can cause mood changes and sexual dysfunction, both of which may respond to androgen treatment. On the negative side, however, androgens are involved in the pathogenesis of both BPH and prostate cancer, may lead to a fall in sperm count, and cause undesirable changes in blood lipids and increased coronary atherosclerotic plaque volume, which may increase the risk of myocardial infarction and stroke. Limited data on safety and effectiveness of androgen replacement are available, and some efficacy that had been anticipated by androgen supplementation has not been shown in controlled trials. For example, administration of testosterone together with sildenafil was not better than sildenafil alone in improving erectile dysfunction. Long-term effects of testosterone therapy on the risk of prostate-related and cardiovascular-related adverse events remain unknown. On the other hand, some evidence suggests that administration of testosterone improves longevity in older men.

> 7% of men in their 40s have low androgen levels. However, the figure rises to 30% of men in their 50s, almost half of those in their 60s, and to 90% of men in their 80s.

Diagnosis

Laboratory testing for partial androgen deficiency generally begins with measurement of serum testosterone. The United States Centers for Disease Control and Prevention (CDC) has led an international effort to improve harmonization of testosterone assays, but those efforts are incomplete, leading to substantial variation in testosterone testing results. Assays based on liquid chromatography/mass spectrometry (LC/MS), rather than immunoassays, are used as the reference and ideal methodology for measuring these steroid hormones, but equivalence and harmonization is challenging even between LC/MS methods. In the recently conducted study with harmonized assays, the normal (2.5%ile to 97.5%ile reference range) in non-obese healthy American and European men age 19 to 39 years was determined to be 264 to 916 ng/dL. Androgen deficiency is unlikely to be present if the total testosterone is >400 ng/dL.

Free testosterone, not bound to proteins, contributes significantly more to the biological effects of testosterone than does protein-bound testosterone. A problem with interpretation of total testosterone levels is that changes in the level of testosterone-binding proteins are common. The major testosterone-binding protein, sex hormone-binding globulin (SHBG), is increased by androgen deficiency, but decreased by obesity, both common problems in older men. Testosterone also binds to a lesser degree to serum albumin. Testosterone bound to albumin may dissociate and become unbound, and thus albumin-bound testosterone contributes partially to the biological effects of testosterone. Reported concentrations of testosterone can thus be total testosterone, free testosterone, or bioavailable testosterone (the free testosterone plus the albumin-bound fraction). All these measures are correlated, but determining the free or bioavailable testosterone may be most helpful in those with testosterone levels between 200 and 400 ng/dL.

Transient decreases in testosterone and gonadotropin levels are commonly seen in persons who are acutely ill. Testing of gonadal function should be avoided in hospitalized individuals for that reason. Certain medications, as well as opiates and ethanol, can cause transient decreases as well. Testosterone secretion has a circadian rhythm, with higher levels in the morning, and lower concentrations in the afternoon and evening. The reference ranges for expected values of testosterone are generally based on morning samples in healthy, non-obese men. If treatment decisions are to be based on androgen concentrations, testosterone blood tests should be drawn in the morning, but fasting is not required. Since testosterone serum concentrations are variable, low concentrations should be confirmed by repeat testing before initiating therapy.

In young men with low testosterone, guidelines suggest measurement of LH. Generally, FSH follows LH and does not add additional information. It is expected that LH levels are usually within the reference range in age-related partial androgen deficiency. Very low levels of LH suggest a pituitary or hypothalamic problem, and require further evaluation of pituitary function, while high levels of LH suggest other causes of a low androgen level.

MALE INFERTILITY

Description

Infertility (defined as a failure to conceive after 1 year of unprotected intercourse) affects about 15% of couples attempting a pregnancy, and most experts agree that male infertility (alone or in combination with female infertility) accounts for about half of these cases. The causes of male infertility range from congenital absence of the vas deferens or incomplete spermatogenesis to subtle pathologies of sperm shape and function. In contrast, female infertility is usually caused by tubal blockage, uterine or endometrial abnormalities, or abnormal levels of reproductive hormones. Female infertility is relatively easily diagnosed by hormone assays, menstrual cycle analysis, and radiologic studies. The male partner in an infertile couple is often overlooked or incompletely evaluated, even though male factors may be a major contributing factor. Endocrine abnormalities (e.g., isolated androgen deficiency) are exceedingly rare (about 1%) among males of infertile couples. Since subtle sperm dysfunctions not obvious by microscopic semen analysis may preclude fertilization, a normal semen analysis is not necessarily predictive of fertility. In fact, a complete lack of sperm in semen (azoospermia) is the only 100% predictive finding for infertility by semen analysis.

Absence of spermatozoa in the semen may be caused by either failure of the testes to produce sperm (i.e., male sterility) or a blockage of the excurrent ducts of the male genital tract. The former is nonobstructive azoospermia (NOA), and the latter, obstructive azoospermia (OA). When azoospermia is discovered by semen analysis, a medical history and physical examination by a qualified physician is recommended. Testicular biopsy may also be performed to differentiate NOA from OA. OA may be congenital or acquired. Vasectomy is usually an elective minor

Infertility (defined as a failure to conceive after 1 year of unprotected intercourse) affects about 15% of couples attempting a pregnancy, and most experts agree that male infertility (alone or in combination with female infertility) accounts for about half of these cases.

surgery leading to azoospermia for contraception, but the vas or epididymis also may become unknowingly blocked after a sexually transmitted infection. Azoospermia may persist after vasectomy reversal. Congenital bilateral absence of the vas deferens (CBAVD) is found in men carrying one of the many cystic fibrosis alleles, as well as in men with clinically apparent cystic fibrosis. In all these cases of OA, spermatozoa are almost always able to be retrieved from the testis by a urologic surgeon. Testicular sperm are not capable of fertilization except by intracytoplasmic sperm injection, in which an individual sperm cell is microinjected into an oocyte in the in vitro fertilization (IVF) laboratory. In the case of a cystic fibrosis carrier, the partner should be checked to determine if she is also a carrier for cystic fibrosis so that the couple understands the risk to the conceived child.

Absence of the vasa deferentia may be determined by palpation on physical exam, and may be suggested by absence of fructose in the semen. Fructose is stored exclusively in the seminal vesicles, and these glands contribute about 60% of the semen volume. Since they are embryonic outgrowths of the vasa deferentia, they are usually absent in men with CBAVD.

Two reasons for NOA are absence of germ cells in the testis (Sertoli-only syndrome) and failure of spermatogenesis (only mitotic cells or no late stages of sperm production). These conditions may be genetic, due to failure of primordial germ cells to migrate to the testis, or acquired through exposure to toxicants. In addition, microdeletions in the Y chromosome in specific regions are associated with NOA or severe oligozoospermia. Testosterone or androgen therapy (see above) for low testosterone or bodybuilding will often result in azoospermia or oligozoospermia due to inhibition of the hypothalamic–pituitary axis, decreased LH, and subsequent lowering of the high intratesticular:plasma ratio of testosterone required for sperm production. Men with testicular and other cancers may exhibit NOA or oligozoospermia. Conversely, men with NOA or oligozoospermia are at increased risk for later development of testicular cancer.

Spermatozoa may not be entirely missing in NOA. A few stem cells throughout the testis may be present, although a random biopsy may not detect any. In such cases, exceedingly low numbers of sperm may be present in the semen, possibly on a cyclical basis. Cryptozoospermia is the presence of very rare sperm in the semen. Often, high levels of FSH are associated with NOA, due to dysfunctional Sertoli cells and lack of the Sertoli hormone inhibin. However, high FSH has not proven to be a good indicator of the absolute absence of spermatogenesis. The surgical technique known as microsurgical testicular sperm extraction has proven to be useful in these cases. Under the surgical microscope, a few seminiferous tubules might be located that have complete spermatogenesis. Highly trained technologists in the andrology or embryology laboratory are needed to identify and recover sperm from the testis in these cases.

In other cases of male infertility, sperm will be present in the semen. The human, unlike almost any other species, produces spermatozoa with numerous defects. "Normal" values for human semen analysis are both surprisingly poorly established and highly variable from one ejaculate to another, and between different men. Although a typical ejaculate contains 200 to 300 million sperm, fertilization only takes 1, and at the time of fertilization there are only about a dozen sperm associated with the egg. If only 1% of sperm are functionally and structurally normal, then the typical ejaculate will contain about 2 to 3 million of these "good sperm." Apparently this is enough to help propagate the human population. Semen analysis helps identify men who have a few "good sperm," and diagnose specific sperm problems that may permit therapy or advanced reproductive techniques, or help guide decisions by the couple.

Diagnosis and Laboratory Test Interpretation

Semen analysis is the cornerstone of male infertility diagnosis, and should be performed early in the evaluation of the infertile couple. The most used laboratory guide for semen analysis is published by the World Health Organization. **Table 19–3** lists the WHO reference/normal values. Semen analysis is performed by many general laboratories and by specialized fertility labs. Home test kits are available, but typically only measure one or two of the semen and sperm values. Collection of a semen sample should take place after 2 to 5 days of sexual abstinence. Longer abstinence is associated with lower motility and higher leukocyte counts, and shorter periods usually lead to lower volumes and sperm counts. A sterile plastic container, known not to be toxic to sperm, is required. Usually a sterile urine collection cup is satisfactory. If the sample is

TABLE 19-3   Semen Reference Ranges Established by the World Health Organization (2010)

Measure	Reference Range	Note
Volume	≥1.5 mL	Ideally measured by weight where 1 g is assumed to be 1 mL
pH	Slightly alkaline	Depends on method and time
Appearance	Opalescent, white or slightly yellowish	Not pink, red, brown, or yellow
Liquefaction	Complete	No masses or strands after at least 20 minutes (incubate up to 1 h if incomplete)
Viscosity	Low	Forms drops or connected drops
Sperm concentration	≥15 M/mL	No upper limit. Do not count separate heads or tails. Note number of tailless heads separately if high
Total sperm number	≥39 M per ejaculate	Volume × sperm concentration
Motility	≥40%	% of tailed sperm
Progressive motility	≥32%	% of sperm swimming either linearly or in a large circle
Percent normal morphology	≥4%	
Viability	≥58% Live	Nonmotile sperm may be alive
Leukocyte concentration	≤1 M/mL	Lower numbers of PMNs may cause sperm dysfunctions
Seminal fructose	≥13 micromol/ejaculate	

Note: These reference ranges were established by using the lower 5th percentile of all values obtained from men whose partners achieved pregnancy during the study. Therefore, interpretation of results lower than these values should be that 95% of men causing pregnancies had higher values. g, gram; mL, milliliter; M, million.

Semen analysis is the cornerstone of male infertility diagnosis, and should be performed early in the evaluation of the infertile couple. If semen analysis is abnormal, it should be repeated after at least 1 month. Semen analysis parameters can vary substantially within an individual. Therefore, a single abnormal specimen should not be used to establish a diagnosis.

not collected in a special collection room near the lab, it should be transported in a tightly sealed collection cup in a sealed plastic bag, protected from light, heat, and cold. A temperature between room temperature and body temperature is adequate. Seminal fluid characteristics are measured after allowing semen to liquefy (due to the enzymatic action of PSA) for 15 to 30 minutes at 37°C or at room temperature. Analysis should be completed within 60 minutes after ejaculation. In vivo, sperm typically swim out of semen into the cervical mucus within a half hour. Semen may contain hepatitis, HIV, and other pathogens. Basic precautions for handling potentially infectious body fluids must be followed.

The main tests in semen analysis are ejaculate volume, sperm concentration ("count"), sperm motility, sperm morphology, and leukocyte count. Aside from azoospermia, findings that may contribute to a couple's infertility include low sperm concentration or total number of sperm (oligozoospermia), poor sperm motility (asthenozoospermia), very poor sperm morphology (teratozoospermia), or any combination of the three. Using odds ratio calculations, it is estimated that a man with defects in all three sperm characteristics is about 9 to 29 times less likely to be able to cause a pregnancy than a man with a normal semen analysis.

A high number of neutrophils or macrophages in the semen (leukocytospermia) may affect sperm function by inducing oxidative stress through the generation of reactive oxygen species. Leukocytes are likely present in all semen samples. There is lack of consensus on the number that is considered abnormal, with authorities suggesting various cutoffs from 200,000 to 1 million per mL of semen.

Component tests of the semen analysis battery include semen viscosity, completeness of liquefaction, appearance, and pH. Spermatozoan motility patterns should be differentiated at least into overall % motility (sperm with beating flagellae) and progressive motility (sperm that are swimming with some direction). Sperm viability is important to determine when motility is very low. Sperm agglutination and the presence of antisperm antibodies may indicate an immunologic basis for infertility.

A semen fructose analysis (a test for functional seminal vesicles) may be considered if there is unexpected azoospermia. Other biochemical tests include neutral alpha-glucosidase for epididymis function; and PSA, zinc, and acid phosphatase for prostate function.

Interpretation of sperm morphology is controversial, largely because of a lack of supporting data relating sperm morphology to fertility. Very few human sperm are "perfect"; in fact, if at least 4% to 5% of sperm have "normal" morphology, then the specimen morphology is generally considered to be normal. The clinical significance of sperm morphology is best understood when most of the sperm have specific defects. The absence of acrosomes (the enzyme-containing structure at the tip of the sperm head) is associated with inability to fertilize eggs, and, sometimes, inability to activate oocytes to complete meiosis. Abnormal midpieces or tails may be associated with poor motility. Most sperm will have abnormal heads. The human spermatozoon is approximately 65 microns long. The tail consists of the midpiece containing mitochondria (3–5 microns long, attached axially to the base of the head), the principal piece (45 microns), and the thin terminal segment (5 microns). The normal head is a smooth oval with a length of 5 to 6 microns, width of 2.5 to 3.5 microns, and containing an acrosomal cap covering about 40% to 60% of the anterior part.

Sperm number, motility and morphology are measures of sperm production in the testis and epididymal function, but provide little information about whether or not sperm can fertilize an egg. Sperm function tests address this question. They include acrosome reaction, hyperactivation (a motility pattern of sperm after some hours of incubation in culture medium), and changes in the surface and signaling pathways in sperm. Sperm DNA fragmentation is a likely cause of failed embryonic development. Electron microscopy may be used to assess ultrastructural features of the flagellum in cases of poor motility. These and other highly specialized tests typically are performed in laboratories certified specifically for semen analysis.

If a semen analysis is abnormal, it should be repeated after at least 2 weeks to 1 month. Semen analysis parameters can vary substantially within an individual. Therefore, a single abnormal specimen should not be used to establish a diagnosis.

LABORATORY TESTING IN TRANSGENDER INDIVIDUALS

A 2016 report estimated that approximately 0.3% of the adult US population, or about 1.4 million people, self-identify as transgender. Using generally accepted definitions, "gender" of an individual refers to the social construct used to classify an individual, whereas "sex" refers to assignment as male, female, or intersex based on at-birth biological factors such as anatomy, chromosomes, and organs. The term "transgender" refers to self and social identification of gender that is not the same as the sex assigned at birth. The term "transgender woman" (also termed "transwoman") is used to designate an individual assigned as male sex at birth who identifies as female (male to female transition). The term "transgender man" (also termed "transman") is used to designate an individual assigned as female sex at birth who identifies as male (female to male transition). (In this context, the term "cisgender" is used to indicate individuals for whom the gender and sex are concordant.) For many transgender individuals, sex hormones are used to modify their appearance, with transmen taking androgens such as testosterone, and transwomen using estrogen derivatives for feminization. Hormone antagonists may also be used to counteract the influence of spontaneously secreted hormones.

There are a number of issues to be addressed in providing laboratory services to transgender people. For clinical laboratories, often the major patient contact is with the phlebotomy staff, who use the laboratory information system and electronic medical record for patient identification and order review. Registration and identification of individuals requires attention to the self-identified name (if changed) and self-identified gender (if changed). Ideally, an individual's preferred pronoun designation (e.g., he or she) should be noted in the record and used by staff in referring to an individual. Access to appropriate information allows the front-end staff to best serve their technical and customer service roles. Furthermore, appropriate information technology needs to facilitate appropriate care. For example, it is possible that some laboratory information systems may not permit or may challenge ordering of tests for PSA in women, but ordering a PSA test may be appropriate for transwomen who still have a prostate gland and therefore are at risk for development of prostate cancer. Whereas androgen antagonists lead to lower concentrations of circulating PSA, the role of estrogens alone on PSA concentrations is unclear. A few cases of prostate cancer developing in transwomen have been reported, and therefore prostate cancer screening may be considered in this population.

The usual reference ranges used for men and women may not be ideal or appropriate for transgender individuals. Limited data are available regarding reference ranges, but for analytes that differ between men and women or that are altered by chronic hormone therapy, reference range adjustments may be advisable.

SELF-ASSESSMENT QUESTIONS

1. Which of the following statements about prostate cancer is not true?
    A. Prostate cancer incidence increases with age.
    B. Most cases of prostate cancer are slowly progressive and do not cause major morbidity or lead to death.
    C. Laboratory testing is available to differentiate the rapidly progressive and fatal forms of prostate cancer from those that do not rapidly progress and do not cause death.
    D. The test for serum prostate-specific antigen concentration has had a significant impact on increased detection of this cancer.

2. Which one of the following statements about the clinical utility of prostate-specific antigen (PSA) is controversial?
    A. It is useful to determine success of treatment.
    B. It is useful as an indicator of the extent of disease, particularly bone metastases.
    C. It is useful for monitoring recurrence of prostate cancer.
    D. It is useful as a screening test for prostate cancer in men older than 50 years.

3. Which of the following choices is not used as a tumor marker for testicular cancer?
    A. CA 19-9
    B. Lactate dehydrogenase (LD)
    C. α-Fetoprotein (AFP)
    D. Human chorionic gonadotropin (hCG)

4. Which of the following statements about male gonadal dysfunction is not true?
    A. Partial androgen deficiency is common in men with advancing age.
    B. Not all men develop low levels of testosterone, while gonadal failure in women is inevitable.
    C. The reference range for testosterone in men is based on the values found in healthy young men.
    D. Routine use of testosterone for hormone replacement, especially in men over the age of 65, is widely accepted.

5. Which of the following statements about testosterone measurements is not true?
    A. Free testosterone, which is not bound to proteins, contributes significantly more of the biological effects of testosterone than protein-bound testosterone.
    B. Testing for testosterone should be avoided in hospitalized individuals because testosterone levels can decrease in persons who are acutely ill.
    C. Testosterone secretion has a circadian rhythm with higher levels in the evening and lower concentrations in the morning and afternoon.
    D. Complete gonadal failure in men is rare, whereas partial androgen deficiency is common.

6. In young men with a low testosterone, a subsequent test to be performed is the test for luteinizing hormone (LH). When the value for LH in a patient with low testosterone is extremely low, which of the following is likely to be dysfunctional?
    A. Testes
    B. Adrenal gland
    C. Pituitary gland
    D. Thyroid gland

7. Which of the following is the least likely cause for male infertility after 1 year of unprotected intercourse among the choices below?
    A. Absence of spermatozoa in the semen
    B. Blockage of a duct within the male genital tract
    C. Absence of the vas deferens
    D. Decreased androgen production in the adrenal glands

8. Which of the following statements is incorrect about the collection of semen for male infertility evaluation?

   A. The ideal specimen for sperm count and volume assessment is one which is collected within 10 hours after a previous ejaculation.

   B. Seminal fluid characteristics should be measured 15 to 30 minutes after ejaculation with the samples stored during that time at 37°C or at room temperature to permit liquefaction of the semen.

   C. Semen analysis should be performed early in the evaluation of the infertile couple.

   D. Semen may contain agents that cause hepatitis or HIV in need to be handled as potentially infectious.

9. Which of the following is not a parameter that is measured as part of the routine semen analysis procedure?

   A. Ejaculate volume

   B. Sperm count and morphology

   C. Sperm motility

   D. Assessment for antisperm antibodies

FURTHER READING

Prostate Cancer:

Carter HB, et al. Detection of life-threatening prostate cancer with prostate-specific antigen velocity during a window of curability. *J Natl Cancer Inst.* 2005;98:1521–1527.

Carter HB, et al. Early detection of prostate cancer, published 2013; reviewed and validity confirmed 2015. American Urological Association (AUA) Guideline. Available at: www.auanet.org/guidelines/early-detection-of-prostate-cancer-(2013-reviewed-and-validity-confirmed-2015)#x2618. Accessed November 1, 2017.

D'Amico AV, et al. Preoperative PSA velocity and the risk of death from prostate cancer after radical prostatectomy. *N Engl J Med.* 2004;351:125–135.

Oesterling JE, et al. The use of prostate specific antigen in staging patients with newly diagnosed prostate cancer. *JAMA.* 1993;269:57.

Qaseem A, et al. Screening for prostate cancer: a guidance statement from the clinical guidelines committee of the American College of Physicians. *Ann Int Med.* 2013;158:761–769.

Thompson IM, et al. Prevalence of prostate cancer among men with a prostate-specific antigen level <4 ng per milliliter. *N Engl J Med.* 2004;350:2239–2246.

US Preventive Services Task Force (USPSTF) Screening for Prostate Cancer website. [Internet]. 2017. Available at: http://www.screeningforprostatecancer.org. Accessed November 1, 2017.

van den Bergh RC, et al. Prostate-specific antigen kinetics in clinical decision-making during active surveillance for early prostate cancer—a review. *Eur Urol.* 2008;54:505–516.

Wyatt AW, Annala M, Aggarwal R, et al. Concordance of circulating tumor DNA and matched metastatic tissue biopsy in prostate cancer. *JNCI J Natl Cancer Inst.* 2018;110:78–86.

Testicular Cancer:

Barlow LJ, et al. Serum tumor markers in the evaluation of male germ cell tumors. *Nat Rev Urol.* 2010;7:610–617.

Salem M, Gilligan T. Serum tumor markers and their utilization in the management of germ-cell tumors in adult males. *Expert Rev Anticancer Ther.* 2011;11:1–4.

Stenman UH. Testicular cancer: the perfect paradigm for marker combinations. *Scand J Clin Lab Invest.* 2005;65:181–188.

Sturgeon CM, et al. National Academy of Clinical Biochemistry laboratory medicine practice guidelines for use of tumor markers in testicular, prostate, colorectal, breast, and ovarian cancers. *Clin Chem.* 2008;54:e11–e79.

Bladder Cancer:

Chou R, et al. Urinary biomarkers of diagnosis of bladder cancer. A systematic review and meta-analysis. *Ann Int Med.* 2015;163:922–931.

Kaufman DS, et al. Bladder cancer. *Lancet.* 2009;374:239–249.

Leiblich A. Recent developments in the search for urinary biomarkers in bladder cancer. *Curr Urol Rep.* 2017;18:100.

Tilki D, et al. Urine markers for detection and surveillance of non-muscle-invasive bladder cancer. *Eur Urol.* 2011;60:484–492.

Male Gonadal Dysfunction:

Bhasin S, et al. Task Force, Endocrine Society. Testosterone therapy in men with androgen deficiency syndromes: an Endocrine Society clinical practice guideline. *J Clin Endocrinol Metab*. 2010;95:2536–2559.

Budoff MJ, et al. Testosterone treatment and coronary artery plaque volume in older men with low testosterone. *JAMA*. 2017;317:708–716.

Dimopoulou C, et al. EMAS position statement: testosterone replacement therapy in the aging male. *Maturitas*. 2016;84:94–99.

Elliott J, et al. Testosterone therapy in hypogonadal men: a systematic review and network meta-analysis. *BMJ Open*. 2017;7:e015284.

Hackett G. An update on the role of testosterone replacement therapy in the management of hypogonadism. *Ther Adv Urol*. 2016;8:147–160.

Spitzer M, et al. Effect of testosterone replacement on response to sildenafil citrate in men with erectile dysfunction: a parallel, randomized trial. *Ann Intern Med*. 2012;157:681–691.

Spitzer M, et al. Risks and benefits of testosterone therapy in older men. *Nat Rev Endocrinol*. 2013;9:414–424.

Travison TG, Vesper HW, Orwoll E, et al. Harmonized reference ranges for circulating testosterone levels in men of four cohort studies in the United States and Europe. *J Clin Endocrinol Metab*. 2017;102:1161–1173.

Male Infertility:

Alvarez C, et al. Biological variation of seminal parameters in healthy subjects. *Hum Reprod*. 2003;18:2082–2088.

Björndahl L, et al. *A Practical Guide to Basic Laboratory Andrology*. Cambridge, UK: Cambridge University Press; 2010.

Guzick DS, Overstreet JW, et al. Sperm morphology, motility, and concentration in fertile and infertile men. *N Engl J Med*. 2001;345:1388–1393.

Krausz C. Male infertility: pathogenesis and clinical diagnosis. *Best Pract Res Clin Endocrinol Metab*. 2011;25:271–285.

Stahl PJ, et al. Interpretation of the semen analysis and initial male factor management. *Clin Obstet Gynecol*. 2011;54:656–665.

World Health Organization. *WHO Laboratory Manual for the Examination and Processing of Human Semen*. 5th ed. Geneva: World Health Organization; 2010.

Transgender Medicine:

Goldstein Z, et al. When gender identity doesn't equal sex recorded at birth: the role of the laboratory in providing effective healthcare to the transgender community. *Clin Chem*. 2017;63:1342–1352.

Gupta S, et al. Challenges in transgender healthcare: the pathology perspective. *Lab Med*. 2016;47:180–188.

Imborek KL, et al. Preferred names, preferred pronouns, and gender identity in the electronic medical record and laboratory information system: is pathology ready? *J Pathol Inform*. 2017;8:42.

Roberts TK, et al. Interpreting laboratory results in transgender patients on hormone therapy. *Am J Med*. 2014;127:159–162.

Velho I, et al. Effects of testosterone therapy on BMI, blood pressure, and laboratory profile of transgender men: a systematic review. *Andrology*. 2017;5:881–888.

Female Genital System

Robert D. Nerenz, Stacy E.F. Melanson,
and Ann M. Gronowski

LEARNING OBJECTIVES

1. Understand the clinical utility of human chorionic gonadotropin (hCG) results in pregnancy, normal and ectopic, spontaneous abortion (miscarriage), and gestational trophoblastic disease.

2. Learn how to diagnose common complications of pregnancy, notably preeclampsia, eclampsia, HELLP syndrome, and fatty liver associated with pregnancy.

3. Understand the causes and the diagnosis of female infertility.

CHAPTER OUTLINE

INTRODUCTION

Clinical laboratory testing is useful for the diagnosis and management of pregnancy and infertility, and such testing is reviewed in this chapter. Gestational diabetes mellitus (GDM) is discussed in Chapter 17, and hemolytic disease of the newborn (HDN) is found in Chapters 7 and 12. Female physiology and biochemistry including amenorrhea are discussed in Chapter 22. The female genital tract is also a common site for infections, which may be sexually transmitted, and it is a common site for tumors. The infections are presented in Chapter 5, and tumor descriptions are found in textbooks of anatomic pathology.

TABLE 20-1   **Routine Testing in Normal Pregnancy**

Test	Comments
Chemistry	
hCG	Should double every 1.5–2 days for the first 8 weeks
First-trimester screen (free beta hCG, PAPP-A)	To screen for trisomy 21
Second-trimester "quad" screen (hCG, AFP, estriol, inhibin A)	To screen for trisomy 21, neural tube defects, and other fetal anomalies
Glucose	To screen for gestational diabetes mellitus
Blood bank	
Type and screen	To assess the risk of hemolytic disease of the newborn; includes blood type (i.e., A, B, AB, O), Rh typing (i.e., negative or positive), and antibody screen
Microbiology	
RPR or treponemal antibody	To screen for syphilis
Hepatitis B surface antigen	To screen for active hepatitis B
HIV antibody	To screen for exposure to HIV
Group B *Streptococcus* (GBS) cervical culture Rubella antibody Toxoplasma antibody CMV antibody HSV antibody	To screen for GBS in the third trimester and if present prevent transmission to fetus during delivery To assess immune status To assess immune status prior to pregnancy or exposure during pregnancy To assess exposure prior to pregnancy or exposure during pregnancy To assess exposure prior to pregnancy

AFP, alpha-fetoprotein; hCG, human chorionic gonadotropin; PAPP-A, pregnancy-associated plasma protein-A.

NORMAL PREGNANCY

Description

Normal pregnancy lasts approximately 40 weeks, as dated from the first day of the previous menstrual period, and is typically divided into three intervals or trimesters each lasting approximately 13 weeks. Approximately 5 days after fertilization, a blastocyst implants in the uterus. Trophoblast cells of the blastocyst invade the endometrium with chorionic villi leading to a placenta and the forming embryo surrounded by amniotic fluid. The placenta nourishes the embryo and produces hormones vital to pregnancy such as human chorionic gonadotropin (hCG), progesterone, estradiol, estriol, and estrone. The amniotic fluid protects the embryo and changes composition as the pregnancy progresses. The embryo undergoes rapid cell division, differentiation, and growth in the first trimester (0–13 weeks). By 10 weeks, most major structures are formed resulting in a fetus. The second trimester (13–26 weeks) is associated with rapid fetal growth. Completion of maturation occurs in the third trimester (26–40 weeks), resulting in a term pregnancy between 37 and 42 weeks.

Diagnosis

Pregnancy has an effect on many laboratory tests, and these alterations should be considered when interpreting laboratory tests from pregnant women.

Once pregnancy has been achieved, several laboratory tests are routinely performed to help ensure an optimal maternal and fetal outcome (**Table 20-1**). Most testing in pregnancy is performed on maternal serum because it is easy to obtain and provides minimal risk to the pregnancy, but maternal urine and amniotic fluid specimens may also be necessary. Of note, pregnancy has an effect on many laboratory tests, other than those used to diagnose and manage pregnancy, and these alterations should be considered when interpreting laboratory tests from pregnant women (**Table 20-2**).

TABLE 20–2   Effects of Pregnancy on Select Laboratory Tests

Test	Result in Pregnancy	Comments
Hematocrit	Decreased	Due to an increased plasma volume
Coagulation factors	Several factors increase; some do not change; Factor XI decreases	The overall effect is an increased thrombotic risk
Lipids (triglycerides, cholesterol)	Increased	
Thyroxine-binding globulin, total T3 and T4	Increased	Patient remains euthyroid
Alkaline phosphatase activity	Increased	Due to production of placental, heat-stable, alkaline phosphatase
BUN, creatinine	Slightly decreased	Due to increased glomerular filtration rate
1,25-Dihydroxyvitamin D	Increased	Due to increased total calcium and transfer of calcium to fetus
Parathyroid hormone	Increased	Ionized calcium remains normal

Serum/plasma or urine hCG measurement is one of the most commonly ordered tests in pregnancy. It is a heterodimer composed of two nonidentical nonconvalently bound glycoprotein subunits, alpha and beta, that is synthesized by the trophoblasts of the placenta. Only the intact molecule is biologically active. A single gene for the alpha subunit of all four glycoprotein hormones (thyroid-stimulating hormone [TSH], luteinizing hormone [LH], follicle-stimulating hormone [FSH], and hCG) is found on chromosome 6. hCG stimulates the LH receptor on the corpus luteum to produce progesterone that helps to prevent pregnancy loss.

Detectable amounts of hCG (>2–5 IU/L, depending on the assay) are present in serum 8 to 11 days after conception. Quantitative serum or plasma testing offers sensitivity as low as 2 to 5 IU/L, and serial measurements may be helpful to reveal problems in a pregnancy. In normal pregnancies, hCG doubles every 1.5 to 2 days for the first 8 weeks (**Table 20–1**) and peaks around 100,000 to 500,000 IU/L. Qualitative urine hCG tests are usually sufficient for screening, but the detection limits of qualitative tests range from 20 to 50 IU/L, limiting their use to the time following a missed menstrual period or greater than 14 days after conception.

Blood and urine contain many hCG variants, including free subunits, and hyperglycosylated and nicked forms. After 5 weeks of gestation the predominant hCG form in urine is the hCG beta core fragment. In addition, the hCG glycosylation pattern changes as the pregnancy progresses. Quantitative hCG immunoassays typically measure total hCG beta concentrations using two antibodies against different regions of the beta subunit. False-negative hCG results can be seen in early pregnancy or when concentrations of intact hCG or hCG variants are very high, causing a hook effect. False-positive results can be caused by heterophile antibodies. Misleading results can be observed in menopausal women when reduced plasma estradiol concentrations permit hCG secretion by the pituitary. These are true results as hCG is present, but the results should not be used as an indicator of pregnancy, as hCG is secreted by the pituitary rather than the placenta.

Other additional routine testing in pregnancy is performed to screen for common and/or treatable pregnancy complications such as gestational diabetes (see Chapter 17), hemolytic disease of the newborn (see Chapters 7 and 12), and infection (see Chapter 5) (**Table 20–1**).

> Detectable amounts of hCG are present in serum 8 to 11 days after conception.

MATERNAL SERUM SCREENING

Description

Maternal serum screening can be performed to identify individuals who need further diagnostic evaluation for fetal anomalies such as neural tube defects, trisomy 21/Down syndrome, and trisomy 18. Neural tube defects result from failure of fusion of the neural plate and failure of complete covering by the 27th day post conception. The extent and location of neural tissue exposed indicates the severity of the defect (i.e., anencephaly, meningomyelocele, and encephalocele).

Maternal serum screening can be performed to identify individuals who need further diagnostic evaluation for fetal anomalies such as neural tube defects, trisomy 21/Down syndrome, and trisomy 18.

The result of a neural tube defect is a direct communication of the amniotic fluid with fetal plasma proteins, and release of alpha-fetoprotein (AFP) into amniotic fluid and maternal serum. Rates of neural tube defects have decreased due to the addition of folic acid to grain, as well as initiation of recommendations for folic acid supplementation prior to conception. Trisomy 21 or Down syndrome is caused by an extra copy of chromosome 21 and is the most frequent chromosomal disorder among live-born children (1/600–1/800 live births). Risk factors for Down syndrome include advanced maternal age, the birth of a previously affected child, and balanced parental structural rearrangement of chromosome 21. Affected children suffer from mental retardation, hypotonia, congenital heart defects, and a flat facial profile. The main phenotypic features of trisomy 18 include hypertonia, prominent occiput, small mouth, micrognathia, short sternum, and horseshoe kidney.

Diagnostic Screening Tests

An additional discussion of maternal screening for Down syndrome is found in Chapter 7.

Screening for neural tube defects is done at 15 to 22 weeks gestation by measurement of serum AFP that is expressed as a multiple of the median (MoM) population of the same gestational age. MoMs greater than 2 or 2.5 are considered abnormal and should be followed up by high-resolution ultrasound or measurement of amniotic fluid AFP and acetylcholinesterase.

Sequential serum screening is performed to screen for trisomies and combines first- and second-trimester testing. First-trimester testing is performed between 10 and 14 weeks and includes measurement of hCG and pregnancy-associated plasma protein-A (PAPP-A) as well as an ultrasound measurement for infant nuchal translucency. Specific training is required of operators for determination of nuchal translucency. This procedure is highly operator dependent. Free beta hCG testing is more accurate than intact hCG testing in the first trimester and is used instead of intact hCG for the first-trimester screen. PAPP-A is a protein produced by the placenta. Elevated hCG, decreased PAPP-A, and increased nuchal translucency are seen in pregnancies affected by trisomy 21.

In the sequential screen, first-trimester screening is followed up with second-trimester screening at 15 to 22 weeks, with measurement of serum AFP, hCG, estriol, and inhibin A (i.e., the quad screen). AFP is the most abundant serum protein in the fetal circulation. Maternal serum AFP is detectable at 10 weeks and peaks at 15 to 20 weeks. Estriol is the predominant estrogen of pregnancy and also the most difficult to measure because of its low concentration and limited stability. Inhibin A, secreted by the ovaries and placenta, is a glycoprotein that inhibits FSH. Concentrations of individual analytes from the first- and second-trimester screens and nuchal translucency measurements are combined into a risk assessment algorithm that adjusts for gestational age, maternal weight, number of fetuses, and presence or absence of diabetes mellitus. The most frequent causes of abnormal results include incorrect dating, the presence of twins, and fetal demise. For this reason, an ultrasound confirming gestational age is the first line of testing in a patient with apparently increased risk. Fetal karyotyping is necessary to confirm chromosomal abnormalities.

Second trimester-only testing can be done and should utilize the quad screen. Elevated hCG, increased inhibin A, decreased estriol, and decreased AFP are seen in pregnancies affected by trisomy 21, while all four analytes in the quad screen are decreased in pregnancies affected by trisomy 18. Patients at risk should undergo further diagnostic evaluation as described with sequential screen.

Recently, new methods have been developed for trisomy 21 screening using circulating fetal DNA. These methods utilize "massively parallel genomic sequencing" (MPGS). DNA fragments are isolated from a sample of maternal blood, which contains a mixture of maternal DNA and infant DNA. The DNA fragments are amplified and then sequenced. The number of sequences that originate from a particular chromosome is counted and tabulated for each chromosome. If a fetus has an extra chromosome, then the percentage of DNA fragments from that chromosome is higher than expected. In a meta-analysis summarizing 37 studies assessing the performance of cell-free fetal DNA to detect fetal aneuploidy in high-risk pregnancies, the sensitivity to detect trisomy 21 was 99.2% and the specificity was 99.9%. For trisomy 18, the sensitivity and specificity were 96% and 99.9%, respectively. For trisomy 13, the sensitivity and specificity were 91% and

99.9%, respectively. Cell-free fetal DNA methods can also detect sex chromosome abnormalities, with a documented sensitivity and specificity for monosomy X (Turner syndrome) of 90% and 99.8%, respectively. A higher rate of false-positive results could be expected in a predominantly low-risk population with a lower prevalence of affected fetuses. However, this is unlikely because a recent large, multicenter trial has demonstrated similar performance of cell-free fetal DNA screening in a routine prenatal population for the detection of trisomy 21 (100% sensitivity, 99.9% specificity). In the same study, the standard screening test group showed a lower sensitivity and specificity of 78% and 94.6%, respectively.

One limitation of cell-free fetal DNA screening is that it does not detect open neural tube defects, such as spina bifida, or placental abnormalities, for which screening usually involves biochemical (not genetic) screening tests. Furthermore, non-diagnostic results may be generated early in pregnancy when the fetal fraction of circulating DNA is low.

The American College of Obstetricians and Gynecologists (ACOG) cautions that these tests are screening tests, not diagnostic tests. They also recommend that DNA-based screening tests be performed only on women who are at increased risk of having a fetus with aneuploidy, including women with maternal age 35 years or older at delivery, fetal ultrasound findings suggesting aneuploidy, a previous aneuploid pregnancy, or abnormal biochemical screening test results. As DNA-based screening tests do not detect open neural tube defects, the ACOG also recommends that women undergoing cell-free fetal DNA screening should be offered maternal serum AFP and/or ultrasound evaluation.

ECTOPIC PREGNANCY

Description

Ectopic pregnancies arise if the fertilized egg implants in a location other than the body of the uterus, primarily in the fallopian tube. Of all reported pregnancies, 1.3% to 2% are extrauterine. The nonuterine location of implantation prevents normal development. Despite increased awareness and improved diagnostic modalities, such as serial hCG and transvaginal ultrasound, ectopic pregnancies are the leading cause of maternal death in the first trimester. Risk factors for ectopic pregnancy include tubal damage from either infection or disease, smoking, infertility, and previous miscarriage.

Diagnosis

Three classic symptoms of an ectopic pregnancy include lower abdominal pain, vaginal bleeding, and an adnexal mass. However, only 25% of women with ectopic pregnancy have these symptoms at the time of presentation, making laboratory testing and transvaginal ultrasound examination essential for diagnosis and management. In ectopic pregnancies, abnormal concentrations of hCG are present (**Table 20–3**). hCG concentrations in ectopic pregnancy range from undetectable to 200,000 IU/L, depending on the size and viability of the trophoblastic tissue. Therefore, the absolute concentration of hCG is not very useful in the diagnosis of ectopic pregnancy. Many utilize a so-called discriminatory zone of hCG in which a fetus should be visible when hCG concentrations are >2000 IU/L. However, recent studies suggest that the discriminatory zone is not very reliable and can lead to misdiagnosis. Instead, serial testing reveals rates of hCG increase as slow as 35% over 2 days in ectopic pregnancy. Medical therapy with methotrexate or surgery is required to prevent rupture and significant hemorrhage.

SPONTANEOUS ABORTION (MISCARRIAGE) AND RECURRENT ABORTION

Description

Spontaneous abortion or miscarriage refers to a pregnancy that ends spontaneously before the fetus has reached a viable gestational age. The most common complication of early pregnancy is spontaneous abortion, and it occurs in approximately 10% to 20% of all recognized pregnancies

Three classic symptoms of an ectopic pregnancy include lower abdominal pain, vaginal bleeding, and an adnexal mass. However, only 25% of women with ectopic pregnancy have these symptoms at the time of presentation, making laboratory testing and transvaginal ultrasound examination essential for diagnosis and management.

TABLE 20–3   Abnormal Pregnancy Conditions

Condition	Laboratory Diagnosis
Ectopic pregnancy	Slow rate of increase in hCG
Gestational trophoblastic disease	hCG concentration greater than that expected for gestational age; rate of increase may be accelerated as well
Preeclampsia	Modest increase in AST and ALT (4–10 × upper limit) >0.3 g/L protein in 24-h urine >1.0 g/L protein in random specimen
HELLP syndrome	Decreased platelets (<100,000/μL) Elevated LDH (>600 IU/L) Elevated ALT and AST (200–700 IU/L)
Fatty liver of pregnancy	Mild increase in AST and ALT (AST > ALT) Serum bilirubin >6 mg/dL Hypoglycemia Increased uric acid Prolonged PT and PTT Low fibrinogen

hCG, human chorionic gonadotropin; PT, prothrombin time; PTT, partial thromboplastin time.

The most common complication of early pregnancy is spontaneous abortion, and it occurs in approximately 10% to 20% of all recognized pregnancies under 20 weeks gestation.

under 20 weeks gestation. The percentage increases if unrecognized or subclinical pregnancies are included. Risk factors include advanced maternal age, previous miscarriage, smoking, and alcohol or drug consumption. Chromosomal abnormalities account for approximately 50% of all miscarriages.

Recurrent spontaneous abortion is defined as three or more consecutive intrauterine pregnancy losses prior to 20 to 24 weeks of gestation. It affects up to 1% to 5% of fertile couples. Primary aborters have had no live births, while secondary aborters were able to achieve at least one successful pregnancy. Assisted reproduction technologies are much less effective in women with recurrent fetal losses compared with those with infertility.

Diagnosis

Women experiencing a miscarriage may present with a history of amenorrhea, vaginal bleeding, and lower abdominal pain. Serial measurements of hCG concentration in conjunction with physical examination and ultrasonography can be helpful in the diagnosis of spontaneous abortion. Decreasing hCG concentrations are consistent with a spontaneous abortion or nonviable pregnancy. Patients with a confirmed miscarriage can be managed expectantly, medically with misoprostol, or surgically. Following treatment, hCG concentrations can be monitored until the concentration is undetectable to confirm complete expulsion of products of conception. It may take 30 to 60 days before serum hCG concentrations are undetectable. The etiology of recurrent loss is often unclear, but can include genetic, anatomic, hormonal, thrombotic, placental, infectious, environmental, or psychological causes. Immunological factors may also play a role. Following a detailed history, physical examination, and radiological studies, additional laboratory tests may be helpful in determining the cause of the recurrent loss (**Table 20–4**). Of all the etiologic factors, only parental genetics has been shown to be a definitive cause of recurrent loss. Although uterine abnormalities, antiphospholipid antibodies, the Factor V Leiden mutation, and other thrombotic risk factors (see Chapter 11) are definitely associated with recurrent loss, there is not sufficient proof of a causative role.

GESTATIONAL TROPHOBLASTIC DISEASE

Description

Gestational trophoblastic diseases are a spectrum of disease processes originating from the placenta that include hydatidiform mole, invasive mole, and choriocarcinoma. Malignant gestational trophoblastic diseases have the potential for local invasion and metastasis.

TABLE 20-4   **Laboratory Evaluation of Recurrent Spontaneous Abortion**

Analysis	Purpose
Parental and fetal tissue karyotype	Tests for chromosomal abnormalities
LH, FSH, TSH, prolactin, cortisol	Tests for endocrine abnormalities
Thrombotic risk factors including protein C, protein S, and antithrombin deficiencies, Factor V Leiden and prothrombin gene 20210 mutations, lupus anticoagulant, anticardiolipin antibodies	Tests for thrombophilic disorders
Antithyroid antibodies	Tests for autoimmune factors
Endometrial biopsy	Tests for luteal phase defect or inadequate endometrial maturation
Glucose, hemoglobin A1c	Tests for diabetes

Hydatidiform moles are the most common and occur in 1 of 600 therapeutic abortions and 1 of 1100 pregnancies. Approximately 20% of patients will be treated for malignant sequelae after evacuation of a hydatidiform mole. Gestational choriocarcinoma occurs in approximately 1 in 30,000 pregnancies.

Diagnosis

Gestational trophoblastic diseases are usually diagnosed early in pregnancy. Patients present with abnormal bleeding and vague complaints. Ultrasound and serum hCG testing are used to make the diagnosis of gestational trophoblastic diseases. Ultrasound findings include the absence of a fetal heartbeat. hCG testing reveals greatly elevated hCG concentrations and shortened doubling time (**Table 20-3**). Dilation and evacuation (D&E) procedures are performed to treat patients. Serial hCG measurements should be performed after treatment to ensure complete removal of tumor and monitoring of disease for recurrence. Chemotherapy may be necessary in cases of malignant transformation.

PREECLAMPSIA AND ECLAMPSIA

Description

Preeclampsia is a multisystem disorder of unknown etiology, and it is a major cause of morbidity and mortality in pregnancy. Patients develop elevated blood pressure and proteinuria. In addition, coagulopathies, impaired liver function, renal failure, and cerebral ischemia may occur. Preeclampsia occurs in 2% to 8% of pregnancies. Eclampsia, in which women with preeclampsia have accompanying seizures, occurs less frequently. Eclampsia is more serious and carries a higher morbidity and mortality rate. Treatment includes controlling symptoms until delivery.

Diagnosis

Preeclampsia is diagnosed by the occurrence of new hypertension and proteinuria in the second half of pregnancy. Hypertension in pregnancy is defined as a persistent systolic blood pressure ≥140 mm Hg and/or a diastolic blood pressure ≥90 mm Hg. Proteinuria in preeclampsia is >300 mg/L protein in a 24-hour urine specimen or >1 g/L protein in a single urine specimen (**Table 20-3**). It should be demonstrated that seizures associated with eclampsia are not explained by a neurological disorder such as epilepsy.

HELLP SYNDROME

Description

The HELLP syndrome involves **h**emolysis, **e**levated **l**iver enzymes, and a **l**ow **p**latelet count. The syndrome can occur during pregnancy, typically between weeks 27 and 36, or in association with preeclampsia; it can also occur postpartum.

Preeclampsia is a multisystem disorder of unknown etiology, and it is a major cause of morbidity and mortality in pregnancy. Preeclampsia is diagnosed by the occurrence of new hypertension and proteinuria in the second half of pregnancy.

Diagnosis

The HELLP syndrome and preeclampsia have similar clinical presentations. A low platelet count and abnormal liver enzymes are important to make a diagnosis of the HELLP syndrome (**Table 20–3**). The hemolysis in the HELLP syndrome is microangiopathic, and this results in schistocytes on the peripheral blood smear, an elevated indirect bilirubin, and an increased lactate dehydrogenase (LD) activity.

FATTY LIVER OF PREGNANCY

Description

Approximately 1 in 13,000 pregnancies is affected by fatty liver of pregnancy. First pregnancies and multiple gestation pregnancies are at a higher risk. Symptoms, which are nonspecific and include nausea and vomiting, right upper quadrant pain, and lethargy, typically begin around the 36th week of gestation. Liver biopsies show accumulation of microvesicular fat, which may be caused by a defect in mitochondrial beta oxidation of fatty acids or a long-chain 3-hydroxyacyl CoA dehydrogenase deficiency. Treatment involves immediate delivery to prevent fulminant hepatic failure requiring liver transplantation. Recurrence in subsequent pregnancies is rare.

Diagnosis

The diagnosis is made using both clinical symptoms and laboratory results. Although liver biopsy is virtually diagnostic in the setting of pregnancy, it is rarely necessary. The laboratory test abnormalities include mild elevations in liver enzymes (AST > ALT), increased bilirubin, hypoglycemia, and hyperuricemia (**Table 20–3**). Abnormal coagulation test results, as indicated by a prolonged prothrombin time, a prolonged partial thromboplastin time, and a low fibrinogen, are found in acute fatty liver of pregnancy, but not in HELLP syndrome, and this helps differentiate the two conditions.

FEMALE INFERTILITY

Description

Infertility is defined as the inability to achieve a successful pregnancy following 1 year of unprotected intercourse. It is estimated that 15% to 25% of couples will experience an episode of infertility. Couples with primary infertility have had no previous successful pregnancies. Couples with secondary infertility had prior pregnancies, but are currently unable to conceive. Both primary and secondary infertility have common causes, most often problems with the hypothalamic–pituitary–gonadal axis. (See the section "Male Infertility" in Chapter 19.)

Infertility is defined as the inability to achieve a successful pregnancy following 1 year of unprotected intercourse. It is estimated that 25% of couples will experience an episode of infertility.

Diagnosis

Factors contributing to female infertility include ovarian, hormonal, tubal, cervical, uterine, psychosocial, iatrogenic, and immunological factors. Ovulatory disorders, such as hypergonadotropic hypogonadism and hypogonadotropic hypogonadism, are the most common and are described in more detail in Chapter 22. Other disorders such as polycystic ovarian syndrome, obesity, thyroid dysfunction, androgen excess, and liver dysfunction can also contribute. Following a detailed history and physical examination, laboratory evaluation of female infertility is performed. Midluteal progesterone concentrations greater than 10 ng/mL indicate normal ovulation while concentrations less than 10 ng/mL suggest anovulation, inadequate luteal phase progesterone production, or inappropriate timing of sample collection. Serum concentrations of FSH and estradiol can be measured on day 3 of the menstrual cycle to indicate ovarian reserve. Serum anti-mullerian hormone (AMH), a dimeric glycoprotein secreted by the granulosa cells of developing follicles, has been proposed as a novel marker of ovarian reserve because serum AMH concentrations directly reflect the number of immature ovarian follicles. In contrast to FSH and estradiol which must be measured early in the menstrual cycle due to fluctuations in concentration, AMH remains relatively stable throughout the menstrual cycle and can be measured anytime. In women undergoing in vitro fertilization (IVF), AMH is frequently measured to tailor the dose of ovarian stimulation to ensure adequate oocyte retrieval in women with low ovarian reserve or to avoid the ovarian hyperstimulation syndrome (OHSS) in women with high ovarian reserve. While AMH accurately reflects ovarian reserve in women over 25 years of age, its utility in younger women is less clear as the relationship between AMH and ovarian reserve is more complex in this age group. Furthermore, long-term oral contraceptive use suppresses ovarian activity and reduces serum AMH concentrations, resulting in an inaccurately low assessment of ovarian reserve. As thyroid and pituitary dysfunction can cause infertility, TSH and prolactin (PRL) should also be measured as part of the infertility workup.

> Midluteal progesterone concentrations greater than 10 ng/mL indicate normal ovulation while concentrations less than 10 ng/mL suggest anovulation, inadequate luteal phase progesterone production, or inappropriate timing of sample collection. Serum concentrations of FSH and estradiol can be measured on day 3 or AMH at any point of the menstrual cycle to indicate ovarian reserve.

SELF-ASSESSMENT QUESTIONS

1. Regarding routine testing in normal pregnancy, which one of the following pairs is an incorrect match?

   A. First trimester screen (free β-hCG, PAPP-A)/Assessment for Down syndrome

   B. Glucose/Assessment for gestational diabetes mellitus

   C. Treponemal antibody test/Assessment for group B *Streptococcus* to prevent transmission to fetus during delivery

   D. Second trimester "quad" screen (hCG, AFP, estriol, inhibin A)/Assessment for Down syndrome, neural tube defects, and other fetal anomalies

2. Pregnancy causes alterations in many laboratory tests such that the reference ranges are different during pregnancy. Which one of the following shows an incorrect change in the reference range during pregnancy?

   A. Hematocrit is increased

   B. Alkaline phosphatase activity is increased

   C. 1,25-dihydroxyvitamin D is increased

   D. Total T3 and T4 are increased

3. Depending on the assay, 2 to 5 IU/L, a detectable amount of hCG, is present in the serum how many days after conception?

   A. 1 to 2

   B. 2 to 4

   C. 5 to 8

   D. 8 to 11

4. For the first 8 weeks of pregnancy, hCG doubles every how many days until it reaches a peak between 100,000 and 500,000 IU/L?

   A. 1.5 to 2

   B. 3 to 5

   C. 7 to 10

   D. 10 to 15

5. Which one of the following is not a characteristic of an ectopic pregnancy?

   A. A transvaginal ultrasound examination consistent with an ectopic pregnancy

   B. A slow increase in the concentration of hCG in the mother

   C. An adnexal mass

   D. Decreased platelets with an elevated LDH, ALT, and AST

6. Which one of the following statements about hCG and spontaneous abortion (miscarriage) is not true?

   A. A spontaneous abortion or nonviable pregnancy is associated with a slow rate of increase in hCG.

   B. hCG concentrations can be monitored after fetal loss until they are undetectable, to confirm complete expulsion of the products of conception.

   C. Up to 60 days may be required after fetal loss before the serum hCG concentrations are undetectable.

   D. Serial measurements of hCG concentration, along with other tests, are often important in the diagnosis of the spontaneous abortion.

7. A pregnant woman has the following laboratory test results: a modest increase in AST and ALT; >0.3 g/L protein in a 24-hour urine specimen; and >1.0 g/L protein in a random urine specimen. She is also markedly hypertensive. Which one of the following abnormal pregnancy conditions does she likely have?

   A. HELLP syndrome
   B. Gestational trophoblast disease
   C. Preeclampsia
   D. Fatty liver of pregnancy

8. Which one of the following choices is unlikely to be part of the laboratory evaluation of a patient experiencing recurrent spontaneous abortions?

   A. Parental and fetal tissue karyotypes to test for chromosomal abnormalities
   B. Endometrial biopsy to test for a luteal phase defect or inadequate endometrial maturation
   C. Hemoglobin A1C to test for diabetes
   D. Exome analysis to identify genetic abnormalities associated with spontaneous abortion

9. Which one of the following is unlikely to be contributory to female infertility?

   A. Hypogonadism, both hypergonadotropic and hypogonadotropic, resulting in defects in ovulation
   B. Polycystic ovarian disease
   C. Elevated midluteal progesterone concentration, resulting in anovulation
   D. Thyroid dysfunction

FURTHER READING

ACOG Committee on Practice Bulletins—Obstetrics. ACOG practice bulletin. Diagnosis and management of preeclampsia and eclampsia. Number 33, January 2002. *Obstet Gynecol*. 2002;99:159–167.

Altman AD, et al. Maternal age-related rates of gestational trophoblastic disease. *Obstet Gynecol*. 2008;112:244–250.

American College of Obstetricians and Gynecologists Committee on Genetics. Committee opinion no. 640: cell-free DNA screening for fetal aneuploidy. *Obstet Gynecol*. 2015;126:e31–e37.

Ashwood ER, et al. Pregnancy and its disorders. In: Burtis CA, Ashwood ER, Bruns DE, eds. *Tietz Textbook of Clinical Chemistry and Molecular Diagnostics*. 5th ed. St. Louis, MO: Elsevier; 2012:1991.

Baek KH, et al. Recurrent pregnancy loss: the key potential mechanisms. *Trends Mol Med*. 2007;13:310–317.

Barton JR, Sibai BM. Prediction and prevention of recurrent preeclampsia. *Obstet Gynecol*. 2008;112:359–372.

Borrelli PTA, et al. Human chorionic gonadotropin isoforms in the diagnosis of ectopic pregnancy. *Clin Chem*. 2003;49:2045–2049.

Brassard M, et al. Basic infertility including polycystic ovary syndrome. *Med Clin North Am*. 2008;92:1163–1192.

Christiansen OB, et al. Evidence-based investigations and treatments of recurrent pregnancy loss. *Fertil Steril*. 2005;83:821–839.

Dashe JS. Aneuploidy screening in pregnancy. *Obstet Gynecol*. 2016;128:181–194.

Dewailly D, et al. The physiology and clinical utility of anti-mullerian hormone in women. *Hum Reprod Update*. 2014;20:370–385.

Doubilet PM, Benson CB. Further evidence against the reliability of the human chorionic gonadotropin discriminatory level. *J Ultrasound Med*. 2011;30:1637–1642.

Farquhar C. Ectopic pregnancy. *Lancet*. 2005;366:583–591.

Frey KA, Patel KS. Initial evaluation and management of infertility by the primary care physician. *Mayo Clin Proc*. 2004;79:1439–1443.

Guntupalli SR, Steingrub J. Hepatic disease and pregnancy: an overview of diagnosis and management. *Crit Care Med*. 2005;33(suppl):S332–S339.

Haymond S, Gronowski AM. Reproductive related disorders. In: Burtis CA, Ashwood ER, Bruns DE, eds. *Tietz Textbook of Clinical Chemistry and Molecular Diagnostics*. 4th ed. St. Louis, MO: Elsevier Saunders; 2006:2097.

Mihu D, et al. HELLP syndrome—a multisystemic disorder. *J Gastrointest Liver Dis*. 2007;16:419–424.

Norton ME, et al. Cell-free DNA analysis for noninvasive examination of trisomy. *N Engl J Med*. 2015;372:1589–1597.

Pandey MK, et al. An update in recurrent spontaneous abortion. *Arch Gynecol Obstet*. 2005;272:95–108.

Papanna R, et al. Protein/creatinine ratio in preeclampsia. *Obstet Gynecol*. 2008;112:135–144.

Rai R, Regan L. Recurrent miscarriage. *Lancet*. 2006;368:601–611.

Rajasri AG, et al. Acute fatty liver of pregnancy (AFLP)—an overview. *J Obstet Gynaecol*. 2007;27:237–240.

Reddy UM, Mennuti MT. Incorporating first-trimester Down syndrome studies into prenatal screening. *Obstet Gynecol*. 2006;107:167–173.

Reddy UM, et al. Infertility, assisted reproductive technology, and adverse pregnancy outcomes. *Obstet Gynecol.* 2007;109:967–977.

Seeber BE, et al. Application of redefined human chorionic gonadotropin curves for the diagnosis of women at risk for ectopic pregnancy. *Fertil Steril.* 2006;86:454–459.

Seki K, et al. Advances in the clinical laboratory detection of gestational trophoblastic disease. *Clin Chim Acta.* 2004;349:1–13.

Shaw SW, et al. First- and second-trimester Down syndrome screening: current strategies and clinical guidelines. *Taiwan J Obstet Gynecol.* 2008;47:157–162.

Smith GCS. Circulating angiogenic factors in early pregnancy and the risk of preeclampsia, intrauterine growth restriction, spontaneous preterm birth, and stillbirth. *Obstet Gynecol.* 2007;109:1316–1324.

Soper JT. Gestational trophoblastic disease. *Obstet Gynecol.* 2006;108:176–187.

Su GL. Pregnancy and liver disease. *Curr Gastroenterol Rep.* 2008;10:15–21.

Breast

Karin E. Finberg and Veerle Bossuyt

LEARNING OBJECTIVES

1. Discuss the tissue- and serum-based biomarkers in breast cancer.

2. Summarize the genes that are associated with highly penetrant forms of hereditary breast cancer, including the hereditary breast and ovarian cancer syndrome.

CHAPTER OUTLINE

INTRODUCTION

This chapter focuses on laboratory testing relevant to breast cancer. Infections of the breast are included in Chapter 5.

BREAST CANCER

Description

Cancers of the breast constitute a major cause of mortality in women of Western countries. In the United States, the lifetime probability that a woman will develop breast cancer is 1 in 8. Breast cancer accounts for 30% of new cancer cases and 14% of cancer deaths in American women. About 1% of breast cancers occur in males. The risk of developing breast cancer is influenced by several factors. These factors include increased age, family history of breast cancer (especially in a first-degree relative), hormonal factors (early age at menarche, older age of menopause, older age at first full-term pregnancy, fewer number of pregnancies, and use of hormone replacement therapy), clinical factors (high breast tissue density and history of prior invasive breast carcinoma, carcinoma in situ, or atypical hyperplasia), obesity, and alcohol consumption. Since 1990, the mortality rate associated with female breast cancer has decreased in the United States, a decline that has been attributed to both therapeutic advances and early detection.

For localized breast cancer, primary treatment typically consists of either breast-conserving surgery and radiation or mastectomy. Most patients with invasive breast cancer subsequently receive systemic adjuvant chemotherapy and/or hormone therapy, both of which have been shown to reduce systemic recurrence and breast cancer-related mortality. However, the fact that some patients who lack lymph node involvement are cured by the combination of surgery and radiotherapy suggests that adjuvant treatment may not be necessary in all cases. Therefore, to rationally administer adjuvant therapy to patients with local disease, several prognostic factors are considered to assess the risk for recurrence. These prognostic factors include tumor size, axillary node involvement, histological type, histologic grade, lymphatic and vascular invasion, and certain biomarkers used as prognostic and predictive markers for breast cancer patients. Predictive markers are used to predict response to a specific therapy.

While adjuvant therapy improves patient outcomes, 25% to 30% of women with lymph node-negative and at least 50% to 60% of women with node-positive disease develop recurrent or metastatic disease. Metastatic breast cancer is currently regarded as incurable. Therapeutic options for metastatic disease include chemotherapy, hormone therapy, and molecularly targeted therapies. In the context of metastatic disease, information gained from serial monitoring of tumor markers detected in the serum may contribute to decisions to continue or terminate a particular treatment.

LABORATORY TESTING

Tissue-based Biomarkers in Breast Cancer

Assessment of biomarkers in tissue obtained from the patient's breast tumor is routinely performed to obtain prognostic information and to guide therapy.

Estrogen Receptor (ER) and Progesterone Receptor (PR)

> Assessment of biomarkers in tissue obtained from the patient's breast tumor is routinely performed to obtain prognostic information and to guide therapy.

ER and PR are intracellular receptors that bind to lipid-soluble steroid hormones that diffuse into target cells. Following ligand binding, two receptor subunits dimerize to form a single, functional DNA-binding unit that binds to specific DNA target sequences to induce transcription of target genes. There are two different forms of the ER, termed ER-α and ER-β, which are encoded by separate genes. Clinical assays assess ER-α, the classical form of the receptor. PR has two isoforms that differ in molecular weight but are encoded by a single gene.

Measurement of the ER and PR status of the tumor is recommended in all patients with breast cancer. ER expression is present in approximately 70% of breast cancers, is associated with a favorable prognosis, and suggests that the growth of the tumor may be estrogen-dependent. The primary purpose of determining ER and PR status in breast cancers is to identify those patients, in both the adjuvant and metastatic settings, who are likely to respond to endocrine treatments. These treatments act by either preventing the formation of estrogen from its precursors or blocking estrogen from binding to its receptors. Endocrine treatments include selective ER modulators (e.g., tamoxifen), ovarian ablation (surgical or chemical), aromatase inhibitors (anastrozole, letrozole, and exemestane), and selective ER degraders (e.g., fulvestrant). In patients with ER-positive tumors, 5 years of adjuvant treatment with tamoxifen significantly reduces annual death rates from breast cancer, while in patients with ER-negative tumors, tamoxifen shows little effect on recurrence or death, and it does not significantly modify the effects of polychemotherapy.

ER/PR status is routinely assessed by immunohistochemistry (IHC) in the clinical setting. IHC evaluates the percentage of cells with nuclear ER/PR and the intensity of staining. The use of validated antibodies is required, and a positive control (i.e., a control tissue with tumor cells known to express the respective receptor) must be examined in parallel. A tumor is scored as positive for either ER or PR if $\geq$1% of tumor cell nuclei are immunoreactive. A tumor is scored as negative for ER or PR if <1% of tumor cell nuclei are immunoreactive. Nuclear staining in adjacent normal breast epithelial cells if present serves as an internal positive control. For optimal results, breast resection specimens should be fixed within 1 hour. Fixation should be performed in 10% neutral buffered formalin for at least 6 hours and for not more than 72 hours in order to preserve ER and PR epitope recognition and thus avoid false-negative results.

HER2

HER2 (also known as *ERBB2* and *NEU*) is a proto-oncogene located at chromosome 17q11 that is a member of the epidermal growth factor receptor (EGFR) family. Like other EGFR family members, HER2 is a transmembrane receptor with cytoplasmic tyrosine kinase activity. Dimerization of the receptor leads to phosphorylation of a variety of substrates, resulting in the activation of intracellular signaling pathways important for cell proliferation and survival.

While normal cells contain two copies of the *HER2* gene (one copy on each chromosome 17), in approximately 10% to 15% of breast cancers *HER2* gene copy number is increased at least two-fold relative to the number of copies of chromosome 17, a phenomenon termed as gene amplification. Gene amplification results in overexpression of the HER2 protein at the cell surface, which in turn promotes tumor cell proliferation and survival. Tumors that overexpress *HER2* behave more aggressively than those lacking overexpression, and they are associated with poorer clinical outcomes.

Assessment of *HER2* status of the tumor is recommended in all patients with invasive breast cancer. The primary purpose of *HER2* testing is to identify those patients with early or advanced breast cancer who are eligible for treatment with trastuzumab, a recombinant monoclonal antibody that recognizes HER2. Although its exact mechanism of action remains to be fully elucidated, trastuzumab has been shown in both in vitro assays and animal studies to inhibit proliferation of human tumor cells that overexpress HER2. In patients with *HER2*-positive early stage breast cancer, the addition of trastuzumab to adjuvant chemotherapy significantly improves disease-free and overall survival. Additionally, in patients with *HER2*-positive metastatic breast cancer, the addition of trastuzumab to adjuvant chemotherapy significantly increases the time until disease progression. Because a small percentage of patients treated with trastuzumab develop cardiotoxicity, the elimination of false-positive *HER2* results is important so that patients are not exposed to this risk unnecessarily.

HER2 status is routinely assessed in formalin-fixed tissues by either fluorescence in situ hybridization (FISH) or IHC. FISH assesses *HER2* status at the DNA level. A fluorescent-labeled nucleic acid probe that recognizes the *HER2* gene on chromosome 17 is hybridized on tissue sections, and the average number of *HER2* signals per nucleus is determined in areas of invasive tumor. In some assay systems, an additional probe that recognizes the centromeric region of chromosome 17 (CEP17) (and which is labeled with a different fluorophore) is included to allow the ratio of the average number of copies of *HER2*:CEP17 (the "FISH ratio") to be calculated. Tumors with intermediate results are considered equivocal for gene amplification; in these cases, IHC for HER2 protein is performed. Chromogenic in situ hybridization (CISH) may be performed as an alternative to FISH. In CISH, the *HER2* probe is visualized by an immunoperoxidase reaction. This enables CISH results to be scored using a conventional light microscope rather than the fluorescence microscope that is required for FISH.

In contrast to the FISH assay, IHC assesses HER2 status at the protein level. The level of HER2 protein expression is scored on a semiquantitative scale. Tumors with 3+ protein expression are scored as positive for HER2 protein expression, while tumors with 0 or 1+ protein expression are scored as negative. Tumors with intermediate staining patterns (e.g., cases showing complete membrane staining that is weak in intensity) are considered equivocal; in these cases, FISH is performed.

Multigene Prognostic Assays

Recently, clinical assays that utilize expression information gathered across a panel of genes have been developed to predict recurrence risk and guide adjuvant chemotherapy decisions in patients with early stage breast cancer. Several assays, which examine different sets of genes, are currently available. Two of the more widely validated testing platforms involve examination of 21 and 70 genes, respectively. Depending on the particular testing platform, fresh frozen tissue or formalin-fixed, paraffin-embedded tissue may be required. While methods used to quantify gene expression vary by platform, one approach involves using the enzyme reverse transcriptase to convert messenger RNA into complementary cDNA; the resulting cDNA then serves as a template for assays such as quantitative polymerase chain reaction or microarray gene expression profiling. While the role for these multigene prognostic assays in the routine clinical management of patients with breast cancer remains to be fully established, several of these assays have

The primary purpose of *HER2* testing is to identify those patients with early or advanced breast cancer who are eligible for treatment with trastuzumab, a recombinant monoclonal antibody that recognizes HER2.

been validated in retrospective and prospective studies. The clinical use of some of these assays is now recommended by expert panels, and these assays are thus increasingly used in clinical practice. Increasingly, treatment recommendations take into account tumor biology as determined by conventional biomarker assays and multigene prognostic assays, as well as clinical factors such as anatomic stage. The most recent American Joint Committee on Cancer (AJCC) staging system (8th edition) includes an anatomic stage group and a prognostic stage group. The prognostic stage group is determined by anatomic stage, tumor grade, and the results of ER, PR, and HER2 testing, as well as multigene panels when available.

Serum-based Biomarkers in Breast Cancer

Serum-based tumor markers may be useful in the identification and management of patients with breast cancer. The ideal breast cancer marker would be both specific for breast cancer and sufficiently sensitive for screening purposes. Unfortunately, no marker identified to date meets these criteria. Candidate protein biomarkers, which can be detected by immunoassays, include CA15-3, CA27.29, and carcinoembryonic antigen (CEA). CA 15-3 and CA 27.29 represent different but overlapping epitopes of the MUC1 protein, a large, complex glycoprotein expressed at the luminal surface of glandular epithelial cells. CEA is a cell-surface glycoprotein involved in cell adhesion that is normally expressed during fetal development. MUC1 and CEA may be overexpressed by malignant cells and shed into the circulation. Due to fairly low sensitivity for detection of early disease, the role of these markers in the management of early stage breast cancer remains unclear. However, in conjunction with history, physical exam, and diagnostic imaging, these markers may have some utility for evaluating the progression of disease after initial therapy and for monitoring subsequent treatment.

When considering the use of serum tumor markers, several points should be kept in mind: (1) none of the currently available markers is elevated in all patients with breast cancer, even in the setting of advanced disease, so that a normal tumor marker level does not exclude a malignancy; (2) these markers are most sensitive for detecting metastatic disease and have little value in the diagnosis of local or regional recurrences; (3) the magnitude of change in marker levels that correlates with disease progression or regression has not been firmly established; (4) tumor marker levels may paradoxically rise after initiation of chemotherapy, a phenomenon attributed to therapy-mediated apoptosis or necrosis of tumor cells; and (5) tumor marker levels may be increased in the setting of certain benign diseases.

HEREDITARY BREAST AND OVARIAN CANCER SYNDROME

Description

Approximately 5% to 10% of breast cancer cases are attributed to a germline mutation in a highly penetrant cancer predisposition gene. A large proportion of these hereditary cases are associated with mutations in two genes, *BRCA1* and *BRCA2*.

While most cases of breast cancer are caused by acquired somatic mutations, approximately 5% to 10% of breast cancer cases are attributed to a germline mutation in a highly penetrant cancer predisposition gene. A large proportion of these hereditary cases are associated with mutations in two genes, breast cancer type 1 and 2 (*BRCA1* and *BRCA2*). Mutations in *BRCA1* and *BRCA2* cause the hereditary breast and ovarian cancer syndrome, an autosomal dominant disorder in which the risk of both breast and ovarian cancer is significantly increased compared with the general population. *BRCA1* and *BRCA2*, which are located at chromosome 17q21 and 13q12, respectively, are tumor suppressor genes that play essential roles in the repair of double-stranded DNA breaks and thus in the maintenance of genome stability. Accordingly, in tumors from individuals with hereditary breast and ovarian cancer syndrome, the wild-type *BRCA1* or *BRCA2* allele is deleted, consistent with a tumor suppressor function for *BRCA1* and *BRCA2*.

A woman's risk for harboring either a *BRCA1* or *BRCA2* mutation is increased by certain factors related to her personal and family medical history. Personal factors include (1) early onset breast cancer (i.e., diagnosis before 50 years of age); (2) bilateral or multifocal breast cancers; and (3) a history of both breast and ovarian cancer. Factors from the family history include (1) breast cancer or breast and ovarian cancer in a pattern consistent with autosomal dominant transmission; and (2) breast cancer in a male relative.

Hereditary breast and ovarian cancer syndrome shows incomplete penetrance. Among women with either a *BRCA1* or *BRCA2* mutation, the lifetime risk of developing breast cancer is 60% to 80%. The lifetime risk of developing ovarian cancer is 15% to 60% for women with *BRCA1* mutations and 10% to 27% for women with *BRCA2* mutations. Mutations in *BRCA1* and *BRCA2* also increase the risk of male breast cancer. Individuals with hereditary breast and ovarian cancer syndrome are also at risk for other tumors, including melanoma and cancers of the prostate (in males) and pancreas.

Determination of *BRCA1* and *BRCA2* mutation status is an important clinical assessment, as the identification of a deleterious mutation may alter clinical management. Interventions available to *BRCA1* and *BRCA2* mutation carriers include intensive screening, chemoprevention, prophylactic mastectomy, and prophylactic oophorectomy. Prophylactic oophorectomy, which reduces the risk of breast cancer as well as ovarian cancer, is recommended for all mutation carriers at the completion of childbearing. Genetic testing for *BRCA1* and *BRCA2* mutations in women diagnosed with breast cancer may also have relevance to selection of targeted cancer therapies. In preclinical and clinical studies, *BRCA*-mutant tumors have been shown to exhibit sensitivity to inhibitors of poly (ADP-ribose) polymerases (PARPs), enzymes that play a key role in DNA repair pathways.

Determination of *BRCA1* and *BRCA2* Mutations

Genetic testing for *BRCA1* and *BRCA2* mutations should be offered to individuals with a personal or family history suspicious for hereditary breast and ovarian cancer syndrome, and to women at risk because of a family member known to harbor a deleterious mutation in one of these genes. It is critical that testing be offered in the setting of appropriate genetic counseling, so that individuals are provided appropriate information regarding the risks, benefits, and limitations of genetic testing. Such counseling should also include consideration of how the results of such testing might affect other family members.

Study of kindreds with hereditary breast and ovarian cancer syndrome has identified hundreds of different deleterious mutations in the *BRCA1* and *BRCA2* genes. Most consist of frameshift or nonsense mutations, which are predicted to result in a loss of function of the encoded gene product. Due to the large number of different mutations described, genetic testing to assess for most of these involves examination of the DNA sequence of the entire coding region of each gene. Additional molecular testing may also be employed to assess for certain large genomic rearrangements that cannot be detected by routine DNA sequencing. In cases where a known deleterious mutation has already been identified in a family member, targeted mutation analysis is performed to specifically assess for the familial mutation.

When possible, genetic testing should be performed on an individual who has been diagnosed with breast or ovarian cancer because this strategy provides the most information for other members of the family. Genetic testing can lead to four possible outcomes: a true-positive result, a true-negative result, an uninformative result, and a variant of uncertain significance. A true-positive result occurs when a deleterious mutation known to be associated with increased cancer risk is identified; such a result confirms the diagnosis of hereditary breast and ovarian cancer syndrome. A true-negative result occurs only when the tested individual is found to lack a specific deleterious mutation already known to run in the family; a true-negative result thus reduces the tested individual's risk of developing breast and/or ovarian cancer to that of general population. An uninformative result occurs when a mutation is not identified in an individual from a family in which a deleterious mutation has not yet been identified; an uninformative result does not exclude the possibility of a *BRCA1* or *BRCA2* mutation that cannot be detected by current testing methodologies, nor does it exclude the possibility of a mutation in another cancer susceptibility gene. Genetic variants of uncertain significance are typically missense variants of unknown functional significance or intronic variants not predicted to disrupt mRNA processing; individuals harboring variants of unknown significance may still be at increased risk for cancer, and their medical management should be based on the known family history. In all cases, posttest genetic counseling should be performed to ensure that individuals fully comprehend the implications of their testing results.

Genetic testing for *BRCA1* and *BRCA2* mutations should be offered to individuals with a personal or family history suspicious for hereditary breast and ovarian cancer syndrome, and to women at risk because of a family member known to harbor a deleterious mutation in one of these genes.

OTHER HIGH-PENETRANCE CANCER PREDISPOSITION GENES

In addition to *BRCA1* and *BRCA2*, highly penetrant forms of hereditary breast cancer have also been linked to mutations in the tumor suppressor genes *TP53*, *PTEN*, serine/threonine kinase 11 (*STK11*), and cadherin 1 (*CDH1*). While mutations in these genes comprise a smaller proportion of hereditary breast cancer cases than *BRCA1* and *BRCA2*, identification of these mutations similarly has profound implications for clinical management and for genetic risks of family members. Genetic testing for mutations in these genes is conducted using molecular approaches similar to those used for *BRCA1* and *BRCA2* and can also lead to the same four possible test outcomes described above. Genetic testing for these mutations should be offered in the setting of appropriate genetic counseling to at-risk family members of an individual with a known deleterious mutation and to individuals with personal or family histories suspicious for these particular syndromes, which are described in detail below.

> In addition to *BRCA1* and *BRCA2*, highly penetrant forms of hereditary breast cancer have also been linked to mutations in the tumor suppressor genes *TP53, PTEN, STK11,* and *CDH1*.

Li–Fraumeni Syndrome

Germline mutations in *TP53* cause Li–Fraumeni syndrome, a rare autosomal dominant condition associated with the development of a variety of tumor types throughout life, including in childhood. *TP53*, located at chromosome 17p13, encodes the p53 protein, which plays key roles in DNA repair, cell cycle control, and the initiation of apoptosis. In addition to breast cancer, tumors associated with Li–Fraumeni syndrome include osteosarcomas, soft tissue sarcomas, brain tumors, leukemias, and adrenocortical carcinomas. In families with Li–Fraumeni syndrome, breast cancer is common and may account for one-third of all cancers.

Cowden Syndrome

Germline mutations in *PTEN* (phosphatase and tensin homolog) cause Cowden syndrome, a rare autosomal dominant condition characterized by an increased risk of certain cancers and the development of multiple skin and mucosal hamartomas (focal malformations that resemble neoplasms but result from faulty development of the tissue). *PTEN*, located at chromosome 10q23, encodes a phosphatase that downregulates the phosphatidylinositol-3-kinase (PI3K) signal transduction pathway, thereby contributing to the regulation of cell growth. The spectrum of cancers seen in Cowden syndrome includes thyroid cancer, uterine cancer, renal cell cancer, and breast cancer. Females with Cowden syndrome have a 25% to 50% lifetime risk of developing breast cancer.

Peutz–Jeghers Syndrome

Germline mutations in *STK11* cause Peutz–Jeghers syndrome, a rare autosomal dominant condition characterized by gastrointestinal polyps and mucocutaneous pigmentation. *STK11*, located at chromosome 19p13, encodes serine/threonine-protein kinase 11 and functions to regulate cell polarity, energy utilization, and apoptosis. Individuals with Peutz–Jeghers syndrome are at increased risk for the development of a variety of cancers, including colorectal, gastric, pancreatic, ovarian, and breast. The lifetime risk of breast cancer reported for females with Peutz–Jeghers syndrome has been estimated at 30% to 50%.

Hereditary Diffuse Gastric Cancer (HDGC) Syndrome

Germline mutations in *CDH1* cause HDGC syndrome, a rare autosomal dominant condition characterized by an increased risk of stomach cancer as well as lobular breast cancer. CDH1, located at chromosome 16q22, encodes E-cadherin, a calcium-dependent cell–cell adhesion protein. Loss of CDH1 activity is believed to contribute to cancer progression by increasing proliferation, invasion, and/or metastasis. The cumulative risk of breast cancer reported for females who carry a pathogenic *CDH1* germline mutation has been estimated at 39% to 52%.

SELF-ASSESSMENT QUESTIONS

1. With regard to biomarkers for breast cancer, which of the following matched pairs is incorrect?

    A. Estrogen receptor/Tissue-based biomarker
    B. Carcinoembryonic antigen (CEA)/Serum-based biomarker
    C. *HER2*/Serum-based biomarker
    D. Progesterone receptor/Tissue-based biomarker

2. Estrogen receptor and progesterone receptor status is routinely assessed by which method in the laboratory?

    A. Fluorescent in-situ hybridization (FISH)
    B. Immunohistochemistry (IHC)
    C. Chromogenic in-situ hybridization (CISH)
    D. Periodic acid-Schiff (PAS) staining

3. One of the following methods is not used to determine *HER2* status. Identify the method which is not used to determine *HER2* status.

    A. Immunohistochemistry (IHC)
    B. Chromogenic in-situ hybridization (CISH)
    C. Karyotype analysis
    D. Fluorescence in-situ hybridization (FISH)

4. Which of the following tumor-suppressor gene mutations is found in the largest number of hereditary breast and ovarian cancer cases?

    A. *TP53* mutation
    B. *PTEN* (phosphatase tensin homolog)
    C. *BRCA1* and *BRCA2*
    D. *STK11*

FURTHER READING

American Cancer Society. Cancer Facts & Figures 2017. Available at: https://www.cancer.org/research/cancer-facts-statistics/all-cancer-facts-figures/cancer-facts-figures-2017. Accessed November 29, 2017.

Amin MB, et al. (eds.) *American Joint Committee on Cancer (AJCC) Cancer Staging Manual.* Vol I. 8th ed. New York, NY: Springer; 2017.

Cobain EF, Milliron KJ, Merajver SD. Updates on breast cancer genetics: clinical implications of detecting syndromes of inherited increased susceptibility to breast cancer. *Semin Oncol.* 2016;43:528–535.

Duffy MJ, et al. Biomarkers in breast cancer: where are we and where are we going? *Adv Clin Chem.* 2015;71:1–23.

Furrer D, et al. Advantages and disadvantages of technologies for HER2 testing in breast cancer specimens. *Am J Clin Pathol.* 2015;144:686–703.

Hammond ME. ASCO-CAP guidelines for breast predictive factor testing: an update. *Appl Immunohistochem Mol Morphol.* 2011;19:499–500.

Hammond ME, et al. American Society of Clinical Oncology/College of American Pathologists guideline recommendations for immunohistochemical testing of estrogen and progesterone receptors in breast cancer (unabridged version). *Arch Pathol Lab Med.* 2010;134:e48–e72.

Kazarian A, et al. Testing breast cancer serum biomarkers for early detection and prognosis in pre-diagnosis samples. *Br J Cancer.* 2017;116:501–508.

Loibl S, Gianni L. HER2-positive breast cancer. *Lancet.* 2017;389(10087):2415–2429.

Markopoulos C, et al. Clinical evidence supporting genomic tests in early breast cancer: do all genomic tests provide the same information? *Eur J Surg Oncol.* 2017;43:909–920.

National Comprehensive Cancer Network. Breast Cancer (Version 3.2017). Available at: https://www.nccn.org/professionals/physician_gls/default.aspx. Accessed November 29, 2017.

Nicolini A, Ferrari P, Duffy MJ. Prognostic and predictive biomarkers in breast cancer: past, present and future. *Semin Cancer Biol.* September 4, 2017. pii: S1044-579X(17)30052-4.

Nicolini A., et al. Mucins and cytokeratins as serum tumor markers in breast cancer. In: Scatena R. (ed.) *Advances in Cancer Biomarkers. Advances in Experimental Medicine and Biology.* Vol 867. New York, NY. Dordrecht: Springer; 2015.

Ohmoto A, Yachida S. Current status of poly(ADP-ribose) polymerase inhibitors and future directions. *Onco Targets Ther.* 2017;10:5195–5208.

Petrucelli N, Daly MB, Pal T. BRCA1- and BRCA2-associated hereditary breast and ovarian cancer. September 4, 1998 [updated December 15, 2016]. In: Adam MP, Ardinger HH, Pagon RA, et al. (eds.). *GeneReviews* [Internet]. Seattle, WA: University of Washington; 1993–2017. Available at: https://www.ncbi.nlm.nih.gov/books/NBK1247/.

Rakha EA, et al. The updated ASCO/CAP guideline recommendations for HER2 testing in the management of invasive breast cancer: a critical review of their implications for routine practice. *Histopathology*. 2014;64:609–615.

Siegel RL, et al. Cancer Statistics, 2017. *CA Cancer J Clin*. 2017;67:7–30.

Valencia OM, et al. The role of genetic testing in patients with breast cancer: a review. *JAMA Surg*. 2017;152:589–594.

Wolff AC, et al. Recommendations for human epidermal growth factor receptor 2 testing in breast cancer: American Society of Clinical Oncology/College of American Pathologists clinical practice guideline update. *J Clin Oncol*. 2013;31:3997–4013.

Xin L, Liu YH, Martin TA, Jiang WG. The era of multigene panels comes? The clinical utility of Oncotype DX and MammaPrint. *World J Oncol*. 2017;8:34–40.

The Endocrine System

Alison Woodworth, Vipul Lakhani, and Michael Laposata

CHAPTER OUTLINE

INTRODUCTION

This chapter on endocrine disorders is divided into separate discussions of each of the endocrine glands. Each section begins with an overview of the physiology and biochemistry of the relevant hormones. In addition, because of the large number of (often complex) laboratory tests in endocrinology, each section has a brief description of the laboratory tests most frequently used to diagnose the disorders in that disease group. Tests for which either serum or plasma is an acceptable specimen for analysis are noted as serum tests. Tests specifically requiring plasma are indicated by inclusion of the word "plasma" before the test name. As with all other chapters, each disorder is presented with a description of the disease and information useful in establishing a diagnosis. **Figure 22–1** shows a general approach to the patient with endocrine disease.

THYROID

Physiology and Biochemistry

Production of thyroid hormones is regulated by the hypothalamic–pituitary–thyroid axis (**Figure 22–2**). Thyrotropin-releasing hormone (TRH) is produced in the hypothalamus and induces thyroid-stimulating hormone (TSH or thyrotropin) production in the anterior pituitary. TSH, in turn, stimulates thyroid hormone production and release by the thyroid gland. TSH production is inversely related to plasma thyroxine (T_4) and triiodothyronine (T_3) concentrations. The two primary hormones synthesized and secreted by the thyroid gland are T_4 and, in lesser quantities, T_3 (**Figure 22–3**). They are transported by plasma proteins—notably thyroid-binding globulin (TBG), transthyretin, and albumin—to various tissue sites where T_4 is deiodinated to the active form, T_3, and the inactive form known as reverse T_3 (rT_3). Thyroid hormones act through nuclear hormone receptors that are transcription factors for numerous genes. These genes regulate a number of critical physiologic functions in development and metabolism.

> A "generational" classification has been applied for TSH assays based on the assay sensitivity. Third-generation assays can accurately measure TSH as low as 0.01 mU/L.

Laboratory Tests

TSH

A "generational" classification has been applied for TSH immunoassays based on the assay sensitivity. Third-generation assays can accurately measure TSH as low as 0.01 mU/L. This allows the physician to distinguish mildly subnormal TSH values from the low values of overt hyperthyroid

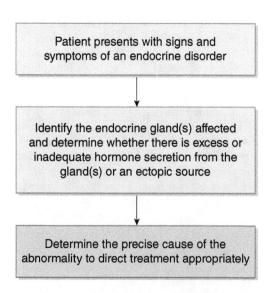

FIGURE 22–1   An approach to the patient with an endocrinologic disorder.

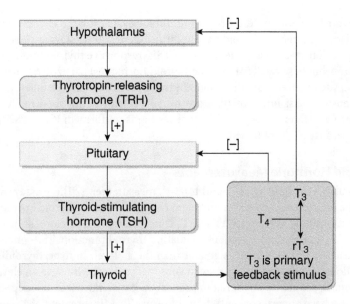

FIGURE 22–2 **Hypothalamic–pituitary–thyroid interactions. [+] Stimulation; [−] inhibition.**

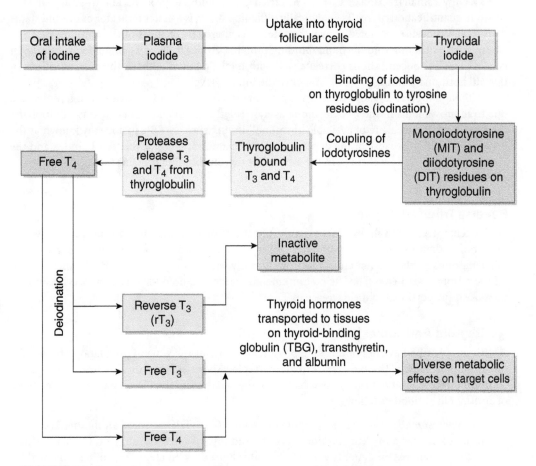

FIGURE 22–3 **The formation, secretion, and transport of thyroid hormones.**

patients. The third-generation tests are also useful for evaluating the effectiveness of the thyroid hormone replacement in hypothyroid patients. Third-generation assays are essential for monitoring TSH suppression therapy in patients with a TSH-responsive thyroid tumor.

The relationship between TSH and the thyroid hormones, particularly free T_4, is an inverse log-linear one, such that very small changes in free T_4 result in large changes in TSH. Thus, TSH is the most sensitive first-line screening test for suspected thyroid abnormalities. If the TSH is within the normal reference range, no further testing is performed. If the TSH is outside of the reference range, a free T_4 is obtained.

Total Thyroid Hormone Measurements

Assays are available for both total T_4 and total T_3 measurements. These assays are quite specific and suffer little interference. However, transient changes in serum thyroid hormone-binding protein concentrations may affect total T_4 and T_3 concentrations. Therefore, an assessment for free T_4 (see below) is usually more helpful in evaluating thyroid function. The concentration of T_4 in the blood is usually 100 to 200 times greater than the T_3 level. In hyperthyroidism, total T_3 and T_4 concentrations correlate in all but a small subset of patients who have an elevation only in T_3. For that reason, T_3 should be measured in the serum of patients clinically suspected to be hyperthyroid and who have normal concentrations of serum T_4. Measurement of T_3 concentrations has limited clinical utility in assessment of hypothyroidism. Significant decreases in total T_3 are seen in euthyroid sick syndrome (ETS), now known as non-thyroidal illness (NTI).

Free Thyroid Hormones and Thyroid Hormone-binding Capacity

"Direct" free thyroid hormone assays, without the need for a preliminary step to separate free hormones from hormones bound to protein carriers, are available for measurement of free T_4 and free T_3. Only a small fraction of T_4 ($<0.1\%$) circulates unbound to proteins, and this has made the accurate quantification of free T_4 analytically difficult. Free T_4 is a better indicator of thyroid status than total T_4 because, as noted above, the total T_4 is altered by changes in the amounts of TBG, albumin, and other thyroid hormone-binding proteins. About 0.3% of T_3 circulates as free T_3. In general, free T_3 concentrations correlate well with total T_3, but as with T_4, the concentrations of thyroid hormone-binding proteins influence the total T_3 level.

Although the free T_4 index offers an approximation of free T_4, this measure is largely obsolete due to improvements in the free hormone assays. The free T_4 index is calculated by multiplying the total T_4 by the measure of available hormone-binding sites on TBG in an assay known as the percent T_3 uptake. Because of the dependence on the amount of TBG, the free T_4 index and the T_3 uptake are affected by changes in the amount of thyroid-binding proteins induced by a variety of stimuli.

Reverse Triiodothyronine

Under acute stress or in illness, there is a shift in the T_4 deiodination in favor of the inactive rT_3 form rather than the active T_3. Numerous immunoassays are available for the measurement of rT_3 using antisera that do not cross-react significantly with T_3 or T_4. rT_3 is markedly increased in ETS syndrome (see below), but its measurement is rarely required for this diagnosis because its increase is proportional to the decrease in T_3.

> Antithyroid antibodies are present in approximately 15% of the general population and are the most common cause of thyroid disease in iodine-replete societies.

Antithyroid Antibodies

Antithyroid antibodies are present in approximately 15% of the general population and are the most common cause of thyroid disease in iodine-replete societies. They are also present in selected autoimmune diseases not usually associated with thyroid dysfunction. Descriptions of three types of antithyroid antibodies follow:

- *Antimicrosomal/antithyroid peroxidase antibodies (anti-TPO)*—These antibodies are directed against a protein component of thyroid microsomes, the enzyme TPO. They are present in almost all patients with Hashimoto thyroiditis, in about 85% of patients with Graves disease (both discussed below), and in some patients with other autoimmune diseases like type 1 diabetes mellitus, celiac disease, and Addison disease. An elevated titer of anti-TPO antibodies in the context of clinical symptoms of thyroid dysfunction and abnormal TSH and free T_4 results is diagnostic for autoimmune thyroid disease. The presence of TPO antibodies before or during pregnancy is a good predictor of those women who will develop postpartum thyroid disease (discussed below). Normal concentrations are not well established because the antibodies may be found in healthy people (up to 12% of the population), and the reference range depends on the method used to perform the test.

- *Antithyroglobulin antibodies*—These are also called colloidal antibodies. They are present in more than 85% of patients with Hashimoto thyroiditis and in more than 30% of patients with Graves disease. Like anti-TPO, antithyroglobulin antibodies also may be found in other autoimmune diseases. In iodine-sufficient areas, the antithyroglobulin antibody test is used less often, in favor of anti-TPO. However, in patients with suspected iodine deficiency, antithyroglobulin antibody is a better indicator of autoimmune thyroid disease.
- *TSH receptor antibodies*—These are a diverse group of immunoglobulins that bind to TSH receptors and influence their action. They are found in most patients with Graves disease and in patients with other autoimmune thyroid disorders. The biological functions of these antibodies vary from thyroid stimulation to thyroid inhibition (by blocking stimulation induced by TSH). Antibodies referred to as thyroid-stimulating immunoglobulins are present in 95% of patients with untreated Graves disease. In vitro bioassays can assess the ability of stimulatory antibodies to induce functional responses in cultured cells by measuring cyclic adenosine monophosphate increases or adenylate cyclase activity. Assays are available that measure the capability of the inhibitory antibodies, called thyrotropin-binding inhibitory immunoglobulins, to block the binding of labeled TSH to its receptors.

Radioactive Iodine Uptake and Thyroid Scans

The radioactive iodine uptake and thyroid scan measurements involve the in vivo administration of radioactive iodine. Accumulated radioactivity in the thyroid is measured at intervals within 24 hours using a gamma scintillation counter. A nuclear imaging scan that examines the anatomic distribution of radioactive iodine uptake within the thyroid gland also may be obtained. Radioactive iodine uptake studies may be helpful when the diagnosis is in question and in differentiating between possible causes of hyperthyroidism.

Thyroglobulin

Thyroglobulin (TG) is stored in the follicular colloid of the thyroid as a prohormone. TG measurements are used to monitor treatment in thyroid cancer. Detection of TG in serum after thyroidectomy is evidence of incomplete ablation or metastatic thyroid cancer. TG measurements should always include measurement of anti-TG antibodies because these autoantibodies may interfere with the TG assay and cause false-positive or negative results. LC/MS or radioimmunoassay methods more accurately detect TG in the presence of anti-TG antibodies.

Calcitonin

Calcitonin is a polypeptide hormone produced by the thyroidal C cells, whose primary function is in regulating calcium homeostasis. It is elevated in patients with C-cell hyperplasia and medullary thyroid carcinoma (MTC). Calcitonin measurements are used to determine when to perform prophylactic thyroidectomy on patients with familial MTC. In addition, it is used to assess prognosis and monitor recurrence of MTC post thyroidectomy.

Fine Needle Aspiration (FNA) Cytology

FNA is the procedure of choice to collect a specimen for microscopic review to distinguish benign from malignant thyroid nodules. The sensitivity of thyroid FNA for detection of thyroid cancer and other disorders varies from 70% to 97%. It depends greatly on the quality of the specimens and the experience of the cytopathologist. TG can also be measured in lymph node FNA aspirates to diagnose and monitor thyroid cancer.

In the presence of a clinical history and physical examination consistent with hyperthyroidism, a diagnosis of hyperthyroidism (but not necessarily its cause) can be established by the demonstration of a low TSH level and a high free T_4.

Hyperthyroidism Overview and Associated Disorders
Description and Diagnosis

Hyperthyroidism, also known as thyrotoxicosis, is a collection of disorders associated with excess thyroid hormone (**Table 22–1**). There are four main causes of hyperthyroidism: (1) overstimulation of the thyroid (elevated TSH, human chorionic gonadotropin [hCG], and/or TSH receptor autoantibodies [TRAbs]); (2) genetic mutations leading to increased synthesis and secretion of thyroid hormone (germline, sporadic, or tumor induced); (3) release of excess hormone from the thyroid (inflammation, infection, injury); and (4) extrathyroidal sources of thyroid hormone (ectopic thyroid tissue or exogenous hormone). Patients with hyperthyroidism demonstrate a spectrum of hypermetabolic features, including nervousness, palpitations, muscle weakness, increased appetite, diarrhea, heat intolerance, warm skin, weight loss, and perspiration. Affected patients also may have exophthalmos, emotional changes, menstrual changes, and a fine tremor of the hands. In the presence of a clinical history and physical examination consistent with hyperthyroidism, a diagnosis of hyperthyroidism (but not necessarily its cause) can be established by the demonstration of a low TSH level and a high free T_4. In uncommon situations, only total T_3 is elevated and the serum free T_4 is normal (T_3 thyrotoxicosis). To determine the etiology of the hyperthyroidism, additional testing is usually necessary. Graves disease, toxic multinodular goiter (TMNG), and toxic adenoma account for the vast majority (>95%) of cases of hyperthyroidism. It should be noted that diffuse or focal enlargement of the thyroid gland, also known as goiter, can be associated with hyperfunction, normal function, and hypofunction of the gland.

Thyroid Storm

Thyroid storm is a relatively uncommon, but life-threatening manifestation of hyperthyroidism caused by excess circulation of thyroid hormones. Thyroid storm is identified by grading a series of clinical signs and symptoms including markedly high fever of 105°F to 106°F, tachycardia, hypertension, congestive heart failure, and neurological and/or gastrointestinal abnormalities. Thyroid storm is precipitated by acute illnesses such as sepsis, diabetic ketoacidosis, and preeclampsia, as well as surgical or other diagnostic or therapeutic actions such as radioactive iodine use, anesthesia, excessive thyroid hormone ingestion, or thyroid palpation. Thyroid storm is associated with a

TABLE 22–1   Laboratory Evaluation of Patients for Thyroid Disease

Disorder	Laboratory Test Results Suggestive of Diagnosis in the Appropriate Clinical Setting
Hyperthyroidism	
Graves disease	TSH low; free T_4 high; in some cases, T_3 is elevated and free T_4 is normal; TRAbs elevated
Toxic multinodular goiter	TSH low; free T_4 and T_3 normal or high; normal or increased radioactive iodine uptake; thyroid scan with multiple areas of increased uptake surrounded by suppressed uptake
Toxic adenoma	TSH low; free T_4 and T_3 normal or high; normal or increased radioactive iodine uptake; thyroid scan with focal increased uptake in tumor surrounded by suppressed uptake in non-tumor tissue
Subacute thyroiditis	TSH low; free T_4 and T_3 high; increased; decreased radioactive iodine uptake
T_3 Thyrotoxicosis	TSH low; free T_4 normal and T_3 high; normal radioactive iodine uptake
Hypothyroidism	
Hashimoto thyroiditis	TSH high; T_4 normal and then low, preceding a decline in T_3; anti-TPO and/or antithyroglobulin antibody positive
Ablative hypothyroidism	TSH high; free T_4 and T_3 low following procedure that ablates thyroid
Infantile hypothyroidism	TSH high; free T_4 low in a newborn or infant
Euthyroid sick syndrome	TSH normal to high; free T_4 normal; T_3 low; rT_3 high; concentrations of TSH and thyroid hormones vary throughout disease course

free T_4, free thyroxine; rT_3, reverse triiodothyronine; T_3, triiodothyronine; TRAbs, TSH receptor autoantibodies; TSH, thyroid-stimulating hormone.

high fatality rate if not identified early. The diagnosis is based on the presence of systemic clinical signs and symptoms of severe thyrotoxicosis in the context of a precipitating cause. In addition, marked elevations in free and total T_4 are common in thyroid storm. Total T_3 is unreliable in this setting because concomitant nonthyroidal illness (NTI) may cause T_3 to decrease significantly.

Graves Disease

Graves disease is a relatively common hyperthyroid disorder occurring more frequently in women. It has a familial predisposition. It is an autoimmune disease caused by TSH receptor antibodies (TRAbs) that bind to and stimulate TSH receptors resulting in autonomous production of thyroid hormone. While many patients have the classic signs and symptoms of thyrotoxicosis, in elderly patients with Graves disease, apathy, muscle weakness, and cardiovascular abnormalities occur more often than hypermetabolic symptoms.

Laboratory tests show undetectable TSH and increased free T_4. In some cases, the T_3 is elevated and the T_4 is normal. The differential diagnosis includes TMNG, toxic adenoma, T_3 toxicosis, subacute thyroiditis, ectopic thyroid tissue, and anxiety states (see below for descriptions). Detection of TRAbs and the results from radioactive iodine uptake and nuclear thyroid scans are helpful in distinguishing among these possibilities. There is usually increased radioactive iodine uptake in Graves disease. The pattern on imaging is diffuse.

> Graves disease is a relatively common hyperthyroid disorder occurring more frequently in women. It is an autoimmune disease caused by TSH receptor autoantibodies that bind to and stimulate TSH receptors resulting in autonomous production of thyroid hormone.

Toxic Multinodular Goiter

The cause of hyperthyroidism in patients with TMNG is an apparent functional autonomy of certain areas within the thyroid gland. The disorder is seen more commonly in elderly patients. The degree of hyperthyroidism is generally less severe than that found in Graves disease. Cardiovascular symptoms are prominent, such as arrhythmias, atrial fibrillation, or congestive heart failure, with weakness and wasting.

Laboratory tests usually show low or undetectable TSH and normal or elevated free T_4 and T_3 concentrations and no evidence of thyroid autoantibodies. Patients with TMNG will have normal to high radioactive iodine uptake, and the thyroid scan shows iodine localized to active nodules.

Toxic Adenoma

Thyroid adenomas that secrete thyroid hormones and cause hyperthyroidism are known as toxic adenomas. Thyroid hormone synthesis by a toxic adenoma is usually independent of TSH regulation, and it results in suppression of TSH secretion. These tumors can usually be distinguished from TMNG and Graves disease by a radioactive iodine uptake study and thyroid scan because there is localized uptake in the adenoma and little or no uptake in surrounding thyroid tissue.

Thyroiditis

Subacute Thyroiditis

Subacute thyroiditis is produced by a viral infection that alters thyroid function. This disease usually lasts for months, with thyroid function eventually returning to normal. The patient often has an associated upper respiratory infection, fever, and local pain mimicking a sore throat or an earache.

Patients in the early stage of this disease may have hyperthyroidism, with elevated T_4 and T_3 concentrations and a low TSH. Laboratory findings also often include a high erythrocyte sedimentation rate or C-reactive protein (CRP) and little to no radioactive iodine uptake. If the disease progresses and the thyroid hormones are depleted, the patient develops hypothyroidism with low T_3 and T_4 concentrations and an elevated TSH.

Postpartum Thyroiditis

Postpartum thyroid disease is a transient inflammatory process that has an onset of 1 to 6 months postpartum. Although the etiology is unclear, it is thought to be caused by a rebound by the immune system in response to the general state of immunosuppression that occurs during pregnancy. This disease can present as either hyperthyroidism or hypothyroidism. The typical disease course begins with a period of hyperthyroidism with elevated free T4, reduced TSH, and little to no radioactive iodine uptake for 3 to 6 months. This is followed by a 3- to 6-month period of hypothyroidism associated with reduced concentrations of free T4 and elevated TSH that completely resolves after

When hypothyroidism occurs during development and in infancy, it results in a condition known as cretinism, which is marked by retardation of physical and intellectual growth. When hypothyroidism first appears in older children and adults, the collection of signs and symptoms is known as myxedema.

1 year. Approximately 20% of women with postpartum hypothyroidism develop permanent disease, requiring lifelong treatment and monitoring. The presence of anti-TPO antibodies prior to and during pregnancy is associated with an increased risk for postpartum thyroiditis.

Painless Thyroiditis

Painless thyroiditis may be induced by numerous drugs including lithium, interferon, and in a small portion of patients on amiodarone therapy. Further, some patients with chronic thyroiditis have a transient painless thyrotoxicosis, of unclear etiology.

Typically, free T_4 and T_3 concentrations are elevated with a low TSH. Patients have a markedly depressed radioactive iodine uptake. Painless thyroiditis can be distinguished clinically from subacute thyroiditis because an elevated erythrocyte sedimentation rate and local pain in the region of the thyroid are more consistent with subacute thyroiditis. A definitive diagnosis can be made by microscopic review of cells obtained by aspiration or biopsy. TG measurements can differentiate among patients with chronic thyroiditis from those with thyrotoxicosis caused by surreptitious thyroid hormone intake.

Hypothyroidism Overview and Associated Disorders

Description and Diagnosis

When hypothyroidism occurs during development and in infancy, it results in a condition known as cretinism, which is marked by retardation of physical and intellectual growth. In 95% of cases, hypothyroidism originates in the thyroid gland itself. If a patient has an increased serum TSH and a decreased free T_4—together with appropriate clinical symptoms—a diagnosis of hypothyroidism is confirmed (**Table 22–1**). In asymptomatic patients, increased TSH, accompanied by a normal free T_4, is known as subclinical hypothyroidism and may be indicative of early stages of primary hypothyroidism. High titers of anti-TPO antibodies suggest Hashimoto thyroiditis (see below) or postpartum thyroid dysfunction in a postpartum woman. While in the United States, autoimmunity is the main cause of hypothyroidism, iodine deficiency is the primary cause worldwide.

Hypothyroidism also may be a result of inadequate stimulation of the thyroid by TSH. This is known as secondary hypothyroidism. A subnormal free T_4 with a decreased or inappropriately normal TSH is suggestive of secondary hypothyroidism from decreased TSH production or production of a biologically inactive form of TSH in the pituitary. It is usually accompanied by other pituitary hormone deficiencies, and it is much less common than primary hypothyroidism.

Clinical pictures of hypothyroidism differ, depending on the age. Congenital hypothyroidism is characterized by low production of thyroid hormones and can result in growth and intellectual delay if untreated. In the United States, all states screen for congenital hypothyroidism by testing for elevated TSH or a combination of elevated TSH and decreased free T_4. Significant changes in thyroid function occur in the neonatal period and throughout childhood. Therefore, TSH and free T_4 concentrations should be assessed using age-specific reference intervals. In particular, T_4 is typically elevated in newborns. In adults, hypothyroidism can have an insidious onset, especially in the elderly. Symptoms are usually nonspecific in the early stage and then progress to more definitive characteristics of hypothyroidism with dry hair, dry skin, periorbital puffiness, dull expression, large tongue, and enlarged heart. If untreated, myxedema coma with respiratory failure may occur. Treatment involves thyroid hormone replacement.

Hashimoto thyroiditis is a common chronic inflammatory disease of the thyroid that accounts for as many as 90% of all cases of hypothyroidism. Patients with Hashimoto thyroiditis carry anti-TPO and anti-TG antibodies.

Hashimoto Thyroiditis

Hashimoto thyroiditis is a common chronic inflammatory disease of the thyroid that accounts for as many as 90% of all cases of hypothyroidism in areas of iodine sufficiency. Hashimoto thyroiditis is often associated with other autoimmune diseases such as Sjögren syndrome and pernicious anemia.

Approximately 90% of patients with Hashimoto thyroiditis express anti-TPO, while 20% to 50% have anti-TG antibodies. Firm thyroid enlargement and goiter is characteristic, but atrophy may also be seen. Patients typically have an increased TSH and a low normal free T_4 and an elevated radioactive iodine uptake in the early stage of the disease. Over time, serum T_4 declines first, followed by a decline in T_3 as hypothyroid symptoms become predominant.

Postablative Hypothyroidism

Postablative hypothyroidism is a relatively common cause of hypothyroidism in adults. Thyroid ablation occurs with total or subtotal thyroidectomy, or following treatment with radioactive iodine for hyperthyroidism.

A history of ablative therapy along with an elevated TSH and a low free T_4 concentration indicates that ablation has produced a hypothyroid state.

Infantile Hypothyroidism

Severe hypothyroidism in infancy is known as cretinism and, as previously noted, is characterized by irreversible mental retardation and growth impairment unless treated promptly. The appearance of symptoms depends on the severity of the disorder. However, even severe hypothyroidism is not usually apparent at birth. Early diagnosis and treatment with thyroid hormone prevents the manifestations of the disease. Elevated TSH and a low T_4 in a newborn or young infant are indicative of infantile hypothyroidism.

Pregnancy-related Thyroid Disease

Normal pregnancy is associated with a number of physiologic changes in thyroid function, resulting in differences in "normal" laboratory values for thyroid function tests. The increase in estrogen stimulates hepatic synthesis of TBG, resulting in a net increase in total T_3 and total T_4 by about 1.5-fold. Significant homology exists between hCG, the pregnancy-associated glycoprotein hormone (see Chapter 20), and TSH. Because of this, hCG can directly stimulate the thyroid to produce thyroid hormone. Excess production of thyroid hormone signals a downregulation of TSH secretion. In the first trimester of pregnancy, increasing hCG concentrations are directly mirrored by decreasing TSH concentrations, which return to low normal in the second and third trimesters. Thus, TSH measurements in pregnancy should be considered in the context of gestational age and a reduced upper limit of normal. Most laboratories now report TSH with trimester-specific reference intervals.

Thyroid dysfunction during pregnancy can result in increased risks for the mother and fetus. Hypothyroidism during pregnancy is associated with an increased risk of miscarriage or preterm delivery and impaired neurological development in the fetus. Although controversial, it is recommended to screen all high-risk and symptomatic pregnant women for hypothyroidism by measuring TSH. An elevated TSH result, evaluated in the context of pregnancy trimester-specific reference intervals, followed by an abnormally reduced fT_4 result, is diagnostic of hypothyroidism. Because of alterations in binding protein expression during pregnancy, fT4 results may vary across assay platforms. While direct measurements via liquid chromatography/tandem mass spectrometry is preferred, automated immunoassays are acceptable as long as results are considered in the context of platform- and trimester-specific reference intervals. The presence of TPO and/or TG antibodies suggests autoimmunity as the etiology. Up to 20% of pregnant, euthyroid women express these antibodies and of these ~20% go on to develop hypothyroidism in pregnancy. Pregnant patients that are TPO and/or TG antibody positive should have TSH measured at initial visit and then once per month for the first half of pregnancy.

Hyperthyroidism in pregnancy is associated with an increased risk of spontaneous abortion, preterm delivery, preeclampsia, and thyroid anomalies in the newborn. A subnormal TSH result, evaluated in the context of trimester-specific reference intervals, should be followed with free T_4 testing. An elevated free T_4 with the presence of TSH receptor antibodies confirms the diagnosis of hyperthyroidism in pregnancy. In mothers with confirmed thyroid disease, fetal thyroid function can be evaluated with ultrasound and amniotic fluid or umbilical cord blood testing for TSH, free T_4, and total T_4. Normal reference intervals are instrument-specific for amniotic fluid thyroid function tests.

Nonthyroidal Illness

Description

It is estimated that 40% of emergency department patients have ETS at presentation. Stress, trauma, and illness can alter thyroid hormone production, transport, and metabolism, and thereby TSH

The condition with altered thyroid hormone levels and no intrinsic disorder of the thyroid gland is called euthyroid sick syndrome or nonthyroidal illness (NTI), of which there are several variants.

production, because of disruption of the normal feedback relationship between TSH and T_3 and T_4. This condition with altered thyroid hormone concentrations and no intrinsic disorder of the thyroid gland is called ETS or NTI, of which there are several variants.

Diagnosis

There is no consensus in the literature regarding the diagnosis and also therapy of NTI. The cause of NTI is different from patient to patient and is dependent on the history and any endocrinologic diagnosis. In moderately ill patients with NTI, serum T_4 concentrations are within the reference range, while serum T_3 is decreased and rT_3 is increased. Serum TSH concentrations are typically normal to low (except for a transient increase that may occur during recovery). However, it is not recommended to measure TSH in hospitalized patients unless there is a strong suspicion for thyroid disease. In seriously ill patients, ETS presents with low-normal T_4 and significantly reduced total T_3 concentrations. Serum rT_3 is increased because of slow thyroid hormone clearance and greater than normal conversion of T_4 to rT_3 rather than to T_3. An elevated rT_3 in the appropriate clinical setting, with appropriately suggestive laboratory test results, points to NTI.

Thyroid Tumors

Description

Masses or "nodules" in the thyroid may be associated with normal function, hyperfunction, or hypofunction, and for that reason, they are considered separately from hyperthyroidism and hypothyroidism. In fact, some studies suggest that 25% to 40% of the population have thyroid nodules. Most solitary masses detected with physical examination are the dominant nodule in a multinodular goiter, a cyst, or an asymmetric enlargement of the gland. Benign thyroid adenomas account for most of the neoplastic nodules. The initial evaluation for a thyroid nodule is to measure TSH and perform a thyroid ultrasound. If the TSH is suppressed, an iodine uptake study/scan should be performed. Hyperfunctioning nodules appear as "hot nodules" by nuclear scan because they take up radioactive iodine while uptake is suppressed in the remainder of the gland. A nonfunctional (cold) nodule carries an increased risk of malignancy and should be followed with ultrasound-guided FNA or biopsy. The morphologic variants of thyroid cancer, diagnosed with histopathologic review of a biopsy specimen or aspirate (in order of frequency), are papillary carcinoma, follicular carcinoma, MTC, and anaplastic carcinoma.

Diagnosis

The diagnosis is established by histopathologic review of a specimen obtained with FNA or biopsy. The accuracy of the diagnosis is increased with the use of guided ultrasound examination for sample collection. Treatment and risk of recurrence of thyroid neoplasms are assessed by periodic measurement of tumor markers, including TG for papillary and follicular carcinomas, and calcitonin and CEA for medullary thyroid carcinoma (MTC). In familial forms of MTC, detection of mutations in the RET gene (RET proto-oncogene) confirms the diagnosis.

ADRENAL CORTEX

Physiology and Biochemistry

The adrenal cortex secretes many steroid hormones that have a wide variety of physiologic effects. The hormones can be grouped into three major categories: glucocorticoids, mineralocorticoids, and sex steroids that include androgens, progestogens, and estrogens. The glucocorticoids and mineralocorticoids are collectively known as corticosteroids. Steroid hormones are cholesterol based and synthesized by the adrenal glands and gonads. They are transported in the blood bound to carrier proteins, such as albumin and hormone-binding globulins, or as free hormone. Steroids may be modified with glucuronate or sulfate to increase their water solubility and permit excretion via the kidneys or the gastrointestinal tract. The percentage of steroid hormone that is bound to protein varies with the hormone affinity for carrier proteins and ranges from 60% to nearly 100%. Quantitatively, the glucocorticoids and mineralocorticoids are the most important group of hormones produced by the adrenal cortex. The major corticosteroids are cortisol (a glucocorticoid) and aldosterone (a mineralocorticoid). The synthesis and metabolism of the steroid hormones are illustrated in **Figure 22–4**. The liver is the main site for conjugation of steroid hormones, and the kidney excretes approximately 90% of the conjugated steroids. Glucocorticoids alter carbohydrate metabolism by increasing gluconeogenesis and decreasing glucose utilization. Additional effects include the inhibition of amino acid uptake and protein synthesis in peripheral tissues. Mineralocorticoids promote sodium conservation and potassium loss and thereby considerably influence the retention or loss of fluid. Among the naturally occurring mineralocorticoids, aldosterone has the highest mineralocorticoid activity followed by deoxycorticosterone and corticosterone.

Secretion of adrenal glucocorticoids and adrenal androgens is regulated by corticotropin (ACTH) that is secreted by the pituitary gland (**Figure 22–5**). ACTH also plays a minor role in aldosterone/mineralocorticoid production. Mineralocorticoid synthesis is primarily controlled by the renin–angiotensin–aldosterone system (RAAS). The hypothalamic–pituitary–adrenal (HPA) axis begins with the episodic release of corticotropin-releasing hormone (CRH) from the hypothalamus. CRH stimulates the episodic release of ACTH from the anterior pituitary. ACTH then stimulates the adrenal cortex to produce cortisol in a diurnal or circadian manner. Cortisol concentrations are highest in the early morning between 4 and 8 AM and about 25% lower in the late evening. Physical and mental stress can elevate cortisol concentrations and blunt the circadian rhythm. ACTH release is under negative feedback control from free (unbound) cortisol. ACTH also stimulates synthesis of two adrenal sex steroids, dehydroepiandrosterone (DHEA) and androstenedione, as well as other hormones including insulin-like growth factor-1 and gonadal steroids. Adrenal androgen production reaches a peak in the second decade, with a rise during late childhood. It gradually decreases to its nadir in the elderly.

The adrenal cortex secretes hormones that can be grouped into three major categories: glucocorticoids, mineralocorticoids, and sex steroids that include androgens, progestogens, and estrogens.

Cortisol concentrations are highest in the early morning between 4 and 8 AM and about 25% lower in the late evening. Physical and mental stress can elevate cortisol concentrations and blunt the circadian rhythm.

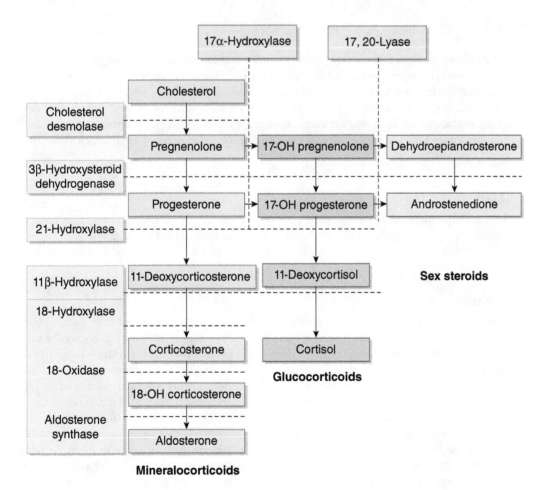

FIGURE 22–4 The synthesis and metabolism of steroid hormones of the adrenal cortex.

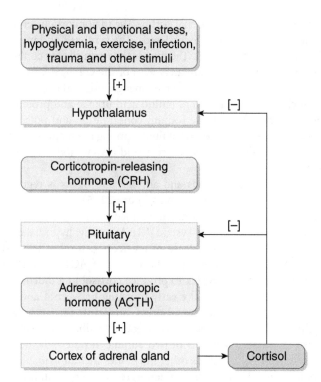

FIGURE 22–5 **Hypothalamic–pituitary–adrenal cortex interactions. [+] Stimulation; [−] inhibition.**

As shown in **Figure 22–6**, aldosterone secretion is primarily controlled by the RAAS. Renin is an enzyme synthesized and stored in cells of the juxtaglomerular afferent arterioles of the renal glomeruli. Renin is released in response to decreased blood sodium, volume, and/or pressure. Circulating renin hydrolyzes angiotensinogen to produce angiotensin I, which is rapidly converted to angiotensin II by angiotensin-converting enzyme (ACE) in the lung. Angiotensin II then stimulates the cells of the adrenal cortex to secrete aldosterone. Angiotensin II is also a potent vasoconstrictor.

Laboratory Tests

The functional status of the adrenal cortex can be evaluated by measuring the circulating concentrations of components of the HPA axis and the RAAS. In addition to measurement of the plasma, serum, or urinary concentrations of these compounds, dynamic stimulation and suppression tests are valuable in identifying certain abnormalities.

Cortisol

Because the secretion of cortisol is diurnal and pulsatile, a single, random serum cortisol measurement is not useful in the diagnosis of adrenal dysfunction. However, a decreased early morning serum cortisol measurement may suggest adrenal insufficiency. The 24-hour urinary excretion of cortisol, an index of plasma-free cortisol during that 24-hour time frame, is a reliable gauge of excess cortisol secretion by the adrenal cortex. This is because taking an average urine cortisol concentration over 24 hours eliminates the need to account for diurnal variation as in a single serum collection. Urinary free cortisol (UFC) measurements should not be used in patients with renal impairment. Late-night salivary cortisol is also a measure of free cortisol since the binding protein does not cross into saliva. Salivary cortisol concentrations correlate well with serum concentrations and are not influenced by changes in cortisol-binding protein concentrations. Measurement of late-night salivary cortisol is an acceptable screening method for hypercortisolism.

Because the secretion of cortisol is pulsatile and diurnal, a single, random serum cortisol measurement is not usually diagnostic for adrenal dysfunction. The 24-hour urinary excretion of cortisol is a reliable gauge of excess cortisol secretion by the adrenal cortex.

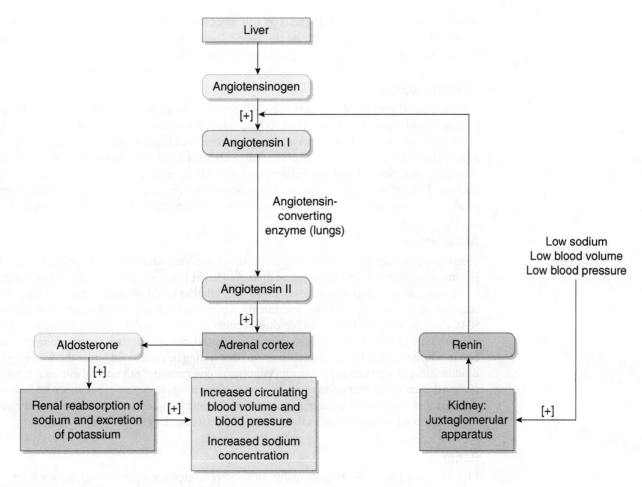

FIGURE 22–6 **The renal and adrenal interactions in the renin–angiotensin system.**

Low-dose Dexamethasone Suppression Tests

Dexamethasone is a synthetic glucocorticoid more potent than cortisol that, when given orally or IV, suppresses ACTH and CRH secretion. It can be administered as 1 mg at midnight in an overnight dexamethasone suppression test, or in a 2-day (i.e., longer) low-dose dexamethasone suppression test (LDDST) by giving the patient 0.5 mg every 6 hours for eight doses. If the dexamethasone is effective, it will suppress ACTH secretion and, thereby, suppress cortisol production. Patients with Cushing disease normally do not show suppression of cortisol synthesis after either dexamethasone administration for the overnight or the LDD suppression test.

ACTH

In patients with an abnormal dexamethasone suppression test, ACTH measurements are important to determine whether Cushing syndrome is ACTH-dependent. The optimum time of day for determination of plasma ACTH concentration in patients with suspected Cushing syndrome is between midnight and 2 AM when the plasma-circulating concentrations of ACTH and cortisol are at their lowest point. At this time, the ability to detect an abnormality in ACTH secretion is the greatest. In patients with suspected adrenal insufficiency, ACTH should be measured in the morning during its peak. Suppressed morning ACTH may indicate excess adrenal cortisol secretion.

ACTH Stimulation Test

The corticotropin (ACTH) stimulation test is the most useful test in diagnosis of adrenal insufficiency. It assesses the secretory response of the adrenal cortex to an ACTH-like stimulus. A 250-mg dose of an ACTH analog, Cortrosyn or cosyntropin, is administered IV or IM to adults and children 2 years or older, and serum cortisol is measured at baseline and 30 and 60 minutes after administration. Normally, ACTH analogs will stimulate production of cortisol to concentrations >18 μg/dL (this varies depending on the assay). Lack of rise in cortisol after ACTH stimulation may indicate primary and secondary adrenal insufficiency.

CRH Stimulation Test

CRH can be administered intravenously to determine the response of the pituitary to stimulation by hypothalamic hormone. The CRH stimulation test can be used to determine the source of adrenal insufficiency in patients with an abnormal ACTH stimulation test. Synthetic CRH is administered IV, and then ACTH and cortisol are measured at 0, 30, 60, 90, and 120 minutes after injection. Normal patients will respond to CRH by stimulating ACTH and cortisol production. Patients with primary adrenal insufficiency will have elevated ACTH, but no cortisol production, while patients with secondary disease will have both low ACTH and cortisol.

Aldosterone

The most important test to establish a diagnosis of hyperaldosteronism or hypoaldosteronism is plasma aldosterone. Aldosterone can be measured in the plasma as the unmodified hormone, and in the urine as the 18-glucuronide conjugated metabolite of aldosterone. Screening for primary aldosteronism should include the determination of the ratio of plasma aldosterone concentration (PAC)/plasma renin activity (PRA) or direct renin concentration (DRC), that is, the aldosterone to renin ratio (ARR). Aldosterone and renin concentrations are affected by numerous conditions and medication. Therefore, it is recommended that testing be performed under the following conditions: patients with normal potassium concentrations, patients with normal salt intake, patients removed from drugs that affect the ARR, and midmorning collection in patients who have been ambulatory for at least 2 hours. In some patients in which it is unsafe to discontinue medications, the ARR should be interpreted in the context of interfering drugs and/or comorbidities.

Renin

PRA is assayed by measuring its ability to convert angiotensinogen to angiotensin I, which is then quantitated by an immunoassay. When primary aldosteronism is present, often because of either resistant or severe hypertension, the ARR will be elevated. Renin mass can also be assessed directly by immunoassay, to determine the DRC. Although the ARR can be calculated using DRC or PRA, fewer studies have investigated the utility of DRC. Renin specimens should not be stored refrigerated or on ice prior to analysis as cold temperatures promote secretion of prorenin, which falsely elevates results. See the section "Aldosterone" for recommended testing conditions.

Steroid Measurements to Identify Enzyme Deficiencies in Congenital Adrenal Hyperplasia (CAH)

CAH represents a spectrum of diseases resulting from enzyme deficiencies that impair normal hormone synthesis in the adrenal cortex. The decrease in cortisol production in most forms of CAH leads to an overproduction and shunting into the androgen synthesis pathway. These disorders are described in the section "Alterations in the Synthesis of Glucocorticoids, Mineralocorticoids, and Sex Steroids: Congenital Adrenal Hyperplasia." The assays used to identify the specific enzyme deficiencies include measurement of 17-hydroxyprogesterone (17-OHP), either unstimulated or after ACTH stimulation, 17-hydroxypregnenolone after ACTH stimulation, deoxycorticosterone, 11-deoxycortisol, and several androgens (androstenedione, DHEA, and testosterone). DNA-based tests also can be used to identify certain gene mutations that result in enzyme deficiencies found in CAH.

> Cushing syndrome is a disorder of excess cortisol production, which is more commonly ACTH-dependent than ACTH-independent.

Hyperfunction Involving Glucocorticoids With or Without Mineralocorticoids: Cushing Syndrome

Description

Cushing syndrome is a disorder of excess cortisol production, which is more commonly ACTH-dependent than ACTH-independent. The early clinical features of Cushing syndrome are hypertension and weight gain. Truncal obesity with a round face, often known as a "moon facies," and an accumulation of fat in the posterior neck and regions of the back close to the neck, known as a "buffalo hump," appear with progression of the disease. Decreased muscle mass and proximal limb weakness occur from atrophy of muscle fibers induced by high cortisol concentrations, which inhibit protein synthesis and uptake of glucose by the cells. Patients with Cushing syndrome often have elevated blood glucose levels with glucosuria. Other clinical signs and symptoms include striae of the skin, osteoporosis, hirsutism, menstrual abnormalities in women, and mental status changes involving mood swings with depression.

Cushing syndrome is separated into three main disease entities, with increased synthesis and loss of circadian rhythm resulting in excess cortisol production by the adrenal cortex as the common theme. Independent of the three naturally occurring forms of Cushing syndrome, the administration of glucocorticoids is a common cause of Cushing syndrome. This should be evident from the medication history. Endogenous forms of Cushing syndrome are described as follows:

- *Cushing* disease is the most common form of Cushing syndrome and is four- to sixfold more prevalent in women. It is caused most often by small ACTH-secreting tumors in the pituitary (<1 cm in size) known as microadenomas. These adenomas can be detected with various radiographic techniques after appropriate hormone tests suggest a pituitary etiology. On rare occasions, the tumors are large macroadenomas.
- *Adrenal Cushing syndrome*—This form of Cushing syndrome is most commonly associated with a benign or malignant tumor in the adrenal cortex. Adrenal adenomas synthesize cortisol efficiently, but adrenal carcinomas often synthesize cortisol inefficiently and overproduce sex steroids, resulting in virilization.
- *Cushing syndrome from ectopic ACTH production*—Small cell lung carcinoma and bronchial carcinoid patients account for most of the Cushing syndrome cases in this category. This form of Cushing syndrome is more common in men because of the higher incidence of lung cancer in men. In the absence of signs and symptoms specifically associated with the lung carcinoma or carcinoid, these patients are clinically indistinguishable from those with pituitary Cushing disease. Because the syndrome often appears in patients with significant clinical manifestations of cancer, the symptoms from ectopic ACTH production often go unrecognized. Another very rare cause of Cushing syndrome with an ectopic focus and high serum ACTH concentrations is a CRH-secreting tumor, most frequently a bronchial carcinoid tumor.

The strategy for the diagnosis of Cushing syndrome, and the subsequent identification of one of the three forms of Cushing syndrome, involves tests to confirm endogenous hypercortisolism and then to determine whether the disease is ACTH-dependent.

Diagnosis

The diagnosis of Cushing syndrome or Cushing disease, discussed below collectively as Cushing syndrome, requires evidence of increased cortisol production and loss of suppression of cortisol synthesis and/or loss of cortisol diurnal variation. Screening for Cushing syndrome is difficult because (1) its prevalence is low; (2) several common conditions can produce biochemical and clinical signs of hypercortisolism in the absence of Cushing syndrome; and (3) the screening is not ideal in all patients, and both false-negative and false-positive results for Cushing syndrome are common. For this reason, it is recommended that a careful clinical history be taken to exclude exogenous causes of hypercortisolism. Only patients with high clinical suspicion, especially those with multiple signs and symptoms, for example, osteoporosis and less than 40 years old, children with a decrease in height and increase in weight percentiles, severe symptoms, or adrenal tumors visualized by imaging, should be screened for Cushing syndrome.

The strategy for the diagnosis of Cushing syndrome, and the subsequent identification of one of the three etiologies of Cushing syndrome, involves tests to confirm endogenous hypercortisolism and then to determine whether the disease is ACTH-dependent. ACTH concentrations are low in patients with adrenal tumors, but normal or elevated with pituitary or ectopic ACTH-producing tumors. **Table 22–2** summarizes the laboratory evaluation for Cushing syndrome.

The following steps to diagnose and differentiate Cushing syndrome can be made using first-line and then second-line diagnostic tests, respectively.

Diagnostic Evaluation

It is recommended that at least one of the following testing strategies be performed to diagnose patients with Cushing syndrome:

1. The 24-hour UFC or late-night salivary cortisol are sensitive screening tests for patients with clinical signs and symptoms of Cushing syndrome. Because of the variability of the

TABLE 22–2   Laboratory Evaluation for Cushing Syndrome

Laboratory Test	Pituitary Cause	Adrenal Cause	Ectopic ACTH Secretion
24-Hour urine-free cortisol or late-night salivary cortisol	Elevated	Elevated	Elevated
Overnight or low-dose dexamethasone suppression test	No cortisol suppression	No cortisol suppression	No cortisol suppression
Plasma ACTH	Moderately elevated or inappropriately normal	Low	Highly elevated
Imaging study	MRI: pituitary tumor	CT: adrenal tumor	Tumor outside pituitary or adrenal glands

ACTH, adrenocorticotropic hormone (corticotropin).

cortisol concentrations, the UFC or salivary cortisol should be elevated on at least two separate occasions in order to proceed with the diagnostic evaluation for Cushing syndrome. If the UFC or salivary cortisol is normal in a high-risk patient, an endocrinologist should be consulted for further studies. A low-risk patient with normal results should be rescreened in 6 months if signs or symptoms persist or worsen. UFC is falsely decreased in patients with renal failure and falsely increased with over collection, excess fluid intake, and/or when cross reacting steroid hormones are present. Late-night salivary cortisol measurements are not accurate in shift workers due to altered circadian rhythm. False elevations are common in smokers as well.

2. In unhealthy, but not critically ill, patients, and/or those with abnormal renal function, or disrupted sleep patterns, physicians should use either the overnight dexamethasone suppression test or the LDDST to screen for Cushing syndrome. If cortisol production is suppressed by a low dose of dexamethasone in an overnight or 48-hour test, Cushing syndrome is ruled out. If the clinical suspicion for Cushing syndrome is still high in the presence of a nonsuggestive result for Cushing syndrome, further evaluation by an endocrinologist may be useful. A lack of cortisol suppression after a low dose of dexamethasone is suggestive of Cushing syndrome. Patients taking oral estrogens should not be screened with the LDDST, as estrogens stimulate the liver to synthesize cortisol-binding globulin (CBG) and elevate serum cortisol concentrations, causing false-positive screening results. Further, critically ill patients synthesize less CBG and albumin, leading to lower serum cortisol concentrations, and possibly false-negative screening results.

3. Other clinical conditions that cause hypercortisolism should be ruled out. These include alcoholism, severe obesity, pregnancy, depression, diabetes mellitus, and glucocorticoid resistance.

Tests to Identify Etiology

Once Cushing syndrome is confirmed, a series of tests can then be performed to locate the source of the hypercortisolism.

1. Plasma ACTH testing should be performed to determine the etiology of the hypercortisolism. If ACTH is suppressed, an adrenal source is suspected. If ACTH is moderately elevated or inappropriately normal, the patient may have a pituitary adenoma.

2. If an ACTH-secreting pituitary adenoma is suspected, MRI of the pituitary gland to identify a mass and/or measurement of ACTH in right and left petrosal sinus blood samples after CRH stimulation can be used to differentiate a pituitary, from an ectopic source. The inferior petrosal sinus (IPS) directly drains the pituitary, and thus ACTH concentrations in IPS samples are significantly higher when an ACTH-secreting pituitary is present. A ratio of IPS ACTH to central venous ACTH above suggested cutoff values before and after CRH administration is consistent with a pituitary cause.

3. If the ACTH is suppressed, a CT of the adrenal glands is likely to be informative to identify an adrenal tumor and indicate an adrenal cause.

Adrenal insufficiency can be either primary, from destruction of the adrenal cortex by a local disease process or a systemic disorder, or secondary from pituitary or hypothalamic disease that reduces stimulation of the adrenal gland.

4. If an ectopic ACTH-secreting tumor is suspected, this can be challenging to locate, but imaging studies are often valuable. Chest, pancreas, colon, and gall bladder carcinomas have been shown to be sources of cortisol secretion.

5. "Pseudo-Cushing syndrome," which can be produced by alcohol abuse and other disorders, mimics both the clinical and biochemical features of the true syndrome.

Hypofunction Involving Glucocorticoids With or Without Mineralocorticoids: Adrenal Insufficiency

Description

Adrenal insufficiency can be either primary, from destruction of the adrenal cortex by a local disease process or a systemic disorder, or secondary from pituitary or hypothalamic disease that reduces stimulation of the adrenal gland. The most common causes of primary adrenal insufficiency, in which all classes of adrenal cortical steroids are deficient, are autoimmune adrenalitis and tuberculosis in endemic regions. In this particular disorder, the adrenal medulla and its catecholamine synthesis are spared. In other primary adrenal insufficiency disorders in which the adrenal gland is damaged, the adrenal medulla may be damaged along with the adrenal cortex. In secondary adrenal insufficiency, in which there is deficient stimulation of the adrenal gland because of pituitary or hypothalamic abnormalities, the adrenal medulla is not affected and aldosterone deficiency is not usually present. Aldosterone secretion is more dependent on angiotensin II stimulation of the adrenal glands than on stimulation of the adrenal cortex by ACTH (as discussed below).

- *Primary adrenal insufficiency*—There are many causes of primary adrenal insufficiency. Dysfunction of one or more sites in the HPA axis is the major cause of the primary adrenal insufficiency. Chronic primary adrenal insufficiency, also known as Addison disease, occurs mostly in adults. The most common causes are autoimmune disease (Western world) and tuberculous adrenalitis (worldwide). Other causes of primary adrenal insufficiency include fungal or viral infections (i.e., histoplasmosis or HIV), and anatomic destruction of the adrenal glands through surgery, hemorrhage, or metastatic carcinomas. Primary adrenal insufficiency is characterized by hyperpigmentation of the skin and mucous membranes. The lack of negative feedback from adrenal cortisol leads to increased ACTH production by the pituitary. A degradation product of ACTH and its prohormone pro-opiomelanocortin is melanocyte-stimulating hormone (MSH). MSH stimulates melanin production and induces melanocyte hyperpigmentation. Hyperkalemia and hypotension may be present if there is deficient aldosterone (see the sections "Primary Hypoaldosteronism" and "Secondary Hypoaldosteronism"). Primary adrenal insufficiency usually has a gradual onset but may occur abruptly with a stressor such as critical illness or surgery. Acute adrenal insufficiency is often the result of adrenal hemorrhage or thrombosis that impairs blood supply to the gland.

  An adrenal (Addisonian) crisis, acute primary adrenocortical failure, can be triggered by a severe infection, sepsis, or abrupt withdrawal of steroids. It is a life-threatening emergency, characterized by abnormal electrolytes (critically high potassium and low sodium), hypotension, and hypoglycemia. Sudden death can occur if it is not treated promptly.

- *Secondary adrenal insufficiency*—A deficiency of ACTH secretion from any cause can lead to adrenal insufficiency. Long-term glucocorticoid therapy can result in prolonged suppression of CRH from the hypothalamus and ACTH from the pituitary and transient adrenal insufficiency. Hypopituitarism as a result of postpartum hemorrhage (Sheehan syndrome), radiation, surgery, or injury may result in decreased ACTH production leading to reduced glucocorticoid synthesis.

> Adrenal insufficiency may involve a deficiency of glucocorticoids or both glucocorticoids and mineralocorticoids. Depending on the extent of adrenal hormone deficiency, patients may have decreased serum cortisol alone or in combination with decreased plasma aldosterone.

Diagnosis

The management of adrenal insufficiency first requires determination of the disease source (i.e., primary or secondary), followed by an identification of the specific cause for the adrenal insufficiency. The tests that are useful in the diagnosis of primary and secondary adrenal insufficiency are shown in **Table 22–3**. Adrenal insufficiency may involve a deficiency of glucocorticoids or both glucocorticoids and mineralocorticoids. Depending on the extent of adrenal cortex damage, patients may have decreased serum cortisol and/or decreased plasma aldosterone concentrations.

TABLE 22–3   **Laboratory Evaluation for Adrenal Insufficiency**

Laboratory Test	Primary Adrenal Insufficiency	Secondary Adrenal Insufficiency
ACTH stimulation test	Synthetic ACTH does not stimulate cortisol secretion because the dysfunctional adrenal cortex is unable to respond to, synthesize, and/or secrete cortisol	Acute and/or mild secondary adrenal insufficiency: cortisol increased Chronic secondary adrenal insufficiency: cortisol is minimally increased due to adrenal atrophy from a long-term lack of stimulation by ACTH
Serum cortisol measured between 8 and 9 AM	Low	Low
Plasma ACTH	Elevated, because feedback inhibition by adrenal cortisol is absent	Low, because the origin of the disorder is in the hypothalamus or pituitary
Plasma aldosterone	Low in cases in which injury to the adrenal gland impacts both cortisol and aldosterone production	Often normal, although it may be depressed if there is significant atrophy of the adrenal glands as a result of chronic lack of stimulation by ACTH
CRH stimulation test	Not necessary	This test can distinguish between ACTH deficiency (from the pituitary) and deficiency of CRH (from the hypothalamus); hypothalamic origin: ACTH is increased and cortisol is minimally increased; pituitary origin: ACTH and cortisol remain low
Adrenal autoantibodies	Serum tests that detect titers of adrenal autoantibodies are available for the confirmation of autoimmune-mediated primary adrenal insufficiency; the most commonly ordered is the 21-hydroxylase antibody test	Not necessary

ACTH, adrenocorticotropic hormone (corticotropin); CRH, corticotropin-releasing hormone.

Adrenal insufficiency should be excluded in acutely ill patients with unexplained symptoms, such as low blood volume, low blood pressure, low sodium, and elevated potassium. The ACTH stimulation test is the most specific test to confirm a diagnosis of adrenal insufficiency in symptomatic patients. Patients with symptoms of adrenal crisis should be treated immediately. In patients with primary adrenal insufficiency, cortisol is typically not upregulated in response to ACTH stimulation due to adrenal gland damage. Baseline ACTH concentrations greater than twofold the upper reference limit in patients with cortisol deficiency confirms primary adrenal insufficiency. Measurement of plasma aldosterone and renin is helpful in determining whether the adrenal medulla is also damaged. Low aldosterone and elevated renin indicate a mineralocorticoid deficiency along with the glucocorticoid deficiency. Patients with mild or recent onset of secondary adrenal insufficiency (and a still viable adrenal cortex) respond to the ACTH stimulation because the defect is not within the adrenal gland. A chronic lack of stimulation of the adrenal cortex by ACTH in secondary adrenal insufficiency can result in cortical atrophy and limited cortisol production following ACTH stimulation. The CRH stimulation test can distinguish between secondary adrenal insufficiency caused by ACTH deficiency and that caused by CRH deficiency. Plasma ACTH and serum cortisol are measured after administration of CRH; increases are observed in hypothalamic disorders, but not in pituitary disorders. A serologic test for antiadrenal antibodies is useful to determine whether autoimmune adrenalitis is the cause of primary adrenal insufficiency.

Hyperfunction and Hypofunction Involving Mineralocorticoids: Hyperaldosteronism and Hypoaldosteronism

Description and Diagnosis

Aldosterone is a mineralocorticoid produced in the adrenal glands. It is largely responsible for regulating sodium retention and water resorption, and thereby control of blood volume. It also promotes excretion of potassium into urine. Aldosterone concentration in the blood is regulated

TABLE 22–4 **Laboratory Evaluation for Hyperaldosteronism and Hypoaldosteronism**

Laboratory Test	Primary Hyperaldosteronism	Secondary Hyperaldosteronism	Primary Hypoaldosteronism	Secondary Hypoaldosteronism
Serum potassium	Usually low, but a low-sodium diet may result in a normal value	Usually low, but a low-sodium diet may result in a normal value	Usually elevated	Usually elevated
Serum sodium	Normal	Normal or mildly elevated	Usually low	Low or low normal
Plasma aldosterone	Elevated in midmorning samples collected from normokalemic patients recumbent 2 h on an unrestricted sodium diet (>100 mmol/day) for at least 3 days, and in the absence of inhibiting medications	Elevated in midmorning samples collected from normokalemic patients recumbent 2 h on an unrestricted sodium diet (>100 mmol/day) for at least 3 days, and in the absence of inhibiting medications	Usually low in the absence of medications that affect activity	Usually low in the absence of medications that affect activity
Plasma renin activity or direct renin	Low for most causes of hyperaldosteronism in normokalemic patients with normal renal function in the absence of medications that affect activity	Elevated when there is decreased perfusion of the kidneys, a common cause of secondary hyperaldosteronism in the absence of medications that affect activity	Normal or elevated in the absence of medications that affect activity	Low renin production disorders—renin is low; other causes of secondary hypoaldosteronism—renin may be normal or elevated
PAC/PRA (DRC) ratio	Elevated (see appropriate collection conditions)	Normal to low	N/A	N/A
Saline suppression or infusion test	Aldosterone is not suppressed by saline	N/A	N/A	N/A

by the RAAS (**Figure 22–6**). In response to decreased blood volume, the juxtaglomerular apparatus of the kidney secretes renin, which converts angiotensinogen to angiotensin I. Angiotensin I is converted to angiotensin II by ACE in the lungs. Angiotensin II is a potent vasoconstrictor and also stimulates the adrenal glands to secrete aldosterone, which then acts to increase blood volume by promoting sodium retention in exchange for potassium that is lost into the urine.

Aldosterone concentrations in disease may be high (hyperaldosteronism) or low (hypoaldosteronism). An abnormal (high or low) PAC may be the result of a defect originating inside (primary disorder) or outside (secondary disorder) of the adrenal gland (**Table 22–4**).

Primary Aldosteronism (PA) formerly Primary Hyperaldosteronism

In this disorder, there is excess secretion of aldosterone as a result of an abnormality within the adrenal gland. Most often, hyperaldosteronism is caused by bilateral hyperplasia of the adrenal glands or by an aldosterone-secreting adrenal adenoma, resulting in a disorder known as Conn syndrome. Less often, PA is a result of primary (unilateral) adrenal hyperplasia or a cancerous tumor. In primary aldosteronism, the PRA is low because aldosterone stimulates sodium retention, leading to increased plasma sodium and an increase in blood volume. Both are triggers that downregulate renin secretion. In patients with hypertension at high risk for PA, the ratio of aldosterone/PRA (also known as the aldosterone to renin ration, ARR), is the recommended screening test. A ratio of greater than 30 when PAC is measured in conventional units (ng/dL) and 750 when PAC is in SI units (pmol/L) is the most commonly used cutoff to identify patients with suspected PA. Because of the effects of numerous drugs, diet, and comorbidities on PAC and PRA concentrations, it is recommended that along with an elevated ratio, patients also have PAC concentrations above 15 ng/dL. Some laboratories use DRC as an indirect measure of renin activity. A few studies have published recommended diagnostic cutoffs for the PAC/DRC ratios for primary hyperaldosteronism, but they have not yet been universally accepted. All abnormal ARR results must be confirmed with one of four stimulation/suppression tests: oral sodium loading test, saline infusion test, fludrocortisone suppression test, or the captopril challenge. Among these, the saline infusion test is preferred. In this test, high doses of saline are given either orally or by infusion. In a normal functioning RAAS, high sodium triggers downregulation of renin and leads to suppression of aldosterone secretion. However, in PA, aldosterone secretion is autonomous and will not

Aldosterone is a mineralocorticoid produced in the adrenal glands. It is largely responsible for sodium retention and water resorption, and thereby control of blood volume. It also promotes the excretion of potassium into the urine.

be suppressed by saline. With an abnormal confirmation test, the next step is to perform adrenal imaging to look for a tumor or adrenal hyperplasia. If the patient is a candidate for surgery, and surgery is desired, the last step is to determine whether the process is unilateral or bilateral through adrenal vein sampling (AVS). Cortisol and aldosterone are measured in the right and left adrenal veins. An elevated aldosterone/cortisol ratio in one adrenal vein compared to the ratio in the inferior vena cava suggests a unilateral process while an elevated aldosterone/cortisol ratio in both adrenal veins compared to a peripheral venous sample is suggestive of a bilateral process. Unilateral processes are treated surgically while bilateral processes and nonsurgical patients are treated with antihypertensive medications.

Secondary Hyperaldosteronism

In this disorder, there is excess secretion of aldosterone as a result of an abnormality outside the adrenal gland. It is much more common than PA. Decreased renal perfusion is the most common cause of secondary hyperaldosteronism. The decreased blood flow into the kidney results in an elevation of the PRA. The elevation in PRA (as shown in **Figure 22–6**) produces the increase in aldosterone. Heart failure, nephrotic syndrome, cirrhosis of the liver, and other hypoproteinemic conditions in which there is chronic depletion of plasma volume can produce an elevation in plasma aldosterone.

> The clinical and laboratory features common to both primary and secondary hyperaldosteronism include hypertension associated with hypervolemia and low or low-normal concentrations of serum potassium.

The clinical and laboratory features common to both primary and secondary hyperaldosteronism usually include hypertension associated with hypervolemia and low or low-normal concentrations of serum potassium. The serum sodium also may be slightly elevated. Additional clinical features include nocturnal polyuria, polydipsia, and weakness from the low potassium concentrations.

Primary Hypoaldosteronism

This disorder is much less common than primary hyperaldosteronism (PA). Primary hypoaldosteronism is most often a result of destruction of the adrenal gland from various causes including autoimmune adrenalitis, adrenal infection by tuberculosis, metastatic tumors to the adrenal, adrenalectomy, CAH associated with low aldosterone production (see the section "Alterations in the Synthesis of Glucocorticoids, Mineralocorticoids, and Sex Steroids: Congenital Adrenal Hyperplasia"), and hemorrhage into the adrenal gland. There is an additional disorder associated with primary hypoaldosteronism, known as pseudohypoaldosteronism, in which the tissues are resistant to the action of aldosterone. Low blood volume and/or sodium due to lack of aldosterone action upregulates renin synthesis, which subsequently upregulates aldosterone. Therefore, these patients have significantly elevated PAC and PRA.

Secondary Hypoaldosteronism

In this disorder, aldosterone hyposecretion results from factors originating outside the adrenal gland. One cause is lack of ACTH production by the pituitary, often accompanied by deficiencies of other pituitary hormones. As noted earlier, the adrenal cortex can become atrophied as a result of a chronic lack of stimulation by ACTH, decreasing aldosterone as well as cortisol production. Another cause is long-term glucocorticoid administration. Long-term glucocorticoid-induced ACTH suppression leads to adrenal atrophy and reduced aldosterone synthesis. Secondary hypoaldosteronism can also occur as a result of deficient renin production due to renal damage or drugs and from inhibition of ACE by drugs. Clinical and laboratory features common to primary and secondary hypoaldosteronism include hypotension, which may be orthostatic, and high serum potassium concentrations. Slightly low serum sodium values also may be present. The clinical signs and symptoms vary significantly and depend on the specific defect leading to the hypoaldosteronism.

Alterations in the Synthesis of Glucocorticoids, Mineralocorticoids, and Sex Steroids: Congenital Adrenal Hyperplasia

Description and Diagnosis

CAH is caused by any one of a group of enzyme deficiencies in the biosynthetic pathways for cortisol and aldosterone. Because cortisol production is decreased, and cortisol provides the inhibitory feedback to the pituitary for ACTH secretion, there is an increase in ACTH and excess

TABLE 22–5 Laboratory Evaluation for Congenital Adrenal Hyperplasia

Enzyme Deficiency	Relevant Laboratory Findings (Focusing on Compounds Most Likely to Be Measured in an Evaluation)
21-Hydroxylase	Elevated: 17-hydroxyprogesterone, androstenedione, DHEA, and its sulfated metabolite (DHEA-S) testosterone; ACTH and plasma renin activity because of the deficiencies of cortisol and aldosterone
	Decreased: aldosterone, cortisol
11-Beta-hydroxylase	Elevated: 11-deoxycortisol, 11-deoxycorticosterone; 17-hydroxyprogesterone, androstenedione, DHEA, DHEA-S, testosterone
	Decreased: aldosterone, cortisol
17-Alpha-hydroxylase	Elevated: aldosterone; deoxycorticosterone
	Decreased: androgens, cortisol
3-Beta-hydroxysteroid dehydrogenase	Elevated: DHEA; ACTH and plasma renin activity because of the deficiencies of cortisol and aldosterone
	Decreased: aldosterone, cortisol
	Assays for 17-hydroxypregnenolone and 17-hydroxyprogesterone, as well as assays for DHEA and androstenedione, are helpful in the differentiation of 3-beta-hydroxysteroid dehydrogenase deficiency from 21-hydroxylase deficiency and 11-beta-hydroxylase deficiency; the 17-hydroxypregnenolone to 17-hydroxyprogesterone ratio and the DHEA to androstenedione ratio in 3-beta-hydroxysteroid dehydrogenase deficiency are extremely high

ACTH, adrenocorticotropic hormone (corticotropin); DHEA, dehydroepiandrosterone.

stimulation of the adrenal glands (see **Figures 22–5** and **22–6** for the regulation of cortisol and aldosterone production). This results in greater flux through pathways around an existing enzymatic defect, producing elevations in adrenal hormones whose synthesis is not affected by the enzyme deficiency. Most of the known enzyme deficiencies in the synthetic pathways for aldosterone and cortisol result in an elevation in sex steroid synthesis, which has a virilizing effect on the patient. The most common of the enzymatic defects is deficiency of 21-hydroxylase. This deficiency accounts for 90% to 95% of the cases of CAH. The clinical manifestations for four of the enzyme deficiencies producing CAH are noted below. **Figure 22–4** shows the intermediate compounds in the synthesis of aldosterone, cortisol, and androgens in the adrenal gland and the enzymes in the pathway, some of which may be deficient. **Table 22–5** presents the laboratory evaluation for CAH.

- *21-Hydroxylase deficiency*—Deficiency of this enzyme is the most common form of CAH. In female infants, a 21-hydroxylase deficiency usually results in hypertrophy of the clitoris and pseudohermaphroditism as a result of disruption in the synthesis pathways for cortisol and aldosterone and shunting of intermediates down the androgen synthesis pathway. In postpubertal females, it results in amenorrhea, infertility, and hirsutism. In males, the virilization results in enlargement of the external genitalia and precocious puberty. As seen in **Figure 22–4**, 21-hydroxylase deficiency will result in a reduced or no synthesis of both cortisol and aldosterone and accumulation of the 17-OHP intermediate. As a result, if infants with this deficiency are not treated with corticosteroids, they can quickly develop life-threatening hyperkalemia, hyponatremia, and hypotension. Because of the severe clinical manifestations, it is recommended that all newborns be screened for 21-hydroxylase deficiency by measurement of 17-OHP. Positive newborn screening results should be followed with sensitive and specific confirmatory testing.
- *11-Beta-hydroxylase deficiency*—This is the second most common enzyme deficiency responsible for CAH. In infancy, the clinical and laboratory features of patients with this abnormality are largely similar to those found in patients with 21-hydroxylase deficiency. However, deficiency of this enzyme causes accumulation of 11-deoxycorticosterone, a potent mineralocorticoid. Thus, these patients develop mineralocorticoid-induced hypertension and hypokalemia.

Most of the known enzyme deficiencies in the synthetic pathways for aldosterone and cortisol result in an elevation in sex steroid synthesis, which has a virilizing effect on the patient. The most common of the enzymatic defects is a deficiency of 21-hydroxylase.

- *17-Alpha-hydroxylase deficiency*—This deficiency is rare and accounts for approximately 1% of all CAH cases. In this deficiency, there is no inhibition of aldosterone synthesis, but there is a block in the synthesis of both cortisol and sex steroids. The elevation of aldosterone results in hyperaldosteronism that produces hypertension and hypokalemia. In females, the androgen deficiency results in a lack of development of secondary sex characteristics because the androgens are biochemical precursors of estrogens. In males, pseudohermaphroditism appears.
- *3-Beta-hydroxysteroid dehydrogenase deficiency*—This is another rare CAH disorder. This enzymatic deficiency results in a metabolic block in the production of aldosterone and cortisol, with no inhibition of the synthesis of DHEA and other androgens. In its severe form, this enzyme deficiency manifests as early masculinization in males and amenorrhea and pseudohermaphroditism in females, as well as life-threatening hyperkalemia, hyponatremia, and hypotension.

ADRENAL MEDULLA

Physiology and Biochemistry

The main sites of production of the catecholamines are the brain, the chromaffin cells of the adrenal medulla, and the sympathetic neurons. The catecholamines include dopamine, epinephrine, and norepinephrine as the most potent of the endogenously produced compounds. Of these, in the adrenal medulla, epinephrine production is quantitatively the greatest. The catecholamines elicit a variety of biological effects. They have a marked impact on the vascular system, and are important in blood pressure regulation. Epinephrine influences many metabolic pathways, especially carbohydrate metabolism. In some tissues, epinephrine and norepinephrine produce opposite effects. Alpha-adrenergic receptors on cells interact effectively with norepinephrine and moderately with epinephrine, while beta-adrenergic receptors respond primarily to epinephrine and norepinephrine.

Catecholamine synthesis and metabolism in the adrenal medulla is illustrated in **Figure 22–7**. The pathway begins when the amino acid tyrosine is metabolized to a catecholamine, dihydroxyphenylalanine (DOPA). DOPA is then converted to dopamine, which is hydroxylated to norepinephrine, which is subsequently converted to epinephrine. Because of their great potency, the catecholamines must be rapidly inactivated through reuptake into storage granules, conversion to metabolites, or excretion. Unlike the steroid hormones, catecholamines are not bound to proteins as they circulate. In plasma, they have a very short half-life of approximately 2 minutes. Urine catecholamines, on the other hand, represent a pool of catecholamines delivered into urine in the preceding hours. There are a number of degradative products of epinephrine and norepinephrine. The compounds noted in **Figure 22–7**—metanephrine, normetanephrine, and vanillylmandelic acid—are the products that are measured in clinical assays to assess catecholamine production and degradation.

Laboratory Tests

Epinephrine and Norepinephrine

Total or fractionated (epinephrine or norepinephrine) catecholamines can be measured in plasma or 24-hour urine samples. The plasma concentration reflects the rate of synthesis and release of catecholamines by the adrenal medulla and their half-life in the circulation. Catecholamines are secreted into the urine as free hormones. Urinary catecholamines are extremely unstable and should be acidified during or right after collection.

Metanephrines (Metanephrine and Normetanephrine)

The preferred screening test for adrenal medullary neuroendocrine tumors is detection of free metanephrines and normetanephrines in plasma. Both metanephrine and normetanephrine undergo conjugation with sulfate or glucuronide. The metanephrines can also be measured in a 24-hour urine specimen. Urine measurements are helpful in cases where plasma metanephrines are marginally elevated. Metanephrines are also unstable in urine and should be acidified during or right after collection.

The catecholamines include dopamine, epinephrine, and norepinephrine as the most potent of the endogenously produced compounds. Of these, in the adrenal medulla, epinephrine production is quantitatively the greatest.

There are a number of degradative products of epinephrine and norepinephrine. Metanephrine, normetanephrine, and vanillylmandelic acid are the ones that are measured in clinical assays to assess catecholamine production and degradation.

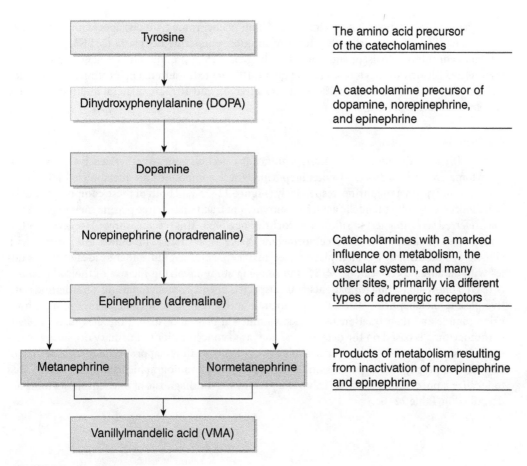

FIGURE 22–7 Catecholamine synthesis and metabolism in the adrenal medulla.

Vanillylmandelic Acid

This compound is the major metabolite of both metanephrine and normetanephrine. It is measured in the urine and, although it is indicative of catecholamine synthesis and metabolism, it is inferior to urinary metanephrine quantitation for this purpose.

Pheochromocytoma

Description

A pheochromocytoma, which may be benign or malignant, is a chromaffin cell tumor of the adrenal medulla or autonomic nervous system that secretes catecholamines. On this basis, it is a cause of hypertension. However, it is a rare cause of hypertension with approximately 5 pheochromocytomas per 100,000 hypertensive cases. Other catecholamine-secreting chromaffin cell tumors are paragangliomas and neuroblastomas. It is essential that a pheochromocytoma be rapidly and accurately identified in patients with hypertension because surgical resection of the tumor, with elimination of the hypertension and its complications, is successful in at least 90% of cases, and the disease may be otherwise fatal. The diagnosis is made most often in patients between the ages of 30 and 60 years. The clinical features of a patient with pheochromocytoma include, most importantly, the presence of sustained or paroxysmal hypertension. The attacks of hypertension occur abruptly and subside slowly, with a total duration of less than 1 hour in approximately 80% of patients. They may be precipitated by palpation of the tumor, postural changes, exertion, anxiety, trauma, pain, intake of foods or beverages containing tyramine (such as certain cheeses, beer, and wine), and the ingestion of certain medications. Headaches are common in patients with pheochromocytoma, and they are usually severe. Generalized sweating and palpitations with tachycardia occur frequently. Other common signs and symptoms are anxiety,

It is essential that a pheochromocytoma be rapidly and accurately identified in patients with hypertension because surgical resection of the tumor, with elimination of the hypertension and its complications, is successful in at least 90% of cases, and the disease may be otherwise fatal.

chest pain, nausea, fatigue, and weight loss. Of all pheochromocytomas, approximately 25% to 30% are familial and coexist with a form of multiple endocrine neoplasia (MEN), von Hippel Lindau, neurofibromatosis, or succinate dehydrogenase (SDH) mutation (see later section); 10% of inherited pheochromocytomas are malignant; 10% are extra-adrenal in location and are called paragangliomas (and therefore 90% are in the adrenal); and 10% are bilateral and most of these are patients with MEN 2A.

Diagnosis

As noted before, the most biologically significant catecholamines synthesized by a pheochromocytoma are epinephrine and norepinephrine. These compounds are metabolized into metanephrine and normetanephrine, respectively (**Figure 22–7**), and both of these compounds can be metabolized to vanillylmandelic acid. Measurement of fractionated, free plasma metanephrines is the preferred screening test to rule out pheochromocytoma. This test measures plasma concentrations of free metanephrine and free normetanephrine as separate compounds. All patients with clinical symptoms and elevated plasma free metanephrines should undergo localization studies with an adrenal CT scan or MIBG (an imaging study involving the use of the radioisotope MIBG). Follow-up testing for patients with suspected pheochromocytoma and a borderline positive plasma metanephrine screening test include measurement of metanephrines in a 24-hour urine sample and then fractionated catecholamines in plasma or urine. The diagnosis of pheochromocytoma is based on the detection of increased concentrations of urinary or plasma metanephrines, and possibly plasma or urinary catecholamines, in the appropriate clinical setting of sustained or paroxysmal hypertension. Adrenal CT or other radiographic techniques can be used to localize a pheochromocytoma. Laboratory tests used for diagnosis of pheochromocytoma are described in **Table 22–6**.

TABLE 22–6   Laboratory Evaluation for Pheochromocytoma

Laboratory Test	Results/Comments
Plasma metanephrines	Measurement of fractionated, free plasma metanephrines is the preferred screening test to rule out pheochromocytoma; low or normal metanephrine and normetanephrine concentrations reliably exclude the diagnosis of pheochromocytoma; several medications as well as caffeine and cigarette smoking may interfere with the plasma metanephrine assay
Urinary metanephrines	More than 95% of patients with pheochromocytoma will have an elevated concentration of metanephrine and normetanephrine in a 24-h urine collection; the measurement of total metanephrines per gram of creatinine can be made in a 24-h urine collection; elevated urinary metanephrines in the presence of clinical signs and symptoms consistent with pheochromocytoma can establish the diagnosis
Plasma catecholamines	Concentrations of plasma catecholamines are elevated in pheochromocytoma; if hypertension is paroxysmal (epinephrine and norepinephrine) rather than sustained, blood must be obtained for catecholamine measurement during a spontaneous or provoked hypertensive episode to demonstrate elevated plasma catecholamines; because plasma catecholamines increase with stress, the sample for plasma catecholamine measurement must be collected with careful regard to minimize stress to the patient; blood is optimally obtained after at least 20 min of rest and drawn through a previously inserted venous cannula; the medications that the patient is ingesting at the time of or immediately prior to the test may also influence catecholamine concentrations
Urinary catecholamines	Catecholamines measured in a 24-h urine collection may be used in the initial assessment of suspected pheochromocytoma; however, the test for urinary metanephrines has a higher sensitivity for detection of pheochromocytoma
Urinary vanillylmandelic acid	Urinary VMA is elevated in the majority of patients who have a pheochromocytoma, but it is less sensitive than the test for urinary metanephrines for diagnosis of the disorder; determination of urinary VMA concentration is not essential to establish the diagnosis; ingestion of tricyclic antidepressants and selected other medications may produce spurious results in this assay

PARATHYROID GLANDS

This section is focused on parathyroid hormone (PTH) and disorders associated with high or low concentrations of this hormone. Most parathyroid disorders alter calcium metabolism, and thereby have an effect on bone. However, there are also a number of disorders associated with hypercalcemia or hypocalcemia, or alterations in bone density, in which a change in the PTH concentration is not a major factor. Therefore, in addition to hyperparathyroidism and hypoparathyroidism, this chapter also briefly describes a few selected disorders associated with hypercalcemia, hypocalcemia, or altered bone density in which PTH does not play a major role.

Physiology and Biochemistry

PTH is a polypeptide secreted from the parathyroid glands. The primary function of PTH is the regulation of the concentration of ionized calcium in extracellular fluids. An increase in secretion of PTH produces a rise in serum ionized calcium and a decrease in the serum phosphorus concentration. A normal or an elevated ionized calcium provides negative feedback to the parathyroid gland to reduce the secretion of PTH (see **Figure 22–8**).

The resorption of bone induced by PTH is mediated by increased activity of osteoclasts. PTH can also promote an increase in the renal tubular reabsorption of calcium.

Vitamin D is an intermediary in the action of PTH to elevate the serum calcium level. It is a fat-soluble hormone required for calcium absorption in the gut, bone metabolism, and development of cells in the immune system. Vitamin D also influences phosphorus metabolism. Vitamin D_2 is known as ergocalciferol, and vitamin D_3 is known as cholecalciferol.

Food can be fortified with either vitamin D_2 or D_3, both of which can be used as vitamin D supplements. Cholecalciferol is ingested in the diet, and it is also synthesized in the skin upon ultraviolet irradiation of 7-dehydrocholesterol. The cholecalciferol is transported to the liver where it is

> An increase in secretion of PTH produces a rise in serum ionized calcium and a decrease in the serum phosphorus concentration. Calcitonin has an opposing action to PTH, but in humans it appears to play a minor role in calcium homeostasis.

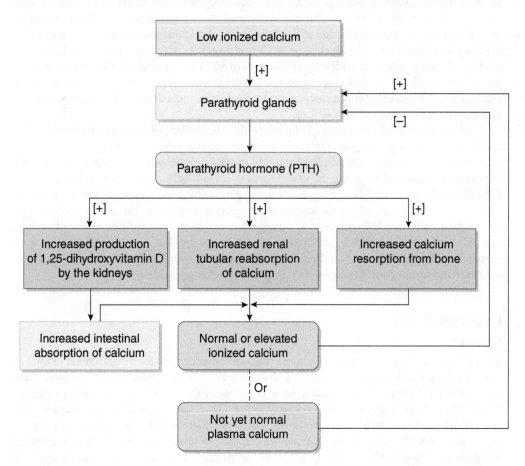

FIGURE 22–8 **The regulation of parathyroid hormone secretion. [+] Stimulation; [−] inhibition.**

hydroxylated to produce 25-hydroxycholecalciferol (25-(OH)D$_3$). The 25-(OH)D$_3$ has limited biological activity, but in the kidney it undergoes further hydroxylation to form dihydroxy metabolites, the most potent of which in calcium metabolism is 1,25-(OH)$_2$D$_3$. An increase in this vitamin D metabolite results in increased intestinal absorption of calcium, mobilization of calcium and phosphorous from the bone, and increased calcium reabsorption in the kidney, all acting to elevate ionized calcium concentrations in blood. The production of this dihydroxy metabolite of vitamin D is regulated by the need for calcium in the circulation. Decreased blood calcium results in a stimulation of the parathyroid glands to secrete PTH that leads to the increased production of 1,25-(OH)$_2$D$_3$ in the renal proximal tubules. Thus, PTH is responsible for maintaining the necessary levels of calcium in the body by extracting sufficient calcium from the diet, resorbing it from bone, or preventing its excretion through the renal tubules. **Figure 22–8** shows the regulation of PTH secretion. Ingested vitamin D$_2$ is hydroxylated into 25-(OH)D$_2$ and follows the same metabolism to 1,25-(OH)$_2$D$_2$.

Calcitonin has an opposing action to PTH, but in humans it appears to play a minor role in calcium homeostasis. As a drug, its pharmacologic action is more definitive. It inhibits osteoclastic bone resorption. It also decreases renal tubular reabsorption of calcium, and by these mechanisms opposes the action of PTH. Calcitonin synthesis occurs in the parafollicular C cells of the thyroid gland.

Approximately 98% of calcium is present in the body within the bones in the form of hydroxyapatite, a crystal lattice composed of calcium, phosphorus, and hydroxide. Of the calcium not within the bones, about half is present in extracellular fluid and the remainder is present in a variety of tissues, particularly skeletal muscle. Only about 1% of the calcium in the bones is exchangeable with the extracellular fluid, and it is this pool that is most significantly affected by changes in PTH concentration. Calcium exists in the plasma in three distinct forms: free or ionized calcium, protein-bound, and complexed with anions. Ionized calcium is the physiologically active form of calcium and accounts for approximately 45% to 50% of the total calcium in the plasma. Another 40% to 45% of calcium in the plasma is bound to plasma proteins. Calcium is primarily bound to albumin, and also binds to other proteins. The remaining 5% to 15% of the total calcium forms a complex with a variety of anions. The most commonly found complexes are calcium phosphate and calcium citrate. The distribution of the three forms of calcium changes with alterations in pH in the extracellular fluid and with changes in plasma protein concentration. In general, the serum ionized calcium increases in acidosis and decreases in alkalosis because calcium more easily binds proteins under alkalotic conditions. An increase in the concentration of plasma proteins that bind calcium results in a corresponding increase in total calcium, and a decrease in the plasma proteins may result in a decrease in total calcium.

> Only about 1% of the calcium in the bones is exchangeable with the extracellular fluid, and it is this pool that is most significantly affected by the level of PTH.

The metabolism of phosphorus is linked to the metabolism of calcium. About 85% of the phosphorus in an adult is present in the bone as part of hydroxyapatite. Most of the remaining phosphorus in the body is within phospholipids, proteins, carbohydrates, nucleotides, and other important biochemical compounds. Phosphorus is present in virtually all foods; thus, dietary deficiencies do not occur. The phosphorus in the extracellular fluid exists primarily as HPO$_4$$^{2-}$ and H$_2$PO$_4$$^-$, which are collectively known as inorganic phosphorus. The amounts of these two phosphate anions are pH-dependent. Food ingestion can alter the serum inorganic phosphorus concentration significantly, with an increase in serum phosphorus concentration following the ingestion of phosphate-rich food. Because of the rapidly growing skeletal system, phosphorous demands and serum concentrations are significantly higher in children.

Laboratory Tests

Calcium

Whole blood, serum, or heparinized plasma specimens can be used for measurement of total and ionized calcium concentrations. Since pH changes may alter concentrations of ionized calcium, careful specimen collection is necessary. Ideally specimens should be measured within 30 minutes of collection without exposure to air to prevent loss of CO$_2$. If specimens cannot be analyzed within an hour of collection, whole blood specimens should be collected and transported on ice or serum specimens should be utilized. Because calcium can bind to several anticoagulants in vacuum collection tubes (notably EDTA and citrate), only heparinized whole blood and plasma specimens are acceptable. In underfilled tubes, heparin may cause falsely decreased ionized calcium results.

Inorganic Phosphorus

About 15% of the inorganic phosphorus, predominantly HPO_4^{2-} and $H_2PO_4^-$, in the plasma is protein-bound, and the remainder is free or complexed to another ion. Organic phosphorus (not measured in the assay for inorganic phosphorus) refers to the phosphorus within phospholipids, proteins, carbohydrates, nucleic acids, and other organic substances.

PTH

The most important test in the differential diagnosis of hypercalcemia is the assay for serum PTH. The biological activity of PTH resides in the first 34-amino terminal amino acids.

The intact hormone (iPTH) with 84 amino acids accounts for much of the circulating PTH, but there are many circulating PTH fragments. The assay for iPTH has largely superseded earlier tests that recognize numerous inactive circulating PTH fragments. One fragment of interest is the fragment of PTH representing amino acids 7-84 that is present in high concentrations during renal disease and capable of antagonizing the PTH receptor. Many newer iPTH assays still recognize the 7-84 fragment, along with the intact molecule, and therefore may be less clinically informative in patients with renal disease. An assay for whole PTH is available that only recognizes the 1-84 amino acid PTH.

Intraoperative PTH Assay

Primary hyperparathyroidism requiring parathyroidectomy is a challenge because of variability in the location and number of parathyroid glands. Of parathyroid adenomas, 15% to 20% are ectopic, and not adjacent to the thyroid gland, and approximately 5% of patients have five parathyroid glands rather than four. Intraoperative PTH measurement has significantly improved success rates in parathyroid surgery. The relatively short half-life of PTH has allowed for surgeons to measure plasma PTH concentrations before and after excision of parathyroid tumors in surgery. A decrease in PTH of >50% suggests complete resection of the tumor. Use of this intraoperative test has resulted in a higher incidence of complete removal of hypersecreting parathyroid gland tissue, reduced the need for extensive exploration of the neck, and decreased the need for repeat surgery.

> The success of parathyroid surgery has been improved by intraoperative PTH measurement. The intraoperative PTH assay is used to detect decreases in plasma PTH levels following excision of parathyroid tumors in surgery.

Vitamin D

The quantitation of selected vitamin D metabolites is useful in assessing vitamin D metabolism. Vitamin D metabolites of greatest relevance to calcium metabolism include $25\text{-}(OH)D_3$ (also known as 25-hydroxyvitamin D) and $1,25\text{-}(OH)_2D_3$ (also known as 1,25-dihydroxyvitamin D). Currently, the most clinically informative screening test for vitamin D deficiency is total 25-(OH) vitamin D, which is the sum of the 25-(OH) vitamin D_2 and 25-(OH) vitamin D_3 concentrations in serum. Recently, tandem mass spectrometry has increased in use and allowed for measurement of vitamin D_2 and vitamin D_3 in either form (i.e., 25-(OH) or 1,25-(OH)) in a single test. 25-(OH) vitamin D is the most abundant metabolite of vitamin D, and it has a long half-life. It is the component measured in most immunoassays for vitamin D. In contrast, $1,25\text{-}(OH)_2$ vitamin D has a much lower serum concentration, and a shorter half-life (4–6 hours).

PTH-related Protein (PTHrP)

This protein, nearly twice the size of PTH, is equipotent with PTH in inducing hypercalcemia. PTHrP is secreted by numerous tumor tissues. Its shared homology allows PTHrP to bind PTH receptors and stimulate renal proximal tubular reabsorption of calcium. The assay to measure PTHrP shows less than 1% cross-reactivity with PTH.

Bone Markers

Markers for bone turnover can be classified into two groups, markers of bone formation and markers for bone resorption. Bone markers should not be used as definitive tests for the diagnosis of osteoporosis. Their primary utility is to monitor response to treatment for bone disease. The markers with the most clinical utility are described below.

Bone Formation Markers

Alkaline Phosphatase. This enzyme is present in a wide variety of tissues, but primarily in bone and liver. Most laboratory assays for alkaline phosphatase (ALP) measure total ALP. The bone-derived fraction of ALP can be differentiated from its isoenzymes in serum by bone-specific ALP immunoassay or based on its instability. Bone ALP is denatured by heat and urea. Falsely elevated results are commonly seen in liver disease.

Osteocalcin. Serum osteocalcin is a moderately specific marker for bone formation. Serum concentrations are highest in adolescence and in the newborn, when bone growth is most active, and in renal failure due to clearance impairment. The serum osteocalcin concentration rises in women from the 4th to the 10th decade as the bone turnover increases. Menopause induces a marked increase in bone turnover, often with an increase in serum osteocalcin. Although not as sensitive as collagen markers, measurement of osteocalcin can help predict bone loss in postmenopausal women. Osteocalcin has limited clinical utility due to significant diurnal variability and accumulation in renal failure.

Procollagen Type I Intact N-terminal Propeptide (PINP). PINP, which is formed during collagen synthesis, is the most sensitive marker of bone formation. Measurement of PINP by radioimmunoassay in serum is recommended for monitoring of therapy to bone disease. It should be measured prior to initiation of therapy and then subsequently 3 to 6 months later. PINP exhibits less intraindividual variability than other collagen markers.

Bone Resorption Markers

N- and C-terminal Telopeptide of Type 1 Collagen (NTx and CTx). NTx and CTx are peptide fragments formed during bone resorption through proteolytic processing of the N- and C-terminal ends of type I collagen, respectively. These can be measured by immunoassay in both serum and urine to assess response to treatment of bone disease. Significant intraindividual variability exists in CTx concentrations because it is affected by diet, exercise, and time of day. NTx should be measured prior to initiation of therapy and then 3 to 6 months later to assess bone disease status.

Pyridinium Cross-links. Pyridinium cross-links, including deoxypyridinoline (DPD), are a group of products formed during bone resorption as a result of collagen breakdown. These can be measured by immunoassay and are useful in monitoring therapy. Urine pyridinium cross-link concentrations can determine efficacy of bone disease treatment after as little as 2 months of therapy.

Primary Hyperparathyroidism

Description

The majority of cases of primary hyperparathyroidism result from a single parathyroid adenoma, with hyperplasia of the parathyroids and parathyroid carcinoma being less common causes. In the diagnosis of primary hyperparathyroidism, the total serum calcium is the initial test.

In primary hyperparathyroidism, there is excess secretion of PTH in the absence of an appropriate stimulus. The disease affects women about twice as frequently as men, and the incidence increases with age. The majority of cases of primary hyperparathyroidism result from a single parathyroid adenoma, with hyperplasia of the parathyroids and parathyroid carcinoma being less common causes. The hypercalcemia in hyperparathyroidism occurs as a result of the direct action of PTH. Primary hyperparathyroidism is often identified in asymptomatic individuals who have an unexpected serum hypercalcemia. Symptomatic patients with primary hyperparathyroidism may present with kidney stones, hypertension, polyuria, chronic constipation, depression, neuromuscular dysfunction, recurrent pancreatitis, peptic ulcer, or an unexplained osteopenia.

Diagnosis

Primary hyperparathyroidism may be suspected in patients with an isolated elevated total calcium. In order to rule out effects of binding proteins, ionized calcium should also be determined, especially in patients with abnormal serum concentrations of total protein or albumin. On demonstration of hypercalcemia, serum PTH and fasting serum phosphorus should be measured.

Assays for PTH can measure the intact molecule, carboxy-terminal, or midregion segments. The use of the intact PTH assay is preferred, especially in patients with renal disease because PTH carboxy-terminal fragments can accumulate with decreased renal function. The diagnosis of hyperparathyroidism is made when both persistent hypercalcemia and elevated serum PTH level are demonstrated. The serum inorganic phosphorus may be low or normal in patients with primary hyperparathyroidism. Patients with severe hyperparathyroidism can have bone pain, skeletal deformities, and even bone fractures (**Table 22–7**).

Secondary Hyperparathyroidism

Description

Secondary hyperparathyroidism occurs when there is chronic hypocalcemia and an excessive compensatory secretion of PTH. Chronic hypocalcemia is often a result of vitamin D deficiency or renal disease with calcium losses into the urine. Inadequate dietary intake of calcium is a rare cause of hypocalcemia. Secondary hyperparathyroidism is often associated with bone disease due to PTH-mediated bone resorption and calcium release.

Diagnosis

In secondary hyperparathyroidism, there is an elevation in the PTH, but unlike primary hyperparathyroidism, the total and ionized calcium in the serum are low or normal. Once established, the etiology of the hypocalcemia should be identified. Vitamin D deficiency is associated with a low total 25-hydroxyvitamin D concentration, while chronic renal disease is identified by abnormal renal function tests and/or a decreased glomerular filtration rate (**Table 22–7**).

Hypoparathyroidism

Description

Hypoparathyroidism occurs most frequently with unintentional removal of the parathyroid glands in the surgical excision of the thyroid gland. Hypocalcemia resulting from the hypoparathyroidism produces characteristic signs and symptoms, including numbness and tingling, and for patients with very low serum calcium levels, convulsions, and muscle spasms.

Diagnosis

In hypoparathyroidism, total and ionized calcium concentrations are low, with a low or undetectable serum PTH concentration. There is an elevation in the serum inorganic phosphorus associated with the decrease in serum calcium (**Table 22–7**).

> Hypoparathyroidism occurs most frequently with unintentional removal of the parathyroids in the surgical excision of the thyroid gland. In hypoparathyroidism, the total and ionized calcium levels in the serum are low, with a low or undetectable serum PTH concentration.

TABLE 22–7 **Laboratory Evaluation for Hyperparathyroidism and Hypoparathyroidism**

Laboratory Test	Primary Hyperparathyroidism	Secondary Hyperparathyroidism	Hypoparathyroidism	Humoral Hypercalcemia of Malignancy
Total or ionized calcium	Elevated	Low or normal	Low	Elevated
Serum intact PTH	Elevated	Elevated	Low or undetectable	Low or normal
Serum PTH-related protein	Undetectable	Undetectable	Undetectable	Detectable in some cancers
Serum 1,25-dihydroxy vitamin D	May be elevated but not usually required for diagnosis	May be elevated, normal, or low depending on the blood concentrations of calcium and phosphorus	Low	Low or normal
Serum phosphorus (inorganic)	Low or normal	Normal	Elevated	Low or normal

PTH, parathyroid hormone.

Pseudohypoparathyroidism

Description

As the name implies, patients with pseudohypoparathyroidism have signs and symptoms that are characteristic of hypoparathyroidism. This disorder results from a resistance of the tissues to the action of PTH and not a PTH deficiency.

Diagnosis

Unlike in patients with hypoparathyroidism, those with pseudohypoparathyroidism have a high concentration of serum PTH, in the presence of a low serum calcium concentration and signs and symptoms of hypoparathyroidism. In addition, patients with pseudohypoparathyroidism do not respond to infused PTH.

Vitamin D Deficiency

Description

Vitamin D deficiency, a major cause of secondary hyperparathyroidism and hypocalcemia, is caused by insufficient sun exposure, decreased intestinal absorption, insufficient intake, renal or liver failure, and numerous genetic disorders with defects in vitamin D processing, receptors, or binding proteins. The National Academy of Medicine defined vitamin D deficiency as total 25-(OH) vitamin D <20 ng/mL (50 nmol/L), but this cutoff is assay-dependent. Based on this cutoff, it is estimated that the prevalence of deficiency ranges from 20% to 100% of the elderly population, and varies among younger individuals by race, age, and sun exposure. Severe vitamin D deficiency in young children results in characteristic skeletal deformities known as rickets. Consistent with secondary hyperparathyroidism, patients with vitamin D deficiency develop bone disease often manifesting in osteomalacia, osteopenia, or osteoporosis. Vitamin D may also have a role in numerous other tissues. Evidence suggests that 1,25-(OH)$_2$ vitamin D may play a direct or indirect role in immune modulation, blood pressure regulation, insulin production, and cardiac muscle contractility. Vitamin D deficiency may be associated with colon, prostate, and breast cancer, autoimmune disease, diabetes, and cardiovascular disease.

Diagnosis

High-risk patients (pregnant women, elderly, or patients with darker skin pigmentation) should be screened for vitamin D deficiency by measurement of total 25-(OH) vitamin D. Concentrations less than 20 ng/mL or a different lab-defined cutoff indicate deficiency. It is not useful to measure 1,25-(OH)$_2$ vitamin D in suspected vitamin D deficiency because of its short half-life and tight regulation by numerous molecules. It is useful in the evaluation of patients with rare forms of inherited rickets. The cause, prognosis, and treatment strategies for vitamin D deficiency can be determined by also measuring PTH, magnesium, and phosphorous in plasma.

Hypercalcemia of Malignancy

Description

The most common cause of severe hypercalcemia in an inpatient population is malignancy. Tumors most often associated with hypercalcemia of malignancy include breast carcinoma, multiple myeloma, and lung carcinoma. The total calcium concentration may be elevated as a result of osteolysis secondary to bone metastases or humoral-induced hypercalcemia. In humoral hypercalcemia of malignancy (HHM), tumor production of PTHrP stimulates the PTH receptors to induce hypercalcemia. Elevated calcium leads to downregulation of PTH. The assay for PTHrP is potentially useful when malignancy is suspected as a cause of hypercalcemia.

> The most common cause of severe hypercalcemia in an inpatient population is malignancy. Tumors most often associated with hypercalcemia of malignancy include breast carcinoma, multiple myeloma, and lung carcinoma.

Diagnosis

HHM must be differentiated from hyperparathyroidism. Patients with hypercalcemia of malignancy will have elevated total and ionized calcium, in the presence of suppressed or low PTH. Low PTH differentiates HHM from primary and secondary hyperparathyroidism, which are both associated with high concentrations of serum PTH (**Table 22–7**). For patients in whom humorally induced hypercalcemia is suspected, the most specific confirmatory test is the assay for PTHrP.

Hypocalciuric Hypercalcemia

Description

Familial hypocalciuric hypercalcemia (FHH) is a rare disease associated with loss of function mutations in the calcium-sensing receptor gene product expressed in the parathyroid glands and kidneys. Normally, this receptor inhibits release of PTH from the parathyroid glands in the presence of high calcium. In the absence of a functioning receptor PTH release is uncontrolled, leading to elevated PTH and hypercalcemia. In the renal tubules, the calcium-sensing receptors inhibit calcium reabsorption in the presence of high calcium. Without this receptor, calcium is continuously reabsorbed and not excreted, leading to high serum concentrations and low urine calcium concentrations (hypocalciuria). Patients who are heterozygous for this mutation typically have asymptomatic hypercalcemia, while homozygotes lack calcium-sensing receptor genes and often require parathyroidectomy in infancy.

Diagnosis

Although rare, clinical and biochemical manifestations of FHH significantly overlap with primary hyperparathyroidism. Thus in cases with hypercalcemia of unclear etiology, a combination of clinical, biochemical, and genetic tests may be necessary. Typically, patients with FHH are asymptomatic, while those with primary hyperparathyroidism have symptoms associated with hypercalcemia as well as decreased bone density. FHH patients usually have a personal and family history of hypercalcemia while those with hyperparathyroidism may not. The laboratory workup for FHH shows elevated total calcium and PTH, and usually a reduced urine calcium. There is variability in urine calcium concentrations. Therefore, the calcium:creatinine clearance ratio (CCCR) is the recommended test for identifying FHH. A CCCR <0.01 suggests FHH, while a ratio >0.02 likely represents primary hyperparathyroidism. For patients with a CCCR between 0.01 and 0.02, genetic identification of mutations in the calcium-sensing receptor gene confirms the diagnosis of FHH.

Osteoporosis

Description

Osteoporosis is the most common metabolic disease of the bone associated with decreased bone mass. The causes of osteoporosis are many and varied. Osteoporosis may be primary or secondary. It can occur in association with hyperparathyroidism as described before, as well as with Cushing syndrome, acromegaly, prolonged use of heparin, excess Vitamin D intake, and immobilization, among other conditions and disorders.

Diagnosis

Bone mineral density (BMD) studies are preferred for diagnosis of primary osteoporosis. BMD estimates obtained by imaging studies are compared with BMD in normal populations to generate a T-score. The WHO defines osteoporosis as a T-score ≤−2.5. T-scores between −1.0 and −2.5 confirm osteopenia. Laboratory testing is preferred for the evaluation of secondary disease. Bone turnover markers can be used to monitor treatment. It is recommended that bone markers be measured every 3 to 6 months to monitor compliance and response to bisphosphonate or other therapy.

Osteomalacia

Description

Osteomalacia is deficient mineralization of bone that results from disturbances in calcium and phosphorus metabolism. It can result from a nutritional deficiency of vitamin D, defects in vitamin D metabolism or action, defects in mineral metabolism, or disturbances of the bone cells in the bone matrix. When osteomalacia occurs before the cessation of growth, it is known as rickets. Skeletal deformities appear in rickets because of the compensatory overgrowth of epiphyseal cartilage.

Diagnosis

Radiographic studies can demonstrate the disorder. The specific cause for osteomalacia, if it is identified, is generally established with laboratory testing. There are many disorders associated with the decreased mineralization of the bone.

Paget Disease

Description

Paget disease is associated with osteoclastic resorption of bone and extensive production of abnormal, poorly mineralized osteoid. This results in a bone that is structurally weak and prone to deformity and fracture. The disorder may involve one bone or may be more generalized.

Diagnosis

In Paget disease, ALP is significantly elevated, which reflects osteoblastic proliferation in the deformed bone. The serum calcium and inorganic phosphorus concentrations are usually normal, but may be increased in some patients.

TESTES AND OVARIES

Male Physiology and Biochemistry

The male testes serve two important functions (**Figure 22–9**). One is the production of sperm, and the other is the synthesis and secretion of androgens. Sertoli cells within the testes secrete inhibin, and this glycoprotein inhibits the pituitary secretion of follicle-stimulating hormone (FSH). FSH acts on the Sertoli cells to stimulate sperm production and the synthesis of inhibin. Leydig cells in the testes are responsible for the production of androgens. The Leydig cells in the testes receive stimulation by luteinizing hormone (LH) to promote the conversion of cholesterol, through many intermediates, to testosterone. Testosterone, one of the androgens, is important for maturation of sperm, production of male secondary sex characteristics, and providing negative feedback to the anterior pituitary and hypothalamus to reduce the stimulation of the male testes. The hormone secreted by the hypothalamus in the hypothalamic–pituitary–gonadal axis is gonadotropin-releasing hormone (GnRH). GnRH stimulates the release of both LH and FSH from the pituitary in pulsatile patterns. Higher values for LH and FSH are found in the early morning hours.

> The androgens are a collection of 19 carbon steroids that produce masculinization and male secondary sex characteristics. The main androgen secreted by the Leydig cells of the testes is testosterone. Other androgens secreted by the testes include androstenedione and DHEA.

The androgens are a collection of 19 carbon steroids that produce masculinization and male secondary sex characteristics. The main androgen secreted by the Leydig cells of the testes is testosterone. Other androgens secreted by the testes include androstenedione and DHEA. These compounds can be metabolized to testosterone and dihydrotestosterone (DHT) in target tissues. Circulating testosterone is a precursor to DHT. As previously noted, a number of androgens are secreted by the adrenal glands, including DHEA, DHEA-sulfate (DHEA-S), androstenedione, and androstenediol. Women also produce testosterone, but only 5% to 10% as much as men. Testosterone, as well as androstenedione, can be converted to estrogens. In men approximately 6% to 8% of the testosterone is converted to DHT, but only about 0.3% to estradiol. Most of the testosterone and DHT in the plasma is bound to plasma proteins. Only approximately 3% is free. The two major proteins that bind testosterone and DHT are sex hormone-binding globulin (SHBG) and albumin. In men, approximately 45% to 65% of protein-bound testosterone is associated with SHBG and 35% to 50% is bound to albumin. Protein-bound testosterone in women is distributed approximately two-thirds on SHBG and one-third on albumin. The bioavailable testosterone includes the small fraction that is free and the portion that is weakly bound to albumin. Testosterone binds less efficiently to albumin, and therefore it is available for tissue uptake when associated with this protein. The main excretory metabolites of testosterone, androstenedione, and DHEA are collectively known as 17-ketosteroids that can be quantitated in the urine.

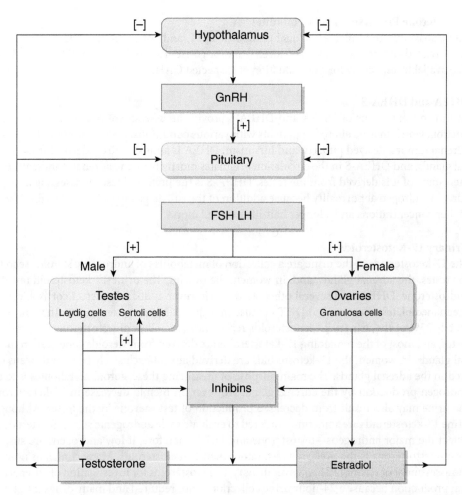

FIGURE 22–9 The hypothalamic–pituitary–gonadal axis in males and females. [+] Stimulation; [−] inhibition.

Laboratory Tests

Total Testosterone

Total testosterone measured by immunoassay is a commonly used first-line test in evaluating a suspected gonadal dysfunction in adult males. Total serum testosterone represents both protein-bound and nonprotein-bound testosterone. Because it is subject to diurnal variation and may be suppressed by food and glucose, specimens for testosterone testing should be collected in the morning from fasting patients. Most contemporary testosterone immunoassays lack specificity in patients with low concentrations of the hormone. Therefore, it is recommended that tandem mass spectrometery based assays be used in females and children.

> Total testosterone measured by immunoassay is a commonly used first-line test in evaluating an adult male for gonadal dysfunction.

Free and Weakly Bound Testosterone

This is the bioavailable pool of circulating testosterone. In cases where total testosterone is abnormal, free testosterone can be assessed as a part of a panel that determines bioavailable testosterone and SHBG. SHBG is measured by immunoassay and total testosterone by immunoassay or tandem mass spectrometry (LC/MS/MS), and concentrations of free and bioavailable testosterone are derived from a mathematical equation based on the constants for the binding of testosterone to albumin and/or SHBG.

SHBG can be measured separately, but the utility is largely in evaluating bioavailable testosterone in men with suspected hypogonadism and women with hyperandrogenism.

Testosterone Precursors and Metabolites

Immunoassays are available for quantitation of DHT, androstenedione, DHEA, DHEA-S, and other related compounds. Panels of adrenal and/or gonadal steroids measured by LC/MS/MS are also available, especially for the evaluation of suspected CAH.

DHEA and DHEA-S

Serum concentrations of DHEA and DHEA-S provide an assessment of adrenal androgen production, which may be altered in patients with various conditions, including adrenal hyperplasia, adrenal tumors, delayed puberty, and hirsutism. DHEA is almost entirely derived from the adrenal glands, and DHEA-S in the circulation originates mostly from the adrenal glands, although in men some of it is derived from the testes. DHEA-S is the preferred test for assessing a suspected adrenal androgen abnormality because addition of the sulfate group stabilizes DHEA, leading to higher concentrations and a longer half-life in circulation.

Urinary 17-Ketosteroids

The 17-ketosteroids in the urine are a collection of metabolites of androgenic steroids secreted by the testes, the adrenal glands, and, in women, the ovaries. The urine 17-ketosteroid test detects androsterone, DHEA, and several other steroids. However, it does not detect cortisol, estrogens, pregnanediol, testosterone, and DHT because they do not have a ketone group. In men, approximately 33% of the urinary 17-ketosteroids represent metabolites of testosterone secreted by the testes, and most of the remaining 17-ketosteroids are derived from steroids generated in the adrenal glands. In women, the 17-ketosteroids are derived almost exclusively from androgens generated in the adrenal glands. The main purpose of measuring these steroid metabolites is to assess androgen production by the adrenal gland. However, in men, a decrease in 17-ketosteroids in the urine may also result from decreased production of testosterone by the testes. Although the urine 17-ketosteroids are sometimes ordered to evaluate male androgenic status, this test does not detect the major androgens—testosterone and DHT. Therefore, if low androgens are suspected, serum testosterone is the preferred test, rather than 17-ketosteroids. Many clinicians now prefer the assessment of serum DHEA-S over urinary 17-ketosteroids for investigation of adrenal androgen production because a 24-hour urine collection is not required and many drugs interfere with the measurement of 17-ketosteroids.

Disorders Affecting Male Reproduction

Description and Diagnosis

Hypogonadotropic Hypogonadism. Hypogonadotropic hypogonadism in males is associated with absent or decreased function of the testes. If this impairment is manifested early in life, sexual development is retarded. In hypogonadotropic hypogonadism, there is a defect in the hypothalamus or pituitary that reduces normal gonadal stimulation. There are many causes for this abnormality, including panhypopituitarism and GnRH deficiency. A deficiency of GnRH in the hypothalamus is responsible for the most common form of hypogonadotropic hypogonadism, Kallmann syndrome. Hypogonadism is diagnosed by measuring fasting morning total testosterone on at least two separate occasions in men with signs and symptoms of androgen deficiency. If total testosterone results are borderline, hypogonadism can be confirmed by measuring free testosterone. Patients with hypogonadotropic hypogonadism have low testosterone and below normal or inappropriately normal serum concentrations of LH and FSH. Because there are many causes for the disorder, there is much heterogeneity in the severity of these hormonal deficiencies. A clinical picture of sexual infantilism and low concentrations of LH, FSH, and testosterone in the serum are characteristic features of hypogonadotropic hypogonadism. In order to differentiate pituitary or hypothalamic sources of this disease, prolactin or other measures of pituitary function or imaging studies may be helpful.

Hypergonadotropic Hypogonadism

This disorder results from a defect in the testes, which may be a result of injury. There is active stimulation of the testes, but they are unresponsive in this disorder. Apart from testicular injury, getting older is among the commonly encountered causes of hypergonadotropic hypogonadism. The disorder can also result from testicular damage from radiation or chemotherapy.

Patients with androgen insensitivity syndrome (AIS) have a severe defect in androgen action, with resistance to the masculinizing effect of the androgenic hormones. This results in a female habitus, with breast tissue and a vagina that ends in a blind pouch, and undescended male testes.

TABLE 22–8 Laboratory Evaluation for Males with Hypogonadism and Complete Androgen Insensitivity Syndrome (AIS)

Disorder	Laboratory Test Results for LH, FSH, and Testosterone
Hypogonadotropic hypogonadism	Low serum concentrations of LH, FSH, and testosterone
Hypergonadotropic hypogonadism	Elevated serum concentrations of LH and FSH with a low serum concentration of testosterone
Testicular feminization syndrome	Elevated or occasionally normal serum testosterone for a male, with an elevated serum LH

Patients with hypergonadotropic hypogonadism have elevated concentrations of LH and FSH in the presence of decreased levels of testosterone. When the source of the gonadal failure is unclear, karyotyping may identify chromosomal anomalies as the cause of the testicular abnormality.

Androgen Insensitivity Syndrome (Testicular Feminization Syndrome)

Patients with androgen insensitivity syndrome (AIS), as it is now called, have a severe defect in androgen action, with resistance to the masculinizing effect of the androgenic hormones. This results in a female habitus, with breast tissue and a vagina that ends in a blind pouch, and undescended male testes.

The circulating concentration of testosterone in patients with AIS (**Table 22–8**) is normal or elevated for a male. An elevation in testosterone can result in estrogen formation in these individuals because testosterone is a precursor for estrogen. The serum concentration of LH is increased, presumably because of resistance to the negative feedback of testosterone within the pituitary and hypothalamus.

Erectile Dysfunction (Formerly Impotence)

There are many causes for the persistent inability to develop or maintain a penile erection sufficient for intercourse and ejaculation. Although psychogenic impotence is the most common (up to 50%), there are many endocrinologic and nonendocrinologic disorders that are associated with impotence. These include vascular disease, diabetes mellitus, hypertension, neoplasms, and adverse drug effects.

An endocrinologic study of the patient may be pursued by measuring the serum testosterone in the early morning, along with LH and FSH, to assess the hypothalamic–pituitary–male gonadal axis for testosterone production. Chapter 19 has additional discussion of this topic.

Female Physiology and Biochemistry

The ovaries function to produce ova and secrete sex hormones, notably estrogens and progestins. Estrogens maintain the female secondary sex characteristics. They are also essential in the regulation of the menstrual cycle, breast and uterine growth, and in the maintenance of pregnancy (see Chapter 20 for a discussion on pregnancy). The estrogens have a major impact on calcium metabolism, and estrogen depletion associated with menopause results in a loss of bone mineral content. Most of estrogens are secreted by the ovarian follicles and the corpus luteum. During pregnancy, estrogen is also synthesized in the placenta. Only minute quantities are synthesized by the adrenals. The normal human ovary produces estrogens, progestins, and androgens, but the primary products are estradiol and progesterone. More than 20 different estrogens have been identified. Those with clinical importance are estradiol, also known as E_2; estrone, also denoted as E_1; and estriol, that is E_3. Estradiol is derived almost exclusively from the ovaries, and for that reason the serum estradiol level is considered a reflection of ovarian function. In the nonpregnant state, most of the estrogen (microgram quantities) is derived from the ovaries. In pregnant women, the major source of estrogen is the placenta, which secretes estriol as the major product in milligram amounts. Like most other steroid hormones, the vast majority of the circulating estrogen is bound to plasma proteins. More than 95% of circulating estradiol is bound with high affinity to SHBG and, less avidly, to albumin.

Progesterone is a member of the progestin family that plays a central role in female reproductive endocrinology. It is involved in regulation of the menstrual cycle and is produced during pregnancy by the placenta. In the nonpregnant state, progesterone is produced largely by the

There are many causes for the persistent inability to develop or maintain a penile erection sufficient for intercourse and ejaculation. Although psychogenic impotence is the most common (up to 50%), there are many endocrinologic and nonendocrinologic disorders that are associated with impotence.

ovary. The adrenal cortex is only a minor source of progesterone production in both sexes, and progesterone is made in very small quantities in the testes in men. More than 90% of progesterone is protein-bound in the circulation to corticosteroid-binding globulin. Progesterone can be metabolized to three groups of metabolites, one of which is the pregnanediols. Urinary pregnanediol concentration can be used as an index of endogenous progesterone production because it correlates with alterations in its synthesis and metabolism.

There is a tightly coordinated feedback system among the hypothalamus, anterior pituitary, and ovaries in adolescent and adult women to regulate menstruation. Each menstrual cycle consists of a follicular and a luteal phase. Day 1 is the first day of menstrual bleeding. The follicular phase is associated with follicle growth and is the first part of the cycle. Ovulation occurs around day 14 of the menstrual cycle, and the luteal phase follows in the last half of the cycle.

> In general, follicular growth in the ovary is stimulated by FSH, and ovulation and progesterone secretion from the developing corpus luteum are driven by LH.

In general, follicular growth in the ovary is stimulated by FSH, and ovulation and progesterone secretion from the developing corpus luteum are driven by LH. During the menstrual cycle:

- FSH increases during the early part of the follicular phase and then declines until ovulation; there is a gradual decrease in FSH through the luteal phase. FSH guides selection of a dominant follicle.
- LH secretion increases around the middle of the follicular phase and just before ovulation; estrogen secretion in the follicular phase stimulates the pituitary to release LH in a surge, with the peak value for LH occurring 3 to 36 hours before ovulation.
- Estradiol concentrations increase as the selected dominant follicle begins to secrete this hormone during midfollicular phase. Its concentrations rapidly rise as the follicle matures. The estradiol concentration then falls abruptly just before ovulation. At ovulation the ovum is released from the follicle. The leftover tissue, called the corpus luteum, is essential for establishing early pregnancy. The corpus luteum secretes estradiol and progesterone to facilitate implantation. If the ovum is not fertilized, the corpus luteum breaks down and estradiol and progesterone synthesis decline after about 14 days. The decline in both hormones signals the beginning of the menstrual cycle.
- Progesterone is at very low concentrations during the follicular phase; with the midcycle surge of LH and ovulation, the corpus luteum secretes progesterone that increases and reaches its peak concentration approximately 8 days after the midcycle LH surge. As the corpus luteum degrades, progesterone concentrations decline to baseline levels at the end of the luteal phase.

Figure 22–9 illustrates the complex relationships in the hypothalamic–pituitary–female gonadal axis.

Laboratory Tests

Estrogens

Serum estrogen concentrations are typically assessed via estradiol (E_2) measurements, because estriol (E_3) in a nonpregnant woman is derived almost exclusively from estradiol. In addition, blood estrone (E_1) and estradiol concentrations fluctuate in a similar manner throughout the menstrual cycle, but E_1 concentrations are lower.

Progesterone

The progesterone concentration in serum is a reflection of progesterone production. Assays for urinary progesterone metabolites are used much less frequently to assess progesterone synthesis than tests for serum progesterone.

FSH and LH

Serum FSH and LH concentrations are useful in determining the cause of reproductive dysfunction in males and females. The gonadotrophs are measured by immunoassay. Reference intervals vary with sex, age, tanner stage, and time of the menstrual cycle. Thus, a carefully documented clinical history and physical exam are essential in order to properly interpret LH and FSH results.

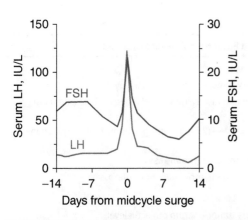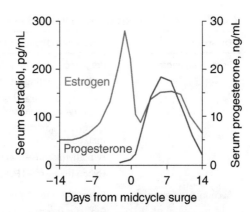

FIGURE 22–10 The changes in LH, FSH, estrogens, and progesterone in menstruating females. Day 1: start of menses; days 5 to 7: estrogen secretion begins; day 13: LH surge; day 14: ovulation; days 18 to 23: increased estrogen and progesterone from the corpus luteum; day 25: decreased estrogen and progesterone with demise of the corpus luteum and breakdown of the endometrium.

Endocrinologic Disorders Affecting Female Reproduction
Description and Diagnosis

Healthy women display considerable variations in the length of the menstrual cycle, but most women have cycles between 25 and 30 days in length (see **Figure 22–10**). The absence of menstrual bleeding is known as amenorrhea. Primary amenorrhea refers to women who have never menstruated, and secondary amenorrhea refers to women in their reproductive years in whom menstruation was present and then ceased for at least 6 months.

Primary Amenorrhea

Primary amenorrhea is established if spontaneous regular menstruation has not begun by the age of 16 years, with or without the presence of secondary sex characteristics. The list of causes of primary amenorrhea is lengthy. They include lower genitourinary tract defects such as imperforate hymen; a host of ovarian disorders—approximately 40% of females with primary amenorrhea have Turner syndrome (45 X karyotype) or pure gonadal dysgenesis (either a 46 XX or XY karyotype); adrenal disorders such as CAH; thyroid disorders, notably hypothyroidism; pituitary–hypothalamic disorders such as hypopituitarism and Kallmann syndrome (which also affects men); and pregnancy.

Because of the long list of possible causes, the workup for primary amenorrhea should begin with a careful history and physical examination to look for anatomic defects, development of secondary sexual characteristics, and/or a personal or family history of short stature, infertility, and/or amenorrhea. The laboratory evaluation for amenorrhea begins with measurement of hCG to rule out pregnancy. If not pregnant, patients should undergo imaging studies looking for a uterus and gonads. Patients with a detectable uterus should be evaluated for hypothyroidism and hyperprolactinemia (discussed below). High TSH and low free T_4 results suggest the amenorrhea is due to primary hypothyroidism. An elevated prolactin result should prompt a physician to perform an MRI in search of a pituitary adenoma. Patients with normal TSH and prolactin should be evaluated for gonadotropic function by measuring LH and FSH. Estrogen measurements may be helpful to determine the cause of disease. Because of the day-to-day variability in estrogen concentrations, the progestin challenge test may be helpful to establish estrogen reserves and/or etiology of primary amenorrhea. Theoretically, if progesterone is given to an estrogen-primed uterus, withdrawal bleeding (menstruation) will occur. Progesterone is given orally for up to 1 week. Bleeding should occur within 1 week of progesterone withdrawal if the woman's ovaries have produced enough estrogen (>40 pg/mL serum) to prime her uterus.

If the patient has congenital anomalies, a karyotype evaluation to look for cytogenetic abnormalities may be helpful (**Table 22–9**).

Primary amenorrhea refers to women who have never menstruated, and secondary amenorrhea refers to women in their reproductive years in whom menstruation was present and then ceased for at least 6 months.

TABLE 22–9   Laboratory Evaluation of Women with Amenorrhea

Disorder	Associated Disorders and Potentially Relevant Laboratory Tests
Primary amenorrhea	Pregnancy—test for hCG
	Prolactin-secreting pituitary tumor—serum prolactin level
	Turner syndrome and pure gonadal dysgenesis—LH and FSH measurements and karyotype analysis
	Congenital adrenal hyperplasia—17-hydroxyprogesterone (adrenal hormone metabolite)
	Hypothyroidism—selected thyroid hormone assays
	Hypopituitarism—LH, FSH, and other pituitary hormone assays
Secondary amenorrhea	Pregnancy—test for hCG
	Prolactin-secreting pituitary tumor—serum prolactin level
	Polycystic ovary syndrome—serum testosterone (free or total), adrenal androgens (DHEA-S), and appropriate radiographic studies
	Cushing syndrome—see the section "Hyperfunction Involving Glucocorticoids With or Without Mineralocorticoids: Cushing Syndrome"
	Nonclassic congenital adrenal hyperplasia—17-hydroxyprogesterone assay
	Hypothyroidism and hypopituitarism—TSH and prolactin

hCG, human chorionic gonadotropin.

Secondary Amenorrhea

Secondary amenorrhea is more common than primary amenorrhea and is the absence of regular menstruation for at least 6 months in a woman who has previously had menses. Oligomenorrhea is present if a woman has less than nine menstrual cycles per year. The causes of secondary amenorrhea include many of those for primary amenorrhea. However, there are a number of conditions associated with secondary amenorrhea that are independent of primary amenorrhea. Most notably, pregnancy is a common cause of amenorrhea and must be considered first in a patient who has stopped menses. An elevated prolactin concentration, which may be induced by a prolactin-secreting tumor, can produce oligomenorrhea or amenorrhea, presumably by inhibition of the release of LH and FSH by the prolactin. Patients with secondary amenorrhea can be divided into those with and without signs of hirsutism and androgen excess. Hirsutism is the excessive growth of terminal hair in women and in children, in a distribution similar to that which occurs in postpubertal men. Causes of hirsutism may be androgen-dependent, with abnormalities often originating in the ovary or the adrenal gland, or androgen-independent, sometimes from antiepileptic medications. Adult women with hirsutism and clinical signs of too much androgen should be further evaluated for androgen excess disorders such as nonclassic CAH (NCCAH), ACTH-dependent Cushing syndrome, an androgen-secreting ovarian tumor, and polycystic ovarian syndrome.

Because the list of disorders associated with secondary amenorrhea is even longer than the list associated with primary amenorrhea (**Table 22–9**), the initial evaluation is very broad until the differential diagnosis is narrowed by the results of physical examination, history, and initial radiographic and laboratory studies. The laboratory workup for secondary amenorrhea begins with measurement of hCG to rule out pregnancy. Hypothyroidism and hyperprolactinemia should next be ruled out as the cause of disease by measuring TSH and prolactin. Patients with normal TSH and prolactin should be evaluated for gonadotropic function by measuring LH and FSH. Estrogen or a progestin stimulation test may be helpful in cases where the cause of amenorrhea is unclear. Women with signs of androgen excess, such as hirsutism, should be further evaluated by measuring total and free testosterone and DHEA-S to confirm hyperandrogenemia. Significant elevations of androgen, combined with a rapid onset of symptoms of hyperandrogenism, may indicate an androgen-secreting neoplasm. Females with androgen excess should be screened for nonclassical CAH (NCCAH) by measuring 17-hydroxyprogesterone. In those with relevant clinical signs, Cushing syndrome should also be ruled out (testing discussed earlier in this chapter). If all other sources of hirsutism have been excluded, a diagnosis of polycystic ovary syndrome (PCOS) should be considered. While not present in all cases, identification of polycystic ovaries on ultrasound in combination with hyperandrogenemia and/or ovulatory dysfunction (amenorrhea) confirms PCOS.

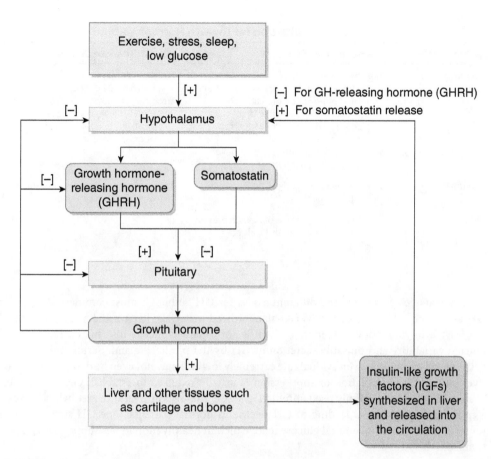

FIGURE 22–11 **The regulation of growth hormone (GH) secretion. [+] Stimulation; [−] inhibition.**

DISORDERS RELATED TO THE PITUITARY GLAND

Growth Hormone/Anterior Pituitary

Physiology and Biochemistry

Growth hormone (GH) is a major product of the pituitary gland. It is a single-chain polypeptide that has structural similarities to prolactin and placental hormones, known as placental lactogens, with which it has overlapping biological activities. GH has secretory spikes, with a half-life of about 20 minutes, which typically occur several hours after meals and exercise. The secretion of GH also rises after the onset of sleep and reaches a peak in deepest sleep. Two hypothalamic factors control the release of GH from the pituitary. Growth hormone-releasing hormone (GHRH) stimulates GH release from the pituitary, and somatostatin (also known as growth hormone-inhibitory hormone [GHIH]) inhibits GH release. The larger influence on the release of GH by the pituitary is the inhibitory action of somatostatin. To promote growth, GH in the circulation binds to target tissues, mostly cartilage, bone, and other soft tissues. GH predominantly exerts its growth effects by stimulating insulin-like growth factors (IGFs) that are produced in the liver and other tissues. Because of its homology to insulin, GH directly affects lipid, carbohydrate, and protein metabolism. IGFs, previously known as somatomedins, also have multiple effects on growth promotion and metabolism. There are a number of IGFs. Unlike most other peptide hormones, IGFs circulate in the blood in a complex with plasma-binding proteins, known as insulin-like growth factor-binding proteins (IGFBPs). The complex physiology of GH signaling is shown in **Figure 22–11**.

> GH has secretory spikes, with a half-life of about 20 minutes, which typically occur several hours after meals and exercise. The secretion of GH also rises after the onset of sleep and reaches a peak in deepest sleep.

Laboratory Tests

Growth Hormone

Most of the assays for GH are performed using serum, because the concentration of GH in urine is approximately 0.1% of that in serum. Human GH exists in the pituitary gland and in the circulation as a heterogeneous mixture of isoforms. The presence of GH variants in serum can lead

TABLE 22–10   Laboratory Evaluation for Growth Hormone Abnormalities

Laboratory Test	Growth Hormone Excess	Growth Hormone Deficiency
Serum growth hormone (GH)	Single measurements of GH are not often reliable because GH secretion is episodic and diurnal and other conditions can increase GH secretion; after administration of an oral glucose load, normal individuals have markedly suppressed GH while patients with acromegaly/gigantism do not have suppressed GH concentrations	Because GH may be low in both normal children and GH-deficient patients, it is necessary to show an inadequate rise of serum GH in response to 2 different provocative stimuli, such as insulin, glucagon, or exercise
Serum IGF-1	IGF-1 is elevated in nearly all patients with acromegaly/gigantism	Low in most deficient patients, but low in many other clinical conditions as well
Radiology	Sellar enlargement in 90% of cases; if present, a pituitary tumor should be localized	

to discrepant results among the different assays for GH, although most commercially available GH assays are calibrated against WHO-standardized materials. Even if the assay problems did not exist, a single random GH measurement is not usually clinically informative because of the diurnal variability and pulsatile secretion of GH by the pituitary gland. Serum concentrations between pulses in healthy individuals are extremely low and may not even be detectable. Provocative testing of its stimulation or suppression is usually required to establish GH abnormalities (**Table 22–10**). A commonly used stimulation test is the insulin tolerance test, which produces a transient hypoglycemia leading to GH release in normal patients. One GH suppression test involves the ingestion of an oral glucose load, which in healthy individuals suppresses GH secretion from the pituitary.

> Provocative testing of its stimulation or suppression is usually required to establish GH abnormalities.

Insulin-like Growth Factors

IGF-1 circulates in much higher concentrations in plasma than GH, and its secretion is not episodic or diurnal. Therefore, IGF-1 is a good screening test for suspected GH abnormalities and for monitoring therapy in patients with known abnormalities. A single elevated IGF-1 in patients with signs and symptoms of GH excess should be followed with an oral glucose tolerance test (GH suppression testing). A single decreased IGF-1 should prompt treatment in patients with known growth deficiency or an insulin tolerance (or other GH stimulation) test in patients suspected to have GH deficiency. There are marked differences in IGF-1 concentration between adults and children. Therefore, it is very important to establish age-specific reference intervals.

Growth Hormone Excess—Acromegaly and Gigantism

Description

The most common cause of excess GH production is a chromophobe adenoma of the pituitary gland. A prolonged excess of GH results in an overgrowth of the skeleton with acral enlargements, as well as overgrowth of the soft tissues. Growth hormone excess in adults is known as acromegaly. Because GH has an action on the cartilaginous portion of the bone, GH excess in children before long bone growth is completed results in gigantism.

Diagnosis

The most important requirement for diagnosis of GH excess is demonstration of unsuppressible GH secretion. Because of the episodic secretion of GH, some patients with active acromegaly have random serum GH concentrations that are within the normal reference interval. An elevated IGF-1 measurement prompts provocative testing and correlates with disease severity. Serum GH concentrations are typically not suppressed by oral glucose loading in patients with acromegaly. Their serum GH concentrations show either no change from baseline or a slight increase. Healthy individuals show marked suppression after oral glucose load. The serum IGF-1 concentration, even as a random test, correlates with the clinical severity of acromegaly better than the test for glucose-induced GH suppression.

> A prolonged excess of GH results in an overgrowth of the skeleton with acral enlargements. In adults, this condition is known as acromegaly. GH excess in children before long bone growth is completed results in gigantism.

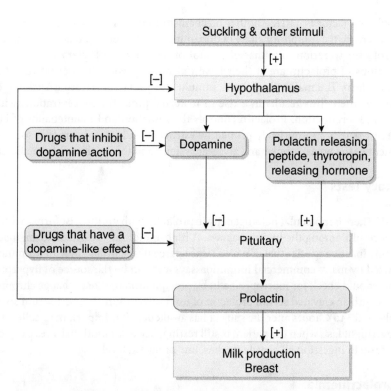

FIGURE 22–12 **The regulation of prolactin secretion. [+] Stimulation; [−] inhibition.**

Growth Hormone Deficiency

Description

A deficiency of GH may be congenital or acquired. Children who have inadequate GH production or action will not grow to full height. It should be noted that growth retardation is not usually caused by GH deficiency. However, children with growth retardation or reduced growth velocity with no obvious explanation should be evaluated for a GH deficiency. In children, causes of GH deficiency include anatomic damage to the pituitary or hypothalamus, isolated GH deficiency in the pituitary, and a combination of pituitary hormone deficiencies from a variety of causes. In adults, the most common causes of GH deficiency are pituitary irradiation and a pituitary adenoma that impairs GH secretion. Since adults are usually at full height, GH deficiency does not change growth velocity. However, it is associated with cardiac abnormalities, increased cholesterol, reduced muscle mass, energy, and bone density, and lean body mass. GH replacement in deficient adults may increase lean body mass and bone density, and reduce cholesterol.

Diagnosis

After ruling out other causes of short stature, patients with signs and symptoms of GH deficiency can be screened by measuring IGF-1; if low, the diagnosis of GH deficiency requires the demonstration of a persistently low GH concentration in two different provocative stimulation tests (**Table 22–10**). The provocations for GH release that are used include vigorous exercise, deep sleep, and treatment with glucagon, L-DOPA, insulin, or arginine. Insulin and glucagon are the most commonly utilized agents.

Prolactin/Anterior Pituitary

Physiology and Biochemistry

Prolactin is secreted by lactotrophic cells in the anterior lobe of the pituitary gland. It is a 198 amino acid polypeptide hormone with some homology to GH. Prolactin production is regulated by stimuli from the hypothalamus, but unlike most other anterior pituitary hormones, its release is primarily controlled by inhibition rather than by stimulation (see **Figure 22–12**). The primary negative stimulus to the pituitary that limits prolactin secretion is provided by dopamine. There are various stimulatory factors for prolactin release, along with the inhibitory compounds.

Prolactin production is regulated by stimuli from the hypothalamus, but unlike most other anterior pituitary hormones, its release is primarily controlled by inhibition rather than by stimulation.

One stimulatory factor is TRH. Another mechanism to increase prolactin release from the pituitary is to decrease the inhibitory effect of dopamine. A number of medications inhibit dopamine action. Prolactin secretion, like that of several other anterior pituitary hormones, is episodic. Concentrations of prolactin are at their lowest at midday, with the highest values shortly after the onset of sleep. The major physiologic stimulus for prolactin release is suckling of the breast in lactating women. This results in a rise in maternal prolactin concentrations within minutes to initiate milk production. Prolactin controls the initiation and maintenance of lactation only if the breast tissue is appropriately primed by estrogens and other hormones for ductal growth, development of the breast lobular and alveolar system, and the synthesis of specific milk proteins.

Laboratory Tests

Prolactin

As with GH, there is molecular heterogeneity in prolactin with multiple isoforms, which can lead to discrepant results among the immunoassays. A high-molecular-weight isoform, macroprolactin, is a clinically inactive species that contains large aggregates of prolactin with immunoglobulins. It is recognized by many commercial immunoassays and can be the source of hyperprolactinemia. Physicians should check for macroprolactin by precipitation or size exchange chromatography in any patient with an elevated serum prolactin of unknown origin. The best serum specimen is one that is collected 3 to 4 hours after the subject has awakened. It is important to collect the specimen after an overnight fast, when the patient is still resting, because emotional stress, exercise, ambulation, and protein ingestion all elevate the baseline prolactin level.

Hyperprolactinemia

Description

There are many causes for an elevated prolactin concentration, one of which is a pituitary adenoma. Pregnancy, chronic renal failure, chest wall trauma, primary hypothyroidism, and a host of medications can also elevate prolactin levels. Elevation of the serum prolactin concentration is associated with many different signs and symptoms. In women, these include anovulation, with or without menstrual irregularity, and amenorrhea. Men with prolactin-secreting pituitary adenomas often present with oligospermia, impotence, or both.

Diagnosis

Because the size of the pituitary adenoma correlates with the amount of prolactin secretion, serum prolactin concentrations are generally higher in patients with a large tumor (macro-prolactinoma) versus a microprolactinoma. A patient with a macroadenoma generally has a higher elevation of serum prolactin than someone with hyperprolactinemia from a different cause. Serum prolactin concentrations of patients with microadenomas are similar to those with prolactinemia secondary to medications, pregnancy, or stress. Therefore, imaging studies and a careful medication history are critical for evaluation of patients with elevated prolactin. Noteworthy medications that can elevate the serum prolactin level include estrogens, dopamine antagonists such as haloperidol, histamine receptor-blocking agents such as cimetidine, and tricyclic antidepressants. Follow-up investigation is warranted in any patient with signs and symptoms of prolactinemia, a pituitary macroadenoma by imaging, and low serum prolactin concentrations (see below). In these cases, repeat testing after specimen dilution can rule out an assay interference, suggesting a low prolactin, due to extremely high prolactin concentrations. This is called the hook effect.

Hypoprolactinemia

Description and Diagnosis

This condition is not detected unless a woman fails to lactate postpartum. A low prolactin level in a woman in this setting is consistent with hypoprolactinemia.

Antidiuretic Hormone (ADH)/Posterior Pituitary

Physiology and Biochemistry

The posterior pituitary secretes oxytocin and ADH, also known as arginine vasopressin (AVP). ADH is a small nine amino acid peptide hormone. Oxytocin has a similar structure. Release of

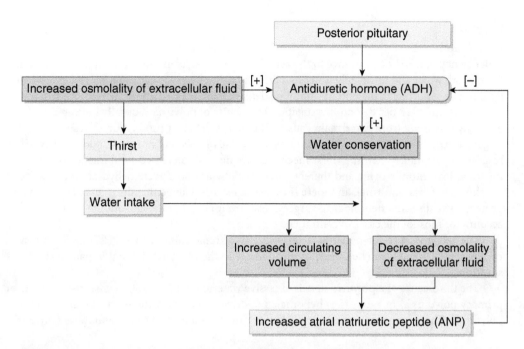

FIGURE 22–13 **The regulation of circulating fluid volume and osmolality. [+] Stimulation; [−] inhibition.**

hormones from the posterior pituitary into the circulation occurs with stimulation of selected neurons. In the circulation, ADH and oxytocin are usually not bound to carrier proteins.

ADH secretion is triggered by elevated plasma osmolality as well as decreased blood volume or blood pressure (**Figure 22–13**). Even a small increase in osmolality causes stimulation of ADH release to increase water retention and decrease the plasma osmolality. ADH induces increased permeability of water in the renal collecting ducts leading to increased water reabsorption and concentration of urine. ADH is also known as vasopressin because it binds to receptors on smooth muscle cells that induce vasoconstriction, thereby increasing the blood pressure and volume. Other nonosmotic stimuli such as pain, stress, sleep, exercise, and a variety of pharmacologic compounds induce ADH secretion from the posterior pituitary as well. Negative feedback for ADH release is provided by atrial natriuretic peptide (ANP). With an increased circulating blood volume or a decreased osmolality, ANP concentrations increase, inducing decreased ADH release. The osmolality of the plasma also impacts the thirst center to coordinate oral intake of water and conservation of water in the kidney.

Laboratory Tests
Antidiuretic Hormone
ADH can be measured using an immunoassay. It is a temperature-sensitive peptide, and plasma testing should be performed within 24 hours after collection. Freezing the specimen stabilizes it for a month. A single ADH measurement is not diagnostic, and the result should be assessed in the context of the results of serum and urine osmolality testing.

Serum and Urine Osmolality
Serum and urine osmolality are measured using a freezing point depression osmometer. Serum osmolality can be calculated with the following formula:

$$2*[Na+]+[glucose]/18+[blood\,urea\,nitrogen(BUN)]/2.8$$

Water Deprivation Test
Patients with suspected diabetes insipidus (DI) are deprived of all fluids until urine osmolality is constant for 3 hours and/or plasma osmolality is greater than the normal range. Once constant, serum osmolality and ADH are measured. ADH (AVP) is then administered, and urine osmolality and volume are measured at 1 and 2 hours post administration.

Polyuria can occur from three main causes. The first is deficient production of ADH, as occurs in central diabetes insipidus. The second cause for polyuria is deficient ADH action in the kidney. The third cause of a polyuric state is excessive water intake.

Polyuria

Description

A deficiency of ADH or resistance to the action of ADH results in the failure of the renal tubules to reabsorb water and ultimately water loss into the urine. Because urine output is dependent on fluid intake, a normal urine output cannot be defined. However, whenever there is more than 2.5 L of urine generated per day, an investigation for a cause of polyuria is usually indicated.

Polyuria arises from three main causes. The first is deficient production of ADH, as occurs in central DI. In this disorder, the pituitary gland fails to secrete normal amounts of ADH in response to stimuli. When the thirst mechanism is normal, increased fluid intake compensates for water loss into the urine and thereby prevents dehydration. Severe dehydration can occur if the thirst center is abnormal, and there is excess water loss. Congenital disorders of the pituitary or neoplastic diseases, neurological surgery, head trauma, ischemia, and autoimmune disorders account for most of the cases of central DI.

The second cause for polyuria is insensitivity of renal tubules to ADH. This is known as nephrogenic DI and it can be caused by any damage to the renal tubules that impairs water reabsorption.

The third cause of a polyuric state is excessive water intake. This is known as psychogenic or primary polydipsia. In rare cases, hypothalamic disease can affect the thirst center and induce polydipsia. There are also many medications that can affect the thirst center and cause polydipsia.

Diagnosis

The differential diagnosis of a polyuric state requires measurements of serum and urine osmolality, serum sodium, urine volume, and plasma ADH concentrations. The first step is to document that polyuria exists by establishing that the urine volume exceeds 2.5 L per day. Glycosuria must be excluded as a cause of the polyuria, as hyperglycemia with diabetes mellitus is a common cause of polyuria. Patients with central DI have hypernatremia, high plasma and low urine osmolality, and low or inappropriately normal plasma ADH concentrations because the pituitary is unable to secrete ADH. Patients with nephrogenic DI also have a high serum sodium and osmolality and a low urine osmolality with polyuria and polydipsia. Renal insensitivity to ADH leads to normal to high plasma concentrations of the hormone because the hypothalamus generates an excess in an attempt to compensate for high plasma osmolality. Patients with primary polydipsia usually have hyponatremia with normal serum and low urine osmolality, and an appropriately low-normal plasma ADH concentration (**Table 22–11**). The diagnosis of DI can be confirmed with a provocative test called the water deprivation test. After dehydration, if the urine osmolality is greater than plasma and ADH is low, DI is suspected. After administration of ADH, an increase in urine osmolality of more than 10% in 1 hour indicates central DI. The excess ADH promotes reabsorption of water by the kidney, resulting in a decreased urine volume and an increased urine osmolality. A high ADH after dehydration, followed by a failure to increase urine osmolality after ADH administration, suggests nephrogenic DI because the defect in this disorder is a failure of the kidney to respond to ADH. After water deprivation, patients with primary polydipsia will have urine osmolality higher than serum and show no increase in urine osmolality after ADH administration.

TABLE 22–11   Laboratory Evaluation for Disorders of Water Uptake and Excretion

Baseline Disorder	Serum Sodium and Osmolality	Urine Sodium and Osmolality	Plasma ADH
SIADH	Low	Normal–high	High
Central diabetes insipidus	Normal–high	Low	Low
Nephrogenic diabetes insipidus	Normal–high	Low	Normal–high
Psychogenic polydipsia	Normal–low	Low	Normal–low

SIADH, syndrome of inappropriate antidiuretic hormone secretion.

Syndrome of Inappropriate Antidiuretic Hormone Secretion (SIADH)

Description

SIADH is an autonomous, sustained synthesis and release of ADH in the absence of stimuli. Thus, plasma ADH concentrations are inappropriately increased relative to the osmolality. There are a number of known causes of SIADH; however, it is common among patients with pulmonary or central nervous system disorders. Another cause is production of ADH by a malignant tumor, especially a small cell carcinoma of the lung. Some medications may also stimulate the production of ADH. The patient's blood volume is modestly expanded, and serum sodium concentrations may be decreased along with serum osmolality. SIADH is a commonly encountered cause of hyponatremia in hospitalized patients.

Diagnosis

Patients with SIADH usually have a low serum osmolality, a urine osmolality greater than that of serum, and an elevated urine sodium concentration (**Table 22–11**). There are many causes for hyponatremia other than SIADH, including congestive heart failure, renal insufficiency, nephrotic syndrome, liver cirrhosis, and treatment with medications that stimulate ADH secretion. Measurement of ADH is not necessary to diagnose SIADH because the diagnosis is made with osmolality and sodium measures alone.

NEOPLASTIC DISORDERS

Multiple Endocrine Neoplasia

Description

MEN is a syndrome most often inherited as an autosomal dominant trait. The MEN syndromes are associated with hyperplasia or tumors in several endocrine glands.

- *Multiple endocrine neoplasia type-1 (MEN 1; Wermer syndrome)*—MEN 1 syndrome involves hyperplasia or neoplasms in one or more of the following: the parathyroid gland, the pancreatic islet cells, or the anterior pituitary in patients with a known family history of MEN 1. In the absence of a family history of the syndrome, however, at least two or more of the primary MEN 1 tumor types must be involved for a diagnosis of MEN 1. The hormonal presentation of MEN 1 is highly variable because the pituitary and the pancreatic islet cells in neoplastic states can secrete many different hormones. Although the prevalence is reported to be 1/30,000, it is likely to be greatly underestimated because the clinical expression of MEN 1 varies and often presents with mild symptoms. Patients with MEN 1 usually present in the fourth decade of life. MEN 1 has been linked to a gene mutation in the MEN 1 (*menin*) gene on chromosome 11. Mutations in the MEN 1 gene are found in ~90% of patients with familial disease.
- *MEN 2 (Sipple syndrome)*—The most commonly found abnormality in the MEN 2 syndrome is MTC that occurs in over 95% of patients with MEN 2. Pheochromocytoma develops in over 50% of patients with MEN 2, and parathyroid hyperplasia or adenoma produces hyperparathyroidism in 15% to 30% of patients with MEN 2. MEN 2 includes three major phenotypes. About 80% of the cases of MEN 2 are MEN 2A that includes risk of developing MTC, pheochromocytoma, and hyperparathyroidism. The familial cases of MEN 2A are most often diagnosed in the third or fourth decade of life. In MEN 2B, parathyroid disease is rare and there are separate developmental abnormalities such as ganglioneuromatosis and marfanoid habitus, in addition to pheochromocytoma and MTC. MEN 2B generally presents 10 years earlier than MEN 2A. It accounts for approximately 5% of all MEN 2 cases. MEN 2B is usually recognized early in life. Children with MEN 2B have a characteristic facial appearance with a failure to thrive, mucosal neuromas, and constipation or diarrhea due to the ganglioneuromatoses in the gut. The diagnosis can be made conclusively by demonstrating the presence of a mutation in the RET proto-oncogene. The RET proto-oncogene product is a receptor tyrosine kinase that transmits growth and differentiation signals. The third form of MEN 2 is familial MTC in the absence of pheochromocytoma and

SIADH is an autonomous, sustained synthesis and release of ADH in the absence of stimuli. Thus, plasma ADH concentrations are inappropriately increased relative to the osmolality.

Multiple endocrine neoplasia type-1 (MEN 1) syndrome involves hyperplasia or neoplasms in one or more of the following: the parathyroid gland, the pancreatic islet cells, or the anterior pituitary. The most commonly found abnormality in the MEN 2 syndrome is medullary thyroid carcinoma that occurs in over 95% of patients.

hyperparathyroidism. This disorder has a later onset than MEN 2A or MEN 2B and usually has a good prognosis. The most common clinical presentation in the patient with medullary carcinoma is a mass in the neck. The diagnosis is most often made by histopathologic review of a specimen acquired by fine needle biopsy.

Diagnosis

Because of the variety of hormonal abnormalities in MEN 1, many different assays are needed to demonstrate hyperplasia or neoplasms of the parathyroid, pancreatic cells, and/or anterior pituitary, all of which may be involved in MEN 1. Genetic mutations in the coding sequence of the RET proto-oncogene are found in the vast majority of patients with MEN 2 (both MEN 2A and MEN 2B) and those with isolated familial MTC. Any first-degree relative of a patient carrying an MEN-associated mutation should also be evaluated. Onset of C-cell hyperplasia and malignancy of the thyroid in patients with a known RET proto-oncogene mutation should be monitored by measuring calcitonin and routine thyroid ultrasounds (see the section "Thyroid").

Carcinoid Tumors

Description

Carcinoid tumors are the most common of the endocrine tumors. They are generally found in the wall of the gastrointestinal tract, but also can be found in the pancreas, rectum, ovary, and lung. Tumors originating from the primitive foregut include carcinoid of the bronchus, the stomach, the first portion of the duodenum, and the pancreas. These tumors often secrete 5-hydroxytryptophan, histamine, and other peptides. Carcinoid tumors originating from the primitive midgut are those found in the second portion of the duodenum, the jejunum, the ileum, and the ascending colon. These tumors secrete serotonin, also known as 5-hydroxytryptamine, and other peptides. They are associated with the development of carcinoid syndrome, which is characterized by cutaneous flushing, gastrointestinal hypermotility with diarrhea, heart disease, bronchospasm, myopathy, and increased skin pigmentation. Tumors originating from the primitive hindgut include those of the transverse colon, descending colon, and rectum. These tumors are typically silent because they are usually nonsecretory. Therefore, functioning carcinoid tumors are more likely to be detected if they secrete a compound that has biological activity. The serotonin-secreting carcinoid tumors arising from the primitive midgut or foregut are the ones most often detected. Silent carcinoid tumors are most often discovered incidentally at surgery for other disorders in the gastrointestinal tract. Patients with silent carcinoid tumors may have vague abdominal pain that is either undiagnosed or attributed to irritable bowel syndrome.

Diagnosis

> 5-HIAA is quantitatively the principal metabolite of serotonin, and the majority of it is excreted into the urine and thus used as an indicator of serotonin production. Platelets contain almost all the serotonin found in the blood and for that reason, the serotonin is measured in whole blood (with platelets) or in platelet-rich plasma.

Serotonin (5-hydroxytryptamine) is transported in the blood by platelets. It is metabolized to 5-hydroxyindoleacetic acid (5-HIAA). 5-HIAA is quantitatively the principal metabolite of serotonin, and the majority of it is excreted into the urine and can be used as an indicator of serotonin production. Patients with serotonin-secreting carcinoid tumors of midgut origin usually have markedly elevated concentrations of urinary 5-HIAA. If there is a borderline concentration of 5-HIAA in a random or 24-hour urine specimen, a repeat collection should be made with an avoidance of foods or medications that might elevate the 5-HIAA concentrations. Only when the 5-HIAA is normal or borderline is the measurement of serotonin needed to document the diagnosis. Platelets contain almost all the serotonin found in the blood and for that reason, the serotonin is measured in whole blood (with platelets) or in platelet-rich plasma.

Functioning foregut tumors may also be detected by the urinary 5-HIAA assay, even though they secrete 5-hydroxytryptophan rather than serotonin. Urinary 5-HIAA is elevated because the 5-hydroxytryptophan released from these tumors is converted to serotonin in other tissues and is subsequently metabolized to 5-HIAA. In addition, urine histamine is generally elevated in patients with functioning foregut carcinoid tumors because these tumors (in contrast to midgut carcinoids) usually produce histamine.

SELF-ASSESSMENT QUESTIONS

1. Which of the following statements about the hypothalamic–pituitary–thyroid axis is not correct?

   A. Thyroid-stimulating hormone (TSH) stimulates the thyroid to produce the thyroid hormones T_3 and T_4.

   B. Thyroid-releasing hormone (TRH) from the hypothalamus stimulates the pituitary to produce TSH.

   C. The primary negative feedback to the hypothalamus and to the pituitary is from T_4, with less negative feedback from T_3.

   D. T_4 is made in much greater quantities within the thyroid than T_3.

2. Which of the following tests is the most sensitive first-line screening test for suspected thyroid abnormalities?

   A. TSH

   B. T_3

   C. T_4

   D. Thyroid-releasing hormone (TRH)

3. Which of the following statements is not true about thyroid hormone measurements?

   A. Changes in serum thyroid hormone-binding protein concentrations may affect total T_4 and T_3 concentrations.

   B. An assessment for free T_4, which represents >0.1% of the total T_4, is more helpful in evaluating thyroid function because it is not affected by changes in the amounts of thyroid hormone-binding protein.

   C. The concentrations of thyroid hormone-binding proteins also influence the total T_3 level.

   D. The T_3 concentration has similarly important diagnostic value in the assessment of both hyperthyroidism and hypothyroidism.

4. Antithyroid antibodies are relatively common. They are present in approximately 15% of the general population, and responsible for much of the thyroid disease in societies that ingest adequate amounts of iodine. Which one of the following antibodies affects the thyroid?

   A. Antitopoisomerase antibodies

   B. Antimicrosomal/Antithyroid peroxidase antibodies (anti-TPO)

   C. Antithyroglobulin antibodies

   D. TSH receptor antibodies

5. All but one of the following disorders is associated with hyperthyroidism. Identify the disorder associated with hypothyroidism among the choices below.

   A. Graves disease

   B. Toxic multinodular goiter

   C. Hashimoto thyroiditis

   D. Toxic adenoma

6. All but one of the following disorders is associated with hypothyroidism. Identify the disorder associated with hyperthyroidism among the choices below.

   A. Postthyroidectomy, total or subtotal

   B. Cretinism in an infant

   C. Hashimoto thyroiditis that is associated with chronic inflammatory disease of the thyroid

   D. Subacute thyroiditis, shortly after a viral infection that affects thyroid function

7. Up to 40% of emergency department patients have nonthyroidal illness (NTI) at the time of presentation. There is a disruption of the normal feedback relationship between TSH and T_3 and T_4. All but one of the following laboratory test results is highly consistent with a diagnosis of NTI. Identify the choice that is unlikely to be found in a patient with NTI.

   A. Reverse T_3 is increased because of slow thyroid hormone clearance and greater than normal conversion of T_4 to reverse T_3 rather than to T_3

   B. Low-normal T_4 levels in seriously ill patients

   C. Markedly elevated total T_3 concentrations

   D. TSH concentrations that are normal or low

8. Masses or nodules in the thyroid may be associated with which of the choices below?

   A. Hypofunction

   B. Hyperfunction

   C. Normal function

   D. Normal function, hyperfunction, or hypofunction

9. Which of the following statements is not true about hypothalamic–pituitary–adrenal cortex interactions?

    A. Corticotropin-releasing hormone (CRH) stimulates the pituitary to release adrenocorticotropic hormone (ACTH).

    B. When the cortex of the adrenal gland is stimulated by ACTH, it secretes cortisol and sex steroids.

    C. The primary negative feedback to reduce stimulation of the pathway is provided by sex steroids, and not cortisol.

    D. Physical and emotional stress are stimuli to activate the hypothalamic–pituitary–adrenal cortex pathway.

10. Which of the following steroid hormones are synthesized in the adrenal medulla, and not the adrenal cortex?

    A. Glucocorticoids, such as cortisol

    B. Norepinephrine

    C. Sex steroids, such as androstenedione

    D. Mineralocorticoids, such as aldosterone

11. Which of the following statements is not true about cortisol?

    A. A single random serum cortisol measurement is useful in the diagnosis of adrenal dysfunction.

    B. A 24-hour urinary excretion of cortisol is an index of plasma-free cortisol during that 24-hour time frame, and it reliably reflects excess cortisol secretion by the adrenal cortex.

    C. Cortisol is synthesized from cholesterol in the adrenal glands and in the gonads.

    D. In the adrenal cortex, the glucocorticoids, including cortisol, and the mineralocorticoids (glucocorticoids and mineralocorticoids are collectively known as corticosteroids) are produced in much higher concentrations than the sex steroids.

12. Which of the following matched pairs is incorrect?

    A. Low-dose dexamethasone suppression test/Patients with Cushing disease do not show suppression of cortisol synthesis after dexamethasone administration.

    B. ACTH measurement/Suppressed morning ACTH may indicate excess adrenal cortisol secretion.

    C. ACTH stimulation test/Lack of an increase in cortisol after ACTH stimulation suggests primary or secondary adrenal insufficiency.

    D. CRH stimulation test/Patients with primary adrenal insufficiency will have low ACTH after CRH stimulation and no cortisol production.

13. Which of the following statements about the renin–angiotensin system is incorrect?

    A. Renin stimulates the conversion of angiotensinogen to angiotensin I.

    B. Angiotensin-converting enzyme in the lungs converts angiotensin I to angiotensin II.

    C. Angiotensin II stimulates the adrenal cortex to synthesize aldosterone, which increases renal reabsorption of sodium and increases circulating blood volume and blood pressure.

    D. When the blood pressure is normal or elevated, a negative feedback signal goes to the liver that results in a generation of renin.

14. Alterations in the renin–angiotensin system can be evaluated with assays for aldosterone and renin. Which one of the following statements regarding the screening for hyperaldosteronism and hypoaldosteronism is incorrect?

    A. Screening for primary hyperaldosteronism includes the ratio of plasma aldosterone concentration to plasma renin activity, also known as the aldosterone-to-renin ratio.

    B. Because both aldosterone and renin concentrations are affected by numerous conditions and medications, it is recommended that the testing be performed when patients have been removed from drugs that affect aldosterone and renin and when the patients have normal potassium concentrations and normal salt intake.

    C. Plasma renin activity is determined by measuring its ability to convert angiotensin I to angiotensin II.

    D. In patients with primary hyperaldosteronism, the aldosterone-to-renin ratio is elevated.

15. There are three forms of Cushing syndrome that occur naturally. Which one of the following is not a naturally occurring form of Cushing syndrome?

    A. Cushing disease, which is caused most often by a small ACTH-secreting tumor in the pituitary

    B. Cushing syndrome resulting from administration of glucocorticoids as a medication

    C. Adrenal Cushing syndrome, which is most commonly associated with a tumor in the adrenal cortex

    D. Cushing syndrome from ectopic ACTH production, often from tumors not present either in the adrenal gland or in the pituitary that are secreting ACTH

16. Which of the following endogenous forms of Cushing syndrome is likely to be present for a patient in which the 24-hour urine-free cortisol or late-night salivary cortisol is elevated, the low-dose dexamethasone-suppression test shows no cortisol suppression, and the plasma ACTH is low?

    A. Pituitary cause

    B. Adrenal cause

    C. Ectopic ACTH secretion

    D. Glucocorticoid induced

17. Chronic primary adrenal insufficiency (the most common causes of which are autoimmune disease in the Western world and tuberculous adrenalitis worldwide) is also known as Addison disease. Primary adrenal insufficiency can be most clearly differentiated from a patient with secondary adrenal insufficiency, resulting from a deficiency of ACTH secretion, by which one of the following laboratory tests?

    A. Serum cortisol measured between 8 and 9 AM
    B. Plasma ACTH level
    C. CRH stimulation test
    D. Adrenal autoantibody tests

18. A patient presenting with an elevated serum potassium, a low serum sodium, a normal or elevated plasma renin activity in the absence of medications that affect plasma renin activity, and a low-plasma aldosterone is most likely to have which diagnosis of the choices below?

    A. Primary hyperaldosteronism
    B. Secondary (renin-mediated) hyperaldosteronism
    C. Primary hypoaldosteronism
    D. Secondary hypoaldosteronism

19. Congenital adrenal hyperplasia is caused by any one of a group of enzyme deficiencies in the biosynthetic pathways for cortisol and aldosterone. This results in an elevation of sex steroid synthesis and a virilizing effect on the patient. Which of the following is the most common of the enzymatic defects in patients with congenital adrenal hyperplasia?

    A. 11-β-Hydroxylase
    B. 21-Hydroxylase
    C. 17-α-Hydroxylase
    D. 3-β-Hydroxysteroid dehydrogenase

20. With regard to catecholamine synthesis and metabolism in the adrenal medulla, which one of the following statements is incorrect?

    A. The amino acid tyrosine is converted to the catecholamine dihydroxyphenylalanine (DOPA).
    B. DOPA leads to the production of dopamine that is the precursor for norepinephrine and epinephrine.
    C. Vanillylmandelic acid (VMA) is a direct metabolite of norepinephrine and can be used as a test in the evaluation for insufficiency of the adrenal medulla.
    D. Norepinephrine is metabolized directly to normetanephrine, and epinephrine is directly metabolized to metanephrine.

21. All but one of the following laboratory test results is consistent with the diagnosis of a tumor of the adrenal medulla or autonomic nervous system that secretes catecholamines, which is known as a pheochromocytoma. Identify the incompatible laboratory test result for a diagnosis of pheochromocytoma among the choices below.

    A. Elevated plasma metanephrine
    B. Elevated urinary metanephrines in a 24-hour urine specimen
    C. Decreased plasma catecholamines
    D. Increased urinary catecholamines

22. Which one of the following statements about the regulation of parathyroid hormone synthesis, secretion, and action is incorrect?

    A. Low-plasma calcium stimulates the parathyroid glands to synthesize and secrete parathyroid hormone (PTH).
    B. The increased concentration of parathyroid hormone results in increased production of 1,25-dihydroxyvitamin D by the kidneys.
    C. The increased concentration of parathyroid hormone results in increased renal tubular reabsorption of calcium.
    D. The increased concentration of parathyroid hormone results in decreased calcium resorption from the bone.

23. What has been the primary impact on the availability of intraoperative parathyroid hormone measurements?

    A. It provides a shorter turnaround time for the test results and permits early calcium supplementation after surgery.
    B. It detects decreases in plasma PTH levels that reflect the success of the excision of parathyroid tumors in surgery, and thereby reduces the need for extensive exploration of the neck and repeat surgery.
    C. It obviates the need for vitamin D testing.
    D. The level of intraoperative PTH provides an early indication of the calcium concentration in the plasma while the patient is still undergoing surgery.

24. A patient with an elevated serum total ionized calcium, an elevated serum intact PTH, a low or normal serum inorganic phosphorus, and an undetectable level of serum PTH-related protein is likely to have which one of the following diagnoses?

    A. Primary hyperparathyroidism
    B. Secondary hyperparathyroidism
    C. Hypoparathyroidism
    D. Hypercalcemia of malignancy

25. Which one of the following statements is incorrect regarding the hypothalamic–pituitary–gonadal axis in males and females?

    A. The hypothalamus synthesizes and releases gonadotropin-releasing hormone (GnRH).
    B. The pituitary gland releases follicle-stimulating hormone (FSH) and luteinizing hormone (LH).
    C. Sertoli cells in the ovaries and granulosa cells in the testes produce estradiol and testosterone, respectively.
    D. Estradiol and testosterone are the primary compounds that provide negative feedback to reduce the stimulation of the pathway.

26. The following series of laboratory test results is consistent with which one of the following diagnoses: elevated serum concentrations of LH and FSH and a low serum concentration of testosterone?

    A. Androgen insensitivity syndrome
    B. Hypogonadotropic hypogonadism
    C. Hypergonadotropic hypogonadism
    D. Hypergonadism

27. Which one of the following laboratory tests is least relevant for a diagnosis of primary amenorrhea rather than secondary amenorrhea?

    A. Adrenal hormone measurements reflective of congenital adrenal hyperplasia
    B. LH and FSH measurements and karyotype analysis for the potential identification of Turner syndrome and pure gonadal dysgenesis
    C. Cortisol measurement and other tests relevant to a diagnosis of Cushing syndrome
    D. hCG measurement as an assessment for pregnancy

28. With regard to the regulation of growth hormone secretion, which one of the following statements is incorrect?

    A. The hypothalamus releases growth hormone-releasing hormone (GHRH) as well as somatostatin.
    B. Upon stimulation of the pituitary, growth hormone is released.
    C. The target tissues for growth hormone include cartilage, bone, and liver.
    D. The negative feedback to the stimulation by GHRH is provided by excess levels of growth hormone.

29. Which one of the following matched pairs is incorrect?

    A. Growth hormone excess in adults/Acromegaly
    B. Growth hormone excess prior to the onset of puberty/Short stature
    C. Growth hormone deficiency/Pituitary irradiation
    D. Growth hormone excess/Chromophobe adenoma of the pituitary gland

30. Which one of the following statements about the regulation of prolactin secretion is incorrect?

    A. The hypothalamus secretes dopamine that has a negative effect on the pituitary and limits the release of prolactin.
    B. Prolactin-releasing peptide is secreted by the hypothalamus and stimulates the pituitary to release prolactin.
    C. Prolactin inhibits milk production by the breast.
    D. Suckling of the breast is a stimulus for the hypothalamus to release dopamine and prolactin-releasing peptide.

31. Which one of the following statements about the regulation of circulating fluid volume and osmolality is incorrect?

    A. The anterior pituitary secretes antidiuretic hormone (ADH).
    B. ADH stimulates conservation of water, leading to an increased circulating fluid volume.
    C. An increase in plasma osmolality of the extracellular fluid is a stimulus for the release of antidiuretic hormone.
    D. The negative feedback signal to reduce the release of antidiuretic hormone is atrial natriuretic peptide (ANP).

32. What is the likely diagnosis from the choices below for a patient with high plasma ADH, low urine sodium and osmolality, and high serum sodium and osmolality?

    A. Syndrome of inappropriate antidiuretic hormone secretion (SIADH)
    B. Central diabetes insipidus

    C. Nephrogenic diabetes insipidus

    D. Psychogenic polydipsia

33. What is the most commonly found abnormality in the multiple endocrine neoplasia type 2 (MEN 2) syndrome?

    A. Medullary thyroid carcinoma

    B. Tumors of the anterior pituitary

    C. Tumors of the pancreatic islet cells

    D. Hyperplasia of the parathyroid gland

FURTHER READING

Alexander EK, et al. 2017 guidelines of the American Thyroid Association for the diagnosis and management of thyroid disease during pregnancy and the postpartum. *Thyroid.* 2017;27:315–389.

Ascoli P, Cavagnini F. Hypopituitarism. *Pituitary.* 2006;9:335.

Ayuk J, et al. Growth hormone and its disorders. *Postgrad Med J.* 2006;82:24.

Bahn RS, et al. Hyperthyroidism and other causes of thyrotoxicosis: management guidelines of the American Thyroid Association and American Association of Clinical Endocrinologists. *Endocr Pract.* 2011;17:456–520.

Baylis PH. The syndrome of inappropriate antidiuretic hormone secretion. *Int J Biochem Cell Biol.* 2003;35:1495.

Bertino EM, et al. Pulmonary neuroendocrine/carcinoid tumors: a review article. *Cancer.* 2009;115:4434.

Bhasin S, et al. Testosterone therapy in adult men with androgen deficiency syndromes: an Endocrine Society clinical practice guideline. *J Clin Endocrinol Metab.* 2018;103:1–30.

Bloomfield D. Secondary amenorrhea. *Pediatr Rev.* 2006;27:113.

Bornstein SR. Predisposing factors for adrenal insufficiency. *N Engl J Med.* 2009;360:2328.

Bornstein SR, et al. Diagnosis and treatment of primary adrenal insufficiency: an Endocrine Society clinical practice guideline. *J Clin Endocrinol Metab.* 2016;101:364–389.

Camacho PM, et al. American Association of Clinical Endocrinologists and American College of Endocrinology clinical practice guidelines for the diagnosis and treatment of postmenopausal osteoporosis—2016. *Endocr Pract.* 2016;22(suppl 4):1–42.

Chen H, et al. The North American Neuroendocrine Tumor Society consensus guideline for the diagnosis and management of neuroendocrine tumors: pheochromocytoma, paraganglioma, and medullary thyroid cancer. *Pancreas.* 2010;39:775.

Fatourechi V. Subclinical hypothyroidism: an update for primary care physicians. *Mayo Clin Proc.* 2009;84:65.

Frazier W. Bone and mineral metabolism. In: Rifai N, Horvath A, Whittwer C, eds. *Tietz Textbook of Clinical Chemistry and Molecular Diagnostics.* 6th ed. St. Louis, MO: Elsevier; 2018.

Funder JW, et al. The management of primary aldosteronism: case detection, diagnosis, and treatment: an Endocrine Society clinical practice guideline. *J Clin Endocrinol Metab.* 2016;101:1889–1916.

Garber JR, et al. Clinical practice guidelines for hypothyroidism in adults cosponsored by the American Association of Clinical Endocrinologists and the American Thyroid Association. *Endocr Pract.* 2012;18:988.

Gordon CM, et al. Functional hypothalamic amenorrhea: an Endocrine Society clinical practice guideline. *J Clin Endocrinol Metab.* 2017;102:1413–1439.

Haugen BR, et al. 2015 American Thyroid Association management guidelines for adult patients with thyroid nodules and differentiated thyroid cancer: the American Thyroid Association guidelines task force on thyroid nodules and differentiated thyroid cancer. *Thyroid.* 2016;26:1–133.

Hindié E, et al. 2009 EANM parathyroid guidelines. *Eur J Nucl Med Mol Imaging.* 2009;36:1201.

Ilias I. A clinical overview of pheochromocytomas/paragangliomas and carcinoid tumors. *Nucl Med Biol.* 2008;1:S27.

Katznelson L, et al. Acromegaly: an Endocrine Society clinical practice guideline. *J Clin Endocrinol Metab.* 2014;99:3933–3951.

Lechan RM. The dilemma of the nonthyroidal illness syndrome. *Acta Biomed.* 2008;79:165.

LeFevre ML; U.S. Preventive Services Task Force. Screening for vitamin D deficiency in adults: U.S. Preventive Services Task Force recommendation statement. *Ann Intern Med.* 2015;162:133–140.

Legro RS, et al. Diagnosis and treatment of polycystic ovary syndrome: an Endocrine Society clinical practice guideline. *J Clin Endocrinol Metab.* 2013;98:4565–4592.

Lenders JW, et al. Pheochromocytoma and paraganglioma: an Endocrine Society clinical practice guideline. *J Clin Endocrinol Metab.* 2014;99:1915–1942.

Majzoub JA, Srivatsa A. Diabetes insipidus: clinical and basic aspects. *Pediatr Endocrinol Rev.* 2006;1:60.

Martin KA, et al. Evaluation and treatment of hirsutism in premenopausal women: an Endocrine Society clinical practice guideline. *J Clin Endocrinol Metab*. 2018. doi:10.1210/jc.2018-00241. [Epub ahead of print].

Melmed S, et al. Diagnosis and treatment of hyperprolactinemia: an Endocrine Society clinical practice guideline. *J Clin Endocrinol Metab*. 2011;96:273.

Minisola S, et al. The diagnosis and management of hypercalcaemia. *BMJ*. 2015;350:h2723.

Molitch ME. Evaluation and treatment of adult growth hormone deficiency: an Endocrine Society clinical practice guideline. *J Clin Endocrinol Metab*. 2011;96:1587.

Nerenz R, et al. Reproductive endocrinology and related disorders. In: Rifai N, Horvath A, Whittwer C, eds. *Tietz Textbook of Clinical Chemistry and Molecular Diagnostics*. 6th ed. St. Louis, MO: Elsevier; 2018.

Practice Committee of American Society for Reproductive Medicine. Current evaluation of amenorrhea. *Fertil Steril*. 2008;90:S219.

Ross DS, et al. 2016 American Thyroid Association guidelines for diagnosis and management of hyperthyroidism and other causes of thyrotoxicosis. *Thyroid*. 2016;26:1343–1421.

Silverberg SJ, et al. Presentation of asymptomatic primary hyperparathyroidism: proceedings of the third international workshop. *J Clin Endocrinol Metab*. 2009;94:351.

Vaidya B, et al. Addison's disease. *BMJ*. 2009;339:b2385.

Walls GV. Multiple endocrine neoplasia (MEN) syndromes. *Semin Pediatr Surg*. 2014;23:96–101.

Winter W, et al. Pituitary function and pathophysiology. In: Rifai N, Horvath A, Whittwer C, eds. *Tietz Textbook of Clinical Chemistry and Molecular Diagnostics*. 6th ed. St. Louis, MO: Elsevier; 2018.

Young DS. *Effects of Drugs on Clinical Laboratory Tests*. 5th ed. Washington, DC: AACC Press; 1990:331.

Zeiger MA, et al. American Association of Clinical Endocrinologists and American Association of Endocrine Surgeons medical guidelines for the management of adrenal incidentalomas. *Endocr Pract*. 2009;15(suppl 1):1–14.

Answers

CHAPTER 1

1. **The correct answer is D.** Answer A is incorrect because the SI units for albumin would be in g/L. Answer B is incorrect because the units are not in molar values. The same is true for answer C.
2. **The correct answer is C.** The blue top tube contains the anticoagulant citrate; the purple top tube contains EDTA; and the green top tube contains heparin—all of which are anticoagulants.
3. **The correct answer is A.** Serum is generated by producing a clot in plasma, with subsequent removal of the clot prior to testing. Cerebrospinal fluid and pleural fluid are not clotted prior to analysis.
4. **The correct answer is C.** Populations that consume large amounts of dietary fat have reference ranges for total cholesterol that are associated with atherosclerotic vascular disease. For that reason, the ranges listed for cholesterol are desirable, borderline, and high. All of the other choices in this question have a reference range established by using the values representing the middle 95% of a healthy population.
5. **The correct answer is A.** The prothrombin time and the vitamin D are not associated with a diurnal variation. Estrogen has ranges that vary with the menstrual cycle, but there is no diurnal variation.
6. **The correct answer is C.** The INR is a measurement of the extent of anticoagulation produced by the drug warfarin. There is no desirable or reference range for gender-specific range for the INR.
7. **The correct answer is A.** When there is overlap between the test results for patients with and without the disease under consideration, 100% sensitivity requires that false-positive results will also be detected. The presence of false positives indicates that the percentage of true positives is *less* than 100%.
8. **The correct answer is C.** Choice A is the definition for specificity for a laboratory test; choice B is the definition of predictive value of a positive test; and choice D is the definition for the sensitivity for a laboratory test.
9. **The correct answer is B.** The precision refers to how tightly the values are clustered. The accuracy refers to how closely the values are to the true value. In this case the values are tightly clustered but they are far away from the true value.
10. **The correct answer is D.** Testosterone is much higher in males, and both luteinizing hormone and estradiol are higher in women.
11. **The correct answer is A.** Glucose can be significantly elevated above its true baseline when the patient presents without fasting. None of the other choices are significantly altered by fasting.
12. **The correct answer is A.** The partial thromboplastin time is often used with the prothrombin time to screen for specific coagulation factor deficiencies. The other choices represent more esoteric laboratory tests not likely to be used to screen for multiple coagulation disorders.
13. **The correct answer is C.** The other three proteins are synthesized in normal-functioning cells and are not released from injured cells. Troponin I and troponin T are released from injured myocardial cells.
14. **The correct answer is C.** The second amino acid listed is the one which replaces the first.
15. **The correct answer is B.** Pharmacogenomic results are often expressed as the version of the gene, that is the allele, that is present.

CHAPTER 2

1. **The correct answer is B.** The test involving fixed cells on glass slides is the antinuclear antibody test.
2. **The correct answer is C.** The test involving an agrose gel and antibodies is imunofixation electrophoresis.
3. **The correct answer is C.** The reason that it is not flow cytometry, used for identification of cell type, is that the sample being tested is acellular.
4. **The correct answer is A.** Carbon dioxide is generated by the growth of microorganisms in the blood culture bottles.
5. **The correct answer is D.** The larger the diameter that is organism free around an antibiotic disk the more likely it is to be an effective drug to treat the infection. Organisms are reported as sensitive or resistant to an antibiotic based upon the value for the diameter.
6. **The correct answer is D.** All other values are directly determined by the instrument.
7. **The correct answer is D.** The others are much more commonly encountered in the United States.
8. **The correct answer is C.** The others are not used as biomarkers of inflammation, even if their blood concentrations change in the presence of inflammation.
9. **The correct answer is B.** They are tests that measure the time until a clot forms in the sample after adding an activator of clot formation.
10. **The correct answer is A.** It shows an immediate correction that prolongs at later time points. Choice B is most suggestive of a lupus anticoagulant. Choices C and D are most consistent with a PTT-related factor deficiency.
11. **The correct answer is C.** Forward typing detects antigens on red blood cells. Reverse typing detects antibodies that can bind to red blood cell antigens. Failure of red blood cells to clump in response to antibody indicates the absence of the corresponding antigen on the red blood cell.

12. **The correct answer is C.** Freshly collected plasma is stored frozen. Packed red blood cells are stored at 1°C to 6°C. Platelets are stored at 20°C to 24°C. Whole blood is stored at 1°C to 6°C.

13. **The correct answer is D.** If IgG or C3d is present on the red blood cells, antibody binds to the red blood cells, resulting in red blood cell agglutination and/or hemolysis.

14. **The correct answer is A.** The other devices are not used for electrolyte measurement.

15. **The correct answer is A.** These are the assays that are best suited to be performed on large automated analyzers and are relatively inexpensive.

16. **The correct answer is C.** The whole blood sample should be transported to the laboratory on ice. Manipulation of the sample with processing steps such as centrifugation will alter the values in the blood present at the time of sample collection.

17. **The correct answer is B.** All the other measurements are performed on the liquid urine rather than the urine sediment, and the values are usually indicated by color changes on pads mounted on a urine dipstick.

18. **The correct answer is D.** The fragments of different masses create the molecular "fingerprint."

19. **The correct answer is B.** Among the four choices in this list, blood glucose is by far used the most. Urine pregnancy point-of-care testing, which is not on this list, is also a commonly used assay, but not nearly as much as blood glucose.

20. **The correct answer is A.** The karyotype is a picture of full-length chromosomes captured in metaphase, and is commonly reviewed in a cytogenetics laboratory.

21. **The correct answer is C.** The molecular assays named in the other choices are all manual with few automated steps and highly expensive.

CHAPTER 3

1. **The correct answer is D.** DiGeorge syndrome is a primary immune deficiency disorder not associated with an antinuclear antibody and does not have an autoimmune etiology, unlike all of the other choices.

2. **The correct answer is D.** The muscle biopsy is more relevant to a different group of autoimmune diseases—the inflammatory muscle diseases that include dermatomyositis, polymyositis, and inclusion body myositis.

3. **The correct answer is D.** The test for antibodies to CCP is both sensitive and specific for rheumatoid arthritis, and these antibodies are absent in patients with Sjögren syndrome. The three appropriate choices are all related to the autoimmune process that leads to dry eyes and dry mouth in Sjögren syndrome.

4. **The correct answer is A.** This patient has one of the four major subtypes of systemic sclerosis/scleroderma. This subtype is limited cutaneous scleroderma in which the disease is limited to the digital extremities and face. CREST syndrome is a variant of this entity, as denoted by the first letter in calcinosis, Raynaud syndrome, esophageal dysmotility, sclerodactyly, and telangiectasia.

5. **The correct answer is C.** Mixed connective tissue disease is commonly associated with a positive result for anti-U1 RNP. Scleroderma is commonly associated with the antibody anti-Scl-70 (antitopoisomerase). SLE is associated with an antibody to double-stranded (ds) DNA that is a marker of active disease. All of these autoimmune diseases show a positive ANA test. The specificity for polymyositis and dermatomyositis resides in the epitopes of double-stranded DNA or U1 RNP or Scl-70.

6. **The correct answer is C.** This assay is more likely to be associated with evaluation of the patient for amyloidosis. C-reactive protein is an acute-phase reactant increased in patients with rheumatoid arthritis and serves as an index of inflammation. Rheumatoid factor is detectable in 70% to 80% of patients with rheumatoid arthritis but is not specific for rheumatoid arthritis. Anticitrullinated α-enolase is a predictor of radiographic progression of disease.

7. **The correct answer is B.** A patient with amyloidosis requires evaluation for renal, cardiac, pulmonary, neurologic, cutaneous, articular, liver, and spleen involvement. For the patient with amyloidosis who has an abnormal PT and/or PTT, performance of an assay for coagulation factor X is indicated.

8. **The correct answer is C.** SCID syndrome is characterized by profound effects in both cellular and humoral immunity. Common variable immunodeficiency affects both males and females equally and is associated with a normal number of B cells that function poorly. DiGeorge syndrome, which is due to deletion of chromosome 22q11.2, is associated with T-cell abnormalities and B-cell dysfunction.

9. **The correct answer is D.** There is strong evidence for complement deficiency state. Factor B deficiency is associated with a normal CH50 result, and C2 deficiency is associated with a normal AH50 result.

CHAPTER 4

1. **The correct answer is B.** The letter A refers to the *HLA-A* gene. The * is a spacer. The number 02 represent an allele group; 101 indicates the specific HLA protein; and 01 shows a synonymous DNA substitution within the coding region.

2. **The correct answer is D.** For liver transplant, no HLA typing is required but ABO matching is necessary. For kidney transplant, HLA matching is preferable but not required (ABO matching is absolutely required). For stem cell/bone marrow transplant, HLA testing is usually a requirement.

CHAPTER 5

1. **The correct answer is D.** Karyotyping of chromosomes is not a diagnostic test for infections. All of the other methods are mainstays in the evaluation for an infectious disease.

2. **The correct answer is A.** Susceptibility testing for the other types of microorganisms is far less common, if they are performed at all.

3. **The correct answer is C.** The result is especially likely to represent a skin contaminant introduced during specimen collection if the coagulase-negative staphylococci are present in only one of multiple blood culture specimens.

4. **The correct answer is D.** All of the other choices are sterile. The sputum is often contaminated from the upper respiratory tract with many other organisms, such as viridans group streptococci.

5. **The correct answer is C.** *Rickettsia*, *Ehrlichia*, and *Anaplasma* are all obligate intracellular bacteria. *Candida* and *Cryptococcus* are yeasts and not intracellular. *Pseudomonas* is a bacterium, but it is not intracellular.

6. **The correct answer is A.** *P. falciparum* can be fatal within days. *P. malariae* is the least virulent species of the four choices.

7. **The correct answer is D.** The causative agent for infectious mononucleosis is Epstein–Barr virus (EBV). The white blood cell differential is important in the evaluation of the patient because there is a mild–moderate leukocytosis and many of the lymphocytes are atypical. Parvovirus is not causative for infectious mononucleosis.

8. **The correct answer is A.** Endocarditis can affect both valvular and nonvalvular endothelium of the heart. The other choices are all correct statements about infectious endocarditis.

9. **The correct answer is B.** Bacterial, viral, and fungal meningitis are all well recognized with multiple species in each of the three groups of organisms known to cause meningitis. Parasites are least likely among the four choices to be identified as causative for meningitis.

10. **The correct answer is B.** The test results shown above are highly consistent with bacterial meningitis. The results are markedly different for cerebrospinal fluid testing from patients with viral, fungal, or tuberculous meningitis.

11. **The correct answer is A.** Of the choices given, the protein concentration of the synovial fluid is the least useful in evaluation for a joint infection.

12. **The correct answer is A.** Osteomyelitis is an infection of the bone and not an infection of the skin or soft tissue. Superficial folliculitis is an infection of the hair follicles of the skin. A furuncle is produced by an infection of the perifollicular skin. A carbuncle is a coalescence of interconnected furuncles with drainage at multiple sites.

13. **The correct answer is C.** Several organisms in the *Bartonella* species are known to cause cat scratch fever and bacillary angiomatosis. Neither causes a rash that has the appearance of erythema migrans. Necrotizing fasciitis is a soft tissue infection with two major subtypes and is also not associated with a distinctive rash.

14. **The correct answer is B.** Rubeola infection produces measles. Rubella infection produces an infection once known as German measles. Herpes simplex virus is associated with multiple infections, but not chickenpox.

15. **The correct answer is A.** Tinea pedis affects the feet rather than the hands, and is also known as "athlete's foot." The corresponding superficial fungal infection of the hand is known as tinea manuum. Tinea cruris is also known as "jock itch."

16. **The correct answer is C.** Conjunctivitis can be viral, bacterial, or chlamydial. Viral conjunctivitis is more common than bacterial conjunctivitis in developed countries. *Chlamydia trachomatis* conjunctivitis is a leading cause of blindness in endemic areas of the world.

17. **The correct answer is D.** Respiratory pathogens are not difficult to assess for antimicrobial sensitivity. This makes testing complex for patients who have a causative agent for a pulmonary infection that is uncommon or not easily detected by laboratory methods. Obtaining a sputum sample originating in the lung and not contaminated with oropharyngeal flora is a well-recognized challenge in the diagnosis of a pulmonary infection which may require multiple tests to identify a pathogenic organism.

18. **The correct answer is B.** Pneumocystis is a well-recognized cause of pulmonary infections in patients with profoundly impaired cell-mediated immunity. It has become much less commonly encountered since the use of antiretroviral therapy for HIV infection.

19. **The correct answer is D.** The other agents can produce a systemic infection, each with its own unique clinical findings.

20. **The correct answer is A.** The other organisms are usually associated with community-acquired diarrhea.

21. **The correct answer is C.** The test for the toxins should only be performed on unformed diarrheal stool.

22. **The correct answer is D.** *Taenia solium* is a helminth. All the other choices are protozoa.

23. **The correct answer is C.** Helminth (worm) infections constitute a significant percentage of the global burden of gastrointestinal infectious diseases.

24. **The correct answer is C.** The enterotoxins in *Bacillus cereus* are commonly found in reheated fried rice.

25. **The correct answer is A.** Botulism is a neuroparalytic disease resulting from blockage of release of acetylcholine at peripheral cholinergic synapses by toxins from *Clostridium botulinum*.

26. **The correct answer is B.** All the other tests are essential in the evaluation of a patient for a urinary tract infection.

27. **The correct answer is D.** Infection of the prostate is associated with different microorganisms than the other three choices. Prostatitis is considered an infection of the male genital tract.

28. **The correct answer is B.** Microscopy after treatment of a vaginal specimen with 10% KOH is commonly used to evaluate a patient for vulvovaginitis caused by *Candida albicans* or *Trichomonas vaginalis*.

29. **The correct answer is D.** The other three choices are commonly recognized to be transmitted by sexual contact.

30. **The correct answer is D.** Unlike males, the urethral swab is not a specimen used for most evaluations of a female suspected of *Neisseria gonorrhea* infection, with the endocervical canal being a much more likely site to reveal infection in a woman. Infants born to untreated mothers can develop ophthalmia neonatorum.

CHAPTER 6

1. **The correct answer is C.** All the other drugs are commonly monitored for patient safety and/or efficacy.

2. **The correct answer is C.** The opposite is true for choice C—that is, an indication for therapeutic drug monitoring is when the prescribed drug has significant pharmacokinetic variability.

3. **The correct answer is B.** With regard to drug metabolism, the liver is the primary site in the body.

4. **The correct answer is A.** Drugs can be eliminated through the kidneys, the liver, the lungs, the skin, the feces, and by other means. However, the elimination of many polar, nonlipophilic drugs is achieved primarily through renal excretion. Reduced drug clearance may occur when a drug that is eliminated by the kidneys is administered to a patient with impaired renal function.

5. **The correct answer is A.** Choice B more likely represents a peak level if 4 hours are required after administration of the drug to reach a peak concentration in the blood. In general, trough levels are used to evaluate the likelihood of a therapeutic effect. Peak levels are drawn at varying times, depending on the particular drug, and are often used to assess toxicity risk.

6. **The correct answer is D.** Methotrexate is not an antidepressant. It is a folate antagonist used in the treatment of a wide variety of neoplasms. Drug-related toxicity is common with high-dose methotrexate therapy.

7. **The correct answer is A.** Excess intake of acetaminophen can be associated with severe liver injury. Alanine aminotransferase is a test commonly used to assess liver function. Blood urea nitrogen is commonly used to assess kidney function, amylase assesses pancreatic function, and troponin assesses cardiac function.

8. **The correct answer is C.** Among the benzodiazepines, diazepam and several other drugs in this class are commonly abused. Among the amphetamines, methamphetamine and its derivative known as MDMA or ecstasy is frequently detected. Oxycodone testing can be used to identify those who are taking the drug in larger amounts than prescribed, and those who are selling the drug for profit when they should be taking the drug as prescribed.

9. **The correct answer is B.** Most drugs and metabolites are concentrated in urine after use, and therefore, urine is appropriate for qualitative analysis and determining recent use of selected drugs of abuse. Plasma, which is derived from the whole blood, is commonly used to determine a quantitative level of the drug to assess for intoxication and toxicity. Although sweat can be used to sample for certain illicit drugs, it is not commonly the sample of choice.

10. **The correct answer is D.** The first three choices are all alcohols, and the most commonly used and abused of the alcohols is ethanol that was not listed. Ethanol is the most common drug of abuse. Methanol intoxication can result in impaired vision up to blindness. Ethylene glycol, which is present in antifreeze, can produce vomiting, seizures, anuria, and even coma. Isopropanol toxicity commonly leads to vomiting with abdominal pain and bleeding from the gastrointestinal tract.

11. **The correct answer is C.** The liver and the pancreas are commonly damaged by excess ethanol intake, and alcoholic cardiomyopathy is also observed in some patients consuming large amounts of ethanol.

12. **The correct answer is D.** In mg/dL, the range for euphoria is 40 to 120; for excitement it is 90 to 250; and for confusion it is 180 to 300.

13. **The correct answer is D.** None of the other choices are associated with oxalate crystals in the urine. The oxalate crystals occur because ethylene glycol is metabolized to oxalate. In addition, hypoglycemia is typically not found with an overdose of isopropanol.

14. **The correct answer is D.** Carbon monoxide poisoning is responsible for up to 4000 deaths per year in the United States. The heart, central nervous system, and lungs are the organs most immediately affected by the toxic effects of carbon monoxide. The principal pathologic consequence of carbon monoxide poisoning is the binding of carbon monoxide to oxygen-binding sites in the hemoglobin molecule.

15. **The correct answer is B.** For patients whose blood lead level exceeds 70 mg/dL, hospitalization is required with commencement of chelation therapy. Oral chelation therapy is also indicated for a level of 45 to 69, with consideration of hospitalization if a lead-safe environment cannot be ensured.

CHAPTER 7

1. **The correct answer is B.** Fetal fibronectin is produced by fetal membranes and appears in the cervix and vagina early in pregnancy as implantation develops, and normally disappears by week 20. Its reappearance in the third trimester often precedes labor and delivery.

2. **The correct answer is A.** Nuchal translucency is in the first-trimester screen along with free β-hCG and pregnancy-associated plasma protein A. The quadruple screen includes AFP, hCG, unconjugated estriol, and inhibin A.

3. **The correct answer is C.** Antibody production by a mother who is Rh negative results from exposure of Rh-positive fetal cells during pregnancy and, to a much greater extent, at delivery. Therefore, the women at greatest risk for delivering infants with hemolytic disease of the newborn are Rh-negative mothers who conceive Rh-positive babies, and are in the second or subsequent pregnancies.

4. **The correct answer is D.** The sweat chloride test is a screening test for cystic fibrosis for patients of all ages. The test for immunoreactive trypsinogen is used to screen newborns for cystic fibrosis. Cystic fibrosis results from mutations in the protein that transports chloride in the cell membrane, known as CFTR. Detection of such mutations is important in the evaluation for cystic fibrosis.

5. **The correct answer is B.** Phenylketonuria results in the accumulation of the amino acid phenylalanine. Therefore, this disorder is an amino aciduria. All of the other choices are correct matches between the category of disease and the named disease with which they are associated.

CHAPTER 8

1. **The correct answer is C.** The apolipoproteins for all of the other plasma lipoproteins are different. In addition, triglycerides are in higher concentration than cholesterol esters in the core of chylomicrons and very low-density lipoproteins.

2. **The correct answer is A.** Low concentrations of LDL, C-reactive protein, and total cholesterol are desirable.

3. **The correct answer is D.** Adenocarcinoma of the lung may be surgically correctable in some patients, but it is not likely to be a cause of hypertension. All of the other cases are causes of hypertension that can be corrected by surgery or changes in medication.

4. **The correct answer is D.** The first three choices provide information about renal, vascular, and adrenal causes of hypertension.

5. **The correct answer is C.** The individual vasculitic disorders can be identified in many cases using the ANCA tests (certain vasculitides are ANCA positive)

along with a marker of inflammation such as C-reactive protein, and also by identifying the vessels associated with inflammation.

6. **The correct answer is A.** The D-dimer test is used to rule out pulmonary embolism when the result is negative. To permit the predictive value of a negative test to approximate 100%, a very high sensitivity test must be used. The manual latex agglutination methods have low sensitivity and cannot be used to rule out pulmonary embolism when the result is negative.

CHAPTER 9

1. **The correct answer is B.** The presence or absence of a pulmonary embolism is unrelated to establishing a diagnosis of myocardial infarction.

2. **The correct answer is C.** All of the other choices have been used as markers of myocardial infarction, but troponin T and troponin I are diagnostically superior to all of them.

3. **The correct answer is A.** BNP monitoring has greatly improved the frequency of correct diagnosis of congestive heart failure over the use of clinical judgment and other diagnostic methods. It is the primary biomarker used for identification of congestive heart failure. It is elevated not only in congestive heart failure, but also increases can occur in inflammatory cardiac conditions, arterial and pulmonary hypertension, chronic renal failure, and liver cirrhosis. Troponin elevations may accompany BNP elevations in congestive heart failure.

CHAPTER 10

1. **The correct answer is C.** The MCV is a measure of red blood cell size. All of the others are measures of red blood cell quantity.

2. **The correct answer is D.** Immune hemolytic anemia does not involve reduced proliferation of red blood cells. Immune hemolytic anemia is produced by antibody-mediated red blood cell destruction.

3. **The correct answer is B.** Iron-deficiency anemia is a very common cause for small red blood cells with a low MCV value. All of the other choices are associated with the presence of a larger than normal red blood cells.

4. **The correct answer is B.** Heinz bodies are gray-black round inclusions, seen only with supravital stains such as crystal violet. They are found in patients with certain unstable hemoglobins. Howell–Jolly bodies are dot-like, dark purple inclusions, unlike Pappenheimer bodies that are more irregular and more gray. Cabot rings are ring-shaped dark purple inclusions. Like Howell–Jolly bodies, they represent residual nuclear fragments.

5. **The correct answer is C.** Spherocytes are red blood cells without central pallor due to decreased red cell membrane. Target cells are red blood cells with a dark circle within the central area of pallor, as a result of redundant membrane. Acanthocytes are red blood cells with circumferential blunt and spiny projections with bulbous tips.

6. **The correct answer is A.** None of the other choices represent red blood cell forms associated with destruction from immune hemolysis. Spherocytes are also found in a rare hereditary condition known as hereditary spherocytosis.

7. **The correct answer is C.** The other three markers are much more likely to be associated with intravascular rather than extravascular hemolysis.

8. **The correct answer is D.** Small bowel resection can result in malabsorption of iron. Chronic blood loss from colorectal cancer leads to loss of iron. A strict vegetarian diet may be poor in iron. Pulmonary embolism is not likely to be associated with iron deficiency.

9. **The correct answer is C.** The serum ferritin value is useful to assess the status of iron stores. The serum iron reflects the status of red blood cell production. When it is low, there is impaired erythropoiesis. The peripheral blood smear shows microcytic red blood cells. The white blood cell count is not particularly informative.

10. **The correct answer is A.** Iron deficiency is the most common causes of anemia globally, but in the United States the most common cause is anemia of chronic disease. The most commonly associated disorders with anemia of chronic disease are rheumatoid arthritis and other collagen vascular diseases, and malignancy.

11. **The correct answer is A.** Choice B represents α-thalassemia minor. Choice C represents hemoglobin Barts. Choice D represents α-thalassemia (silent) carrier state.

12. **The correct answer is B.** Malabsorption from the gastrointestinal tract can lead to vitamin B_{12} deficiency, most commonly from pernicious anemia. Pernicious anemia results from a deficiency in gastric intrinsic factor, which is reduced as a result of an autoimmune effect on the gastric mucosa.

13. **The correct answer is C.** Choice A represents sickle cell trait. Homozygous hemoglobin C disease is milder than sickle cell anemia represented by the correct choice (C). Hemoglobin E is relatively benign in both heterozygous and homozygous forms.

14. **The correct answer is B.** IgG antibodies bind to red blood cells at body temperature to produce hemolysis in patients with warm autoimmune hemolytic anemia (WAIHA).

15. **The correct answer is A.** The other three choices are well known to be associated with drug-induced hemolytic anemia.

16. **The correct answer is D.** The father is not immunized in this process, and in fact, he provides the red blood cell antigens to the fetus that are not present in the mother. This accounts for the immune response to the fetal red blood cells by the mother.

17. **The correct answer is B.** The peripheral blood smear shows most prominently a combination of red blood cells with Heinz bodies and "bite cells." All the other statements about the anemia associated with G6PD deficiency are true.

18. **The correct answer is A.** Choice B refers to anemia from pyruvate kinase deficiency in red blood cells. Choice C is descriptive of paroxysmal nocturnal hemoglobinuria (which is paroxysmal but not nocturnal, despite the name). Choice D is a description of, among other entities, pure red blood cell aplasia.

19. **The correct answer is B.** The other mutations are associated with disorders other than polycythemia vera. *btk* is associated with X-linked agammaglobulinemia. The prothrombin 20210 mutation is associated with venous thrombosis. Mutations in the α-globin gene can lead to different forms of α-thalassemia.

20. **The correct answer is D.** Hemoglobin electrophoresis separates whole hemoglobin molecules and not the separate chains that compose the hemoglobin molecule, such as the α or β chains. Hemoglobin A_2 represents only 2% to 3% of hemoglobin in a normal electrophoretic pattern.

21. **The correct answer is B.** The osmotic fragility test assesses red blood cell lysis in progressively hypotonic solutions. Enhanced lysis, when compared with controls, is a positive test. Spherocytes lyse at a faster rate than normal biconcave red blood cells.

CHAPTER 11

1. **The correct answer is C.** The other choices are all associated with bleeding and not thrombosis. Note that factor V deficiency and the factor V Leiden mutation are associated with bleeding and thrombosis, respectively.

2. **The correct answer is A.** Hemophilia A is a deficiency of only factor VIII. Vitamin K deficiency produces deficiencies in factors II, VII, IX, and X. Liver disease, when severe, produces some decrease in all factors from baseline, except factor VIII. DIC when severe can also produce deficiencies of most of the coagulation factors, including factor VIII.

3. **The correct answer is C.** All of the others are thrombocytopenias in which the platelets are lost by a consumptive process within the circulation. For posttransfusion purpura, in more than 90% of cases, there is an antibody directed against the platelet antigen known as HPA-1a.

4. **The correct answer is A.** Qualitative platelet disorders are associated with a normal platelet count but impaired platelet function. Choices B and C are thrombocytopenic disorders. Choice D is a disorder with an increased number of platelet in the circulation.

5. **The correct answer is B.** A deficiency of factor VII would prolong the PT rather than the PTT. A deficiency of factor XIII prolongs neither the PT nor the PTT. A deficiency of fibrinogen should prolong both the PT and the PTT.

6. **The correct answer is C.** All of the other factors, when markedly deficient, predispose the patient to bleed. Factor XII deficiency markedly prolongs the PTT, without prolonging the PT, but has no effect on bleeding risk.

7. **The correct answer is D.** Hepatitis does not lead to malabsorption of vitamin K. Warfarin therapy reduces the amount of active vitamin K. Malabsorption results in decreased uptake of vitamin K, which is fat soluble. Antibiotic therapy can reduce the number of vitamin K-producing bacteria in the gastrointestinal tract and impair vitamin K metabolism in the liver.

8. **The correct answer is B.** Choices A, C, and D are all well-known stimuli for the development of disseminated intravascular coagulation.

9. **The correct answer is A.** DIC results in consumption of coagulation factors and platelets. Thrombi appear in smaller blood vessels, but the thrombi rarely block the larger blood vessels and result in poor perfusion of the tissues. As a result of the consumption of coagulation factors and platelets, the patients are predisposed to bleed. It is for this reason that clinically, patients in DIC, especially when it is severe, present with bleeding.

10. **The correct answer is B.** The coagulation factors are made in hepatocytes that are decreased in number in patients with cirrhosis. Thrombocytopenia can occur from sequestration in an enlarged spleen or from decreased platelet production. Increased D-dimer levels are found because these fibrin breakdown products are cleared by the liver that is dysfunctional in cirrhosis.

11. **The correct answer is D.** ITP is much more common in females, with a ratio of 2:1 to 3:1 relative to males. All of the other statements about ITP are correct.

12. **The correct answer is D.** The other choices are well-known causes of drug-induced thrombocytopenia. Aspirin impairs platelet function but does not reduce the platelet count.

13. **The correct answer is A.** Although von Willebrand prevalence rates vary, decreased levels of von Willebrand factor may be present in as much as 1% of the population. Factor V deficiency is one of the rare factor deficiencies. Essential thrombocythemia is a relatively rare quantitative platelet disorder. Platelet storage pool deficiency is a rare qualitative platelet disorder in which one or more granule types within the platelet are deficient.

14. **The correct answer is D.** A standard panel for von Willebrand testing includes the tests listed in choices A, B, and C. The white blood cell count is rarely altered.

15. **The correct answer is C.** An abnormal form of von Willebrand factor is present in patients with Type 2B, and the abnormal von Willebrand factor binds to platelets when it should remain unbound. This makes the platelets hypersensitive to aggregation with the agonist ristocetin.

16. **The correct answer is A.** The mean von Willebrand factor levels per blood type are as follows: type O—76%; type A—106%; type B—117%; and type AB—123%. Several hypotheses exist as an explanation. Because the baseline value for von Willebrand factor is lower in patients with blood type O, patients with this blood type are found much more frequently among those with a diagnosis of low von Willebrand factor.

17. **The correct answer is B.** Glanzmann thrombasthenia is associated with decreased functional glycoprotein IIb/IIIa. Platelet storage pool disease involves the absence of granules in the platelets. Cyclooxygenase deficiency is a disorder affecting platelet function (and other cells) as a result of a reduction in the intracellular enzyme cyclooxygenase.

18. **The correct answer is C.** The factor V Leiden mutation is present in approximately 5% of Caucasians, and its incidence is far higher than any of the other choices.

19. **The correct answer is C.** Warfarin decreases the synthesis of coagulation factors II, VII, IX, and X. In addition, warfarin also decreases the production of the natural anticoagulants, protein C and protein S.

20. **The correct answer is A.** All of the other choices are phospholipids and not proteins. The function of β2 glycoprotein 1 is still not clearly established.

21. **The correct answer is D.** "Antiphospholipid antibodies" is a general term that encompasses choices A, B, and C.

22. **The correct answer is D.** Warfarin inhibits the synthesis of coagulation factors II, VII, IX, and X. Heparin inhibits the activated forms of all the coagulation factors. Dabigatran is a selective inhibitor of coagulation factor IIa (thrombin).

23. **The correct answer is D.** The INR measures the anticoagulant effect of warfarin. The INR is derived from the prothrombin time and is used to minimize the impact of the differences in thromboplastin reagents used in the prothrombin time assays.

24. **The correct answer is D.** The effect of aspirin is the inhibition of platelet function. All of the other choices are anticoagulants that slow down the coagulation cascade without a noteworthy effect on platelet function.

25. **The correct answer is B.** Like ibuprofen, aspirin inhibits platelet cyclooxygenase. However, the inhibition produced by aspirin is irreversible for the lifetime of the platelets exposed to aspirin in the circulation. The inhibition by ibuprofen is essentially fully reversed within 1 day. Therefore, platelet function studies will be affected by aspirin for a longer period of time than by ibuprofen. Clopidogrel is metabolized to a clopidogrel metabolite that binds to the ADP receptor of a platelet. Eptifibatide blocks the fibrinogen receptor that is glycoprotein IIb/IIIa.

CHAPTER 12

1. **The correct answer is B.** The steps are in the order—B, A, C and then D.

2. **The correct answer is B.** There is a small amount of plasma in packed red blood cells and in random donor platelet products. Cryoprecipitate contains a very limited number of plasma proteins. Fresh frozen plasma contains all of the proteins found in normal human plasma.

3. **The correct answer is C.** Platelets are stored at 20°C to 24°C. Packed red blood cells are stored at 1°C to 6°C. Fresh frozen plasma can be stored at less than –18°C for 1 year or at less than –65°C for 7 years. The same is true for cryoprecipitate.

4. **The correct answer is B**, with the assumption that it has been processed correctly and frozen within 8 hours of blood collection. This preserves the labile coagulation factors, particularly factor V and factor VIII. Cryoprecipitate contains the coagulation factor fibrinogen, and coagulation factor VIII along with von Willebrand factor. The other coagulation factors are missing or in very low concentration in cryoprecipitate. The coagulation factors are not preserved at 1°C to 6°C, the storage temperature for packed red blood cells, or at 20°C to 24°C, the storage temperature for platelets.

5. **The correct answer is D.** Recombinant VIIa is approved for treatment of patients with bleeding from a factor VIII inhibitor. It has also been used widely for patients with massive bleeding. Recombinant VIII is a treatment for patients with hemophilia A. Recombinant IX is used for treatment of patients with hemophilia B. Recombinant IIa is used to create a product known as "fibrin glue," which can be used to physically connect tissues in vivo, and can be used topically to reduce bleeding, especially in patients with hemophilia A or hemophilia B. However, bovine factor II is also used for this purpose. As a result, recombinant IIa is the least used of the four choices.

6. **The correct answer is B.** Although Ebola virus infection has high mortality, testing for it in donated blood is not mandatory. Presumably, individuals who are contagious with Ebola virus would be excluded because of their clinical symptoms. All of the other choices have long been required for testing of donated blood products.

7. **The correct answer is C.** Blood type O is the universal donor. Blood type AB is the universal recipient. For choice C, the anti-A antibodies in type B blood would cause a severe reaction when infused into a patient who has type A antigen on red blood cells.

8. **The correct answer is C.** The indirect antiglobulin test identifies antibodies in the circulation that can bind to red blood cells, unlike the direct antiglobulin test that measures IgG or complement already bound to the red blood cell surface. The red blood cell crossmatch is a compatibility test to determine if a donated red blood cell product is suitable for a particular recipient. The test described in choice D is one in which antibodies to specific red blood cell antigens, such as Kell, Kidd, and Duffy, are detected, if present.

9. **The correct answer is D.** All of the other choices are accepted indications for transfusion. Fresh frozen plasma is not indicated for patients who have an INR value of less than 1.5.

10. **The correct answer is B.** Delayed hemolytic transfusion reactions are generally less severe than their acute counterparts. They are known to occur when a patient is reexposed to an antigen to which he or she was sensitized in the past by a previous transfusion or a pregnancy. Exposure to the antigen can stimulate an anamnestic response, even if the antibody to this antigen is no longer detectable prior to transfusion. Delayed hemolytic transfusion reactions may also occur when the transfusion recipient mounts a primary immune response to alloantigens on transfused RBCs, that is, alloimmunization. The most severe acute hemolytic transfusion reactions are due to ABO incompatibility.

11. **The correct answer is A.** Lewis (Le) antigens on red blood cells can be either Le^a or Le^b. Antibodies to Le^a have not been implicated in hemolytic disease of the newborn and in only in a few cases of hemolytic transfusion reactions. Anti-Le^b has not been implicated in either hemolytic disease of the newborn or hemolytic transfusion reactions. All of the other choices listed above are clearly implicated in hemolytic disease of the newborn and hemolytic transfusion reactions.

12. **The correct answer is D.** Rh-negative individuals lacking the D antigen, another name for the Rh antigen, are vulnerable to development of an alloantibody to the D antigen. This is a highly immunogenic antigen on human red blood cells. Anti-D is the most common cause of severe cases of hemolytic disease of the newborn. Approximately 85% of Caucasians express the D antigen.

13. **The correct answer is B.** Febrile nonhemolytic transfusion reactions are among the most common transfusion-related complications. Approximately 1% to 3% of transfusions of cellular components are associated with a febrile nonhemolytic transfusion reaction. These reactions are the product of antileukocyte antibodies present in the recipient's plasma that react with the white blood cells in the transfused product.

14. **The correct answer is A.** TRALI is associated with antibodies in the donor's plasma rather than the recipient's plasma. It is characterized by acute respiratory distress, hypoxia, and infiltrates on the chest x-ray, along with fever and hypertension within about 6 hours of completion of the transfusion.

15. **The correct answer is D.** Depletion of 2,3 DPG occurs with increased storage time of red blood cells. There is no active transfer of this component to platelets. After red blood cells depleted of 2,3 DPG are transfused, they restore their levels toward normal over a period of 24 to 48 hours.

16. **The correct answer is C.** The ABO and Rh type of the posttransfusion specimen is determined to confirm that the pretransfusion specimen was indeed from the patient. It is not the Kell and Duffy antigens that are evaluated in this test.

17. **The correct answer is D.** Immune thrombocytopenia is a category IV indication for therapeutic apheresis. Category IV indicates a demonstrated lack of therapeutic efficacy of apheresis and that controlled studies or case reports failed to show a clinical benefit with apheresis.

CHAPTER 13

1. **The correct answer is A.** Lymph node biopsy is more relevant to the initial evaluation for lymphoma than a bone marrow biopsy. An initial evaluation for autoimmunity is an antinuclear antibody test, with no indication at initial presentation for a bone marrow biopsy. Recurrent infections in the presence of a normal white blood cell count direct an initial evaluation to white blood cell function.
2. **The correct answer is D.** Acute lymphocytic leukemia is associated with large amounts of lymphocytes with no excess of eosinophils. All of the other choices have strong associations to eosinophilia.
3. **The correct answer is D.** In Hodgkin lymphoma, proliferating cells spread by contiguity, mesenteric lymph nodes are rarely involved, and there are fewer types than in non-Hodgkin lymphomas.
4. **The correct answer is D.** Acute lymphocytic leukemia is very common in young children, with a high cure rate.
5. **The correct answer is A.** Chronic lymphocytic leukemia is the most common of the non-Hodgkin lymphomas. There is a slight male predominance and the neoplastic cells are mature B cells. It is an indolent disease with a highly variable life expectancy.
6. **The correct answer is B.** Plasma cell neoplasms are disorders in which there is an expanded single clone of immunoglobulin-secreting cells. The immunoglobulin is monoclonal and is commonly detected as an extra band in a protein electrophoresis test.
7. **The correct answer is B.** Bence–Jones proteins are free light chains present in the circulation that may also be excreted into the urine. They are incomplete immunoglobulins produced in certain plasma cell neoplasms.
8. **The correct answer is B.** There are rare cases of plasma cell myelomas in which the monoclonal protein produced is IgM. However, such patients typically have lytic bone lesions, and patients with Waldenström macroglobulinemia do not.
9. **The correct answer is B.** Approximately 15% to 20% of patients with MGUS develop myeloma, macroglobulinemia, amyloidosis, or lymphoma.
10. **The correct answer is A.** The lineage of the Reed–Sternberg cell has for many years been controversial. Current evidence indicates that it is an abnormal malignant B cell.
11. **The correct answer is B.** A uniform classification for acute leukemias was developed in the 1970s by a cooperative French–American–British group (FAB classification). The types of leukemias in this classification were based primarily on the morphology of the leukemic blast cells and, to a lesser extent, on cytochemical staining. The WHO system defines specific leukemias by their molecular pathology for those with recurrent chromosomal abnormalities and contains categories for leukemias that evolve from myelodysplastic syndromes and leukemias arising from chemotherapy from prior malignancies.
12. **The correct answer is B.** Myelodysplastic syndromes are a group of bone marrow disorders with dysplastic (i.e., not normal) but not neoplastic changes of cells in the myeloid series. Also, the myeloblasts must represent less than 20% of all nucleated marrow cells. If more than 20% of myeloblasts are found, a diagnosis of acute leukemia is made.
13. **The correct answer is D.** Production of a monoclonal immunoglobulin identified by serum protein electrophoresis is more likely to be included in the evaluation for plasma cell dyscrasias.
14. **The correct answer is D.** Myeloproliferative neoplasms are those with a clonal neoplastic proliferation of a multipotent myeloid stem cell. Therefore, this excludes multiple myeloma in which there is a proliferation of antibody-producing plasma cells.
15. **The correct answer is D.** In chronic myeloid leukemia, the white blood cell count is markedly elevated. The other disorders typically have normal white blood cell counts but impaired white blood cell function.

CHAPTER 14

1. **The correct answer is D.** The anatomical portion of the lung affected in chronic obstructive pulmonary disease is the airways.
2. **The correct answer is B.** The partial pressure of nitrogen is not used diagnostically.
3. **The correct answer is D.** The anion gap is the difference between the major free cations (sodium and potassium) and free anions (chloride and bicarbonate). Calcium is not included in the calculation of the anion gap.
4. **The correct answer is A.** Patients with uncontrolled diabetes have increased ketoacids, lowering the arterial pH, and producing an increased anion gap.
5. **The correct answer is B.** The patient has respiratory acidosis because of decreased partial pressure of carbon dioxide, resulting in an increase in carbonic acid, which lowers the arterial pH.
6. **The correct answer is C.** Patients with a substantial amount of vomiting lose stomach acids and thereby experience an increase in the arterial pH.
7. **The correct answer is D.** Hyperventilation results in increased excretion of carbon dioxide, which results in a decreased concentration of carbonic acid. This causes an increase in the arterial pH.
8. **The correct answer is A.** A transudate is an ultrafiltrate of plasma with a relatively low protein concentrations and relatively low pleural fluid LDH.
9. **The correct answer is D.** Patients with congestive heart failure have an increase in their systemic venous pressure and pulmonary capillary pressure. This is a result of the diminished effectiveness of the heart as a pump. This results in the leakage of transudate fluid into the pleural space.
10. **The correct answer is D.** Hemoglobin AIc is generally used for assessment of diabetes mellitus. All of the other three choices are directly relevant to the diagnosis of chronic obstructive pulmonary disease.
11. **The correct answer is B.** The appropriate test is a qualitative assay for detection for phosphatidylglycerol, not phosphatidylcholine. All of the other choices are available tests for fetal lung maturity.
12. **The correct answer is D.** Smoking induces a variety of mutations that result in lung cancer. A mutation in cystathionine β-synthase can result in extremely elevated homocysteine levels that damage the blood vessel wall and cause thrombosis. It is not known to cause lung cancer.

CHAPTER 15

1. **The correct answer is A.** Asthma generally causes airway obstruction without prominent symptoms in the gastrointestinal tract. All of the other choices affect the stomach and the esophagus.
2. **The correct answer is B.** Infection with *H. pylori* is most likely to occur in childhood, more common in low socioeconomic conditions, and its prevalence increases with age.

3. **The correct answer is B.** *H. pylori* is able to split urea, and, therefore, active infection with *H. pylori* can be detected by metabolism of urea. The urea breath test involves ingestion of a substance containing urea that is labeled with radioactive carbon. Urease splits the urea into ammonia and carbon dioxide, and the radioactivity in the breath correlates with urease activity. Choices A and C are based on urease activity. A molecular test for *H. pylori* also detects the presence of active *H. pylori*. Serologic tests can remain positive for years, even if the disease is treated, and therefore active infection is not required for a positive test result.

4. **The correct answer is C.** The fecal immunochemical test is a stool-based test to detect bleeding in the colon. It is used as a screening test for colorectal cancer. All of the other tests are relevant to an evaluation for celiac disease. Small bowel biopsy, which requires endoscopy, is expensive and invasive, but a reliable test in the assessment of a patient for celiac disease.

5. **The correct answer is D.** Choices A, B, and C are all related to dietary gluten which is the dietary compound that triggers celiac disease. Glycine is an amino acid that is irrelevant to celiac disease.

6. **The correct answer is B.** Patients with IgA deficiency, which is not uncommon, are likely to have a false-negative test result for the IgA tissue transglutaminase antibody assay. Therefore, evaluation of such patients should involve the use of the test for IgG tissue transglutaminase antibodies.

7. **The correct answer is C.** Choices A, B, and D are all true statements about the two commonly available screening tests for colon cancer. Choice C is correct because the fecal immunochemical test is more expensive than the guaiac fecal occult blood test.

8. **The correct answer is C.** One genetic profile for colon cancer involves the analysis of 63 mutations involving seven different genes that include *BRAF, KRAS, PIK3CA, AKT1, SMAD4, PTEN*, and *NRAS*.

CHAPTER 16

1. **The correct answer is C.** Alkaline phosphatase is associated with the plasma membrane of the hepatocytes which are adjacent to the biliary canaliculi. An increased concentration of alkaline phosphatase occurs in the circulation when there is obstruction or inflammation of the biliary tract. It should also be noted, however, that LD is not favored for routine evaluation of hepatocellular disease because this enzyme is released with cell injury from many different tissues.

2. **The correct answer is A.** Choices B, C, and D are all tests indicative of biliary tract disease. Elevations in alkaline phosphatase can occur for many reasons other than biliary tract disease. Therefore, it is common to select the GGT and/or 5′-NT along with the alkaline phosphatase in the assessment for biliary tract disease.

3. **The correct answer is A.** Hemochromatosis is an inborn error that leads to hepatocellular disease which progresses over time.

All of the other choices produce hepatocellular disease abruptly, and, therefore, represent acute causes of damage to the liver.

4. **The correct answer is B.** Bilirubin is derived from myoglobin in the muscle but to a much lesser extent than from hemoglobin in red blood cells. Senescent red blood cells are destroyed in macrophages, primarily in the spleen, and within the phagocytes, hemoglobin is metabolized to bilirubin. Neither transferrin nor iron is a precursor compound for bilirubin.

5. **The correct answer is B.** Unconjugated bilirubin is poorly soluble in water. The color of the skin and sclerae with an increase in the concentration of circulating bilirubin is yellow, not pink. Conjugated bilirubin is transported into the biliary tract, but the biliary tract is not anatomically connected to the genitourinary tract. Patients with a significantly elevated plasma bilirubin are commonly found to have bilirubin in the urine.

6. **The correct answer is A.** The impairment in hepatocyte function is the cause for decreased transport unconjugated bilirubin into the bile canaliculi. There is no evidence for any of the other processes to explain the elevation in conjugated bilirubin in a patient with acute viral hepatitis.

7. **The correct answer is D.** When the ratio of conjugated to total bilirubin is greater than or equal to 0.4, a conjugated hyperbilirubinemia is present. For a neonate, the cutoff ratio is approximately 0.2, because unconjugated bilirubin is higher in neonates than in children or adults. The 3-year-old child should metabolize bilirubin as an adult and therefore has cutoff of 0.4. Therefore, only choice D is a predominantly unconjugated hyperbilirubinemia.

8. **The correct answer is D.** Impaired transport of conjugated bilirubin into the bile ducts will result in a conjugated hyperbilirubinemia. All of the other choices result in an increase in unconjugated bilirubin.

9. **The correct answer is D.** The first three choices all represent causes of intravascular hemolysis. Vitamin B_{12} deficiency with ineffective erythropoiesis results in intramarrow hemolysis rather than hemolysis within the circulation.

10. **The correct answer is C.** Crigler–Najjar syndrome, type I, causes marked elevations in unconjugated bilirubin because the enzyme to conjugate bilirubin, UDP-glucuronyl transferase, is severely deficient. Type II of this syndrome is a much milder deficiency of the UDP-glucuronyl transferase enzyme. All of the other choices are associated with hemolysis.

11. **The correct answer is B.** Biliary atresia would present in a neonate. Both pancreatic adenocarcinoma and parasitic infections from organisms such as helminths can compress the bile duct and produce extrahepatic obstruction, but the most common cause of biliary obstruction outside the liver is a stone in the bile duct. This is known as cholelithiasis.

12. **The correct answer is D.** Immunoglobulins are products of B cells and plasma cells. Their concentration in the circulation is higher than most plasma proteins, but not albumin. The other two proteins are synthesized in the liver, but are not nearly as abundant in the plasma as albumin.

13. **The correct answer is B.** The coagulation factor with the shortest half-life is factor VII. However, the PT, and the INR that is derived from it, is greatly influenced by the circulating concentration of factor VII. Virtually every clinical laboratory can produce a PT/INR value, but many laboratories are not able to perform a quantitative assessment for factor VII. Therefore, the PT/INR is commonly used as an assessment of liver synthetic function. The PTT is not influenced by a deficiency of factor VII, nor is the fibrinogen concentration.

14. **The correct choice is C.** An increase in coagulation factor VIII is likely to decrease the risk of bleeding rather than increase it. All of the other choices are potential causes of bleeding in a patient with severe liver disease.

15. **The correct answer is B.** Hepatitis B surface antigen indicates acute or chronic hepatitis B virus infection; hepatitis A virus IgM antibody indicates acute infection with hepatitis A virus; and hepatitis D virus antibody indicates present or past infection with hepatitis D.

16. **The correct answer is C.** α-fetoprotein is a marker of hepatocellular carcinoma. Antismooth muscle autoantibodies are a marker of autoimmune hepatitis. The liver disease associated with α_1-antitrypsin is a deficiency of this protein, and not an elevation in the production and plasma concentration of α_1-antitrypsin.

17. **The correct answer is D.** Wilson disease is associated with elevated concentrations of copper in the circulation with copper deposition in the brain, liver, kidneys, and cornea. Hepatocellular carcinoma is unrelated to iron deposition. Glycogen storage disorders result from impaired glycogen breakdown.

18. **The correct answer is B.** The plasma or serum ferritin is increased in hemochromatosis, although the elevation in ferritin is not specific for iron overload. Ferritin is released from the liver with disease or injury, and it is also elevated as an acute-phase reactant. Percent transferrin saturation is the recommended screening test and the earliest biochemical marker of hemochromatosis.

19. **The correct answer is C.** Liver disease occurs because of copper overload in the liver. The Kayser–Fleischer rings are a result of increased copper deposition at the corneo–scleral junction (the limbus). Urinary copper is a useful noninvasive test to evaluate a patient for possible Wilson disease. The ceruloplasmin level is decreased, not increased, in >90% of patients with Wilson disease.

20. **The correct answer is D.** Because of defects in conjugation and excretion of bilirubin, there is an elevation in concentrations of both conjugated and unconjugated bilirubin in the circulation. The elevated concentrations of ammonia result from an impairment in the urea cycle. The blood glucose is low because of impaired gluconeogenesis in the fasting state after glycogen stores in the liver have been depleted. The increased prothrombin time is a result of decreased production of clotting factors, malabsorption of vitamin K, and decreased clearance of fibrin split products.

21. **The correct answer is A.** The approximate percentage of cases of cirrhosis from the other choices are viral hepatitis—10%; biliary tract diseases—5% to 10%; and hereditary hemochromatosis—5%.

22. **The correct answer is B.** Patients with primary biliary cirrhosis have elevated concentrations of conjugated hyperbilirubinemia. The alkaline phosphatase is higher than the alanine aminotransferase or aspartate aminotransferase levels. The condition is most common among women between the ages of 40 and 50 years. Primary sclerosing cholangitis affects the larger bile ducts in men more commonly than in women. Patients with primary sclerosing cholangitis generally have a negative test result for antimitochondrial antibodies, unlike those with primary biliary cirrhosis. Hepatic encephalopathy occurs in patients who have extremely high concentrations of circulating ammonia, which occurs in patients with severe liver disease. Cholestasis of pregnancy is associated with elevated serum bile acid concentrations in pregnant women.

CHAPTER 17

1. **The correct answer is D.** In addition to the first three choices above, which are well-known causes of acute pancreatitis, other causes include hypercalcemia, selected infections, obstructing pancreatic tumors, and trauma to the pancreas. Hypercholesterolemia is not known to be causative for acute pancreatitis.

2. **The correct answer is C.** The calcium may be altered in acute pancreatitis, but when it is, it generally is lower than normal rather than elevated. The two primary markers for acute pancreatitis are serum amylase and serum lipase. In acute pancreatitis, the clearance of amylase into the urine may be higher than the clearance of creatinine into the urine. This creates an increase in the (amylase/creatinine clearance) ratio.

3. **The correct answer is C.** In about 50% of patients with chronic pancreatitis, the serum amylase level is normal. In patients who do have an increased amylase level, the value may be borderline or only slightly elevated. The amylase level is far more important diagnostically for acute pancreatitis than it is for chronic pancreatitis.

4. **The correct answer is D.** CA 19-9 may be elevated in pancreatic and several types of gastrointestinal cancers, and even in some nonneoplastic disorders. Therefore, it is not specific to pancreatic cancers.

5. **The correct answer is A.** Tumors of the δ cells of the endocrine pancreas are somatostatinomas. Glucagonoma are tumors of the α cells of the pancreatic islets. Patients with Zollinger–Ellison syndrome have peptic ulcer disease and should be evaluated for a gastrinoma. Islet cell tumors known as VIPomas induce a syndrome of watery diarrhea, hypokalemia, hypochlorhydria, and acidosis, also known as the WDHHA syndrome.

6. **The correct answer is C.** The random plasma glucose threshold is 200 mg/dL, not 150. All the other choices are current criteria for the diagnosis of diabetes mellitus. Only one of the criteria has to be met for a diagnosis to be made.

7. **The correct answer is B.** Type 1 diabetes represents in most cases an immune-mediated destruction of β cells, resulting in absolute deficiency of insulin secretion. Type 2 diabetes occurs as a result of varying degrees of insulin resistance, such that increased plasma insulin may be insufficient to compensate for the resistance.

8. **The correct answer is C.** A hemoglobin A1C value of 3% to 5% in an otherwise healthy individual is not concerning for diabetes. One of the criteria for a diagnosis of diabetes mellitus is a hemoglobin A1C value greater than or equal to 6.5%. A hemoglobin A1C value >5.7% but lower than 6.5% identifies high-risk individuals for whom diabetes mellitus screening is recommended.

9. **The correct answer is B.** It is permissible for patients to drink water while fasting. All of the other statements about the patient preparation prior to obtaining a blood sample for a fasting blood glucose level are correct.

10. **The correct answer is D.** The range of plasma glucose representing impaired glucose tolerance is greater than 140 mg/dL but less than 200 mg/dL.

11. **The correct answer is C.** Hemoglobin A1C is primarily used for monitoring glycemic status over the long term. It is also used to determine whether a diabetic patient has adequate control of blood glucose levels. It reflects the blood glucose levels over the preceding 8 to 12 weeks.

12. **The correct answer is A.** In diabetic patients, with hemoglobin A1C values below 6.5%, there is a very low prevalence of retinopathy.

13. **The correct answer is C.** Gestational diabetes is much more common than 1 in 1000 pregnancies in the United States. Currently, approximately 1 in 25 pregnancies in the United States is complicated by gestational diabetes mellitus. Some ethnic groups show an even higher incidence, with one in seven native American pregnant women affected.

14. **The correct answer is D.** The laboratory evaluation for gestational diabetes mellitus does not involve any testing for the offspring. Most women will be normal glycemic after pregnancy.

15. **The correct answer is C.** When an insufficient amount of insulin is administered to a patient with diabetes, the patient is more likely to be hyperglycemic than hypoglycemic. Choice A describes reactive hypoglycemia. An insulinoma secretes large amounts of insulin to produce hypoglycemia. Surreptitious insulin injection lowers the plasma glucose. Importantly, the insulin used for injection, unlike native insulin, has the C-peptide of the insulin moiety removed. Therefore, the C-peptide is not present in patients with surreptitious insulin injection because the insulin found in their blood is not synthesized from the proinsulin synthesized in the pancreas.

16. **The correct answer is A.** There is no consideration of the hemoglobin A1C value in the diagnosis of hypoglycemia.

CHAPTER 18

1. **The correct answer is B.** Oliguria is defined as <500 mL of urine produced per day. Anuria is essentially absent urine production defined in adults with a threshold of <100 mL of urine produced per day. Dysuria refers to pain upon urination. Hematuria refers to red blood cells in the urine.

2. **The correct answer is A.** Choices B and D are both examples of renal azotemia because the diseases are intrinsic to the kidney. Choice C is an example of postrenal azotemia because the problem is related to urine flow out of the kidney.

3. **The correct answer is C.** Choice A is the definition for chronic renal failure. Choice B is the definition of azotemia. Choice D is the definition for oliguria or, if more severe, anuria.

4. **The correct answer is B.** Decreased production of erythropoietin results in decreased synthesis of red blood cells and, subsequently, anemia. Untreated renal failure can result in dysfunctional platelets, but not thrombocytopenia. All of the other choices are correct matches.

5. **The correct answer is B.** Because the creatinine concentration is directly related to skeletal muscle mass, and skeletal muscle mass is greater in men than women, creatinine is higher in males than females.

6. **The correct answer is C.** The basic formula for creatinine clearance is as follows (serum creatinine and plasma creatinine are interchangeable in the formula):

(urine creatinine/serum creatinine) × (urine volume in milliliters/collection time in minutes)

When corrected for body surface area, the formula for creatinine clearance is:

(urine creatinine/serum creatinine) × (urine volume in milliliters/collection time in minutes) × (1.73/body surface area in meters squared)

7. **The correct answer is A.** The formula for eGFR is 186 (serum creatinine)$^{-1.154}$ × (Age)$^{-0.203}$ × F, where F equals 0.742 for females and 1.210 for African Americans. Therefore, the value for urine creatinine is not necessary.

8. **The correct answer is C.** Values between 60 and 89 mL/min/1.73 m^2 are associated with evidence of mild kidney damage. Values >90 are associated with normal kidney function when there is no proteinuria. Therefore, eGFR values that are >60 could reflect mild kidney disease or the absence of kidney disease.

9. **The correct answer is A.** Microalbuminuria is often found in association with renal damage from diabetic nephropathy and hypertension. Microalbuminuria can be determined using a spot urine collection, a timed urine collection, or a 24-hour urine collection. The amount of albumin excreted by patients with nephrosis far exceeds the range of urinary albumin in patients with microalbuminuria.

10. **The correct answer is C.** Overflow proteinuria is the likely explanation because high concentrations of plasma monoclonal immunoglobulin, when present, can "spill over" from the plasma into the urine.

11. **The correct answer is B.** Dipstick positivity for blood occurs whether red blood cells, hemoglobin, or myoglobin are present. Myoglobin does not result in a positive microscopic examination for red blood cells or red blood cell casts. Trauma can release large amounts of myoglobin from skeletal muscle. This myoglobin can appear in the urine. When saturated ammonium sulfate is added to urine, the hemoglobin is precipitated, but not the myoglobin. Therefore, the compound present in the urine responsible for the markedly positive test for heme is myoglobin. Infection in the kidney would likely have produced hematuria or bacteriuria or both. Advanced bladder cancer could also result in red blood cells in the urine. Severe liver disease is not associated with a positive test for heme unless it is associated with a bleeding disorder. It is highly unlikely to be associated with myoglobin in the urine.

12. **The correct answer is A.** All of the findings on urinalysis are consistent with an infection in the kidney. Neutrophils contain leukocyte esterase enzyme activity, which can be detected by urinalysis, even if the neutrophils are disrupted. The white blood cell casts originate in the renal tubules, similar to the red blood cell casts. The nitrite test on a urinalysis reagent strip is sensitive to the presence of clinically significant numbers of certain bacteria (such as *Proteus*) in the urine.

13. **The correct answer is D.** Bilirubin is not a normal component of urine. When present, liver dysfunction and biliary obstruction are likely possibilities. An elevated urinary urobilinogen can be produced in a patient with liver disease because of the failure of the liver to remove urobilinogen from the blood, resulting in higher blood concentrations and subsequently higher concentrations in the urine. The dark yellow color of the urine is associated with the presence of urine bilirubin and/or urine urobilinogen.

14. **The correct answer is C.** Patients with poorly controlled diabetes often have ketones in the urine. Although urine glucose is not present in all patients with diabetes mellitus, if it is present, diabetes should be considered among the diagnostic possibilities. The hypertensive renal damage in a diabetic patient can lead to minimal but persistent amounts of albumin in the urine.

15. **The correct answer is D.** Calcium oxalate and calcium phosphate stones can result from an elevated concentration of calcium in the urine. Patients with Crohn disease have an increased absorption of oxalate from the ileum, and this can result in the formation of urinary stones. Gout is associated with high concentrations of uric acid in the urine, and these patients are predisposed to form urate stones, particularly when the pH of the urine is <5.4.

CHAPTER 19

1. **The correct answer is C.** Currently, there are no laboratory tests to differentiate rapidly progressive prostate cancer that leads to death from the indolent forms. A man who has been diagnosed with prostate cancer, therefore, is unable to know whether prostatectomy will be lifesaving or relatively unnecessary. This is a major dilemma at the current time because of the complications of impotence and incontinence, which may arise from prostatectomy.

2. **The correct answer is D.** The use of the PSA level as a screening test for prostate cancer is highly controversial. PSA levels correlate with the size of the prostate, and, therefore, a larger gland results in a higher PSA value even if there is no prostate cancer. Men with benign prostatic hyperplasia (BPH) can also show elevations in serum PSA.

3. **The correct answer is A.** More than 90% of testicular cancers arise from germ cell tumors. These tumors produce substances, which include choices B, C, and D, that can be used as tumor markers. All of these markers are most useful to evaluate the patient for complete removal of the tumor and detect cancer recurrence, as well as monitor the effects of treatment to eliminate the testicular cancer.

4. **The correct answer is D.** Treatment of deficiency of androgens in young men with primary gonadal failure is clearly beneficial. However, it is a much more controversial issue for middle aged and older men. Androgen supplementation increases the likelihood of both benign prostatic hyperplasia and prostate cancer, may lead to a decreased sperm count, and causes undesirable changes in blood lipids that increase the risk of myocardial infarction and stroke.

5. **The correct answer is C.** Testosterone secretion does have a circadian rhythm, but the higher levels are present in the morning and the lower concentrations are found in the afternoon and evening. The reference ranges for the expected values of testosterone are generally based on morning samples. Therefore, collection of a blood sample for testosterone measurement in the afternoon or evening is problematic because the value obtained is being compared to a reference range generated by the results from samples collected in the morning when the testosterone is highest.

6. **The correct answer is C.** When a man with low testosterone levels is also found to have a very low level of luteinizing hormone, it is likely that the pituitary or the hypothalamus is not functioning correctly. The follicle-stimulating hormone (FSH) follows the LH. Therefore, there is no additional information provided by the results of the test for FSH.

7. **The correct answer is D.** All the other choices are well-known causes of male infertility. Nonobstructive azoospermia may occur as a result of the absence of germ cells in the testes or failure of spermatogenesis.

Obstructive azoospermia may follow from a vasectomy reversal because it may persist after reversal of a vasectomy. Obstructive azoospermia can also result from a sexually transmitted infection. The absence of the vas deferens may be a congenital defect in men carrying one of the many alleles for cystic fibrosis, even if the cystic fibrosis is not clinically apparent.

8. **The correct answer is A.** The semen sample should be collected 2 to 5 days after sexual abstinence. When this fact is not taken into consideration, the semen presented for evaluation is usually of a lower volume and a decreased sperm count.

9. **The correct answer is D.** Antisperm antibodies may indicate an immunologic basis for infertility. However, this is a highly specialized test and not part of a routine semen analysis.

CHAPTER 20

1. **The correct answer is C.** The treponemal antibody test is to screen for syphilis, and not group B streptococcal infection. A group B *Streptococcus* cervical culture is important in the third trimester. If the test is positive, treatment is provided to prevent transmission to the fetus during delivery.

2. **The correct answer is A.** The hematocrit is decreased during pregnancy because there is an increase in the plasma volume. For that reason, the percentage of red cells relative to the entire blood volume is decreased. Alkaline phosphatase activity is increased due to the production of placental, heat-stable alkaline phosphatase. 1,25-Dihydroxyvitamin D is increased as a result of increased calcium and transfer of calcium to the fetus. Total T_3 and T_4 are increased, but the patient remains euthyroid.

3. **The correct answer is D.** An increase in hCG, when measured with a quantitative assay and a serum sample, is detectable 8 to 11 days after conception. On the other hand, qualitative urine hCG tests (that produce a yes or no answer) have detection limits that range from 20 to 50 IU/L and become positive 14 or more days after conception, usually after a missed menstrual period.

4. **The correct answer is A.** Serial measurements of hCG may reveal problems in a pregnancy. For example, there is a slow rate of increase in hCG in a woman with an ectopic pregnancy. hCG concentrations greater than expected for gestational age can be present in a woman with gestational trophoblast disease.

5. **The correct answer is D.** Decreased platelets with elevated liver function tests are characteristic of pregnant women suffering from the HELLP syndrome. These values are not associated with ectopic pregnancy.

6. **The correct answer is A.** A spontaneous abortion or non-viable pregnancy is associated with a faster than expected rate of increase in serum/plasma hCG concentrations.

7. **The correct answer is C.** Preeclampsia is a major cause of morbidity and mortality in pregnancy. Patients with preeclampsia develop elevated blood pressure and proteinuria along with impaired liver function. Women with preeclampsia can develop eclampsia with accompanying seizures. Eclampsia has a higher morbidity and mortality rate than preeclampsia. Proteinuria is not a major feature of any of the other choices.

8. **The correct answer is D.** Data from an exome analysis provide information about genetic alterations in thousands of genes. Although this may one day become routine, it is not a part of the laboratory evaluation for recurrent spontaneous abortion.

9. **The correct answer is C.** Midluteal progesterone concentrations <10 ng/mL suggest anovulation (a value >10 is expected with normal ovulation). Thus, it is a decrease, not an increase, in the midluteal progesterone concentration that is associated with female infertility.

CHAPTER 21

1. **The correct answer is C.** *HER2*, which is also known as *ERBB2* and *NEU*, is a tissue-based marker. *HER2* is a transmembrane receptor with cytoplasmic tyrosine kinase activity.

2. **The correct answer is B.** The IHC method evaluates the percentage of cells with nuclear estrogen and progesterone receptors. A tumor is scored positive for either of the receptors if >1% of the tumor cell nuclei are immunoreactive.

3. **The correct answer is C.** FISH assesses *HER2* status at the DNA level with a fluorescent-labeled nucleic acid probe that recognizes the *HER2* gene. In the CISH method, an alternative to FISH, the *HER2* probe is visualized by an immunoperoxidase reaction. Immunohistochemistry assesses *HER2* status at the protein level, and the result is presented on a semiquantitative scale with higher numbers representing more *HER2* protein expression. There is no role for karyotype analysis in the determination of *HER2* status.

4. **The correct answer is C.** All of the choices listed represent highly penetrant forms of hereditary breast cancer. However, the *BRCA1* and *BRCA2* mutations represent a much larger proportion of hereditary breast cancer cases than the other choices.

CHAPTER 22

1. **The correct answer is C.** The primary negative feedback to the hypothalamus and to the pituitary is from T_3. All of the other statements about the thyroid axis are correct.

2. **The correct answer is A.** If the TSH is within the reference range, no further testing is performed. However, if the TSH is outside the reference range, a free T_4 measurement is typically performed.

3. **The correct answer is D.** In hyperthyroidism, the concentrations of total T_3 and total T_4 correlate in the vast majority of patients. However, measurement of T_3 concentration is of limited diagnostic value in the assessment of hypothyroidism.

4. **The correct answer is A.** Antitopoisomerase antibodies are used to establish a diagnosis for the autoimmune disease scleroderma. Anti-TPO antibodies are directed against the enzyme TPO. They are present in almost all individuals with Hashimoto thyroiditis and in approximately 85% of patients with Graves disease. Antithyroglobulin antibodies are present in >85% of patients with Hashimoto thyroiditis and are antibodies to colloid in the thyroid gland. These antibodies may also be found in patients with other autoimmune diseases. Antibodies to TSH receptors are found in most patients with Graves disease and may either stimulate the thyroid or inhibit the thyroid by blocking stimulation from TSH. The antibodies that are thyroid-stimulating immunoglobulins are present in up to 95% of patients with untreated Graves disease.

5. **The correct answer is C.** Hashimoto thyroiditis is associated with an elevated TSH and a positive test for antithyroglobulin antibodies. The T_4 value is initially normal and then becomes low with disease progression, and this decline precedes the decline in T_3. All of the other choices are associated with low values for TSH, and commonly, high values for free T_4, free T_3, or both.

6. **The correct answer is D.** Patients in the early phase of subacute thyroiditis are typically hyperthyroid, but if the disease progresses and the thyroid hormones are depleted, hypothyroidism may ensue. All of the other choices are associated with elevations in TSH and at some point in the process, low values for T_4 and/or T_3.

7. **The correct answer is C.** With the increase in reverse T_3, there are significantly reduced concentrations of total T_3. An elevated reverse T_3 in the appropriate clinical setting and other suggestive laboratory test results are consistent with NTI.

8. **The correct answer is D.** The evaluation for a thyroid nodule is to measure TSH and perform a thyroid ultrasound study; if the TSH is suppressed, a nuclear scan is performed to identify "hot" nodules that take up radioactive iodine while iodine uptake is suppressed elsewhere in the gland. Hyperfunctioning nodules appear as hot nodules. A nonfunctional (cold) nodule carries a higher risk of malignancy than a hot nodule. Histopathologic review of the biopsy specimen from the nodule is then required to determine if the patient has thyroid cancer.

9. **The correct answer is C.** The negative feedback to reduce stimulation is provided by cortisol. Cortisol has a negative feedback effect upon both the pituitary and the hypothalamus.

10. **The correct answer is B.** Norepinephrine is synthesized in the adrenal medulla, and it is metabolized to compounds that can also be measured to assess function of the adrenal medulla. There are a variety of compounds generated in the adrenal cortex in each of the three correct categories—glucocorticoids, sex steroids, and mineralocorticoids.

11. **The correct answer is A.** Cortisol concentrations are at their highest level between 4 and 8 AM in the morning. Because cortisol secretion is diurnal and pulsatile, a single, random serum cortisol measurement is not useful in the diagnosis of adrenal function.

12. **The correct answer is D.** Patients with primary adrenal insufficiency will develop an increased ACTH in response to CRH stimulation because the pituitary gland is still functionally intact. However, there should be no cortisol production because of the adrenal insufficiency.

13. **The correct answer is D.** Renin is synthesized and secreted from the juxtaglomerular apparatus in the kidney, and not in the liver. The other points regarding negative feedback in choice D are correct.

14. **The correct answer is C.** Renin stimulates the conversion from angiotensinogen to angiotensin I. The enzyme activity that converts angiotensin I to angiotensin II is angiotensin-converting enzyme that is present in the lungs.

15. **The correct answer is B.** The administration of glucocorticoids as a medication is a common cause of Cushing syndrome. However, it is not a naturally occurring form of the disease but instead is a complication of glucocorticoid therapy.

16. **The correct answer is B.** The distinguishing factor is the low value for ACTH that is a result of cortisol suppression of ACTH synthesis in the pituitary, particularly when there is an adrenal adenoma rather than an adrenal carcinoma. The ACTH level is elevated or inappropriately normal for the pituitary cause, and the ACTH is elevated when there is ectopic ACTH secretion as a cause for Cushing syndrome.

17. **The correct answer is B.** In primary adrenal insufficiency, the plasma ACTH is elevated because feedback inhibition by adrenal cortisol is absent. In secondary adrenal insufficiency, the plasma ACTH is low because the origin of secondary adrenal insufficiency is in the hypothalamus or the pituitary. The serum cortisol levels are low for both primary and secondary adrenal insufficiency. The CRH stimulation test is generally not necessary in the laboratory evaluation for primary adrenal insufficiency. Similarly, adrenal autoantibody tests are not performed in the evaluation for secondary adrenal insufficiency.

18. **The correct answer is C.** The low-plasma aldosterone rules out hyperaldosteronism in this patient. The plasma renin activity level in secondary hypoaldosteronism is usually low.

19. **The correct answer is B.** The virilizing effect in females results in hypertrophy of the clitoris, and in postpubertal females, there is infertility and hirsutism as well. In males, the virilization results in precocious puberty with enlargement of the external genitalia. The biochemical impact of 21-hydroxylase deficiency is a reduced or absent synthesis of both cortisol and aldosterone.

20. **The correct answer is C.** Vanillylmandelic acid is a metabolite of metanephrine and normetanephrine. It is inferior to the measurement of urinary metanephrines to establish a diagnosis of adrenal medulla insufficiency.

21. **The correct answer is C.** The concentrations of plasma catecholamines are elevated in patients with pheochromocytoma, along with the increase in urinary catecholamines.

22. **The correct answer is D.** Parathyroid hormone stimulates an increase in calcium resorption from the bone, which, along with the other effects of parathyroid hormone, results in normal or elevated plasma calcium. The normal or elevated calcium level provides negative feedback to the parathyroid gland to reduce the production of PTH.

23. **The correct answer is B.** The success of parathyroid surgery to remove parathyroid adenomas, which are small, has been improved by intraoperative PTH measurement. There is a relatively short half-life of PTH, and this has allowed surgeons to measure plasma PTH concentrations before and after excision of parathyroid tumors in surgery. Complete resection of the tumor is indicated by a decrease in PTH of >50%.

24. **The correct answer is A.** The combination of an elevated intact serum PTH and an elevated total or ionized serum calcium, along with an undetectable serum PTH-related protein, which is detectable in some cancers, are all consistent with a diagnosis of primary hyperparathyroidism.

25. **The correct answer is C.** The Sertoli cells are contained within the testes, and the granulosa cells are within the ovaries. Their anatomic locations are reversed in choice C.

26. **The correct answer is C.** The elevations in LH and FSH indicate that the hypogonadism is hypergonadotropic. The low testosterone differentiates hypergonadotropic hypogonadism from androgen insensitivity syndrome, which has an elevated or occasionally normal serum testosterone for a male.

27. **The correct answer is C.** Cushing syndrome may result in amenorrhea, and, therefore, the amenorrhea in patients with Cushing syndrome is secondary. The measurement of hCG would be relevant to an evaluation for both primary and secondary amenorrhea.

28. **The correct answer is D.** The negative feedback is provided by insulin-like growth factors (IGFs) synthesized in the liver and released into the circulation.

29. **The correct answer is B.** Growth hormone excess long before bone growth is completed results in gigantism. Short stature is associated with growth hormone deficiency.

30. **The correct answer is C.** Prolactin stimulates, rather than inhibits, milk production by the breast.

31. **The correct answer is A.** Antidiuretic hormone is secreted from the posterior pituitary, not the anterior pituitary.

32. **The correct answer is C.** The high level for plasma ADH differentiates nephrogenic diabetes insipidus from central diabetes insipidus, which is characterized by a low-plasma ADH. SIADH is associated with a low serum sodium and osmolality, and a normal or high value for urine sodium and osmolality. Psychogenic polydipsia should be identifiable by a history of excess water intake.

33. **The correct answer is A.** MEN 1 syndrome involves hyperplasia or neoplasms in the parathyroid, the pancreatic islet cells, and/or the anterior pituitary. The correct choice for MEN 2 syndrome is medullary thyroid carcinoma that is present in over 90% of patients with MEN 2.

Index

Page numbers in bold indicate figures and tables.